DRUGS AFFECTING THE PERIPHERAL NERVOUS SYSTEM

Volume 1

MEDICINAL RESEARCH:
A SERIES OF MONOGRAPHS

VOLUME 1: *Drugs Affecting the Peripheral Nervous System*
VOLUME 2: *Drugs Affecting the Central Nervous System*
VOLUME 3: *Pharmacological Testing Methods*

edited by Alfred Burger

DRUGS AFFECTING THE PERIPHERAL NERVOUS SYSTEM

VOLUME 1

Edited by ALFRED BURGER
DEPARTMENT OF CHEMISTRY
UNIVERSITY OF VIRGINIA
CHARLOTTESVILLE, VIRGINIA

1967

MARCEL DEKKER, INC., New York

MARCEL DEKKER, INC.
95 *Madison Avenue, New York, New York* 10016

LIBRARY OF CONGRESS CATALOG CARD NUMBER 66-22491

PRINTED IN THE UNITED STATES OF AMERICA

INTRODUCTION TO THE SERIES

The first two volumes of this series present surveys of major topics in the area of pharmacodynamic agents which affect both the peripheral and the central nervous systems. Reviews of neuropharmacological drugs have been written at various intervals, and from various points of view. A few individual subjects have been dealt with as chapters in monographs devoted to either the chemistry or the strictly biological and medical aspects of the drugs concerned. However, the whole field has not been considered before on a fundamental biochemical-pharmacological basis. This has now been attempted in this series.

The contributors, originally approached by the late Professor F. W. Schueler of Tulane University, were chosen because their interpretation relies on fundamental rather than applied facets of their fields. Some of the contributors have critically reviewed existing data; others have ventured into predictive speculations but always building on the solid background of observed facts. Together, they have presented a picture of the relation of the chemistry and biological action of neuropharmacodynamic agents that answers many questions of the past and present, and opens the doors to future queries.

The editor is grateful to the contributors for the time and devotion they have given of their busy lives in order to make these volumes possible. He will be obliged to the readers of these books for pertinent comments and corrections.

Alfred Burger

November 1966
Charlottesville, Virginia

PREFACE TO VOLUME I

Most drugs that affect the peripheral nervous system have been considered by classical pharmacologists to be either adrenergic or cholinergic in nature. Although the overt manifestations of their actions may be understood on this basis, there remain many examples of autonomic drug action which require clarification. Few drugs affect only one of the major divisions exclusively; since the extent of adrenergic-cholinergic crossover is generally unknown, seemingly unpredictable results are often obtained, particularly in the intact animal. Some additional factors contribute to the problem; among these are the difficulties in access of a drug to its receptors, and its removal at various sites of loss, for example, by reaction with "silent receptors." There is little one can do about these factors, although the use of isolated tissues or organs for studies of drug action may lessen the influence of at least some of these extraneous circumstances. Molecular modification, by equipping a drug molecule with hydrophilic or hydrophobic groups, may well promote its desired absorption and distribution, but then one deals with a new compound, whose complementarity with the biomacromolecule with which it reacts in exerting its biological action is no longer assured. Nevertheless, structure-activity studies involving systematic modifications of a "lead" molecule provide the cornerstone for understanding drug action at the molecular level and offer the greatest promise for determining the relationship between chemical constitution and biological activity of many types of agents. Several contributors to this volume have drawn heavily upon these kinds of studies, particularly when carried out in a quantitative fashion on isolated preparations. Such experiments are of considerable use in attempts to explain in depth the mode of action of the vast numbers of different types of compounds known to alter autonomic activity.

The central interest of pharmacology has been, and continues to be, the description and interpretation of events which occur at receptor sites. Definitive theories are still lacking although an attack on the molecular level is in progress in a number of laboratories. A few bold attempts to isolate receptors have even been made in recent years. Progress in the precise localization of at least some receptors has been achieved through the use of newer, highly sophisticated techniques. What yet escapes us completely is the exact way in which agonist-receptor interaction initiates the complex series of events which lead to an overt response. It is suspected that this process combines tranformations highly dependent on stereochemically controlled anchimeric assistance with ionic mechanisms in a manner not yet encountered in simpler chemical reactions. For this reason, the "lock-and-key" concept given us by Ehrlich so many years ago may no longer be applicable to the receptor, although a more adequate description has not been offered in its stead. There is perhaps some justification for this dilemma: we do not yet know the chemical nature of any receptor substance. The problem with the receptor is thus of far greater magnitude than that encountered in the elucidation of the mechanism of catalysis by even simple, well-defined enzymes—and receptors probably do resemble enzymes at least in terms of specificity of interaction. The hope has materialized that X-ray crystallographic analysis for the study of the tertiary structure of proteins can be applied successfully to those enzymes whose complete amino acid sequence is known. Detailed information about the three-dimensional topography of active sites of enzymes may well shed light upon active sites of receptors. However, we must not lose sight of the fact that the receptor substances almost undoubtedly are membrane components, and that as such their reactivities may be modified greatly by adjacent membrane constituents such as lipids, proteins, etc. Thus even the detailed understanding of the mechanism of enzyme catalysis may still only provide the merest glimpse into basic mechanisms of receptor reactions. It has been the intent of at least some of the contributors to suggest ways in which our horizons may be broadened along these lines.

In a very few instances, it has been pointed out that the active site of a soluble, though membrane-associated, enzyme may be almost identical with a receptor for a particular neurohormone. This has been pursued most steadfastly in the case of cholinesterase and the cholinergic receptor since there is little doubt that so simple a molecule as acetylcholine should interact with both enzyme and receptor in a similar manner. The discussion in Chapter 2 in which the actual identity of enzyme and receptor is proposed is therefore especially timely, even if the details of the concepts presented have to be refined or amended in the next few years. No analogous comparisons have been made with the adrenergic receptors, perhaps because of the intracellular localization of the enzymes which serve in part to remove adrenergic amines from the vicinity of the receptor sites. For various reasons there is perhaps less justification for considering the receptor for these compounds to be related to an enzyme than in the case of the cholinergic system. However, the exquisite degree of specificity exhibited by the adrenergic receptors, for example, their ability to discriminate between *d* and *l* forms of the same substrate, suggests enzyme-like properties.

If a single author were to write a book on autonomic pharmacology which at every turn reflects uncertainty and yet-to-be-done experiments, a somewhat biased view could be expected at best. In a multiauthor cooperative volume, this may be avoided; but in its place we are faced with a divergence of approaches, some in opposition to each other, others overlapping one another. An attempt could have been made to unify these facets, but in this case the individuality of thought provided by each author might have suffered. In this volume, therefore, the editor has felt it to be of advantage to have each contributor present his unencumbered views on how various chemical agents influence autonomic events, permitting each free rein to describe his own unique approach to the question of how chemical constitution can be correlated with biological activities in this field. These approaches are in fact quite varied; they range from the use of in vitro reactions of drugs with purified, well-characterized macromolecules and enzymes, or tissue components, to reactions with isolated tissues and experiments with intact animals. Other contributors have made a valuable and almost exhaustive compilation of the literature of their field, and have evaluated it critically. Thus, there is presentation of the old and the new—classical pharmacology as well as the newer problems of molecular pharmacology, with its emphasis on the use of chemical, biochemical, and physicochemical techniques.

Equally tantalizing has been the distribution of emphasis on details, and on the description of different shades of similar experiments. In some areas of autonomic agents interest has been intense, and there are large numbers of drugs which have been studied in detail. Their biological main and side effects, and the investigation of their chemical, biochemical, and physical behavior in diverse environments, have contributed handsomely to the definition of their pharmacodynamic mode of action. In other autonomic areas only a few drugs have become known, and these have not provided all the answers one could ask; chapters concerned with such areas are shorter. In a few areas, for instance, the inhibitors of acetylcholinesterase, such a diversity of drugs is available that inclusion of all of them would have been unwise; the authors have preferred to assume that the experienced reader would not wish to scan endless tables, and have instead concentrated on underlying theories based on the rich experimental material.

It could be anticipated that the final answers to the all-important question of what really constitutes the underlying factors governing the relationship between chemical constitution and biological activity may well lie within the realm of physical chemistry or perhaps even in quantum chemistry. One of the earliest exponents of this approach is the late F. W. Schueler, whose untimely death has taken from us the man who was responsible for the inception of this series. It is our fond hope that the information presented herein may provide the stimulus for someone who has Schueler's breadth of vision and knowledge to find the answers to the important questions which still remain unsolved in autonomic pharmacology.

A. Burger
S. Ehrenpreis

IN MEMORIAM: FRED W. SCHUELER

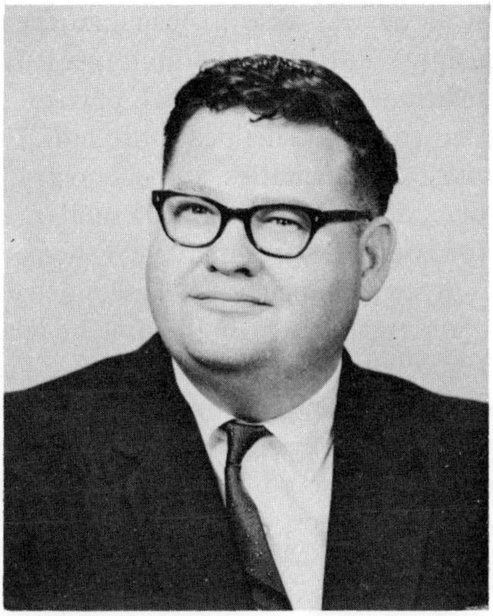

FRED W. SCHUELER, 1921–1964

In 1963 Fred Schueler undertook the editing of the Dekker series in Medicinal Research as a welcome opportunity to focus interest on this branch of pharmacology, in which he had invested so much time, labor, and thought. This project, together with many others, was left unfinished, owing to his untimely death at the age of 43 on Labor Day, September 7, 1964.

Fred Schueler was born in 1921 in Fort Collins, Colorado, at the foot of the Rocky Mountains. Of his childhood he remembered little, except the sound of Bach preludes, an open campfire, a lead pencil which he tried to melt and which almost put out his eye, and later a chemistry set, which started him on his life-long career.

At twelve, Fred worked his way through an old chemistry text, trying every experiment in the book, and a lot that weren't in the book. He used to scrounge around for leftover chemicals at the drugstore and at the "College," and one of the chemistry teachers there took an interest in him. He found he needed to know more than eighth-grade arithmetic, and systematically worked his way through elementary mathematics. This renewed his interest in music and composition; he studied harmony and counterpoint, practiced the piano diligently, and at the age of sixteen started to write a symphony which was performed two years later by the Long Beach Symphony Orchestra in California. Fred never heard this symphony except in his mind's "ear." He could "hear" both the orchestra as a whole and each instrument separately at the same time, just as he was able to visualize special configurations of mathematical relationships. This ability simultaneously to "orchestrate" or "visualize" complex relationships both in each particular and as a whole had its counterpart in his approach to chemical problems.

Of his three loves, music, mathematics, and chemistry, Fred chose chemistry upon entering the University of Colorado in Boulder, in 1939. Having been left without funds at the end of his freshman year, he peeled potatoes, cleaned the rat house, and was given a chance to teach chemistry in the Navy Training Program while still an undergraduate. By the time he received his B.A. degree, in 1943, Fred was organizing laboratory sessions and giving lectures in organic chemistry with a tremendous outpour of formulas with which he covered the board with great flourish. He had an almost uncanny ability to keep students spellbound, discovered he could hypnotize almost anyone, and became fascinated with the effects of hypnotism, of mescaline, and other hallucinatory agents.

There followed a long succession of days and nights in the lab, since rats needed inspection every four hours, either for injections or for smears. Fred solved his domestic problem by marrying an undergraduate with a foreign accent, and for all practical purposes, moving his bride into the lab with him. The lab furnished warmth, inspiration, entertainment, and nourishment (rabbit and chicken experiments, and an icebox to preserve same). Neither the birth of a daughter, nor one of his first attacks of illness, kept Fred from his experiments. He simply pulled on his suit over his pajamas, roused a friend in the middle of the night to drive him to the animal house, and installed a cot for future emergencies.

In 1954, Fred was offered a Lederle Fellowship in Pharmacology at the University of Chicago, which defined the course of his professional career, and allowed him to complete his Ph.D. in two years of concentrated work uninterrupted by teaching assignments. While still at Boulder, he had begun to study the effect of chemical structure on chemical activity. He now refined, sharpened, and revised his thinking on structure-activity relationships in terms of the concept of an activating moiety. He became intrigued with a variety of techniques borrowed from the gamut of scientific disciplines, with statistics and probability theory, and in turn with their effect on the design of experiments. Fred perfected his own animal-operating techniques, took great pride in a "clean" operation, was an expert glassblower, made much of his own equipment, and in general loved all manner of apparatus and machinery. Certainly at this time he had already priced and stocked in his mind a great part of his future laboratories.

In 1947, Fred Schueler received his Ph.D. and was appointed instructor at the State University of Iowa, where he plunged into a program of medical and graduate education in pharmacology, with a block of free time set aside for his own research. For the first time, he now had a laboratory of his own, and he worked in it until late every night, expecting his students to do the same. He could not stay away from the lab for any length of time. Weekends and holidays out of town were cut short just because he simply had to try out something new. He would wake up in a tent several hundred miles from home at three in the morning, hurriedly scribble some structures on the back of an envelope, and start packing.

One of Fred's tasks at Iowa was to write a syllabus for the student laboratory, which he organized in terms of subject disciplines in ascending order of complexity, and out of which grew the groundwork for his book on chemobiodynamics. Fred prepared his lectures with a great deal of care, but usually delivered them "live" without notes. In truth, he needed his audience to help him crystallize his thoughts. He often came home as enthusiastic as if he had been a student listening, because he had gained a completely unexpected insight while on the lecture platform.

Fred gave numerous talks to professional and civic organizations, in which he presented the science of pharmacology to the public and tried to divorce its meaning from that of pharmacy in the layman's mind. More and more, he came to speak simply of the "design of drugs" or "drug design."

By 1952 he became associate professor and applied for a Fulbright grant in Italy to work in Professor Daniel Bovet's laboratory at the Istituto Superiore di Sanità the following year. Fred felt somewhat handicapped by his youthful appearance, being at thirty-two the youngest ranking scientist at the Istituto, and tried to grow a beard. He bought a Lambretta, upon which he transported three-fourths of his family (his wife, a girl, and a boy) in various combinations, darting through traffic Italian-style, and thoroughly enjoying the sun-bathed scenery. Unlike other onlookers, Fred was incapable of absorbing impressions without acting upon them, and started painting to work out his thoughts in yet another medium. His year in Rome gave him freedom from academic responsibilities and the necessary distance and perspective to view his own work in a larger context. In spite of the constant ribbing about a year's "holiday" in Rome, he did in fact put in his full share of work: to everyone's consternation, he even worked through the siesta. The result was a paper entitled "A New Group of Central Nervous System Paralyzants," which he published with Dr. Vincenzo Longo of the Istituto.

Upon his return from Italy, Fred Schueler was honored by receiving the Ebert Prize in Pharmaceutical Chemistry and the Abel Award in Pharmacology in quick succession. He now resumed an ever-increasing load of out-of-town lectures, industrial consultantships, and medical-school committee work, and began to lay plans for the department he hoped some day to direct.

Fred had completed a major portion of his experimental work at Iowa. In particular he designed a compound which he defined as a "hemicholinium" (HC-3) and which gave rise to a family of drugs that he watched grow in scope and variety with eager parental interest. His family had long been used to Fred's detailed descriptions of highly toxic materials, but he never took their impunity for granted. A usual remark was: "If I breathed any of it in I should be dead: there is no antidote." One evening, he patiently sat down at the kitchen table to wait for effects, but since he was still alive in the morning, he put on his coat and went back to work.

In 1956, he was offered the chairmanship of the pharmacology department at Tulane University in New Orleans, which was to be his home for the next eight years. Fred had taken a long weekend off to move his family south from Iowa City. After three days of unbearable August heat, with the children and a grown German shepherd dog in a packed car, he drove straight home through the heart of town to the Medical School, parked the car, and with children and dog in tow went up to the pharmacology department on the third floor, which was mercifully air-conditioned and literally shining and gleaming in its unused newness. Fred explained what he called his first "five-year plan" for the department; as it is today, vastly expanded and humming with activity, the department was as much of a reality to him then as it became in fact, largely through his efforts.

For some time, Fred had read through a not-inconsiderable library in the humanities, philosophy, history of science, and a fairly detailed literature in the behavioral sciences. He now proceeded to apply the results of his informal study to his new administrative duties. Above all, he approached his new responsibilities with a fresh outlook and characteristic energy, and became deeply involved in the problems of medical education. Time in the lab was now almost a personal luxury. More and more of his time was spent in committees, raising funds, consulting, interviewing, and traveling about the country. He moved closer to the airport and kept his flight schedules posted by the telephone. Yet he could no longer put off writing the book that was on his mind. For several years, Fred had worked out a philosophical approach to his subject matter and developed what he called a "rational basis for drug design." Over a period of two years, from 1956 to 1958, at the same time that he organized his new department, he wrote his book on chemobiodynamics, mostly at night, and into it he poured the best of himself. At the end of it, he rewarded himself with a summer in Colombia on the Tulane Colombia Project, came home sun-tanned and loaded down with Indian artifacts, tales of adventure in the jungles of the Amazon, and a program for furthering training in pharmacology in Colombia.

Fred had arrived in Bogota minus his suitcase, which flew on to Ecuador by mistake. After that, he never packed more on any subsequent trips than would fit into an oversized briefcase. For travel by car, he put handles on a sturdy box, his travel library, stuffed the trunk with more books, and took clothes as an afterthought. He loved to hunt, fish, watch birds, and generally just loaf—his loafing was usually productive of original thought and apparently essential to it. Fred all his life longed for the mountains, was addicted to "westerns," and was perfectly capable of sustaining himself in the wilderness. In his thinking and in his work, he was always drawn to unchartered territory, while he managed to imbue the ordinary, the familiar, and the commonplace with an intensity of meaning which sprang from his own vitality and trained imagination. He loved every kind of animal and over the years his home was host to a long succession of pets, wild, domesticated, winged, and otherwise. A small dachshund, a long-haired cat, and a green parakeet were permanent companions. A squirrel monkey had to make his home in the lab, where he has become the departmental mascot and resides in a palatial cage in the hall.

Fred always found time to read, to play, to have fun, and to relax, no matter how crowded his schedule, usually by the expedient of doing several things at the same time, yet being able to devote his full attention to the need of the moment no matter how many other thoughts might be pressing for attention. He would listen to a Mahler symphony, keep an eye on a "western" without sound, work on a differential equation, and read Schopenhauer, alternately, while in the back of his mind he was solving some technical problem.

He was curious about everything; whether at home, on the road, or on the beach, he watched stars, birds, fish, insects, flowers, trees, and stones; he read up on the details of their various structures and anatomies, and in general had an infinite capacity for keeping amused. A pebble in his hand came magically to life, as did everything else around him. Fred used to divide the world into "those that just live in it" and "those that help make it," and with every resource at his command he strove to be part of that ever-growing, changing world.

The summers of 1962 and 1963 Fred Schueler spent in Bethesda at the NIH Laboratories for Infectious Diseases. This was his idea of a perfect vacation: once more free to work in the lab undisturbed by administrative responsibilities.

The department at Tulane was to be expanded by a new building addition, and Fred planned his own two laboratories, one for pharmacology and one for organic synthesis, with almost childish enthusiasm. In anticipation of all his plans to work there, he had given up several of his former commitments, in particular his long association with the Pharmacology Training Grant Committee of the NIH. Except for a short period in the summer of 1964, Fred had had almost no chance to work in his new laboratories.

Sunday afternoon, September 6, Fred had gone to the office as usual. He took care of some correspondence, "checked on the lab," discussed work with an assistant, and left on his desk two papers for publication.

The next day, suddenly, he was gone.

Julia Schueler

New Orleans
February 1965

CONTRIBUTORS TO VOLUME I

Theodore G. Brown, Jr., *Sterling-Winthrop Research Institute, Rensselaer, New York*

Joseph G. Cannon, *Department of Chemistry, College of Pharmacy, State University of Iowa, Iowa City, Iowa*

N. B. Chapman, *Department of Chemistry, The University of Hull, Hull, England*

S. Ehrenpreis, *Department of Pharmacology, Georgetown University Schools of Medicine and Dentistry, Washington, D.C.*

C. J. Evans, *Department of Pharmacology, College of Medicine, State University of Iowa, Iowa City, Iowa*

Harris L. Friedman, *Lakeside Laboratories, Division of Colgate-Palmolive Company, Milwaukee, Wisconsin*

James D. P. Graham, *Pharmacology Department, The Welsh National School of Medicine, The Parade, Cardiff, Wales*

Laszlo Gyermek, *Syntex Research Center and Department of Pharmacology, School of Medicine, Stanford University, Palo Alto, California*

A. M. Lands, *Sterling-Winthrop Research Institute, Rensselaer, New York*

J. J. Lewis, *Division of Experimental Pharmacology, Institute of Physiology, University of Glasgow, Scotland*

J. P. Long, *Department of Pharmacology, College of Medicine, State University of Iowa, Iowa City, Iowa*

T. C. Muir, *Division of Experimental Pharmacology, Institute of Physiology, University of Glasgow, Scotland*

Cedric M. Smith, *Department of Pharmacology, State University of New York at Buffalo, Buffalo, New York*

Irwin B. Wilson, *Department of Chemistry, University of Colorado, Boulder, Colorado*

CONTRIBUTORS TO VOLUME 2

L. G. Abood, *Center for Brain Research and Department of Biochemistry, University of Rochester, Rochester, New York*

R. Banziger, *Research Division, Hoffmann-La Roche, Inc., Nutley, New Jersey*

John H. Biel, *Aldrich Chemical Company, Milwaukee, Wisconsin*

Maynard B. Chenoweth, *Biochemical Research Laboratory, The Dow Chemical Company, Midland, Michigan*

Edward F. Domino, *Department of Pharmacology, The University of Michigan, Ann Arbor, Michigan*

Hugh B. Donahoe, *Department of Chemistry, St. Louis University, St. Louis, Missouri*

Albert Hofmann, *Sandoz A.G., Basel, Switzerland*

Roy D. Hudson, *Department of Pharmacology, Brown University, Providence, Rhode Island*

Paul A. J. Janssen, *Research Laboratoria, Janssen Pharmaceutica, Beerse, Belgium*

Kazuo K. Kimura, *Atlas Chemical Industries, Inc., Wilmington, Delaware*

Eric R. Larsen, *Halogens Research Laboratory, The Dow Chemical Company, Midland, Michigan*

H. Lehr, *Research Division, Hoffmann-La Roche, Inc., Nutley, New Jersey*

L. O. Randall, *Research Division, Hoffmann-La Roche, Inc., Nutley, New Jersey*

L. H. Sternbach, *Research Division, Hoffmann-La Roche, Inc., Nutley, New Jersey*

Cyriel A. M. Van der Eycken, *Research Laboratoria, Janssen Pharmaceutica, Beerse, Belgium*

Russell A. Van Dyke, *Biochemical Research Laboratory, The Dow Chemical Company, Midland, Michigan*

George Zografi, *Department of Pharmacy, The University of Michigan, Ann Arbor, Michigan*

CONTENTS

CHAPTER I

MOLECULAR ASPECTS OF CHOLINERGIC MECHANISMS*

S. Ehrenpreis

DEPARTMENT OF PHARMACOLOGY
GEORGETOWN UNIVERSITY SCHOOLS OF MEDICINE AND DENTISTRY
WASHINGTON, D.C.

1.1. INTRODUCTION

The effects of most drugs on the body are due primarily to interaction with a receptor substance. Usually, the exact chemical or molecular nature of the receptor is completely unknown, although in the cholinergic system there is certainly a close similarity between receptor and cholinesterase (ChE). One of the primary aims of pharmacologists is to elucidate the nature of receptors and ultimately to isolate and identify them. This chapter will discuss some of

* This work was supported in part by Grants NB-03695 and HE 08597 from the Public Health Service, Bethesda, Maryland, and Grants GB-148 and GB-3190 from the National Science Foundation, Washington, D.C.

the studies that have been made in an effort to characterize the receptor in situ and to isolate the cholinergic receptor.

Among the most important aspects of the receptor system, from the molecular standpoint, are the organization and localization of its components. Molecular organization is essential for the precise evaluation of transmission phenomena within the framework of the two chief current hypotheses, those concerning neurohumoral and electrical transmission. The localization of the system is essential to a complete understanding of the mechanism by which cholinergic drugs produce their effects, because it is now recognized that such compounds have pronounced activity at sites other than the postsynaptic membrane where, it is generally agreed, the cholinergic receptor exists. Two of these sites are the conducting membranes of nerve and muscle; the question of whether these membrane components are indeed identical with the receptor at junctions will be discussed in detail.

Although many aspects of the cholinergic system on the molecular level will be considered, emphasis will be placed on the two members of the system most directly concerned with drug effects, ChE and the receptor. It is intended to examine in detail the generally accepted concept that the enzyme acts exclusively as a regulator of acetylcholine (ACh) action, particularly since a number of major discrepancies have emerged, which cast some doubt upon this role. If this function can be shown to be inoperative under physiological conditions, then the way may be paved for equating enzyme with receptor. The actions of the potent inhibitors of ChE will be discussed in detail from this standpoint, and the mechanism by which they produce their effects will be reinterpreted. Although the idea of equating enzyme and receptor is not novel, having been proposed by Župančič (*1*, *2*), Wurzel and Sapeika (*3–5*), and Belleau (*6*), the precise way in which the enzyme participates in membrane phenomena has not been defined. A proposal will be made which attempts not only to do this but also to provide a molecular mechanism for unifying cholinergic drug effects. These suggestions are of necessity speculative, although some supporting evidence has been obtained.

1.2. LOCALIZATION AND FUNCTION OF THE CHOLINERGIC RECEPTOR SYSTEM

A. Relationship to Neurohumoral Theory

Most physiologists and pharmacologists accept the theory that the normal function of ACh is an intercellular one; that is, ACh is released from nerve cells and acts upon a receptor located in the second structure with which the nerve endings are intimately associated. This reaction sets up the series of events that greatly increases permeability of the postsynaptic membrane to ions. In the case of striated muscle, this gives rise to the end-plate potential which, when it reaches a critical level, causes depolarization of the conducting membrane of the muscle. It is generally considered that cholinesterase is the agent mainly responsible for the transient effect of ACh, hydrolyzing the ester with great rapidity to inactive choline and acetate.

To understand fully how these events occur in an orderly and continuing fashion and to account for the effects that many compounds produce on the system it is essential to consider the localization and molecular characteristics of the various components of the system.

Although there is only conjecture about the chemical nature of the receptor molecule, some attempts have been made to determine its precise location at junctions. Of these the electrophoretic jet technique has been the most successful (*7, 8*). On the basis of the elegant studies made it was concluded that the receptor of striated muscle must be present on the outer extremity of the postsynaptic membrane. Thus, when a micropipette was placed a small distance below the postsynaptic membrane, there was complete lack of effect of ACh and *d*-tubocurarine (*7*). This conclusion was substantiated by two entirely different types of experiment (*9*). When a single electroplax of the electric organ of electric eel was mounted and bathed in 1 mg/ml of ^{14}C-labeled *d*-tubocurarine (1,000,000 counts/min/ml), not a trace of the drug had penetrated into the cell in 1 hr. Under these conditions the drug rapidly blocks electrical activity by combining with the receptor. In another type of experiment it was shown that the highly basic proteins protamine and lysozyme could block the electrical activity of electroplax, presumably by combining with the receptors. It is unlikely that these high-molecular-weight substances penetrated the cell when they had produced their effects. Protamine has at times been found to react with receptors of other tissues, such as heart, as shown by its ability to block the effect of added ACh (*9*).

Attempts have been made to localize the receptor more directly by "tagging" it in situ with compounds with which it is known to combine; these studies will be discussed below (Section 1.3).

The precise localization of cholinesterase has proved to be a difficult matter. Although there are excellent histochemical methods of determining the enzyme in situ (*10*), somewhat conflicting results have been obtained. One possible reason is that it is extremely difficult to regulate the degree of diffusion of the product of enzymatic hydrolysis; another is the specificity of the substrate used. Thus, for example, the enzyme has been shown by Barrnett to be present within nerve terminal particles (*11*), a finding that is consistent with results of analyses of vesicles isolated from nerve tissue (*12–14*). However, in the Barrnett experiment the substrate used was thiolacetic acid, a fairly nonspecific esterase substrate, and since the vesicular enzyme was extremely resistant to inhibition by both diisopropyl fluorophosphate (DFP) and physostigmine (it was totally inhibited only at 10^{-4} *M*), there is some doubt that this enzyme represents true cholinesterase activity.

A most promising approach to the more precise localization of ChE was introduced by Ostrowski and Barnard through the use of tritiated DFP (*15*, *16*) in conjunction with radioautography. In this way the problem of diffusion is eliminated, although there is still the possibility that the compound reacts with esterases other than ChE. Perhaps the ideal method would involve the use of some irreversible highly specific ChE inhibitor that could be visualized with the electron microscope.

There is no doubt that ChE is present within nerve axons, although its precise location in regions away from the terminals has not been determined. As to the possible function of axonal ChE, perhaps the most generalized proposal has been set forth by Nachmansohn (*17*), who implicates the enzyme directly in the nerve-action potential; this will be discussed later (Section 1.2B). Koelle has suggested a more restricted function at certain ganglia, principally the superior cervical, where the enzyme has been shown to be present mainly at presynaptic sites. On the basis of this finding and much pharmacological evidence, Koelle has proposed that presynaptic ChE is involved with the normal function of preganglionic neurons (*18*). It is suggested that ACh released from preganglionic terminals causes an additional liberation of ACh from the terminals, thereby amplifying the effect of the initial amount released. Under ordinary circumstances presynaptic ChE serves to limit the degree of autoliberation. When DFP was administered and the presynaptic nerve briefly stimulated, a repetitive postsynaptic firing of long duration was observed; the regulating influence of ChE on presynaptically released ACh had apparently been eliminated. Additional details of this attractive hypothesis have recently been reviewed (*18*).

Another complication with regard to the enzyme is the fact that the ChE present at junctions is now known to be nonuniform, in that both true and pseudo ChE have been shown to exist side by side at many types of junction (*19–21*). The full significance of this finding has not been explored.

Despite the disagreement concerning the precise localization of ChE, isolation and histochemical studies show unequivocally that the enzyme is associated with membranous structures (*10*, *12–14*). The fact that it is very difficult to solubilize the enzyme from tissue homogenates implies a very strong binding of the enzyme with membranes although, interestingly enough, lecithinases are quite effective in liberating ChE from structural material (*22*). Tissues such as intact nerve (*23*), heart, or stomach (*24*, *24a*) may be washed repeatedly for many days at 32°C with no indication that the enzyme is solubilized. However, cobra venom lecithinase, even at very high concentrations, failed to liberate this bound ChE from intact atria (*25*).

ChE has been stated to be one of the fastest-acting enzymes in hydrolyzing

ACh (*26*). The turnover number for a single molecule of eel ChE has been calculated to be about 4×10^7/min (*26*), assuming a molecular weight of 3,000,000 (*27*),* and this high activity is consistent with the generally accepted role of the enzyme as a regulator of ACh action at junctions. The activity of axonal ChE also is considered sufficiently high to enable the enzyme to inactivate endogenously released ACh with sufficient rapidity (i.e., within milliseconds) to be consistent with the postulated role of the ester in initiating and propagating the action potential (*17*). However, the kinetic properties of the enzyme and its accepted role as a regulator of ACh action may require revision in view of the following recent findings.

The turnover number frequently quoted is calculated on the basis of hydrolytic activity of ChE at the optimal ACh concentration, about 3×10^{-3} *M*, where the reaction is zero-order. However, it is apparent from the shape of the substrate–activity curve (*33, 34*) that the hydrolytic rate falls rapidly as the concentration of ACh is decreased, and this fact raises a question about the catalytic activity of the enzyme at physiological concentrations of the ester. Using a bioassay, various workers have observed that enzyme activity is indeed very low at 10^{-6} *M* ACh (*5, 35*). Using even more sensitive bioassay procedures, Ehrenpreis and co-workers (*24*) found that purified true ChE (electric eel or red blood cell) hydrolyzes ACh at an extremely low rate when the ester concentration is much below 10^{-6} *M*.† This was demonstrated by adding the enzyme to an ACh solution bathing rabbit atria (ACh concentration, 10^{-7} *M*) or rat stomach strips (10^{-8} *M* ACh). In neither instance was there evidence of hydrolysis of ACh, even when the mixtures were permitted to stand for 1 hr. According to the assay made at optimal ACh concentration the amount of enzyme used was sufficient to hydrolyze all of the ACh within seconds. As far as pseudo ChE is concerned, incubation of 2×10^{-6} *M* ACh with serum (final dilution, 1:1) revealed a complete absence of hydrolysis over a period of 30 min at 25°C.‡

At concentrations of ACh that act upon atria or stomach muscle the tissue enzyme itself fails to hydrolyze ACh to any significant extent over a prolonged period of time (*24*). This was shown by allowing ACh solutions to remain in contact with the particular tissue for varying periods of time and determining

* This value, given by Nachmansohn, apparently was based on the total hydrolytic activity of purified ChE. However, as pointed out by Dixon and Webb (*28*), the turnover number must refer to the number of molecules hydrolyzed per minute per catalytic site. Ultimately it was determined (*29*) that the minimal molecular weight is about 100,000 and that, in fact, the turnover number is in the range of 7×10^5. This value is more in line with other determinations of the turnover number (*30, 31*).

† The turnover number of red blood cell ChE at 32°C is about 10,000 times greater at 5×10^{-3} *M* ACh than at 10^{-7} *M*.

‡ These findings contradict results obtained by Dzoljic (*36*), who reported that under similar conditions ACh was destroyed by serum ChE within 5 min.

the ACh by bioassay. Even when 2 μg ACh was in contact with these tissues for about an hour, there was no evidence of hydrolysis of the ester. At 4×10^{-3} *M* ACh, the ChE of intact atria from a single rabbit heart or a strip from a single rat stomach hydrolyzes ACh at the rate of about 8 μg./min.

These findings raise a question about the general concept that ChE ordinarily regulates ACh activity by rapidly breaking down the ester after its action. According to various calculations (*35*, *37–39*), the concentration of ACh liberated upon nerve stimulation is about 6×10^{-7} *M* in the vicinity of the postsynaptic membrane. It is apparent from these experiments that the enzyme fails to hydrolyze its substrate at a significant rate when the latter is at this concentration. In view of this finding, it is obvious that the mechanism of action of the inhibitors of ChE must be revised. Additional evidence to support such a contention will be discussed below (Section 1.5).

As for the precise localization of ACh, evidence has been accumulating that it is present within vesicles located primarily, but not exclusively, at nerve endings. The first proposal that a relationship might exist between vesicles and transmission was made by de Robertis and Bennett (*40*) and Palay (*41*), who showed that a distinct reduction in the number of vesicles followed the stimulation of splanchnic nerve with supramaximal pulses. Subsequently, vesicles having the same size and shape as those observed at nerve endings were isolated from brain homogenates by centrifugation in density gradients (*12–14*). Although there is disagreement between the two major groups of workers in this field about the method of isolation and the type of particle which is obtained, there is no doubt that at least some vesicles contain ACh. Vesicles containing other neurotransmitters (for example, serotonin or norepinephrine) also have been isolated, but they apparently differ from the ACh vesicles (*42*).

More recent work has indicated that the state of ACh present in homogenates may be quite complex. In fact, according to Whittaker et al. (*14*) there are three forms of ACh in nerve tissue: a fraction that is released upon homogenization in iso-osmotic medium, a particulate-bound fraction, which is somewhat labile (i.e., released by hypotonic solution), and a much more stable bound fraction, which requires such drastic treatment as boiling before release is achieved. These investigators feel that at least some of the ACh shown to be present in bound form may arise from the cytoplasm and that during the isolation procedure ACh shifts from one compartment to another.

Evidence that this is a possibility was obtained by Burton, who showed that the vesicular fractions isolated according to procedures of Whittaker and co-workers can accumulate large amounts of exogenous ACh (*43*, *44*). This uptake correlated well with the ganglioside content of the subcellular particles and led to the conclusion that this may be the component involved with ACh binding or as part of the wall of the vesicle. The fact that neuraminidase released a good portion of the bound ACh seems to fit in with these suggestions. Burton has presented the only molecular formulation of how nerve stimulation can give rise to the release of ACh. The formulation is presented in Figure 1.1 and is described as follows (*43*):

> ACh is contained in synaptic vesicles which may be composed of a (protein?) matrix with holes which are "plugged" with lipids—especially the gangliosides. The gangliosides are attached to the matrix by non-covalent bonds, i.e., bonds hydrophobic in nature. . . . These bonds are formed and stable in aqueous media, but are rapidly broken in non-polar solvents. As the nerve terminal depolarizes, the negatively charged synaptic vesicle moves into a lipid area of the presynaptic membrane, . . . the gangliosides dissociate from the other gangliosides and lipids in the vesicle matrix leaving ACh in a lipid phase of the membrane. Since the highly polar ACh will be repelled by the lipid phase it will be expelled into the synaptic cleft.

Experimental verification of this hypothesis is completely lacking and depends on, among other things, the correctness of the assumption that the vesicles are released during nerve activity—a view that is not universally accepted (*45*) but appears to be quite reasonable.

Aside from their strategic localization, the vesicles apparently are sufficiently

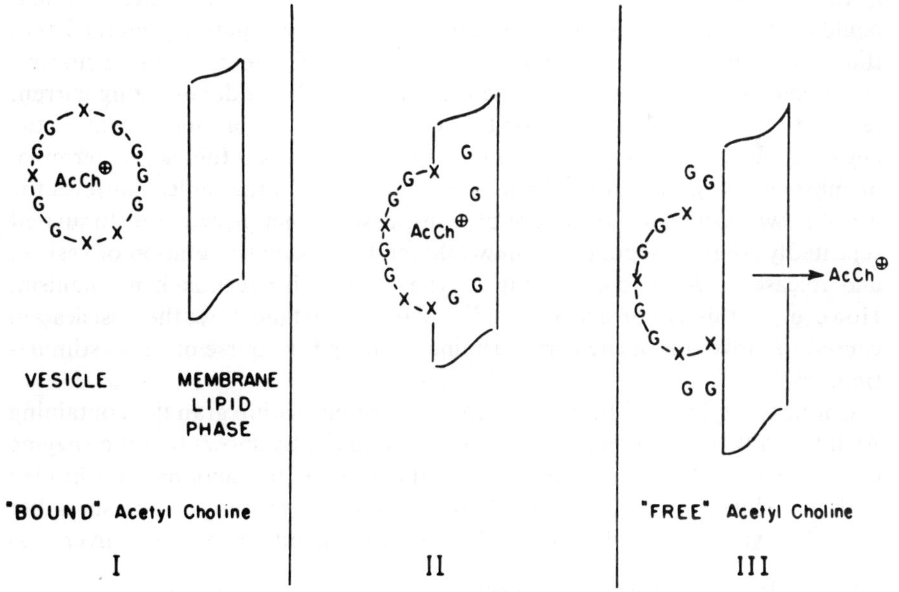

Fig. 1.1. Hypothetical mechanism for acetylcholine release involving gangliosides. G represents gangliosides in noncovalent bonding with the synaptic vesicle membrane matrix, X, and other lipids, X. [From Ref. (*43*).]

large to contain about 45,000 molecules of ACh (*46*),* which is approximately the amount of ACh liberated per nerve impulse, according to Acheson's calculations (*37*). Krnjevic and Miledi (*47*), using the electrophoretic jet technique, determined that the minimal amount required was actually 10 times Acheson's value, suggesting that 10 vesicles must be mobilized simultaneously to stimulate an end plate.

One of the difficulties with the vesicle concept concerns the weight of the particle, assuming these calculations are correct. The contribution of ACh would be about one million; regardless of whether the vesicle wall is comprised primarily of polypeptide material (*46*) or ganglioside (*43*, *44*), the molecular weight of a vesicle would be several million. The rate of movement of such a particle even under the influence of an electric field would undoubtedly be extremely slow, particularly since it may be embedded in the highly viscous nerve-terminal cytoplasm.

Another problem with regard to the vesicular concept concerns the question of the link between electrical events at the nerve terminal and movement of the vesicles. This question was investigated by Hubbard and Willis (*48*), who used the direct approach of electrical stimulation of nerve terminals. They had previously observed (*49*) that hyperpolarization of nerve terminals (rat phrenic nerve) led to an increase in the end-plate potential, an effect which was attributed to an increase in ACh quanta released. This increase, they felt, could be explained by assuming that the vesicles were negatively charged and, thus, their outward movement was accelerated by the hyperpolarizing current. In agreement with this it was subsequently found that a depolarizing current reduced the end-plate potentials; this was explained by a "movement of the negatively charged vesicles of transmitter away from the nerve terminal membrane" (*48*). Such a mechanism could explain on the molecular level the well-known occurrence of failure of transmission when nerves are stimulated repeatedly; that is, depolarization would tend to prevent migration of vesicles and release of ACh, constituting a type of negative feedback mechanism. However, if this is correct, it is difficult to understand how the vesicles are caused to move out of the nerve terminals during the course of nerve stimulation.

Cholineacetylase has been reported to be present within granules containing ACh (*14*, *50*), although another report (*51*) apparently shows that the enzyme is found primarily in the supernatant of the particulate fractions. This has led to the conclusion that "ACh is synthesized in the nerve ending cytoplasm rather than the synaptic vesicles" (*51*). On the other hand, Hebb and Silver (*52*)

* This calculation is based on the volume of an ACh molecule in the crystalline state which, Canepa believes, might actually be the form in which ACh exists within a vesicle. This proposition is difficult to reconcile with recent indications that ACh might be bound to a considerable extent inside vesicles and so would not be present in the crystalline state.

reported that the enzyme is entirely membrane-bound and that the observed axonal movement of the enzyme is a reflection of translocation of entire structural regions of the axon. At this writing these seemingly contradictory findings have not been resolved.

One apparent discrepancy in the neurohumoral theory stems from the finding that after denervation and the concomitant disappearance of the miniature end-plate potential the electrical silence may be broken with the resumption of spontaneous activity at most of the denervated end plates. The question was raised how this can occur when neural elements are absent, because it is considered that ACh liberated continuously from nerve terminals is responsible for these end-plate potentials. The work of Birks et al. (*53*) has gone a long way toward clearing up this mystery through the finding that the Schwann cell apparently can take over the function of the motor nerve ending in synaptic regions and produce not only ACh but synaptic vesicles as well.

B. The Nachmansohn Concept of Cholinergic Function and Localization of the Receptor System

For many years the neurohumoral transmission theory has been steadfastly rejected by Nachmansohn and his co-workers. In their view, ACh has an exclusively *intracellular* action rather than a function of transmitter between cells, as neurohumoral theory demands. In this view ACh "forms an integral part of the elementary processes by which bioelectric potentials are generated in the axon, in the nerve terminal, and in the postsynaptic membrane, but the electric currents are the propagating agent in transmission as well as in conduction" (*54*). In other words, Nachmansohn considers events within axons to be mediated by chemical reactions involving the ACh system, while he maintains that transmission between cells is produced not by ACh but rather by electric currents emerging from nerve terminals.

Nachmansohn has presented a precise description of how he considers the ACh receptor system to function in the initiation and propagation of the action potential at all sites, including junctions (*55*). His mechanism may be summarized briefly as follows: An electrical stimulus which is above threshold intensity produces a liberation of ACh from its bound form. The liberated ACh reacts locally with a specific ACh receptor that is present within the membrane, either at postsynaptic sites or in conducting membranes. The combination of ACh and receptor results in a change in configuration of the latter; this change alters the local structure of the membrane resulting in the passage of sodium ions through it. This in turn causes a local depolarization, which stimulates an adjacent region of the membrane, and additional ACh is liberated and reacts with the receptor, and so forth. In this way the disturbance is propagated down the axon or along the conducting membrane of a muscle. The free ACh liberated from the bound form is considered to be rapidly hydrolyzed by ChE, which is present in close proximity to the receptor. This results in a shift of the ACh-receptor equilibrium; the complex dissociates and eventually all the substrate is hydrolyzed. The receptor is thereby restored to its initial configuration, and the localized region of the membrane returns to its initial degree of impermeability to sodium ions. The stores of ACh are said to be constantly replenished by metabolic activity involving acetylcoenzyme A, choline, and cholineacetylase.

The effects of drugs are explained primarily by their reaction with the ACh receptor or with ChE. A compound would be expected to mimic the action of ACh if it had a similar chemical structure and could penetrate to the receptors within the membrane;* such a compound also would be expected to cause depolarization. The term "receptor activator" is given to such a compound. Other compounds, particularly tertiary ammonium derivatives, would be expected to block by reacting with the receptor in such a way as to prevent the action of liberated ACh; such compounds are termed "receptor-inhibitors," and they block without depolarization. Finally, inhibitors of ChE block nerve activity by preventing the cycle of events leading to the restoration of the membrane to its initial state. Theoretically, inhibition of axonal ChE should lead to membrane depolarization because of accumulated ACh.

It may be noted that Nachmansohn has never presented a model of how the proposed cholinergic system is organized within a membrane. Karlson (*56*) has attempted such a pictorial representation (Figure 1.2) based on his interpretation of Nachmansohn's written description of the mechanism. We consider this a reasonable picture, although Nachmansohn has not commented upon it. Nevertheless, Karlson's formulation could prove useful in an attempt to understand the action of various types of compound within the framework of the Nachmansohn hypothesis.

The major experimental support for this hypothesis, as it relates to conducting membranes, has been obtained from studies of the effects that many different types of cholinergic compounds have on the electrical activity of isolated nerves and single electroplax. The following is an analysis of some of the major results obtained and includes a discussion of the data published subsequent to a detailed critique of the theory which the author recently presented (*57*).

It should be stressed that Nachmansohn's concept of transmission between

* Penetration is an important consideration since the active membrane of most nerves is not very accessible to externally applied compounds because of the presence of such barriers as the myelin sheath or the Schwann cell (a discussion of how the barriers serve to complicate drug action will be presented in the text).

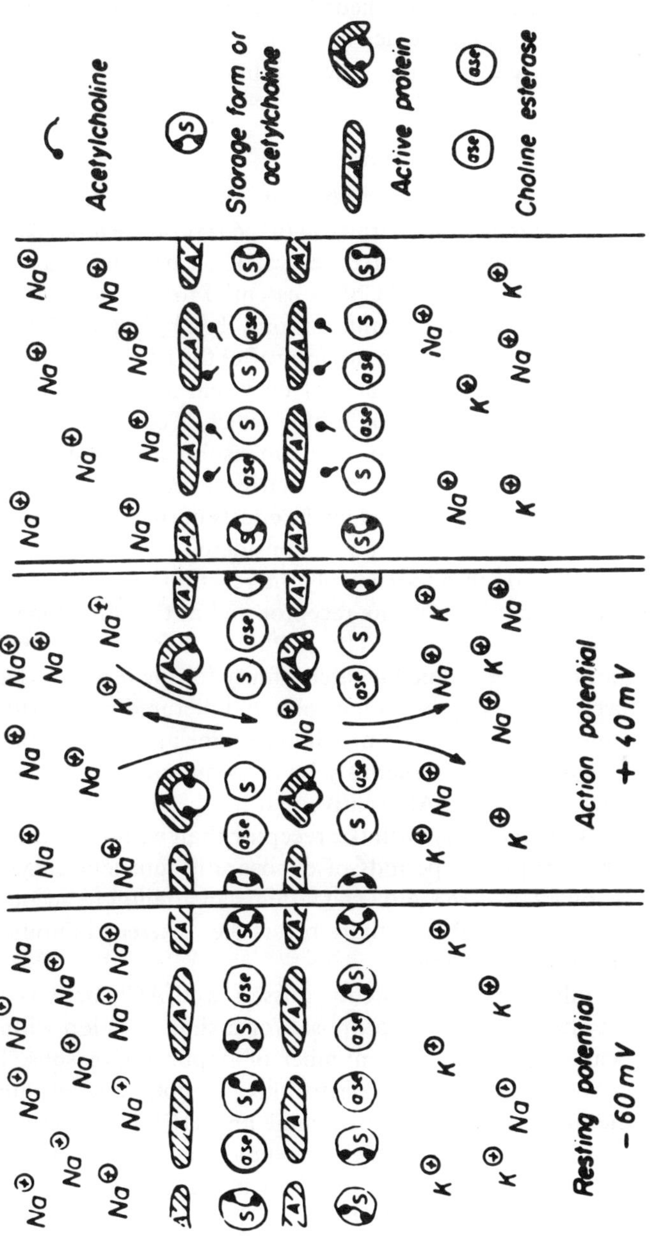

Fig. 1.2. According to Nachmansohn's hypothesis of permeability changes in nerves. The diagram shows three phases: left, the resting state; middle, the influx of Na^+ with concomitant reversal of potential; right, the state after hydrolysis of acetylcholine. S, A, and ase represent storage protein, receptor, and cholinesterase respectively. [From Ref. (*56*).]

cells is a necessary consequence of the theory that ACh action is strictly "intramembranous"; he and his colleagues have presented no evidence of a direct nature that would refute the theory of neurohumoral transmission.

1. CHOLINESTERASE INHIBITORS

There is no doubt that the very potent inhibitors of ChE, such as DFP (*58–60*), physostigmine (*59, 61–64*), and paraoxon (*65, 66*) produce a blockade of electrical activity when applied to isolated nerves. The early findings were originally interpreted as being proof that ChE is essential for nerve function. If ChE is indeed essential for bioelectric manifestations, then by implication so, too, is ACh, its natural substrate. However, not long after the first observations were made, it was recognized that blockade of electrical activity occurred without the expected depolarization (*60*), a finding which is contradictory to the theory. This led to the suggestion by Nachmansohn and co-workers (*67, 68*) that both DFP and physostigmine act primarily as receptor-inhibitors on nerves, a mode of action that was justified by the effects of these compounds on electroplax (*67, 69*). In other words, it was considered that the primary effect of these compounds is to inhibit selectively the reaction of ACh (postulated to be released during activity) with its receptor and at the same time to react only minimally with the tissue's ChE. This sort of mechanism necessarily implies that the compounds have a much greater affinity for the receptor than for the enzyme because, as stated by Nachmansohn and pictured by Karlson, receptor and enzyme must coexist in close proximity to one another and both would be reached more or less simultaneously by any compound capable of penetrating to the active membrane. Alternatively, it has been suggested that DFP in particular reacts *more rapidly* with the receptor than with the enzyme and that only after very prolonged periods of exposure is sufficient enzyme inhibited to permit depolarization (*68, 69*). The latter is an attempt to account for the fact that blockade by DFP is initially reversible, whereas inhibition of ChE by DFP is certainly irreversible.

Although the ChE inhibitors undoubtedly possess anti-ACh actions at established cholinergic sites (*70–73*), the proposal for a similar action within nerves does not appear to be valid for a number of important reasons. In virtually every other system examined (electroplax, smooth and striated muscle, and heart) the first action of physostigmine and DFP is to facilitate or potentiate the actions of ACh, whether the compound is added exogenously or is released by nerve stimulation. It is only when the concentration of inhibitor is greatly increased that the anti-ACh effect becomes manifest (*70–73*). Not only do these compounds not have a similar effect on the action potential of nerve (*62, 63*)—that is, a prolongation of the descending phase suggestive of a preservation of endogenously released ACh—but they even *inhibit* the weak effects of the ester on those few nerves in which it has now been shown to act (see below). Thus, there is no analogy between the action of these compounds at junctional regions, where ACh has a clear physiological role, and that at nerve axons.

Although kinetic factors may be involved in the effects produced by the ChE inhibitors, these do not appear important at junctions where these compounds act very rapidly in very low concentrations. Moreover, kinetics of reaction may not be nearly as essential as the comparative affinities of a compound for its target macromolecule, whether it be enzyme or receptor. It is evident from the preceding discussion that the affinity for the enzyme of a compound such as physostigmine would almost certainly be far greater than its affinity for other tissue components, including the proposed receptor. This would be even more pronounced in the case of DFP, a compound which bears no charged group or other substituent that would enable it to form a strong reversible bond. In the case of the ACh system those compounds which combine strongly with the receptor almost always have a positive charge, and therefore a high affinity for DFP would be most unlikely. With regard to physostigmine, it is now stated by the Nachmansohn group that this compound actually has a *low* affinity for the ACh receptor (*74*, *75*), in contradiction to earlier statements that its affinity may be very great (*67*, *76*, *77*).

The proposed mechanism of action of the inhibitors of ChE is further confused by the fact that the results obtained with these compounds were originally construed to indicate the essentiality of the enzyme. In fact, this was the original basis for explaining the irreversibility of DFP blockade of nerve activity and the complete reversibility of the effect of physostigmine, the latter being considered a freely reversible inhibitor of the enzyme. Thus, we are faced with the predicament of attempting to ascertain which aspect of the action of these compounds is consistent with the theory: if they block by inhibiting the enzyme, why is depolarization not observed, and if they block by inhibiting the receptor, where is the evidence that ChE is essential in controlling axonal events? This dilemma has never been satisfactorily resolved although whenever depolarization is observed (*65*) it is described as having been "expected" in terms of the theory. Moreover, despite the emphasis that organophosphates initially act as receptor-inhibitors, it has now been reported that paraoxon produces a rapid depolarizing block (*65*) which is claimed to occur exclusively through inhibition of ChE (*66*).

Another aspect of the problem with the ChE-inhibitors (in particular, DFP and physostigmine) is their obviously weak effect on nerves as compared with their great potency in altering cholinergic events at junctions. The concentration of DFP, physostigmine, or paraoxon required to affect nerve activity (by whatever mechanism this may occur) is generally several milligrams per milliliter, whereas junctional effects occur at concentrations several thousand-fold lower. This disparity has been countered with the argument that the presence of barriers, lipid in nature, prevents the penetration of these compounds to the active site in the conducting membrane; although this site is unspecified, it presumably is ChE itself but, as indicated above, there is considerable uncertainty on this point.

This explanation gives rise to an obvious paradox: highly potent lipid-soluble cholinergic compounds are still rather inert on nerves. The paradox appeared to be resolved by evidence purportedly demonstrating that even a compound like DFP encounters barriers of some sort that restrict its penetration into nerve. This was shown by the fact that, when externally applied, DFP penetrated into the axoplasm of squid nerves at a very small fraction of its initial concentration (*78*). On the basis of this result and others involving ACh (*79*), it was concluded that for a drug to affect axonal conduction it must somehow penetrate into the interior of the axon. Thus, DFP and physostigmine act upon nerves because they can penetrate into axoplasm, whereas ACh is inert because it is completely excluded. DFP acts only weakly, however, because it is in very low concentration in axoplasm, having encountered barriers on the way into the nerve. Accordingly, Nachmansohn suggested that various cholinotropic compounds should be highly effective if injected directly into the axoplasm, enabling the compounds to approach the active membrane from the inside and thereby circumventing external barriers (*80*). Indeed, when *d*-tubocurarine was so injected, it was reported to block conduction at extremely low concentrations (*81*). However, this finding could not be confirmed either for *d*-tubocurarine (*82*) or for many other cholinergic compounds injected in a similar way at very high concentrations (*83*, *84*).

There is some question about the validity of the concept that a compound must pass not only through external barriers but through the conducting membrane itself (and thus all the way into the axoplasm) in order to have an effect on membrane-associated events. Karlson's picture leads one to expect that the determinant of action would depend, rather, upon the ability of a compound to penetrate to, and *combine* with, some element in the conducting membrane. The combination might well serve to hold back the compound, and therefore its concentration in the "interior" would give no indication of its ability to react at the membrane. Certainly, at neuromuscular or other junctions a lack of penetration through the postsynaptic membrane is no hindrance to activity, as is shown by the action of various compounds ejected electrophoretically in the experiments of Del Castillo and Katz (*7*, *8*). In fact, these studies showed that only when the compound is confined to the membrane *surface* does it produce its effects. In carrying this argument further and showing its lack of applicability to nerve activity, it has been stated (*85*) that dimethylaminoethyl acetate (DMAEA) is able to penetrate readily and, because this compound is a very close analogue of ACh, it would be expected to have very profound effects upon nerves; yet DMAEA is singularly ineffectual in this regard (*86*, *87*).

Lack of penetration into axoplasm could certainly not be invoked to explain the very weak effects of physostigmine, particularly since it was shown earlier that another tertiary amine, trimethylamine, penetrates axoplasm very rapidly (*79*). As a rationalization of the low potency of physostigmine it is stated that "at pH 7.2 only 5% (of physostigmine) are neutral molecules and this is the only form likely to penetrate through lipid material" (*88*). From this statement it is evident that the barrier now is considered to be of an external nature, yet as is indicated above other tertiary compounds do penetrate very well. It is clear that DMAEA must penetrate readily to the active membrane, this being the basis of its use in assaying ChE in intact nerves for the purpose of correlating enzyme activity and nerve function (*89*). If the same difficulties in penetrating were encountered by DMAEA, then the concentration of the ester in the vicinity of membrane ChE would be very low, and the compound would be of no value as a substrate for the enzyme. Moreover, other types of tertiary amines, such as local anesthetics and chlorpromazine, have very potent effects on nerve activity. They should have the same difficulties in penetrating as are now suggested for physostigmine, since their p*K*'s are all about the same. In most instances, however, these tertiary amines are far more potent in blocking nerve activity than are the ChE inhibitors. If it is argued that all these compounds encounter the same barriers in penetrating to the active membrane, then the following situation obtains. DFP and physostigmine are considered to penetrate only to a small extent, say about 0.1%, a value given for DFP (*85*); in other words, there is a factor of 10^3 in the ratio of external to effective internal concentrations. On squid axon dibucaine and chlorpromazine have a minimal effective blocking concentration of about 5×10^{-5} *M* (*87*). By analogy with the ChE inhibitors, this means that the inhibiting concentration at the active site is about 10^{-8} *M*, implying that these compounds have an extraordinarily high affinity for membrane receptors. Accordingly, dibucaine and chlorpromazine should be among the most potent anti-ACh agents; however, this is not borne out by their affinity for cholinergic receptors of electroplax (*90*), striated muscle (*91*), and heart (*92*). On the other hand, atropine, which is an extremely potent anti-ACh agent, is particularly weak in its effects on nerve (*63*, *65*, *87*) despite its high lipid solubility and anticipated high degree of penetration.

It is now known that external permeability barriers are almost minimal under certain conditions, since even highly lipid-insoluble quaternary ammonium compounds are able to penetrate to the active membrane. The preparations include detergent-treated (*93–95*) and venom-treated nerves (*87*, *96*), desheathed vagus nerve (*62*, *63*), and denervated muscles (*97*, *98*). In no instance is there evidence of marked increase in the potency of the ChE inhibitors

(*62*, *63*, *74*, *87*, *99*), despite the ability of such compounds as *d*-tubocurarine, chlorisondamine, and even protamine (molecular weight, 6000) to block conduction (*87*).

2. CORRELATION BETWEEN ENZYME ACTIVITY AND NERVE FUNCTION

In an early study Wilson and Cohen (*89*) reported that the action potential of crab leg nerves failed when the ChE activity fell below 20% under the influence of DFP. This was considered by Nachmansohn to be the level of ChE below which nerve activity, being intimately related to enzyme activity, could not be sustained (*59*). More recent studies have shown that this apparent correlation between enzyme activity and function does not hold. Nachmansohn and co-workers recently reported (*66*) that 0.01 *M* paraoxon could completely obliterate the action potential of lobster nerves in about one minute. Prolonged washing failed to restore electrical activity, whereas function returned almost immediately in the presence of 0.05 *M* pyridine-2-aldoxime methiodide (2-PAM), a potent reactivator of organophosphate-inhibited ChE. It may be noted that the Nachmansohn group expected 2-PAM, a quaternary ammonium compound, to be an effective reactivator, because "this preparation is apparently poorly protected against lipid-insoluble compounds since curare and ACh are capable to block its axonal electrical activity" (*66*). These experiments on lobster nerve are reminiscent of earlier ones (*99*), in which action potentials of paraoxon-inhibited denervated muscle were apparently restored by means of a 2-PAM derivative. These results were interpreted as proof of the involvement of ChE in the function of conducting membranes of nerve and muscle: the inhibition of electrical activity was accomplished "by a well-defined chemical reaction, namely the phosphorylation of a serine molecule in the active site of ChE by paraoxon," whereas 2-PAM restored electrical activity by a specific reactivation of the inhibited enzyme (*66*).

Although the experiments appear to be rather convincing, they are lacking in certain important respects. First, no evidence was presented, nor was it even stated, that blockade of lobster nerve by paraoxon under the conditions described was accompanied by depolarization. This omission is somewhat surprising in view of the fact that the sucrose gap technique was used and, therefore, the membrane potentials could have been monitored readily. In fact, the one figure showing action potential data reveals that the blockade was *not* of the depolarizing type. This finding was completely ignored in interpreting the data solely in terms of ChE inhibition.

Second, and perhaps even more importantly, no data on ChE activity during the experiment were presented; in other words, it was *assumed* that the ChE had been completely inhibited by the paraoxon and that the 2-PAM had increased enzyme activity. When Ehrenpreis and co-workers (*23*) did enzyme assays under conditions as nearly as possible like those described in the Nachmansohn experiment, it was found that the paraoxon inhibited the enzyme to the extent of 75% and, moreover, there was no evidence of an increase in enzyme activity in the presence of 0.05 *M* 2-PAM. The latter finding was actually expected, because at that very high concentration 2-PAM strongly *inhibits* the enzyme of intact lobster nerves.* In another experiment it was shown that, when lobster nerves were bathed in 5×10^{-3} *M* physostigmine, 100% inhibition of the enzyme was achieved and that this was very difficult to reverse by merely washing the nerves.† Yet action potentials of nerves that were blocked by the drug at this concentration were rapidly restored after washing (*65*). Both of these results reveal that there is, indeed, a lack of correlation between responsiveness of lobster nerve and its ChE activity.

Another recent example of this lack of correlation was provided by other experiments from Nachmansohn's laboratory (*103*). In this study it was shown that 5×10^{-4} *M* DFP had no effect on the electrical activity of isolated vagus nerve (rabbit), whereas 5×10^{-2} *M* DFP invariably abolished the action potential. Yet there was essentially no difference in the extent of ChE inhibition at these two concentrations; in fact, some nerves (Figure 1.3) showed greater enzyme activity at the higher DFP concentration than at the lower. Nevertheless, functioning of the nerves was attributed to the small amount (average, about 10%) of residual enzyme present at the lower DFP concentration although it was admitted that the enzyme activity at the higher concentration (average, about 7%) was not significantly different.

It may be noted that, even when bathed in 0.05 *M* DFP, enzymatic activity attributable to ChE was in evidence. To explain this resistance of ChE to DFP, the authors invoked the often repeated conclusion that "the most likely explanation for this is the presence of a barrier to DFP in the intact nerve" (*103*). However, in the same paper they reported that, in fact, desheathed vagus nerve presented no detectable barrier to methacholine, because they obtained the same enzyme activity in intact and in homogenized nerves (Figure 1.4). Thus, one would be led to the contradictory conclusion that these barriers had excluded DFP but not methacholine, because residual enzyme was

* It had previously been shown (*99a*) that at the neuromuscular junction even 0.0076 *M* 2-PAM does not restore enzymatic activity of organophosphate-inhibited ChE. The interpretation given was the same as that proposed by Ehrenpreis and co-workers (*23*), that even though reactivation occurs, the 2-PAM effectively inhibits the reactivated enzyme. This inhibition does not, of course, become manifest except at very high concentrations of PAM, that is, above about 0.001 *M*.

† This effect was to be expected, because physostigmine inhibition is not strictly reversible; that is, the compound actually carbamylates the enzyme (*100–102*). Thus, the rapid reversibility of blockade of nerve (*65*) may not be attributed to the rapid restoration of enzyme activity, decarbamoylation being a fairly slow process.

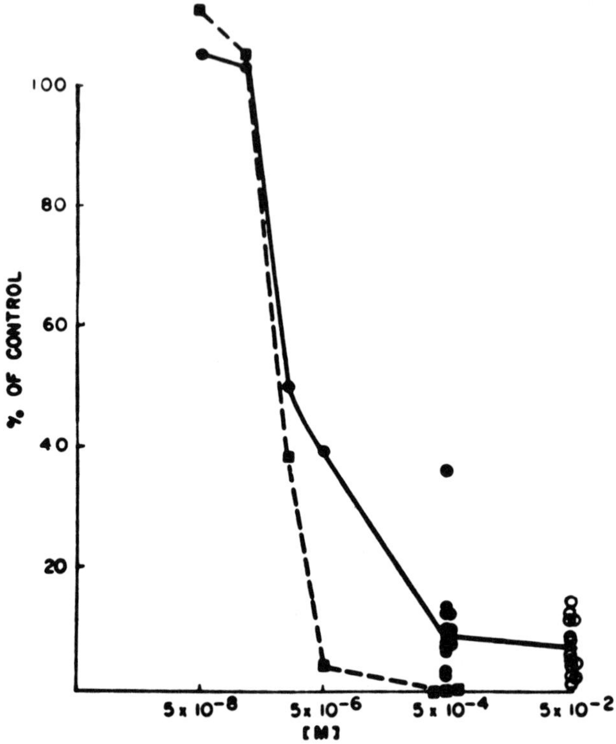

Fig. 1.3. Comparison of acetylcholinesterase activity in homogenized (---) and intact (—) nerves exposed to various concentration of diisopropylfluorophosphate. Conduction was blocked in all nerves exposed to 5×10^{-2} *M* DFP (○) but was not blocked in any of the other concentrations. [From Ref. (*106*).]

detected through the use of this substrate. It had been repeatedly stated that such barriers were very probably of a lipid nature and hence should be much more effective in excluding methacholine than DFP.

One alternative explanation of this observation stems from the recent findings that nerve tissue contains several varieties of enzyme having ChE properties (*104*, *105*). A ChE is present which is extremely resistant, for some reason, to the inhibiting properties of DFP and eserine (*105*). It may be that this highly resistant enzyme accounts for the last traces of ChE activity, obviating the need to invoke barriers. In fact, the data of Dettbarn and Rosenberg (Figure 1.3) showed that at all concentrations of DFP but one, the amount of enzyme in intact and homogenized nerves differed by less than 10% and strongly suggested, once again, the absence of true barriers to penetration of DFP.

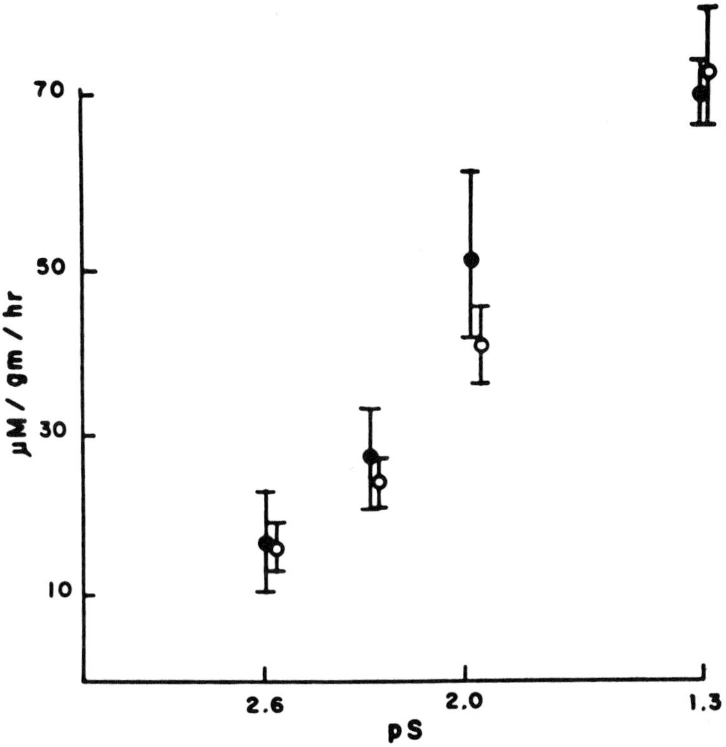

Fig. 1.4. Acetylcholinesterase activity of intact and homogenized nerve with acetyl-β-methylcholine as substrate. Homogenized nerve (●), intact nerve (○); pS = log reciprocal of the molar concentration of substrate. Vertical bars indicate ±1 standard error. [From Ref. (*106*).]

3. LIPID-SOLUBLE QUATERNARY AMMONIUM COMPOUNDS

Lipid-soluble quaternary ammonium compounds were recently used by the Nachmansohn group in an attempt to demonstrate the essentiality of ACh in the functioning of several tissues that are insensitive to externally applied ACh. Some of the limitations in the use of these compounds have been discussed in detail elsewhere (*57*) and so will only be summarized here.

Although the compounds can at times produce an ACh-like depolarizing effect in such tissues as electroplax (*106*, *107*), nerves (*76*, *86*, *108*, *109*), and striated muscle (*110*), the effect is certainly not what might be considered highly specific. Thus, *N*-(β-acetoxyethyl)-*N*,*N*-dimethyl-*N*-*n*-dodecylammonium, *N*,*N*-dimethyl-*N*-*n*-dodecyl-*N*-(β-hydroxyethyl)ammonium,* pyridine dodeciodide (PDI), and pyridine-2-aldoxime dodecyl iodide (2-PAD) are all about

* These compounds are known as noracetylcholine 12 and norcholine 12, respectively.

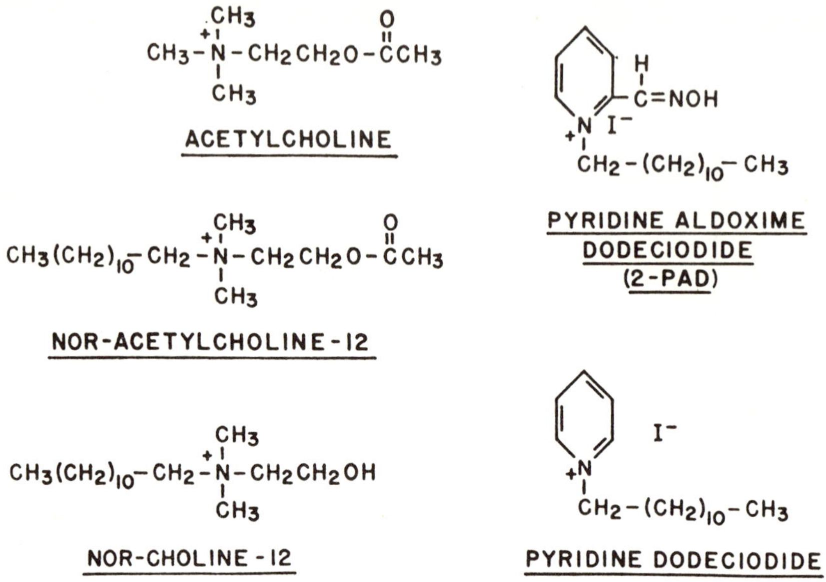

Fig. 1.5. Chemical formulas for ACh and some lipid-soluble quaternary ammonium compounds.

equally potent in producing an effect on nerves that is said to "mimic the physiological action postulated for the ester" (*109*) when it is released internally and produces an action potential. This property was thought to account for their ability, not only to depolarize, but also to produce an "overshoot" (*106*), just as is ordinarily observed during the passage of an action potential. In other words, the compounds caused a reversal in the sign of the resting potential, which became positive under their influence. This finding was considered by the Nachmansohn group to be very significant and led them to write "noracetylcholine dodeciodide, and other lipid-soluble quaternary ammonium ions, block conduction at low concentrations and produce an overshoot which is a striking feature of conduction . . . this first demonstration of a direct action . . . appears at this writing to be a striking confirmation of the theory that ACh is intrinsically connected with conduction" (*106*). The fact that compounds of such diverse chemical structure as 2-PAD and PDI acted in what appeared to be such a similar manner should have indicated that the proposed mechanism of action with respect to faithfully mimicking ACh encounters many difficulties. Indeed, it was subsequently reported that the initial finding of an overshoot could not be confirmed when the experiments were repeated (*111*).

Actually, these compounds were recently shown to have a fairly nonspecific action upon aortic smooth muscle, in the sense that they quite effectively inhibit responses of this tissue to norepinephrine, histamine, serotonin, and KCl (*112*). No evidence of an ACh-like activity was observed; in fact, the compounds were extremely potent *inhibitors* of ACh-induced contractions. These results strongly suggest that these compounds do not have a highly specific effect on the cholinergic receptor system.

4. ACTION OF ACETYLCHOLINE AND OTHER CHOLINOTROPIC AGENTS UPON NERVE

In any inquiry into the question of a functional cholinergic system in nerves, the effect of ACh and related compounds that react strongly with junctional receptors must be considered. However, the situation is rather complicated since most of the compounds are quaternary ammonium derivatives and, hence, would not be expected to penetrate readily to the active membrane of most nerves because of external lipoid barriers. This has been given as the reason for the very weak action of these compounds on such nerves as giant squid axon and frog sciatic (*113*). Nachmansohn and co-workers appeared to have obtained experimental verification of this proposal by demonstrating the apparent lack of penetration of ^{15}N-labeled ACh into squid axoplasm (*79*). However, other workers completely failed to confirm this finding (*114*, *115*); indeed, Clark reported that not only ACh but other quaternary ammonium compounds can penetrate rapidly into squid axoplasm (*115*). Clark makes the rather pointed remark that "a compound may lack activity (to block conduction) because it lacks structural features and not necessarily because of its ability to distribute into the axon." More recently evidence of a different sort, which substantiates Clark's statement, has been obtained by Rosenberg and Dettbarn (*116*): they showed clearly that 5×10^{-3} *M* ACh penetrates extremely well to the ChE of intact squid nerves, the difference in activity between intact and homogenized nerves being less than 20%. Since in Nachmansohn's view the ChE of squid nerve is associated with the active membrane (*34*), it is evident that externally applied ACh should indeed have some effect on electrical activity. This has not been shown to be so, even when 0.1 *M* ACh was used (*87*).

In recent years it has been reported that ACh and related compounds do have effects on nerves, but the question remains whether their action is similar to that at junctions. In most instances this seems not to be the case as indicated in the following discussion.

The effect of the ChE inhibitors, particularly DFP and physostigmine, is to inhibit rather than potentiate the weak effects of ACh on desheathed vagus (*62*, *63*) or lobster nerves (*65*). The effect of physostigmine as an anti-ACh agent is manifest even when the concentration is very low, 5×10^{-5} *M* (*65*).

The ChE inhibitors also counteract depolarization by carbamoylcholine, pilocarpine, and arecoline (*63*). Furthermore, Armett and Ritchie made the important finding that when the ChE inhibitors were blocking the effects of externally applied ACh, they failed to alter electrical activity. They made the cogent point that this finding provides further negation of the ACh hypothesis, since the compounds had evidently penetrated at a sufficiently high concentration to antagonize the reaction of externally applied ACh molecules with some receptor while at the same time there was no significant alteration in nerve function, which is presumed to depend entirely upon the reaction of internally liberated ACh with the same receptor.

As previously indicated, lobster nerves are considered to present very limited barriers to the penetration of quaternary ammonium compounds, and yet Dettbarn and Davis reported that 0.05 *M* carbamoylcholine and methacholine at a concentration less than 0.01 *M* had no significant effects on these nerves (*65*).

Following the pioneering work of Walsh and Deal, who used detergents to reduce barriers surrounding sciatic nerve (*93–95*), Rosenberg and Ehrenpreis used snake venoms for the same purpose (*87*, *96*). The treated nerves show the interesting property of being reversibly blocked by *d*-tubocurarine. Other lipid-insoluble compounds, totally without effect on intact nerves, become active following venom treatment. Among these are chlorisondamine and protamine (*87*); that the latter acts at all strongly suggests a considerable breakdown of barriers. However, even very high concentrations (0.1 *M*) of ACh, carbamoylcholine, decamethonium, and neostigmine failed to produce significant effects on nerves that had previously responded to *d*-tubocurarine (*87*). In studies with detergent-treated nerves, these various compounds were shown to block conduction (*94*), but at the concentration used (0.1 *M*) choline was equally effective; this suggests that the specificity of "receptor" involved is entirely different from the specificities of junctional receptors.

In a similar study, Rosenberg and Dettbarn (*116*) showed that cotton-mouth moccasin venom apparently completely breaks down the barriers of squid nerve, since ACh was now able to penetrate to all the ChE present. Yet the potency of ACh, decamethonium, or carbamolycholine acting on the same venom-treated axons was not remarkable, the minimal concentrations needed being 2×10^{-4} *M* or greater. Despite the evident ability of ACh to penetrate to the enzyme, physostigmine at 2.4×10^{-4} *M* (about 0.07 mg/ml) failed to change the action potential (*74*).

The Nachmansohn group recognizes the contradictory nature of the effect of the ChE inhibitors in blocking the action of ACh on lobster nerve, venom-treated nerves, and desheathed vagus; this effect "was difficult to reconcile with the well known anticholinesterase action of physostigmine" (*74*). They attempt to rationalize this on the basis that such a compound "is at the pH used, to a large part cationic. The pathways for cationic molecules, even after venom treatment, are limited . . . the cationic molecules if present in sufficiently high concentrations, may compete with ACh for these pathways and prevent ACh from reaching the active sites" (*74*). This statement completely ignores the fact that these "channels" are at times sufficiently large to accommodate the protamine molecule (*87*). Moreover, the same inhibition was observed with physostigmine on desheathed vagus nerve, which does not require venom treatment to permit an effect of ACh; the uncharged molecule DFP acts in similar fashion. An alternative and also implausible explanation has been suggested by Dettbarn, who now considers that there may be "a competition of these two compounds [ACh and physostigmine] for constituents of the outside structure rather than for those in the membrane" (*117*). With this statement the Nachmansohn group appears to have given up the attempt to explain the action of physostigmine within the context of the ACh hypothesis.

The node of Ranvier is a region of myelinated nerve that has been shown by electron miscroscopy to be surrounded by only mimimal external barriers. This has been given as the explanation of the fact that *d*-tubocurarine can block conduction when applied at this site (*118*). However, ACh itself has no appreciable effect at the node (*119, 120*). Moreover, the report by Dettbarn that physostigmine blocks the node rapidly at low concentrations (0.03 to 0.04 mg/ml) (*121*), could not be confirmed by Whitcomb and Friess (*122*), who found that even about 1 mg/ml of physostigmine produced only minimal effects in one hour. Moreover, the latter workers have shown that compounds that were 100 to 1000 times weaker as inhibitors of ChE than physostigmine were far more potent in blocking the node.

Of some interest is Bloom and Schoepfle's demonstration (*123*) that an antagonism exists between procaine and ACh at the node of Ranvier. This was manifested by the ability of ACh to overcome the blockade of nodal conduction by procaine. Thus, ACh evidently is able to penetrate to the site of action of procaine; this site is considered by Nachmansohn to be the ACh receptor of the conducting membrane. However, as indicated above, ACh itself produces no effect at the node, regardless of the concentration used.

Where resting potentials have been measured, ACh at times produces weak depolarization (*62, 63*), although at other times it blocks without depolarizing the nerve significantly (*74*). In this connection it may be noted that despite the now demonstrated ability of ACh to penetrate to the active membrane there is no evidence that it can itself produce an action potential. Although it is perhaps true, as stated by Nachmansohn (*124*)* that an externally applied

* It is interesting that this statement was made in reference to the action of the lipid-soluble quaternary ammonium compounds shortly after it had been claimed that these same compounds, when externally applied, could produce effects that constituted direct proof of the correctness of the ACh hypothesis (Section 1.2, B, 3).

compound is unlikely to "be able to mimic exactly the action of the ester [ACh]" liberated internally, the problem does not seem to be a significant one at junctions, for there externally applied ACh apparently faithfully mimics ACh liberated by nerve stimulation. If, indeed, ACh acts only intramembranously, as postulated by Nachmansohn, the same difficulties in approaching and acting upon the active site should be encountered at junctions as at conducting membranes. Moreover, it is well known that some compounds totally unrelated to ACh in structure are able to fire nerves; examples are aconitine and veratrum alkaloids (*125*, *126*). Simply reducing the calcium ion concentration also is quite effective in producing spontaneous firing. Davis and Dettbarn recently attributed this effect to release of ACh within the nerve (*127*), but they do not attempt to explain the fact that physostigmine effectively stopped the depolarization observed with low calcium.*

In recent years the interesting finding has been made that stimulation of a tissue by ACh either exogenously applied or released during nerve activity can lead to the rapid incorporation of ^{32}P-labeled phosphate into tissue lipids, particularly phosphatidyl inositol (*129*). The effect is so specific as to pinpoint those sites where ACh acts in what might be considered a truly physiological manner. Although Larrabee and co-workers were able to show this ACh effect upon the superior cervical ganglion when preganglionic nerves were stimulated, they could not find any phosphate incorporation when the sciatic nerve itself was stimulated repeatedly over long periods of time. This might be taken as additional and rather subtle evidence that ACh is not involved in reactions connected with the stimulation of elements within the axon.

5. REINTERPRETATION OF CHOLINERGIC DRUG EFFECTS ON NERVES

The fact does remain that many cholinotropic compounds alter the electrical activity of nerves and other tissues; there is even good evidence of an important presynaptic component in the action of such compounds as *d*-tubocurarine and succinylcholine at some neuromuscular junctions suggesting a reaction with some element in the nerve terminals. Some attempts have been made to elucidate the nature of drug-binding macromolecules in nerve by direct isolation (*130*, *131*). The attempts have proved somewhat successful, in that Neet and Friess (*130*) demonstrated that a certain macromolecule extracted from rabbit sciatic nerve has the property of precipitating with *d*-tubocurarine in a way similar to components of the electric organ of electric eel, as described by Ehrenpreis (*132*). Ehrenpreis and co-workers (*131*, *133*) have extended these studies and demonstrated that many neurotropic compounds,

* A similar antagonism of veratrine-induced depolarization and firing of skeletal muscle by physostigmine has been reported by Sandow and Kiebel (*128*).

including *d*-tubocurarine, chlorisondamine, gallamine triethiodide, chlorpromazine, protamine, and local anesthetics, react with some macromolecular component or components present in extracts of rabbit sciatic nerve. That the drug-binding component could not be similar to the ACh receptor was indicated by the extremely weak binding of ACh and carbamoylcholine. Ehrenpreis has speculated about the possible role such macromolecules play in axonal activity and in the action of neurotropic agents on the molecular level (*57*, *131*, *134–136a*). In this proposal physostigmine emerges as a type of weak local anesthetic (*134*). Nerve endings as such are not considered, but it is conceivable that the presence of the drug-binding components at this site could account for the now established presynaptic actions of *d*-tubocurarine and related compounds. It must be emphasized, however, that the mechanism of the presynaptic actions is probably very different from that of the postsynaptic; that is, in the former there is no evidence that the blockade occurs by competition with endogenously released ACh. It should be stressed that these recently proposed molecular mechanisms of presynaptic action of cholinotropic compounds require that the ACh system does not have a physiological role in electrical activity of nerves.

A word of caution might be interjected at this point concerning the use of very high concentrations of various compounds on nerve or other tissues. Although plausible explanations may be offered to rationalize such use, the possibility remains that the effects observed may be nonspecific and not related to ChE inhibition or specific receptor reactions. Among these effects may be included both the initial blocking action (nondepolarizing) and the depolarization that may occur on exposure to very high concentrations of organophosphates or physostigmine. Evidence of such nonspecific actions has been unequivocally obtained with aortic smooth muscle (*112*). On this tissue, 0.01 mg/ml of DFP irreversibly abolishes all ChE activity. Strips subsequently immersed in 0.3 mg/ml of DFP can be made to contract under the influence of high concentrations of physostigmine (0.5 mg/ml.). The same strips contract when the concentration of DFP is raised to about 1 mg/ml. It is evident that the production of contractions by DFP and physostigmine, which might be considered analogous to nerve depolarization, is totally unrelated to inhibition of ChE and thus must be attributed to some as yet undefined action of these compounds.

Once the aortic smooth muscle is exposed to very high concentrations of DFP (2 to 4 mg/ml), the tissue no longer responds to any stimulating compound. The situation is analogous to the later phase of DFP action upon nerves, when the action potential is irreversibly abolished, presumably by inhibition of ChE. However, in the case of aortic smooth muscle this irreversible phase has been conclusively shown to be unrelated to inhibition of ChE (*112*). It would appear that very high concentrations of DFP have a nonspecific destructive action on tissues, yet these are precisely the concentrations required (*59*) to block nerve activity by a mechanism said to involve specific inhibition of ChE. It may be noted that Hinterbuchner and Nachmansohn observed that paraoxon produced irreversible damage of striated muscle, an effect evidently not related to its ChE-inhibiting action. In fact, they stated that it was "only a very short step from an irreversibly inhibited preparation to one irreparably damaged" (*99*).

6. LOCALIZATION OF ACETYLCHOLINE AND CHOLINESTERASE IN RELATION TO NERVE ACTIVITY

The foregoing discussion of the role of the cholinergic receptor system in nerve raises an important point about the concept that high enzymatic activity (in this case ChE) in conjunction with a substrate having the requisite physiological activity (ACh can, of course, produce depolarization) necessarily implicates the components in the function of the particular tissue. Nerve tissue evidently possesses all the readily identified components of the cholinergic system, and thus it may be logical to propose that the system is essential to nerve activity. However, the finding that ACh in particular has a vastly asymmetric distribution, being concentrated primarily at the nerve endings, is one of the greatest deterrents to considering it a mediator of membrane depolarization throughout the nerve. Furthermore, the distribution of ChE is far from uniform, being rather sparse in axons and abundant in cell bodies and nerve terminals. Perhaps even more important is the finding that the enzyme is present primarily within granules; it therefore could not be associated with events at conducting membranes (*12*, *13*). In truth, however, in rejecting the ACh hypothesis of nerve function one is still faced with the need to explain the very existence of neural ChE and also the fact that the enzyme may be synthesized not only in the cell body but throughout the axon (*137*). Certainly, it may be almost totally inhibited without any striking effect on electrical activity.*

C. Cholinergic System in Denervated Muscle

It is well known that upon prolonged denervation a striated muscle becomes extremely sensitive to ACh injected intra-arterially; moreover, as shown by electrophoretic jet technique, the entire muscle responds to ACh, whereas in normal muscle the area of sensitivity falls rapidly at small distances (200 to

* The function of the ChE of aorta—which may also be totally inhibited without significantly affecting responsiveness of the tissue to contracting agents (*112*)—has recently been considered to be that of regulating endogenously released substrates, such as butyrylcholine, which could have a detrimental effect on the tissue (*138*). Perhaps this is the role which at least some of the ChE in nerve also subserves.

400 μ) from the junction (*139*). Although there has been some question about the actual state of responsiveness of the junctional receptors themselves, the indication is that their sensitivity to ACh does not increase appreciably (*140*), despite an earlier report by Kuffler (*141*) which indicated that the junctional receptors reacted with remarkably greater sensitivity to ACh. The fact that the entire muscle becomes sensitive to ACh appears to support Nachmansohn's hypothesis concerning the ubiquitousness of the ACh system, which is said to be masked under ordinary circumstances but becomes accessible during denervation, perhaps because of the breakdown of the barriers to externally applied compounds (*98*). Such a proposal could be justified on the basis of the rather profound changes in the muscle which become apparent in the electron microscope (*53*), but this has not been considered to explain the extended area of sensitivity. Thesleff (*98*) has discussed in detail the various hypotheses concerning the spread of sensitivity; the most widely held notion is that the receptor system spreads throughout the muscle, perhaps through actual de novo synthesis of the components. Many aspects of the action of compounds at these new sites appear to agree with such a mechanism; among them are the potentiation of ACh action by the inhibitors of ChE, blockade of applied ACh by *d*-tubocurarine, production of an action potential by ACh applied locally, etc. In fact, the number of molecules of ACh required to stimulate these extrajunctional receptors was almost identical with that required to stimulate normal end-plate receptors (*140*). However, there is considerable evidence that this "receptor" system is not physiologically functional in the sense described by Nachmansohn. First, although the local application of ACh does give rise to an action potential, it is nonpropagated (that is, localized) and therefore would not be conducted throughout the muscle to produce a contraction, as demanded by the Nachmansohn formulation. Second, although ACh is potentiated by neostigmine, the potentiation extends to only a limited region of the muscle fiber (*142*); thus, as the micropipette is moved farther and farther from the end-plate region, the extent of potentiation diminishes. This finding clearly shows that, as in the case of nerve, the distribution of ChE is not uniform throughout the muscle, as is required if the cholinergic system is to function in initiation and conduction of the action potential. This type of pharmacological evidence is fully substantiated by results using histochemical electron-microscope techniques for localizing ChE in denervated muscle.

The great sensitivity of denervated muscle to ACh is manifested most readily when the compound is injected intra-arterially. In this case ACh produces an increase in discharge frequency and contraction of the muscle. Evidence of a pharmacological nature, obtained by Bowman and Raper (*143*), clearly showed that the extrajunctional membrane sites that give rise to the increased activity are not stimulated by ACh released internally, that is, within the conducting membrane. Thus, the ACh-induced discharge was only slightly affected by an injection of physostigmine which was at a sufficiently high dose to cause a significant increase in tone of the innervated contralateral muscle. Moreover, the injection of doses of *d*-tubocurarine which blocked end-plate effects of the innervated muscle failed to abolish the increase in discharge produced by injected ACh. Presumably both drugs should have reached the conducting membrane at sufficiently high concentration to have affected any ACh liberated at this point.

I.3. UPTAKE OF CHOLINOTROPIC COMPOUNDS BY TISSUE RECEPTORS

That an ACh receptor actually exists at the precise site at which ACh acts (namely, the postsynaptic membranes) has long been accepted despite the lack of definitive molecular evidence. Such evidence is extremely difficult to obtain, because until recently no specific technique was available for tagging receptors. In recent years attempts have been made to label the cholinergic receptor in situ as well as to determine the extent of uptake of cholinotropic compounds in various tissues. These experiments were intended not only to establish the existence of the receptor but, hopefully, to determine the number of molecules of this component in tissues. Such information is basic in terms of the ultimate objective, namely, the isolation of the receptor substance in solution. Moreover, the effect of certain variables on specific uptake could provide insight into the molecular nature of the receptor substance itself.

It is evident that the difficulties of this approach are considerable, if for no other reason than that junctional regions abound with components that conceivably could react with almost any cholinotropic compound used. Furthermore, since none of the compounds binds irreversibly with the receptor, the site of reaction must be detected by a method that does not disturb the equilibrium of complex formation.

A. Studies with Labeled Curarine, Muscarine Derivatives, and Decamethonium

Perhaps the most extensive attempt to localize the receptor in situ has been made by Waser, who investigated the in vivo fixation of radioactive compounds considered to react with a high degree of specificity with the cholinergic receptor (*144–147*). After the injection of ^{14}C-labeled calabash curarine, mouse diaphragms were removed and subjected to autoradiography, a procedure which permits the in situ localization to be determined under equilibrium conditions and with a fair amount of precision. Not only was the curarine found to be located almost exclusively in end-plate regions, but by counting silver grains it was estimated that the number of molecules bound per synapse was about 10^7. This value was obtained even after many lethal doses had been injected, indicating that saturation of the binding sites had occurred. The finding is of great importance, because it indicates that curarine, which undoubtedly can combine with a diverse group of macromolecules (as has been shown for *d*-tubocurarine (*148–151*)), is fixed with a high degree of specificity at a limited number of sites. Of considerable interest was the finding that the distribution of radioactivity correlated well with the localization of ChE as determined by concurrent histochemical techniques. ChE and the ACh receptor obviously are in close proximity to each other, and a precise mapping of the cholinergic receptor system for this particular synapse appears to have been achieved.

The work produced several very interesting additional results which may have an important bearing on a number of related problems. For example, the quantity of labeled decamethonium (C_{10}) fixed to end-plate regions was about ten times greater than that of curarine when comparable degrees of paralysis had occurred (*145*, *147*). Moreover, the binding of C_{10} apparently did not reach saturation, as did that of curarine, nor was the compound localized as discretely as the curarine. Similar results were obtained with labeled muscarone. The question arises: Do the receptors have a greater capacity for binding decamethonium or muscarone than curarine, or does the accumulation occur by some other mechanism? Certainly, on the basis of affinities for molecules such as proteins, nucleic acids, and acidic polysaccharides (*148–150*), it would be predicted that curarine would be bound to a greater extent than the decamethonium type of molecule; that is, curarine would be expected to have a greater affinity for a larger number of sites. The differences in uptake and distribution may be explained by the findings of Taylor and co-workers (*152*, *153*), who studied the relative rates and degrees of uptake* in mouse diaphragm. In this experiment the diaphragms were soaked in the radioactive compounds. The results indicated that the decamethonium type of molecule is able to diffuse much further into the muscle than *d*-tubocurarine. In fact, the uptake appears to proceed for several hours, whereas with curare it apparently reaches a stable value very quickly. Such results are in complete agreement with Waser's localization data, which show a much more diffuse region of uptake for decamethonium than for curarine. An indication that some sort of receptor mechanism is involved is apparent from the finding of Taylor et al. (*153*) that the prior application of a low concentration of *d*-tubocurarine (10^{-6} *M*) was very effective in suppressing the entry of decamethonium into the muscle. The finding strongly implies that decamethonium and, perhaps, other depolarizers alter receptor structure in such a way as to enable them to bypass the postsynaptic membrane and

* *d*-Tubocurarine was used in these studies, but the results almost undoubtedly would have been the same as with calabash curarine.

accumulate in interior regions. Nastuk has presented the uppermost limit in the size of molecules that can penetrate in this way (*154*).

The full significance of the finding that a decamethonium type of molecule can readily penetrate beyond the postsynaptic membrane is not as yet appreciated, but it has been suggested (*153*) that the behavior may somehow be related to the dual action of such compounds (*155*). The following proposal on the molecular level may explain not only the dual action but the pronounced differences in uptake between the decamethonium and curarine types of molecule. Decamethonium and the majority of depolarizing compounds are very weakly bound to all types of macromolecules in solution (*149*, *150*). They are probably in only fleeting contact with the receptor, as postulated by Paton (*156*, *157*). The transient contact produces the initial stage of their action, the activation of the receptor; this not only opens the membrane to various cations but also promotes penetration of the activator itself. The concentration of the compound builds up rapidly in the interior and eventually surpasses that of the external solution; that is, there appears to be a mechanism within the muscle that promotes the accumulation of the compound at high concentration (*153*). As a result, the concentration in the vicinity of the receptor increases and so, therefore, does the tendency of the molecules to remain associated with the receptor—a situation that would be considered to cause blockade (see Section 1.4).

d-Tubocurarine, on the other hand, is a molecule that has a high affinity for many types of macromolecule and can form complexes that are stabilized by several types of bond, such as hydrophobic, electrostatic, and hydrogen bonds (*148–150*). With some tissue components the bonds are so strong that the drug can be dissociated only with concentrated urea or salt (*25*, *150*). A similar type of complex could well occur when tubocurarine combines with the receptor. Stable complex formation at the receptor site may be viewed as a self-limiting process: once formed, it prevents tubocurarine in the external medium from penetrating into the interior. This type of association might account for the prevention of the passage of decamethonium into the muscle, as was actually found by Creese et al. (*153*).

It is apparent that the large uptake of decamethonium must be attributed to at least two factors: a certain amount actually complexed with the receptor but the bulk in a more or less free state in equilibrium with the bound form. This conclusion is based on the finding that the uptake of the decamethonium type of molecule is 3 μg per gram of tissue, an amount far in excess of that expected to combine with the cholinergic receptors present.* It would be very

* This amounts to approximately 5×10^{-9} *M* per gram of tissue. Assuming 1000 synapses per gram, the number of molecules per synapse would be 10^{11}, about 4 orders of magnitude greater than that calculated from Waser's data on curarine. Unfortunately, similar studies with *d*-tubocurarine were not made by Taylor.

interesting to attempt to elucidate the mechanism of this accumulation, which may not involve actual binding to components of the muscle but, rather, some process of active uptake.

Several additional features of Waser's work require clarification and amplification; the following suggested studies could contribute greatly to our understanding of many aspects of the receptor problem on the molecular level and would strengthen the conclusion that the observed binding has occurred exclusively with the receptor. One question is whether inert or relatively inert quaternary ammonium compounds, such as choline, are bound by the curarine receptors. On the basis of the pharmacological action observed it has long been considered that choline is far less potent than ACh because it combines weakly with the receptor, but this very logical explanation is based exclusively on in vivo findings and thus is subject to all the uncertainties with regard to receptor affinity. It is conceivable, as an alternative explanation, that choline and ACh are bound with equal affinity but that only the latter possesses the intrinsic activity (*158*) required to activate the receptor strongly. This proposal is not without some foundation, inasmuch as both compounds have fairly similar affinities for ChE. The question could be answered more unequivocally by comparing the fixation of choline and that of the highly active carbamoylcholine by the Waser technique. If choline is not at all, or very poorly, bound, then intrinsic activity is not the likely explanation. The difference in activity between ACh and choline would be attributed exclusively to large differences in binding to the receptor, and some special features of the ACh molecule must then be sought in order to explain the very profound differences in affinity. If, on the other hand, choline is indistinguishable from carbamoylcholine in terms of fixation, then two alternatives must be considered: the differences in physiological effect are due to an intrinsic ability to activate the receptor, or the fixation of these compounds does not actually reflect binding with the cholinergic receptor. Experiments must be devised to distinguish between the two possibilities, but until uptake of choline is determined, definitive conclusions from these interesting results may not be possible.

Another question remaining unanswered is the extent of fixation, if any, of cholinotropic compounds with components other than the receptor. Other binding sites may include those present on ChE, which is known to combine with *d*-tubocurarine (*159*), decamethonium (*159*), and muscarone (*160*). Another possibility is that fixation occurs with elements in the nerve endings, a plausible suggestion in view of the recent pharmacological evidence (*161–164*) that this may be an important site of action of the compounds. That these are real possibilities is indicated by Waser's studies with denervated diaphragms. In this preparation the amount of bound curarine first rose markedly, then diminished progressively, and finally returned to normal (Figure 1.6).

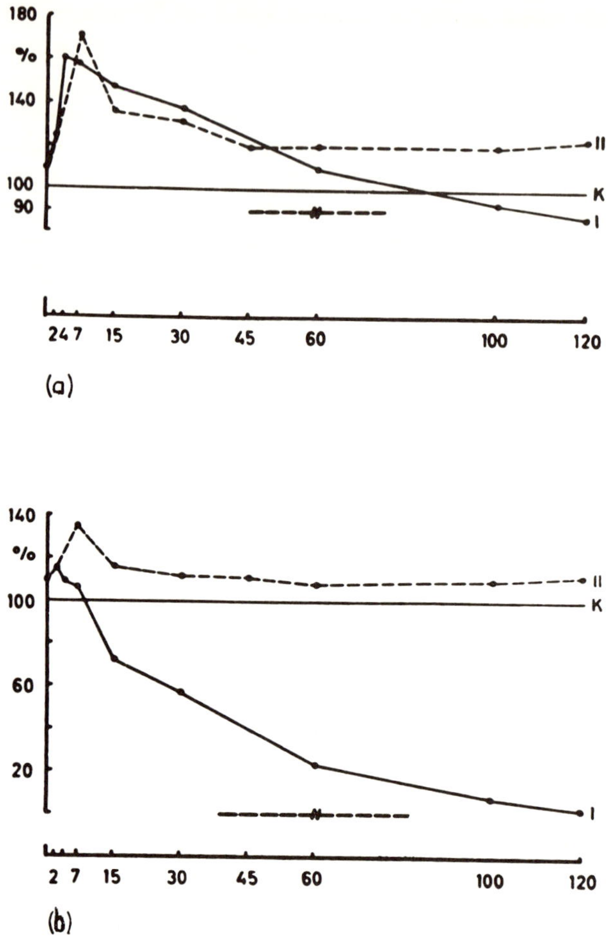

Fig. 1.6. (a) Radioactivity of end-plate band by ^{14}C-curarine fixation after total phrenicotomy (I) and coagulation of phrenic nerve with regeneration (II). K is normal control side (right part of diaphragm), and N is radioactivity of muscle. (b) Cholinesterase activity of end-plate band determined with densitometer after histochemical staining. [From Ref. (*147*).]

Of considerable interest is the exact parallelism between the time course of degree of fixation and the ChE activity as determined histochemically (Figure 1.6).* This may well indicate that binding with the enzyme does occur to a considerable extent. Binding to presynaptic elements would be consistent

* The profound decrease in ChE activity observed by Waser in denervated diaphragm is usually not found in other denervated preparations. Although there is some disagreement in the literature concerning this point, it is generally agreed that changes in enzyme upon denervation generally do not exceed 50%.

with some of the observed changes in degree of uptake, particularly since re-innervation would undoubtedly occur after long periods of time. As indicated previously, macromolecules having the property of combining very strongly with *d*-tubocurarine may be isolated from peripheral nerve (*136a*).

Last, there is the somewhat surprising result that even fairly large doses of neostigmine failed to reduce the extent of curarine fixation despite the relief of block of transmission (*144*, *145*, *147*). This finding indicated to Waser (*144*) that "the cholinergic receptors blocked by curarine and the ChE blocked by neostigmine are located at different sites, since both molecules cannot be at the same place (at the same time)." The fact that transmission did occur was interpreted in terms of "a large reserve of cholinergic receptors" (*144*), but this would mean that the number of receptors involved in transmission was extremely small; otherwise, the degree of curarine binding would have been significantly reduced by the accumulated ACh. On the other hand, when a tenfold lethal dose of neostigmine was given (*144*, *145*), the amount of curarine fixed was significantly reduced. Although Waser does not so state, this result could be interpreted in terms of the established direct competition between neostigmine and *d*-tubocurarine for receptor sites (*165*). An alternative and perhaps equally valid explanation may be that the neostigmine was displacing the curarine from its complex with ChE or from presynaptic sites where, as Masland and Wigton have shown, neostigmine has a distinct action (*166*).

In conclusion, the autoradiographic approach to the precise localization of macromolecules involved in the action of cholinergic compounds is a notable one and has probably demonstrated the presence of the specific receptor substance itself. The findings contain a number of important inconsistencies, and the possibility that a fraction, if not the bulk, of binding occurs with ChE or with presynaptic elements, or both, has not been ruled out. Until this is done, Waser's contention that the results demonstrate the existence of the cholinergic receptor as an entity completely unique and distinct from all known cellular components, including ChE (*144*), must be regarded with some reservation.

B. Atropine Binding by Smooth Muscle

Atropine is another drug that has an extremely high affinity and specificity for cholinergic receptors; the affinity constant is about 10^{-9} *M*, judging from the in vivo antagonism of ACh (*167*).* Paton and Rang have discovered that atropine can bind to a smooth-muscle component (guinea pig ileum) with an affinity in the range of that expected for the receptor (*167*). Inactive compounds, such as tropic acid, are not bound, whereas compounds known

* I am indebted to Dr. Paton and Dr. Rang for permitting me to read their manuscript prior to publication.

to block the receptor compete with atropine for the strong binding sites. This work appears to be the most direct evidence of the existence of a receptor substance as a discrete molecular entity having the correct binding properties.

The situation is, however, complicated by a number of factors. First, there seem to be several tissue components that are capable of binding atropine; their affinities are perhaps 500 times lower than what is calculated for the constant of binding to the receptor itself. Paton and Rang attribute the weaker uptake to "silent receptors," nonspecific binding, or "sites of loss." It is suggested that even the weaker binding is not very nonspecific, because its constant is still less than 10^{-6} *M*, while the affinity constant of atropine to known macromolecules (bovine serum albumin, other proteins, and acidic polysaccharides) is in the range of 10^{-4} to 10^{-3} *M* (*25*, *168*). Second, the rate of uptake appears to be somewhat too slow in relation to the fairly rapid rate of inhibition of ACh shown by atropine. Third, a potent smooth-muscle stimulant (methylfurthrethonium) failed to alter the uptake of atropine; ACh behaved similarly. Nevertheless, Paton and Rang present numerous convincing arguments for considering that the component with the highest affinity for atropine does have the properties expected for the cholinergic receptor.

Of particular interest is the finding that even homogenates of smooth muscle have the same high affinity for atropine as do components of intact tissue. This strongly suggests that disruption of the cell had little effect on the native properties of the receptor. When a homogenate of smooth muscle that had previously taken up atropine was centrifuged, all the atropine appeared in the supernatant. Paton and Rang attributed this fact to the rapid dissociation of the atropine from the receptor, but it could just as easily be that the binding component or components were solubilized upon homogenization. It may, therefore, be possible to extract the atropine-binding component (receptor?) from smooth muscle, but one would still be faced with the enormous problem of selectively removing very minute amounts of active material from the vast bulk of inactive components. The amount of receptor was calculated by Paton to be about 2×10^{-10} moles per gram of tissue, assuming a 1:1 molar relationship between bound atropine and receptor. Assuming a molecular weight of 100,000 for the receptor molecule, 1 g of tissue would contain about 10^{-5} g of receptor substance.*

* Recent studies (*168a*) suggest that the situation with regard to atropine and related compounds is far more complex than previously thought. Evidence has been obtained that even *l*-hyoscyamine, long considered to be a competitive inhibitor of ACh (*168b*), may not react at the same site as ACh. The anti-ACh action of *l*-hyoscyamine on isolated rabbit atria lasts for many hours. The time course for reversal of blockade was unaltered even if the compound was added in the presence of very high concentrations of ACh plus benzoylcholine, the latter being a rapidly reversible, competitive inhibitor of ACh on this tissue. Additional evidence against a truly competitive mechanism of action for these compounds was presented by Ehrenpreis (*168c*) and by Ariëns (*168d*) at a New York Academy of Sciences Conference on Cholinergic Mechanisms held in May, 1966.

Although a number of other studies have been concerned with the binding and uptake of cholinergic compounds, they were made in connection with attempts to isolate the cholinergic receptor in solution. These studies will be discussed in the next section.

I.4. ATTEMPTS TO ISOLATE THE CHOLINERGIC RECEPTOR

Despite the vast number of in vivo experiments performed with ACh and related compounds there seems to have been little interest until recently in isolating the cholinergic receptor from any tissue. This is, perhaps, somewhat surprising in view of the fact that most workers in the field would agree that having the receptor in solution is a requirement for fully understanding mechanisms of cholinergic drug action. The reasons, however, are not difficult to perceive. First, the most rudimentary calculations indicated that the amount of receptor substance present in even the most favorable tissue constitutes only the minutest fraction of the total material. Although the first realization of this was, perhaps, intuitive (in other words, that the reaction of ACh was limited to only a few active sites in a cell), Waser's experiments on the fixation of labeled curarine provided the first direct evidence; as previously indicated, his values of receptor content may even be much too high. Second, even greater difficulties were in store for those intrepid enough to attempt to isolate what Schueler termed "that shadowy anonymity" (*169*). For example, although the chemical or molecular nature of the receptor substance could not be elucidated on the basis of in vivo studies, the general consensus was that a receptor substance had to be a macromolecule of some sort; however, there is a school of thought that dissents even from this view (*170*). Even the assumption that the receptor is a macromolecule is of little help since it may be shown that quaternary ammonium compounds can combine with some degree of specificity with many types of macromolecule (*132*, *148–150*). Many considered that only a protein could possess the necessary specificity of binding required of a receptor. The question still remained: How might a receptor be identified, even assuming that it could be extracted in the native state?

A. Studies of Chagas and Co-workers

The first major attempt to isolate a receptor substance was made by Chagas and co-workers (*171–176*), using the electric organ of the electric eel as a source of receptor material. This tissue appears to be most suitable for the purpose, because each cell (electroplax) has 30,000 to 50,000 synapses and weighs only about 30 mg. This is, perhaps, the greatest synaptic density of any tissue, and thus the amount of receptor per unit weight is probably the highest. Moreover, the bulk of the tissue is water, and the protein content is only about

2%. Therefore, in terms of total extraneous material the amount of specific receptor would be favored over that of almost any tissue. From Waser's data it may be calculated that the amount of receptor present is about 50 mg per kilogram of tissue, a very considerable amount considering the composition of the electric organ.

The approach used in these studies was quite simple. A radioactively labeled compound, gallamine triethiodide (TRIEG), known to have a high affinity for cholinergic receptors in electric organ, was injected into eels in the hope of tagging the receptor. After the compound was allowed to fix to the receptors, excess radioactivity was flushed out, and the tissue was homogenized. It was considered that the label would remain attached to the receptor even during the extraction procedure. After dialysis the label was retained in several fractions, although one fraction showed a significantly greater specific activity than the others. The component bearing the label was initially said to be a protein (*172*) but subsequently was shown to be a type of hyaluronic acid (*173*, *175*, *176*). Evidence was presented that a number of cholinergic compounds could compete with TRIEG for the binding sites (*172*), and from this it was concluded that the binding properties were sufficiently specific to justify the claim that the molecule plays a key role in cholinergic mechanisms. In other words, there appeared to be the same type of competition between a blocking compound (TRIEG) and depolarizing agents as that which had been documented in in vivo studies. Another report (*176*) apparently demonstrated that the "receptor" could bind ACh and succinylcholine at low concentrations, thereby reinforcing the validity of the interpretation.

Unfortunately, these studies involved a number of incorrect assumptions that led to many contradictions, and ultimately the interpretation was completely altered, to the extent that the isolated macromolecule was no longer considered to have ACh-receptor activity (*175*). Since the approach used appears to be the most direct one, it is necessary to examine the reasons for the lack of success.

Perhaps the chief reason was the incorrectness of the primary assumption that the labeled TRIEG or other receptor-bound molecule would remain associated with the receptor throughout the extraction procedure. This assumption is not valid because the combination between these compounds with the receptor is highly labile, primarily by electrostatic bonds that would be rapidly broken once equilibrium conditions were disturbed. The rapid reversibility of the anti-ACh effects of TRIEG is well known. Thus, homogenization of the tissue necessarily causes a redistribution of the label. The questions remain: Why was the label found associated mostly with hyaluronic acid, and why did this component subsequently prove to have the greatest capacity to bind quaternary ammonium compounds? The answer to both is that a procedural error had been made. Although the various fractions obtained upon homogenization were dialyzed, the label was retained only when dialysis was carried out in distilled water. Since in this tissue hyaluronic acid constitutes the largest amount of macromolecules with the highest density of negative charges, it is evident that fractions in which it was present would show the greatest degree of retention of the highly cationic TRIEG molecule in distilled water.

Subsequent studies were carried out with components of the various extracts isolated by alcohol precipitation or trichloroacetic acid precipitation and by column chromatography. The components were then examined for their ability to bind labeled TRIEG in the following way. Mixtures of TRIEG solution and the macromolecular binding substance were prepared "in such proportions as to obtain saturation conditions. The mixture [was] then dialyzed against continuously renewed distilled water at low temperature" (*173*). It was found that under these conditions the amount of "binding" correlated with the uronic acid content of the various fractions. As expected, other polysaccharides, including chondroitin sulfate A, B, and C, kerato sulfate, and heparitin sulfate, showed an even greater capacity for retaining the label than did the hyaluronic acid "receptor" (*173*, *174*, *176*).

The competition studies were carried out in a similar way. TRIEG plus the presumed competitor (for example, tetramethylammonium) were mixed with the extract and dialyzed against large volumes of distilled water.

We have shown that hyaluronic acid has a high retention capacity for many types of drugs if dialysis is carried out in distilled water (*177*). However, this "binding" is completely nonspecific, all the cationic substances examined having been retained indiscriminately. For example, ACh and 2-PAM were retained to the same extent, yet 2-PAM is singularly inactive on the electroplax. Thus, although the procedure may give an indication of the number of negative charges or binding sites on a macromolecule (its binding capacity), affinity constants cannot be determined in this way nor can information be obtained about interactions occurring under physiological conditions of pH and ionic strength. This was clearly shown by the fact that, when examined by equilibrium dialysis in dilute salt (0.1 *M* tris, pH 7.5), binding of *d*-tubocurarine by hyaluronic acid was virtually absent (*177*) although under the conditions employed by Chagas and co-workers the hyaluronic acid retained large amounts of the drug.

In view of these facts it is apparent that the competition experiments of Chagas and co-workers, also carried out in distilled water, could not give results that may be attributed to specific interactions.

Chagas has recognized the difficulty of considering that hyaluronic acid or other polysaccharides are concerned directly with the actions of cholinotropic compounds at junctions. As he stated recently, "The role attributed to the mucopolysaccharide fraction is that of a non-specific receptor, and it may be further considered as a protective one in which the polymer acts as a barrier to an increase of concentration of free drug which would lead to rapid, systemic intoxication" (*175*). This, too, seems unlikely in view of the demonstrated lack of affinity of cholinergic compounds for hyaluronic acid at physiological pH and ionic strength. It is conceivable, of course, that the polysaccharide isolated by the Chagas group has different properties from the purified hyaluronic acid used in our study (*177*). However, until true affinity constants for the electric eel component are determined, the role of hyaluronic acid in any phase of the action of cholinergic compounds remains uncertain.

B. Studies of Ehrenpreis and Co-workers

The early reports of Chagas and his colleagues were followed by studies along two broad lines by Ehrenpreis and co-workers. Investigation into the combination of cholinotropic compounds and various well-characterized macromolecules was carried out and, concurrently, an attempt was made to isolate the cholinergic receptor from the electric organ of eel by an entirely different approach from that of Chagas.

1. COMBINATION OF CHOLINOTROPIC COMPOUNDS WITH PURIFIED MACROMOLECULES

It was hoped that the use of model systems would give information about the molecular nature of the cholinergic receptor as well as the basic mechanism of interaction of various cholinergic compounds with this receptor. The reasoning went as follows. If a compound such as *d*-tubocurarine combines with many types of macromolecule in nearly the same way, then it is highly probable that its reaction with the receptor in vivo occurs by a similar mechanism. The first studies along these lines were aided greatly by the observation that *d*-tubocurarine can form a precipitate with a number of macromolecules (for example, chondroitin sulfate (CSA), nucleic acids (NA), casein, pepsin, and insulin) at neutral pH and in 0.1 *M* salt solutions. Analysis of precipitated complexes revealed that a single *d*-tubocurarine molecule can become attached simultaneously to two negative charges on CSA and NA (*148*). Furthermore, complex formation with CSA, NA, and proteins is salt-sensitive (*150*), indicating the importance of electrostatic factors in the interaction. Of considerable interest was the finding that the *d*-tubocurarine reaction was also highly urea-sensitive, suggesting that hydrogen-bonding contributes materially to stabilizing the complex. The fact that binding of dimethyl *d*-tubocurarine, which cannot form such hydrogen bonds, is invariably weaker than binding of *d*-tubocurarine confirms this contention. Moreover, this effect of urea was not observed in interactions involving compounds such as stilbamidine or cetylpyridinium chloride (*149, 150*), which evidently react solely by urea-insensitive electrostatic and hydrophobic bonds.

An additional piece of information concerning the possible configuration of the *d*-tubocurarine molecule in solution was deduced from these studies. As indicated previously, *d*-tubocurarine fails to bind to hyaluronic acid, although it reacts very strongly with CSA. On the other hand, stilbamidine reacts strongly with *both* macromolecules (*177*), also by a two-point attachment. These results suggest that the interquaternary distances in *d*-tubocurarine and stilbamidine are probably different, and that the distance in *d*-tubocurarine must be far less than that in stilbamidine. According to a molecular model, the intercationic distance in stilbamidine is about 14 A, the same as has been long proposed for *d*-tubocurarine. However, the intercationic distance in *d*-tubocurarine was questioned by Loewe and Harvey (*178*), who made a model of the molecule and found the distance to be only 7 A; Ehrenpreis and co-workers confirmed this possibility also by using models. If these distances are correct, then the different reactivities of *d*-tubocurarine and stilbamidine with the acidic polysaccharides may be readily understood. *d*-Tubocurarine is visualized as binding with each successive carboxyl and sulfate group of CSA, but stilbamidine binds to every other anionic group; that is, the molecule overlaps adjacent sugar moieties. The intervening sulfate in CSA is missing in hyaluronic acid, and therefore *d*-tubocurarine can combine by only a single point with each carboxyl group resulting in very weak binding. On the other hand, the stilbamidine molecule can bridge the distance between successive carboxyl groups and thus shows strong binding.

These results demonstrated for the first time that two-point binding of *d*-tubocurarine with macromolecules is possible, and they thereby strengthened the widely held concept that this drug combines simultaneously with two anionic groups on the cholinergic receptor. However, these findings do not favor the view that the distance between the anionic groups is 14 A; indeed, such a distance is contrary to the fact that many bisquaternary compounds with far smaller interquaternary distances are highly potent, a fact which implies a two-point attachment with the cholinergic receptor (*179–181*). Even the interquaternary distance in decamethonium and succinylcholine is almost certainly less than 14 A in solution, as deduced from the binding of related compounds to hyaluronic acid (*177*). The proposed 7 A interquaternary distance in *d*-tubocurarine (and, by extrapolation, a corresponding inter-anionic distance on the receptor) appears to be more in line with known structure–activity relationships among bisquaternary compounds. This distance is precisely in the range of that proposed by Gill (*182*) to account for the observed ganglionic blocking potency of various bisquaternary compounds.

The possibility that *d*-tubocurarine can combine strongly with many different types of naturally occurring macromolecules has raised a number of problems concerning the nature of the cholinergic receptor substance, particularly since the binding sites on CSA and NA apparently are exactly complementary to the *d*-tubocurarine molecule. How, then, could it be ruled out that these macromolecules are directly involved in the effects, not only of *d*-tubocurarine, but of other cholinergic compounds? The question is extremely difficult to answer; for example, the binding of *d*-tubocurarine by CSA can be overcome with carbamoylcholine (*183*). However, two important aspects of the interacting properties of these macromolecules make it unlikely that they could function as the specific cholinergic receptor.

First, the number of binding sites for cholinotropic drugs is evidently very great, one *d*-tubocurarine molecule combining with every two nucleotide groups on nucleic acid and with every two sugar residues on CSA, whereas most other cholinergic compounds can combine with every negative group. It might be expected that the receptor molecule has only a limited number of active sites for compounds such as *d*-tubocurarine or ACh. In fact, Waser has suggested that there is only a single curarine binding site on each receptor molecule.

Second, the binding strength of flexible bisquaternary ammonium compounds is no greater than that of the corresponding monoquaternary compound (*148*), and this fact is contrary to the observed in vivo potency of such compounds. These and other considerations (*132*) strongly suggest that the receptor is constituted at least in part of protein material since only a protein could exhibit the high degree of specificity and limited number of binding sites required. In many respects the receptor even resembles an enzyme, having the property of distinguishing between optical isomers. Nevertheless, arguments that other types of molecule may be involved in the primary action of ACh have been presented; they are discussed below.

Evidence has been obtained that the mechanism of the reaction of *d*-tubocurarine with the receptor in vivo may be similar to that which occurs with macromolecules in the test tube. For example, Quilliam and Taylor have shown (*184*) that blocking by *d*-tubocurarine is potassium-sensitive, and although they attributed this fact to the competition for binding sites on the receptor, it might be interpreted in terms of an ionic-strength effect. Moreover, on the electroplax the blocking of electrical activity by *d*-tubocurarine is somewhat urea-sensitive (*9*) and, according to an old observation made by Feng (*185*), action of this drug at neuromuscular junction can be relieved by guanidine, a compound that breaks hydrogen bonds. Finally, dimethyltubocurarine is considerably weaker on the electroplax than *d*-tubocurarine itself and, as Kalow observed, the effectiveness of *d*-tubocurarine at the neuromuscular junction diminishes with increasing pH (*186*). These observations all indicate that the reaction of *d*-tubocurarine with its receptor is mediated by electrostatic and hydrogen bonds.

2. CRITERIA FOR IDENTIFYING AN ISOLATED COMPONENT AS A RECEPTOR

The information from model systems has been considered essential to any attempt at isolating the cholinergic receptor from the electric organ or any tissue since even a highly specific cholinotropic compound, such as *d*-tubocurarine, can combine strongly with many types of macromolecule. Certain rigid criteria of receptor activity must be set up to identify a given macromolecule as the receptor; among them the following are considered the most important.

a. Criterion 1

It is not sufficient to demonstrate that a given tissue component combines with compounds known to react with the receptor, although the fact that they do is, of course, essential. The affinity for such compounds must parallel the in vivo receptor affinity as determined by their potency in influencing some response of the tissue (electrical activity, contractility, etc.). This criterion itself contains another important assumption, because it implies that drug effects obey mass-action laws. Although receptor-blocking compounds may well obey these laws, there is some doubt whether this is true for agonists. In the case of agonists, as pointed out by Paton (*156, 157*), the kinetics of dissociation in vivo from the receptor may be of prime importance, but how to measure this parameter in a system in solution is not immediately apparent. Moreover, the receptor undoubtedly exists as an integral part of the membrane, and therefore such factors as surface phenomena and influence of adjacent components could greatly alter not only the affinities but the kinetics of interaction.

Further, in measuring the in vivo affinities for the receptor one must be certain that all compounds act by the same mechanism. However, the structure of the electroplax and, indeed, of any tissue possessing a cholinergic receptor system is such that a given compound could alter the response by one or more of the following mechanisms: (a) reaction with the receptor substance itself, preventing the action of ACh either liberated by nerve stimulation or exogenously applied, (b) reaction with a component or components in the nerve terminals, preventing the release of ACh, (c) reaction with a component or components in the conducting membrane, leading either to a blockade of electrical activity or to depolarization, (d) combination with nonreceptor elements in the postjunctional membrane, (e) promoting release of ACh.

Very few compounds exhibit only a single site of reactivity; ACh, carbamoylcholine, decamethonium, succinylcholine, and *d*-tubocurarine on the electroplax probably react chiefly by a receptor mechanism, although multiple sites of action have been discerned at neuromuscular junctions (*161–164*). The many other compounds that act on electroplax probably do so by mechanisms (a), (b), and (c), given above. They include the lipid-soluble quaternary ammonium compounds and local anesthetics, which alter events in the conducting membrane as well as produce receptor-mediated effects (*75*, *107*). It is of some interest that local anesthetics depress both the direct and indirect responses of electroplax about equally, and this is further indication that they paralyze the nerve endings and thereby prevent the release of ACh through neural stimulation. Such blockade, however, may yet result from a receptor reaction, because this parameter is frequently measured in terms of the ability of a compound to inhibit the response elicited by nerve stimulation. Thus, although local anesthetics very probably combine with the cholinergic receptor, as a result of a multiplicity of actions, it is extremely difficult, if not impossible, to determine their affinity for it. It is possible to measure the competition between the compound under consideration and externally applied ACh as a means of determining the affinity constants—the approach used by Jenkinson with *d*-tubocurarine and skeletal muscle receptors (*187*)—but even when this was done, Higman and Bartels (*75*) could not arrive at any definitive value for the binding constant of tetracaine and the cholinergic receptor of electroplax.

The dose–response relationship for determining affinities in the manner described by Ariëns et al. (*158*) also could entail a number of difficulties with all but a few compounds. As the concentration of a compound is increased, the site of its reactions and, hence, the mechanism of action could well be drastically changed; regions of the cell that were inaccessible to the compound in low concentration might be reached to a significant extent at high concentrations, and macromolecules that failed to react to low concentrations might begin to react. These difficulties probably would become more pronounced as the members of a series of compounds increased in complexity and in lipid solubility; this may explain in part why chemical modification of agonists produces antagonists. Perhaps the best way to measure these ancillary reactions of an inhibitor would be to determine the extent to which the anti-ACh action could be reversed by ACh, since such reversal probably would be brought about only through reactions taking place at the receptor site.

Thus, the most fundamental criterion upon which identification of any isolated receptor rests contains many pitfalls.

b. Criterion 2

The amount of receptor substance isolated should be consistent with the amount expected to be present in the tissue. This criterion poses considerable difficulties, because there is a great paucity of knowledge about the receptor content of any tissue. Waser's data on the fixation of labeled curarine has provided what may be an upper limit for the number of receptors present at the synapse of mouse diaphragm. But, as previously discussed, his value may be several orders of magnitude too high. Moreover, there are no similar data for other tissues, and so it may not be correct to assume that all junctions contain the same number of receptor molecules.

Because Waser's figures refer to the number of binding sites at junctions and not to the total number of receptor molecules, it is essential to know both the binding *capacity* of any proposed receptor as well as the amount isolated.

c. Criterion 3

Any molecule satisfying the criteria given above must be shown to originate from regions of the cell where the receptor would be expected to exist, namely, the postsynaptic sites. Localization of any isolated tissue component poses considerable technical difficulties which may be overcome, at least in part, by means of immunohistochemical techniques, as shown by Ehrenpreis (*188*). However, even these methods may not be sufficiently precise for one to ascertain whether a given component originates from the exact point where the receptor exists in the cell.

d. Criterion 4

The isolated receptor substance should aid in understanding the molecular basis of the action of ACh and other cholinergic compounds, including an explanation of the fundamental difference which exists between agonists and antagonists. Combining ACh with an isolated receptor might cause some discernible alteration in molecular structure, which would afford insight into how the union in vivo gives rise to change in membrane structure and resultant depolarization. Such an effect should be opposed by *d*-tubocurarine and other antagonists.

3. ISOLATION OF DRUG-BINDING COMPONENTS FROM THE ELECTRIC ORGAN OF THE ELECTRIC EEL

In the isolation studies of Ehrenpreis (*132*, *136*, *189*, *190*), *d*-tubocurarine interaction was used as the primary guide to possible receptor activity; this was coupled with semiquantitative studies of the binding of various cholinotropic compounds with components extracted from the electric organ.* The approach promised some success, because protein components that actually

* For binding-constant determination, equilibrium dialysis is the method of choice, but very large amounts of macromolecule are required (several hundred milligrams for each drug). Although the various fractions may be used over and over again, they deteriorate fairly rapidly. Hence these studies represented a compromise: fewer points with many compounds, rather than many points with a few compounds. It is felt that identification of receptor activity is more feasible by the former approach than the latter.

precipitated with *d*-tubocurarine could be extracted. *d*-Tubocurarine precipitation was then used as a means of selectively removing the "receptor" from the remainder of thc extracted material. Although, as previously indicated, both CSA and NA also precipitate with this compound, a portion of the tissue component-curare complex appeared to be unlike the other complexes, in that prolonged dialysis at neutral pH failed to produce complete solubilization. The clue to dissociating the complex was provided by the observation that precipitation could be suppressed by urea, implicating hydrogen bonds in the reaction. Thus, when dialysis was carried out at pH 9, at which the phenolic hydroxyl groups of *d*-tubocurarine are ionized, dissociation was promoted and the precipitate dissolved. The fraction insoluble at pH 7.5 was considered to be the receptor material.

Fig. 1.7. (a) Free electrophoresis (Spinco) of purified receptor protein of electric organ of electric eel. Photographs are of ascending boundary and were taken 30, 60, and 90 min after start. Run was made at pH 7.5 in 0.1 *M* tris buffer.

Of particular interest was the observation that binding of *d*-tubocurarine to the isolated "receptor" was many times greater than that to the residue remaining after extraction (*132*). This finding provided evidence that the major material binding *d*-tubocurarine was present in extractable form. However, even this seemingly conclusive evidence has a pitfall: it does not unambiguously preclude the possibility that a small amount of highly active material was present in the residue and would completely escape detection.

The "receptor" isolated by precipitation with *d*-tubocurarine was found to be essentially protein in nature, to be as much as 90% homogeneous* in free electrophoresis (Figure 1.7a) (confirmed by Dr. S. Beychok, personal communication) but completely homogeneous in gel electrophoresis (Figure 1.7b), to sediment in the ultracentrifuge essentially as a single peak, and to contain about 10% lipid comprised of lecithin, cholesterol, and sphingomyelin. The protein was found to combine with a large number of drugs known to affect the

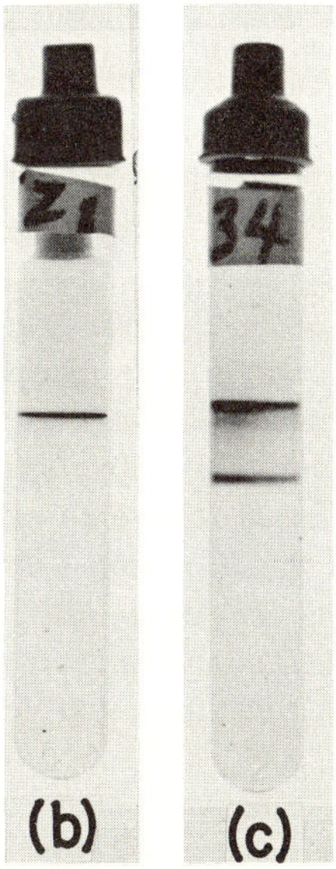

Fig. 1.7. (b). Polymethacrilide gel electrophoresis patterns for purified drug-binding protein from electric organ of electric eel and (c) for total curare precipitate of extract of electric organ (*183*).

* Trams et al. (*191*) reported disagreement with the stated homogeneity of this protein, claiming that when it was chromatographed on diethylaminoethyl cellulose, three components were obtained. However, their preparation consisted of the entire *d*-tubocurarine precipitate, whereas the protein of Ehrenpreis and associates was fractionated by means of dialysis at pH 7.5 (*132*). When the total *d*-tubocurarine precipitate was examined by gel electrophoresis, it was indeed found to be quite heterogeneous (Figure 1.7c).

electrical activity of electroplax (*132, 134, 189, 190*). Interestingly, some of these drugs also yielded precipitates with the protein; among them were chlorpromazine, diphenhydramine, methantheline, chlorisondamine, several local anesthetics, and a large number of monoquaternary and diquaternary ammonium compounds (*132, 134*). The precipitation reaction could be quantitated by dissolving the precipitates and determining the optical densities in the UV. From the extensive study conducted with this method as well as with equilibrium dialysis, it was concluded that the protein isolated as previously described showed the highest affinity for the greatest number of cholinotropic compounds of any component present in electroplax (*132, 134*). The number of binding sites on the protein for the various drugs was limited, being about 10 per 100,000 molecular weight. The amount isolated appeared to be in the range of that expected from Waser's data. On the basis of the available data, it was proposed that this drug-binding protein was identical with the ACh receptor (*132*). No reasonable alternative explanation of its properties could be offered despite the fact that the binding of ACh appeared too weak to be consistent with that expected on the basis of in vivo affinity for electroplax receptors.

When the protein was localized in sections of individual electroplax by means of the fluorescent antibody technique (*188*), it was found to be situated within or near both the innervated and noninnervated membranes of the cell and completely excluded from the interior (Figure 1.8). It was, in fact, strategically located at sites where it could react with drugs known to affect electrical responses of electroplax. However, a major contradiction was apparent in that the ACh receptor was expected to be restricted to the innervated membrane alone. Evidently, the role the protein might play in the pharmacological actions of drugs on electroplax was different from that originally proposed.

A new possible function of the protein was suggested (*57, 134, 136*) by results obtained with detergent-treated (*93–95*) and venom-treated nerves (*87, 96*). These studies revealed that some component of conducting membranes can combine with many of the drugs that react with the drug-binding protein of the electric organ. For example, *d*-tubocurarine and chlorisondamine, formerly thought to combine exclusively with junctional receptors of ACh, were now shown to react with some sort of extrajunctional "receptor" which is ordinarily "masked" and that this combination could lead to a blockade of electrical activity. The low activity of ACh, carbamoylcholine, decamethonium, and succinylcholine on treated nerves (*87, 94*) is consistent with their weak binding to the protein (binding constants greater than 10^{-3} *M*). The affinity constants of *d*-tubocurarine and carbamoylcholine (2×10^{-4} and 4×10^{-3} *M*, respectively) for the drug-binding protein (*183*) are well in line with the potencies of these compounds on conducting membranes (*63, 87*). It is now proposed that the drug-binding protein is an important constituent of the conducting membrane of the electroplax and that blockade of the propagated

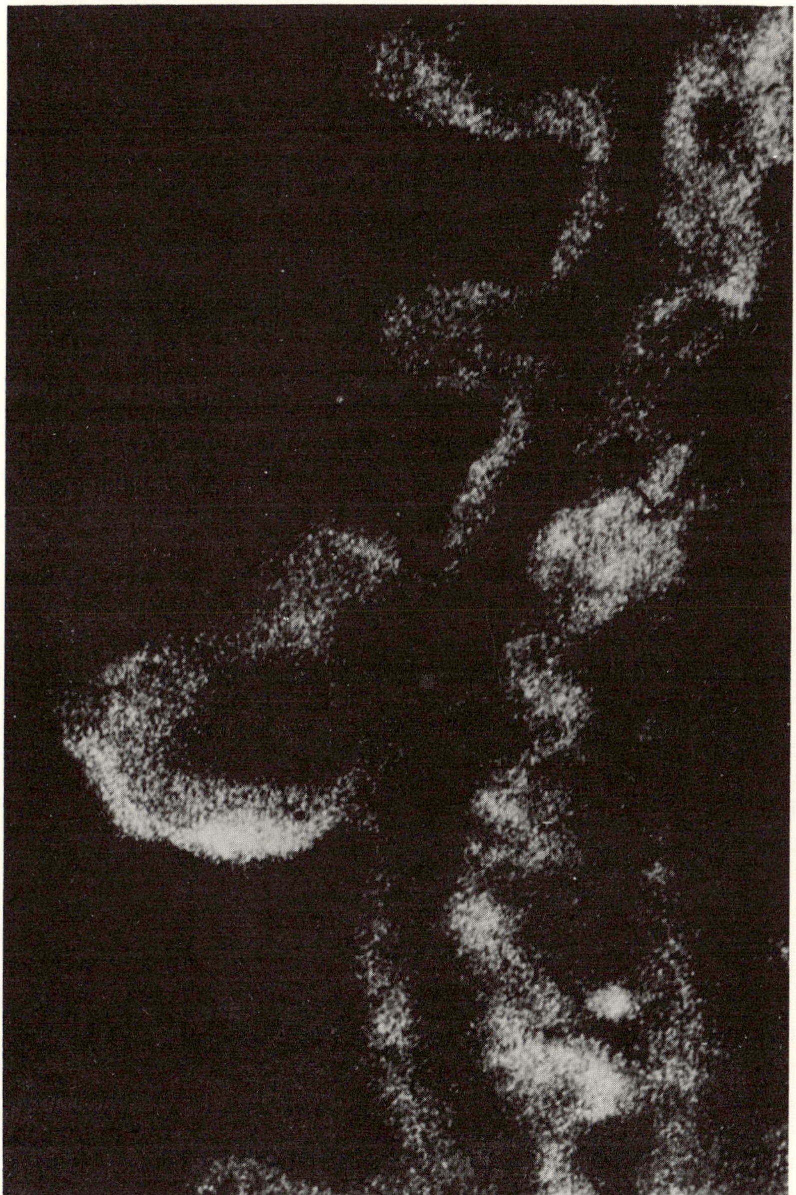

Fig. 1.8. Localization of drug-binding protein in the electroplax of electric eel. Areas where the protein is present are white. Specific staining may be seen at both the innervated (bottom) and noninnervated membrane (top), as well as in the loose connective tissue on the innervated side. [From Ref. (*188*).]

impulse by various drugs is brought about by their combination with this component. As such, the component has an important function in this cell, one which is intimately concerned with ion movements, perhaps in the manner described elsewhere (*57*, *136a*). It should be noted that such reactions would occur only with those drugs which are able to penetrate through the barriers to the conducting membrane, and this includes essentially only those compounds which are fairly lipid-soluble, such as local anesthetics, chlorpromazine, diphenhydramine, and lipid-soluble quaternary ammonium compounds. The protein is not considered to be involved with the effects upon the electroplax of ACh, carbamoylcholine, decamethonium, or *d*-tubocurarine, because their action is presumed to be limited to the true ACh receptors in the synaptic region.

Although no macromolecule having ACh receptor activity has yet been isolated in solution from electric organ, such a molecule almost certainly does exist. It might be present as a small contaminant in the protein fraction isolated by *d*-tubocurarine precipitation, although, as previously stated, the best preparations are extremely homogeneous in polymethacrylide gel electrophoresis. However, evidence has been accumulating that the ChE molecule may be part of the receptor apparatus and, if that is so, the lack of success in demonstrating receptor activity for other tissue components is understandable. Such evidence will be discussed below (Sections 1.5 and 1.6).

C. Binding of Dimethyl-*d*-Tubocurarine to a Microsomal Fraction of the Electric Organ

Trams (*192*) recently reported that some electric organ components bind dimethyltubocurarine at very low concentrations, that is, in the range of 10^{-8} to 10^{-9} *M*, and this was considered evidence that the material represented the receptor substance. However, the ligand material consisted of "microsomal proteins" of an unknown nature. No information was presented concerning the number of components in the preparation or how many are involved in the binding. Moreover, the degree of binding actually appeared to be quite negligible: at 5×10^{-8} *M* of dimethyltubocurarine, 1 g of protein material bound about 3×10^{-9} moles of drug. If it is assumed that the average molecular weight of the proteins present was 100,000, then one drug molecule was distributed among 3000 protein molecules. Even when the concentration was increased to 2.5×10^{-6} *M*, the binding ratio of drug to protein was 1:500. Saturation of the binding sites was not achieved even at the highest dimethyltubocurarine concentrations used. It is difficult to see how these results "substantiate the author's skepticism regarding the isolation of receptors by methods such as proposed by Ehrenpreis." The methods referred to by Trams involved the use of *d*-tubocurarine or other drugs as a means of isolating tissue components involved in their pharmacological effects. Presumably, this skepticism was prompted by a belief that the particulate components bound *d*-tubocurarine "significantly" and had, therefore, much higher affinities for the drug than that of any solubilized components. The inference was clearly made that the latter could not possibly have an important role in the effects of *d*-tubocurarine on electroplax. Although the supposition may be correct and was pointed out even earlier by Ehrenpreis (*136*, *188*, *189*), the results obtained by Trams could hardly be used to substantiate this contention.

D. Studies of Woolley and Co-workers

Woolley and his associates have attempted to isolate and identify the receptors for ACh and serotonin (*170*, *193–197*) by an entirely different approach. In their view the key to the problem is that the reaction of these and other agonists with the receptor is directly responsible for facilitating the transport of calcium into the cell and promoting contraction of muscle. This is said to come about as follows (*170*): "Serotonin and other hormones which cause contraction...do so because they cause this flow of Ca^{++},...because ionized Ca is not soluble in fats, these ions can pass into the cell only by 'leakage' through the non-lipoidal part of the membrane or by some sort of active transport." The latter is said to occur in several ways: "One of these was for serotonin [or ACh] to combine with a constituent of the cell membrane and the complex so formed to form a fat-soluble Ca^{++} salt or chelate." After diffusing through the membrane to the interior, an enzyme would cleave some group, disintegrating the complex and liberating calcium and serotonin. The various hormones, including ACh, would be expected to combine with their own specific substances (receptors) in a similar way, thus providing several mechanisms for transporting calcium into the interior. In accordance with this concept of the function and nature of the receptor it was decided to attempt to isolate a substance that "should cause serotonin (or ACh) to join with it and become soluble in fat solvents in the presence of Ca^{++} ions and at physiological pH" (*170*). A simple assay was devised, in which the measure of "receptor" activity was the ability of a tissue component to render serotonin or ACh soluble in a benzene–butanol mixture in the presence of Ca^{++}. Although such materials were shown to be present in most of the tissues examined (*170*), it is doubtful that the findings provide insight into either the nature of the receptor substance itself or the mechanism of action of ACh, serotonin, or other contracting substance, for the following reasons.

First of all, it has been shown that this tissue "receptor" is essentially lipid in nature and as such could scarcely possess the characteristics necessary for specificity of interaction with the many compounds known to affect receptor systems. Indeed, lipids other than those present in the tissues seemed to be far more active in transporting biogenic amines into the lipid phase (*195*). Vogt in examining phosphatidic acid found that this, too, could form a complex with ACh that could be extracted from aqueous solution by a mixture of isobutyl alcohol and benzene (*198*). He was even able to demonstrate that atropine was bound to this lipid and that its affinity was greater than that of ACh. On the other hand, the affinity of calcium for this "receptor" also was greater than that of ACh, and it was, perhaps, for this reason that Vogt concluded that "phosphatidic acid does not meet the requirements of an ACh receptor as designed by Woolley." It may be noted that although this seems a reasonable conclusion, there is some doubt that affinities alone can be used as justification because, as discussed elsewhere, there are many problems in the mechanism by which ACh and atropine produce their effects.

A second point concerns the basic postulate that the transport of Ca^{++} proceeds stoichiometrically with a given hormone; that is, one ACh molecule is considered to be responsible for the movement of one calcium ion. All the evidence indicates, rather, that ACh and other agonists are catalytic, in the sense that very small amounts promote the transport of a very large amount of calcium (*199*). Potassium chloride can readily produce a contraction of most muscles, even when ACh participation can be ruled out through the use of such potent anti-ACh compounds as atropine and *d*-tubocurarine. This contraction involves membrane depolarization which, as discussed before, probably does not proceed by an ACh mechanism. Similarly, smooth or striated muscle may be contracted by direct electrical stimulation, and there is no evidence of the participation of ACh in the response produced. Thus, the primary premise upon which Woolley and co-workers based their attempt at receptor isolation and identification lacks experimental justification. Aside from this, Woolley did not determine the affinity constants for ACh or serotonin or present any evidence that other cholinergic compounds could combine with the component and influence the reaction of ACh in accordance with their known in vivo action.

E. Studies of Grob and Namba

Grob and associates (*200–204*)* have been attempting to isolate the cholinergic receptor of striated muscle by using essentially the same procedure of precipitation with *d*-tubocurarine as that devised by Ehrenpreis (*132*). Their isolated "receptor" proved to be a nucleoprotein, which was about one third nucleic acid and two thirds protein had a molecular weight of about 300,000, and seemed to originate primarily from the microsomal fraction of the muscle (*203*). It was noted early that this component was able to bind various cholinergic compounds and that apparently a competition took place between

* I am indebted to Dr. Namba and Dr. Grob for allowing me to read their manuscript (*203*) prior to publication.

d-tubocurarine and ACh, decamethonium, and succinylcholine (*201*). However, this study was carried out in distilled water and therefore is subject to the criticism previously set forth. Later studies using equilibrium dialysis in buffer of 0.1 ionic strength revealed that the binding constant for dimethyl-*d*-tubocurarine is actually greater than 10^{-4} *M* (*203*). Although binding of acetylcholine was apparent, the results were complicated by the fact that the purified material was contaminated with ChE. The binding sites for ACh could not be highly specific, because both choline and ACh were about equally effective in inhibiting the reaction with *d*-tubocurarine.

Namba and Grob calculated that the number of isolated "receptor" molecules originating from each end plate of the muscle they used was about 2×10^9. As they recognize, this value is somewhat high in comparison with Waser's directly determined number (discussed previously), but when the *binding capacity* of their receptor is taken into consideration, then the amount isolated becomes almost astronomically high. The nucleoprotein receptor probably has a capacity for binding *d*-tubocurarine of at least 50 per molecule, because multiple binding to the nucleic acid part certainly occurs. The number of binding sites at an end plate, then, would be about 10^{11}, if this macromolecule were involved in binding of *d*-tubocurarine at the synapse. This may be why Namba and Grob (*203*) more recently suggested that their material "is not confined to the endplate, and is more widely distributed throughout the muscle fiber" and may, in fact, be involved in the extra-junctional effects of ACh and *d*-tubocurarine on denervated muscle. This is an intriguing possibility since, as they point out, "it is unlikely that synthesis or transportation of receptor protein occurs this rapidly [i.e., during denervation]. It is probable that receptor protein normally exists in an inactive state in the entire muscle fiber, and is physiologically active only in the endplate region." However, the properties of this nucleoprotein, together with the fact that it originates primarily from the microsomal fraction, suggest that it does not participate directly in events at either the postsynaptic or the conducting membranes. Nevertheless, it is very interesting that fluorescent-labeled antibodies to this component were found to be fixed in synaptic regions (*204*). Possibly, these antibodies were directed against ChE, which appears to be a significant contaminant in the preparations isolated by *d*-tubocurarine precipitation.

I.5. CHOLINESTERASE AND THE CHOLINERGIC RECEPTOR

It is apparent from the studies described in the previous section that no isolated tissue molecule, large or small, satisfies even a few of the requirements of a receptor substance. Although undoubtedly a number of tissue components react with many compounds that have a high affinity for the receptor in vivo, the affinities of ACh and other depolarizing compounds appear to be far too small to be compatible with their in vivo potencies. This statement assumes a direct correlation between affinity and potency, an assumption that may not be applicable to receptor–agonist reactions because of the additional element of "efficacy." Efficacy has no obvious counterpart in other interacting systems, but it might conceivably endow a weakly interacting molecule with great potency. Unfortunately, "efficacy" has escaped definitive formulation on the molecular level, and thus is a property that virtually defies measurement in an in vitro system. Perhaps the only suggestion of a basis for efficacy has been the concept of change in molecular configuration, and as regards ACh the only molecule capable of undergoing molecular reorientation appears to be ChE itself (*205*, *206*). For these reasons we must re-examine ChE as a possible model for the receptor, since it appears to be the only tissue component having the specificity and at least some of the affinity properties expected of the receptor.

There is no doubt that most, if not all, of the compounds having actions attributable entirely or in part to combination with the receptor also react with the enzyme in solution. Among them are choline esters of various kinds, (*33*, *208*, *209*), *d*-tubocurarine, TRIEG (*159*), and a host of other monoquaternary, diquaternary, and tertiary nitrogen compounds (*6*, *7*, *33*, *159*, *207*). It is somewhat gratifying to have a macromolecule, particularly an enzyme, for which association constants of cholinergic compounds or rates of hydrolysis of substrates may be determined and correlated with reactivity with the receptor in situ. Moreover, the effect of many of these compounds is to inhibit hydrolysis of ACh by the enzyme, and this has its counterpart in their anti-ACh action with the receptor. On the basis of studies of this type, several workers have suggested (*1–6*) that ChE functions as the cholinergic receptor, although no attempt has been made, with the exception of Belleau (*6*), to define precisely the manner in which the enzyme may participate directly. However, even Belleau's very elegant molecular perturbation theory fails to come to grips with some of the fundamental problems involved in equating enzyme and receptor. Among these are the following: How the potent inhibitors of ChE potentiate ACh action in vivo while seemingly preventing their reaction with the enzyme; how to reconcile the great potency of the atropine-type compounds and of ACh with their fairly low affinity for the enzyme; how the reaction of ACh with an active catalytic site can be "productive"; how to distinguish agonists and antagonists among compounds that all seem to combine similarly with the enzyme; and how an agonist causes the change in membrane that increases ion permeability. Of the last mentioned Belleau states that the change comes about through the release of bound water resulting from agonist interaction; this interesting proposition does not seem specific enough for agonist reactions alone.

Although it is qualitatively true that the enzyme and the receptor combine with many of the same compounds and that at times the correlation between affinity and potency is quite satisfactory, it is equally true that in a number of important instances great discrepancies are apparent. For example, the atropine-type compounds are very weakly bound by the enzyme (*33*) but these are the most potent inhibitors of ACh action; this has been an important reason for rejecting the concept that receptor and enzyme are identical. However, recent work by Ehrenpreis and co-workers (*168a*, *c*)* shows that the receptor for ACh and atropine-type compounds may not be the same or, if it is, then the binding sites on the molecule are different. Thus, this objection is considered invalid.

Another important factor, all too frequently overlooked, is the fact that ACh itself has a rather low affinity for ChE, the binding constant, according to kinetic studies, being about 10^{-4} *M*, whereas its apparent affinity for the receptor is of the order of 10^{-7} *M* (*158*, *187*). The same is true of other potent choline esters, such as methacholine and carbamoylcholine, which are weakly bound yet very potent agonists. Although Wilson (*211*) has calculated on the basis of bond energies that it is possible that the constant for the binding of ACh to the receptor can be about 10^{-7} *M*, the fact remains that an increase in the chemical complexity of the ACh molecule usually is accompanied by a *decrease* in its ability to stimulate receptors (*158*). This occurs even when the modification results in compounds which would be anticipated to have a much higher affinity. As pointed out by Wurzel (*3–5*), the *hydrolytic activity* of a tissue's ChE toward various substrates (ACh, butyrylcholine, benzoylcholine, acetylthiocholine) seems to be in excellent correlation with the potency of these esters as agonists on the tissue. This may imply that *substrate specificity*, rather than *affinity*, is the important determinant of agonist activity (why this may be so will be discussed in the next section). Of course one must not lose sight of the fact that many agonists are not substrates of ChE and, conversely, many substrates of the enzyme are not agonists at all (*210*).

One of the most effective arguments against the identity of ChE and the receptor is the fact that the most potent inhibitors of ChE (physostigmine, neostigmine, and DFP) are strong potentiators of the action of ACh. It would be anticipated that these compounds, by combining with the active site on the enzyme-receptor, would only *block* subsequently added ACh, just as they block the hydrolysis of the ester. As Schild pointed out, atropine (and other receptor inhibitors) and physostigmine should produce similar effects if enzyme and receptor were identical (*212*). Although the potent inhibitors of ChE do have an action attributable to blockade of ACh (*70–73*), this action occurs only at concentrations that are much greater than those required to potentiate ACh. However, the inhibitors of ChE may exhibit a multitude of actions at cholinergic sites. At the lowest concentrations, at which ChE

* See also footnote, p. 34.

inhibition is minimal, or perhaps even undetectable, "sensitization" of the receptor may occur (*165*, *213–216*), an effect which may be the underlying and primary cause of the potentiation of ACh (a mechanism of this sensitization will be presented below). At higher concentrations, where a significant degree of ChE inhibition is observed, sensitization would be reinforced. As the concentration is increased, anti-ACh effects predominate, and at still higher concentrations some compounds may again cause stimulation, an effect totally unrelated to inhibition of ChE (*99*, *112*) whereas others (DFP and other organophosphates) cause tissue destruction (*99*, *112*).

The question of the identity of ChE and receptor appears to revolve upon two interrelated problems: the exact mechanism by which the potent ChE inhibitors combine with the enzyme and potentiate ACh and the function of the enzyme as a regulator of ACh action at sites where the ester produces a physiological effect. The following discussion is intended to point out why recent studies may have indicated the need of a re-evaluation of current concepts regarding these two problems. It is suggested that the evidence strengthens the possibility that the enzyme is involved in receptor function.

It was long considered that the ChE inhibitors, particularly neostigmine and physostigmine, are truly reversible inhibitors of ChE, combining simultaneously with esteratic and anionic sites on the enzyme (*217*) and in this way preventing hydrolysis of ACh. It is now known (*211*, *218*, *219*) that this mechanism is incorrect and that these compounds, like DFP, are substrates of the enzyme. The intermediates produced, the carbamates or phosphates, remain associated with the esteratic site of the enzyme and are only slowly removed by hydrolysis. However, this still leaves the anionic site free to combine with ACh and other quaternary ammonium compounds. In fact, the binding strength may actually be enhanced. Župančič has shown that the affinity constant of ACh for DFP-treated ChE is about 10^{-6} *M* (*219*), whereas from kinetic data the affinity constant for intact ChE is calculated to be only about 10^{-4} *M*.

That the inhibitors of ChE can promote the in vivo actions of ACh by a mechanism attributable only in part to a decrease in enzyme activity has been observed in a number of instances; the important aspect of these studies is the fact that intact tissues (not homogenates) were used to correlate the inhibition of enzyme with the potentiation of ACh. Thus, Rosenberg and co-workers reported that physostigmine (3×10^{-5} *M*) potentiates ACh action on the electroplax 1000-fold (*220*). Based on the value of about 10^{-8} *M* for the K_i of physostigmine for ChE, the concentration used would have been expected to inhibit all of the enzyme, yet when assays were performed on intact single electroplax only about 50% inhibition was observed (*221*). It is thus evident that the profound potentiating action of physostigmine cannot be due to inhibition of the enzyme alone.

Other examples of a similar nature have emerged from studies of the heart and stomach smooth muscle (*24, 24a, 168c*). Neostigmine (0.1 μg/ml) and physostigmine (0.2 μg/ml) potentiate the effect of ACh on isolated rabbit atria 8-fold and 15-fold, respectively, and potentiation is maintained even after several washings of the tissue. However, under the conditions used, there is no discernible inhibition of ChE in the intact atria. DFP potentiates ACh 300-fold on this tissue, an effect which is accompanied by only 50% inhibition of ChE. Physostigmine and neostigmine (0.1 μg/ml) produce a contraction of stomach smooth muscle and potentiate ACh several fold after washing. In accordance with current concepts, this smooth-muscle stimulation would be attributed solely to an accumulation of endogenous ACh through the suppression of enzyme activity. Such a mechanism is probably invalid for at least three reasons: there was no evidence of actual diminution of enzyme activity in the intact tissue when stimulation occurred; the contraction occurred very rapidly (within seconds) and so resembled a "receptor" reaction, in contradistinction to the rate of ChE inhibition, which is very slow (*211*); and potentiation of exogenously applied ACh was observed following washout of physostigmine and neostigmine. The last would imply a continuing inhibition of ChE, but the muscle was in its normally relaxed state, contrary to what would be expected if endogenous ACh were accumulating in the vicinity of the receptor under the influence of such inhibition.

The next important point concerns the rate of hydrolysis of ACh and the role of the enzyme as a regulator of ACh action through its ability to reduce the free concentration of the ester in equilibrium with the receptor.

It is well recognized that purified ChE hydrolyzes ACh very rapidly, the turnover being about 7×10^5 molecules per minute per catalytic center (*29–31*). In fact, the rapidity has been used by Nachmansohn as an argument for the essential role of the enzyme and, by implication, of ACh in bioelectric mechanisms in nerve (*34*). Furthermore, the rapidity of action fits in well with the proposed role of the enzyme in terminating ACh action at various cholinergic sites. However, some recent findings (*5, 24, 24a, 35*) may have cast doubt on the validity of the concept of the purely regulatory action of ChE and are perhaps suggestive of some other role of the enzyme in ACh action. The newer experiments have been designed to examine the hydrolytic activity of ChE at very low concentrations, as close as possible to the concentrations required to produce a physiological effect. For this type of study a bioassay is required, e.g., rectus abdominus (*5*) or the even more sensitive, isolated atria (rabbit) and rat stomach strip (*24, 24a*). In one examination of the concentration dependence of hydrolysis of ACh with purified ChE it was shown that the rate of hydrolysis at 10^{-6} *M* is very low (*5*) although at a somewhat higher concentration, about 10^{-5} *M*, hydrolysis is quite rapid (*5, 35*). In other studies the following facts were found. Adding ChE (red blood cell or purified electric eel enzyme) to the bath containing ACh at 10^{-7} or 10^{-8} *M* in no way affected the response of atria or stomach strip to the ester. Incubating ACh at these concentrations with purified ChE in solution gave a rate of hydrolysis many orders of magnitude lower than was expected on the basis of enzyme activity as determined at optimal substrate concentration. Reusing ACh solutions after they had been in contact with the isolated atria or stomach strip for long periods of time (up to 45 min.) revealed essentially no hydrolysis of the ACh by the tissue enzyme. Even when the enzymatic activity was checked by the Hestrin method with ACh at 4×10^{-3} *M*, the half-life of ACh in the presence of intact atria from a single heart was found to be about 1 hr at 32°C.

These findings reveal that at extremely low concentrations of ACh (10^{-7} *M* or lower) neither ChE in situ nor the purified enzyme in solution hydrolyzes the ester at a significant rate; thus, the concentration of solutions surrounding these intact organs fails to be reduced to any sensible extent even over long periods of time. This finding has a distinct bearing on the concept of the role of ChE in normal transmission events, because the concentration of ACh released upon nerve stimulation is about 5×10^{-7} *M* in the vicinity of the postsynaptic membrane (*35*). A regulatory role of ChE would require that the enzyme turn over ACh at such a rapid rate that the concentration of free ester in equilibrium with receptor would be reduced within milliseconds; clearly, this does not occur at physiological concentrations of ACh, because the enzyme is not sufficiently active to hydrolyze the ester in the time required to account for its transient effects, either when ACh is liberated or when it is applied to isolated organs.* Thus some role other than a regulatory one must be invoked for ChE in terms of ACh action, since there is no doubt that the enzyme has an important function at cholinergic sites.

In view of the evident stability of ACh at low concentration in the presence of tissue ChE, there is no immediate reason for attributing the potentiating action of the inhibitors of ChE solely to a reduction in enzyme activity.

I.6. PARTICIPATION OF CHOLINESTERASE IN CHOLINERGIC RECEPTOR ACTIVITY: A NEW CONCEPT

A new proposal implicating ChE in receptor function will now be presented in detail. The mechanism differs from others in the sense that it attempts to show on the molecular level how the reaction of ACh and other agonists can

* It has been calculated (*31*) that the concentration of ChE at an endplate must be 10^{-5} *M* in order for the rate of hydrolysis of liberated ACh to be sufficiently rapid to account for the time course for the endplate potential. It remains to be determined whether this extraordinarily high density of enzyme is actually present at this site.

be translated into a change in membrane permeability, how certain structure–activity relationships among quaternary ammonium compounds can be explained, why *d*-tubocurarine blocks without altering the resting potential, how certain compounds initially stimulate and then competitively block the action of ACh, and how inhibitors of ChE potentiate ACh even though they may react at the active site on the enzyme.

The model is based in part on some concepts recently developed by Watkins,* who attempted to explain depolarization of ACh on the molecular level.

It is considered, in agreement with Watkins, that the receptor is an integral part of the bimolecular leaflet of which the postsynaptic membrane is composed. The area covered by the receptor is evidently only a small fraction of the total surface. The active site on the receptor is so constituted and localized that it controls the movement of ions through the postsynaptic membrane. This site is considered by Watkins to be composed partly of protein and partly of phospholipid (Figure 1.9). The protein is considered to contain both an anionic and esteratic site, and is assumed to be attached in the resting state to the phosphorylcholine portion of lecithin, which, of course, is highly complementary to most of the ACh molecule.

In Watkins' formulation the protein part of the receptor is of an unspecified nature although distinct from ChE. In our modification this is considered to be the active site of a ChE molecule. This obviates the need of postulating two types of protein with sites exactly complementary to the ACh molecule and which can combine with the many cationic substances known to alter cholinergic activity. Such sites are evidently present on the ChE molecule. As pictured by Krupka (*32*), the imidazole group of histidine† and the hydroxyl of serine may be part of the esteratic site (Figure 1.10). Although the exact nature of the anionic site is unknown, it may be a carboxyl (*32*) or phosphate group.

In the Watkins mechanism, attachment of ACh or other agonist to the protein portion of the receptor site disrupts the protein–lecithin bonds (Figure 1.9); this dissociation of the active site opens the membrane and enhances the rate of ion flux into the interior. Although not stated, it is presumed that the ACh is then hydrolyzed by adjacently located ChE thereby permitting the membrane to be restored to its original state.

In our modification, the site of attachment of ACh is a hydrolytic center on the enzyme but, because the site is complexed with lecithin, it is initially not

* I am indebted to Dr. J. C. Watkins for permitting me to quote from his work (*221a*) prior to its publication.

† In Watkins' formulation a divalent metal ion bridges the lipid phosphate group with a second anionic group of the protein (Figure 1.9). In our picture we would have the phosphate group bind directly with a positively charged group (possibly the histidine) at the esteratic site of ChE.

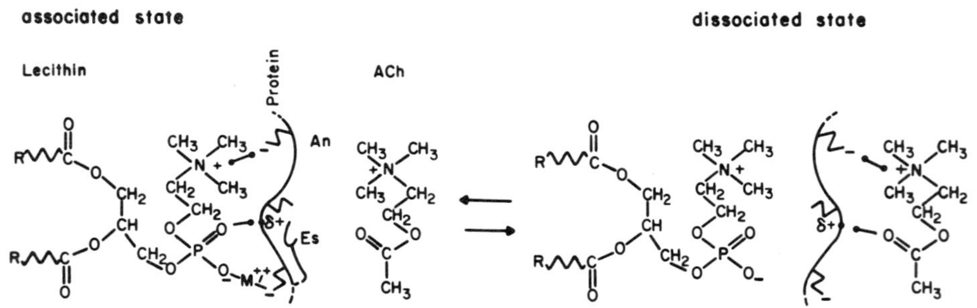

Fig. 1.9. Watkins' formulation of the receptor site and its dissociation by ACh. Lecithin is complexed to a protein with an anionic site (An) and an esteratic site (Es); the latter has two subsites, bearing a positive charge and a negative charge. The phosphate of lecithin is postulated to be linked by two points to the esteratic site as shown. A metal (M) is believed to be split off following the reaction of ACh with the anionic site and (+). As indicated in the text, we do not feel that the metal is an essential part of the active site and that the negatively charged oxygen of the phosphate is linked to the + of the protein (ChE in our formulation). [From Ref. (*221a*).]

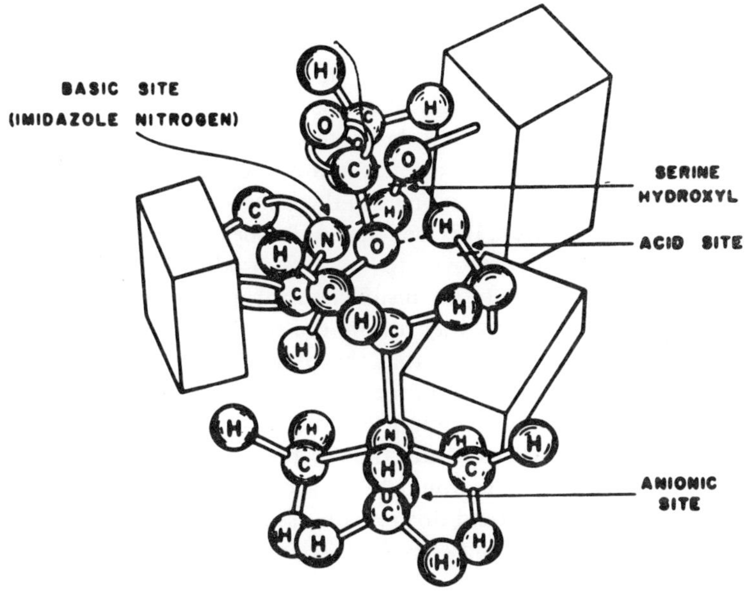

Fig. 1.10. Suggested arrangement of functional groups at the active center of AChE, showing the substrate in position in the enzyme-substrate complex. The dotted lines indicate electrostatic attractions and also bonds formed during the acetylation process; the three bonds broken are marked on the diagram. [From Ref. (*32*).]

catalytically active. After attachment of ACh and subsequent dissociation from the lecithin, a number of events may ensue: (a) The lecithin moiety is now free to undergo internal zwitterion formation, which further increases the size of the opening and also neutralizes the positive charge on the lecithin which ordinarily would repel cations. (b) A change in configuration could occur with the enzyme part of the active site leading to additional opening of the membrane. Changes in structure have been reported when ACh combines with ChE (*205*, *206*). (c) Once the active site of the enzyme is freed of its lecithin attachment, it becomes activated, thus ensuring the hydrolysis of the particular ACh molecule with which it had reacted or of any other ACh molecules which might impinge upon this site. Alternatively, diffusion of ACh or other agonist away from the site would lead to a return to the resting state.

The reassociation phase is considered to be fairly slow, which could account for the phenomenon of receptor desensitization that occurs following prolonged application of agonists. This is clearly shown on isolated atria:

Adding successive amounts of ACh without washing the atria results in progressively diminishing effects.

What should be made clear is that this formulation postulates that the direct combination of ACh with an appropriate enzyme-receptor site is the primary step in triggering membrane depolarization. In the model suggested (Figure 1.9), dissociation of the lecithin-catalytic site is accompanied by hydrolysis of the interacting ACh molecule. Thus, both steps—initiation of the increase in membrane permeability as well as inactivation of the interacting ACh molecule—are considered to occur at one and the same site rather than in two stages, as is generally considered. It is true that ACh does react at nonreceptor hydrolytic sites, resulting in turnover to inactive products, but the latter reaction has now been shown to be insufficiently rapid to reduce the free concentration of ACh and in this way restore the receptor to its initial state by shifting the equilibrium. It is felt that the bulk of ACh liberated upon nerve stimulation rapidly diffuses from the postsynaptic membrane and that this diffusion constitutes one of the important means by which ACh concentration is reduced. Diffusion away from the receptor could not occur in an isolated organ, because the ACh would be at a constant concentration; in this case the ACh molecules would not remain associated with the receptor because of their basically low affinity (see below). It is, rather, the momentary contact of a few agonist molecules with the limited number of active sites (as described above) which begins the chain of events leading to an overt effect.

It is well known that a molecule of ChE contains many hydrolytic sites. At a given time only a fraction of such sites probably is involved in the receptor function described. Complexing with lecithin is visualized as a mobile equilibrium, so that a fraction of the sites may be complexed with lecithin and another fraction may be free at any given time. Impingement of ACh on a site that is momentarily free would result in a nonproductive effect, namely, hydrolysis. Moreover, only a small fraction of the total number of ChE molecules present in a given tissue may actually function as receptor; evidence for this will be presented in the discussion of the ChE inhibitors.

The type of ChE that may be involved in receptor function depends on the individual tissue. Those tissues most sensitive to ACh and methacholine would have true ChE participating as receptor; those responding best to butyrylcholine, such as frog rectus abdominus (*4*), would have the pseudoenzyme as part of the receptor apparatus. Since it is now apparent that many junctions contain both types of enzyme, one or the other may be in a reserve form in order to eliminate any ACh which may increase in concentration under unusual circumstances. It should be stressed, however, that our current concept does not attribute such a role to the enzyme under ordinary circumstances because, as indicated in Section 3.5, the rate of hydrolysis of free ACh is too low under physiological conditions.

In considering the finer details of the mechanism, it should be noted that agonist activity requires that the compound *not* remain associated with the active site. Agonist activity may be viewed as resulting from a hit-and-run type of reaction, in the sense implied in Paton's kinetic theory (*156, 157*). Obviously, the agonist must show some binding with the active site but, once the binding becomes too strong, inhibition rather than stimulation probably occurs. Agonist activity is thus viewed as being determined strictly in terms of "efficacy," which in turn is considered to be a reflection of the ability to dissociate the lecithin–enzyme complex. For example, ACh and other highly potent agonists show high complementarity for the active site, particularly for the enzyme surface part, and so are highly effective in dissociating the complex without necessarily being strongly bound. Quaternary ammonium compounds which are weak agonists are weakly bound and also lack complementarity with the enzyme surface. Once a molecule is strongly bound, the activity would change to that of an antagonist in the manner described below. At present, it is evidently impossible to state the magnitude of the affinity constants that characterize "strong" and "weak" binding to the receptor. In the absence of such knowledge the binding constants determined for the purified enzyme in solution, for lecithin, or for other macromolecules could give trends of affinities in series of compounds which might clarify structure–activity relationships in a qualitative way on the molecular level. However, it must be recognized that neither the enzyme nor lecithin in solution is entirely satisfactory, because the receptor site visualized in the model contains points for binding that are not present on either molecule alone. Cooperative binding between sites could greatly influence affinity, as could complexing of the active site on the enzyme with lecithin. It is felt that only by studying the interacting properties of the enzyme in situ can affinity constants be correctly correlated with potency. However, even this approach would entail considerable difficulties, if it is true that only a limited number of enzyme molecules are actually involved in receptor function. These are the molecules which may be considered to be situated in the "biophase," and their properties may well be different from those of the bulk of the enzyme. Somehow or other methods must be devised to distinguish these enzyme-receptors from extraneous enzyme.

Perhaps the greatest utility of any receptor hypothesis is its ability to account for structure–activity relationships among a number of different series of compounds. It is evident that with regard to the cholinergic system this would be virtually impossible, since there are too many different types of compound that have been examined in in vivo systems. For detailed discussions of the actions of many series of quaternary ammonium compounds from a physico-organic standpoint, the reader is referred to the extensive reviews by Cavallito and Gray (*222*) and Stenlake (*223*). As regards molecular mechanisms, unfortunately their analyses are based mainly on whole-animal experiments and, as such, involve many unknown factors superimposed upon receptor affinity. Among these are binding of drugs to plasma proteins (*224*), combination with serum ChE, reactions with sites other than the receptor as exist in presynaptic nerve terminals (*161–164*), biotransformation, and excretion. These factors would all combine to render knowledge of the concentration of an injected compound at the active site virtually impossible; they would change progressively as the members of a given series of compounds are altered chemically, but the extent of the changes would be extremely difficult, if not impossible, to assess.

From the standpoint of molecular pharmacology, it is clear that the isolated organ or tissue offers the greatest number of advantages, even though drug actions under these conditions are far from uncomplicated. Perhaps the finest collection of data along these lines has been compiled by Ariëns and his collaborators (*158*). Use of their approach in conjunction with drug reactions with tissue components and purified macromolecules can, it is felt, provide the type of information needed to gain insight into the molecular aspects of receptor reactions. Studies in which such correlative data have been acquired are the major source of material for the discussion that follows.

A. Detailed Mechanism of Action of Various Cholinergic Compounds

1. CHOLINE ESTERS AND OTHER MONOQUATERNARY AMMONIUM COMPOUNDS

ACh is the compound with the best fit for the active site on the enzyme and therefore is the most effective in dissociating the lecithin complex. Since the affinities of ACh for both true and pseudo ChE are quite similar, the ester clearly would be highly effective at all types of junction. As far as other esters are concerned (methacholine, butyrylcholine, etc.), their effectiveness depends on the type of enzyme functioning as receptor at a particular junction. This may be the true significance of the parallelism between the rates of hydrolysis of several esters and their abilities to stimulate various tissues, as shown by Wurzel (*3–6*); but this in itself may not always indicate the type of enzyme actually involved as receptor. For example, the predominant enzyme of intact atria is pseudo ChE, yet butyrylcholine is fairly inactive whereas methacholine is quite potent. Therefore the receptor-enzyme would be considered to be true ChE.

The lipid-insoluble simple monoquaternary compounds, such as tetramethylammonium, may actually react at two subsites of the active site: the phosphate group of the lecithin part and the anionic site of the enzyme. These simple molecules are essentially not strongly bound to either site, but the momentary attachment is sufficient to cause dissociation of the complex. Their effects would be terminated by diffusion from the active site.

The situation with regard to quaternary ammonium compounds in which more than one of the alkyl groups on the nitrogen are modified is very complex, because these compounds may be incomplete agonists or even competitive antagonists of ACh (*158*, *225*). According to the present formulation, the partial agonists of this group cannot fully dissociate the complex perhaps because they combine with only one of the two anionic sites, whereas a complete agonist, such as tetramethylammonium, reacts with both sites. The antagonists of this group, such as tetrabutylammonium, interact at the same site as the agonists but fail to cause dissociation of the receptor complex; rather, they stabilize the complex against the dissociating action of ACh or other agonists. Although the inhibiting potency of such compounds would be expected to increase as the size of the four alkyl groups is increased, the reverse appears to be the case as shown by Collier and Exley (*225*). This is explained in terms of charge delocalization; that is, as the size of the alkyl chain increases, its electron-releasing activity also increases, thereby diminishing the charge density around the quaternary nitrogen. However, as pointed out by Stenlake (*223*), there are certain obvious exceptions to this rule, and it is most likely that steric factors also play an important role in the reaction of these compounds with the anionic sites on the receptor. Although this may explain in a qualitative way the order of potency of this series of compounds, there has been no suggestion as to why such compounds are not agonists but rather antagonists of ACh. It is conceivable that, just as in the case of the trimethylammonium compounds, these derivatives also combine with both negative groups on the receptor site resulting in the formation of intramolecular hydrophobic bonds which stabilize the complex and thereby hinder the dissociating action of ACh (Figure 1.11). Although it might be expected that the larger the group the greater the tendency to form such bonds, the competing factors of charge delocalization and steric hindrance may outbalance the formation of hydrophobic bonds. Furthermore, some of these compounds may promote the release of ACh, a factor which could influence their apparent affinity for the receptor.

We shall now consider compounds of the tetramethylammonium type in which the length of a single alkyl substituent is increased progressively. Although alteration of chain length might appear to be the ideal way to study structure–activity relationships, many complexities arise particularly when the number of carbon atoms in the alkyl group is greater than eight. For example, in a whole-animal experiment cholinomimetic activity reaches

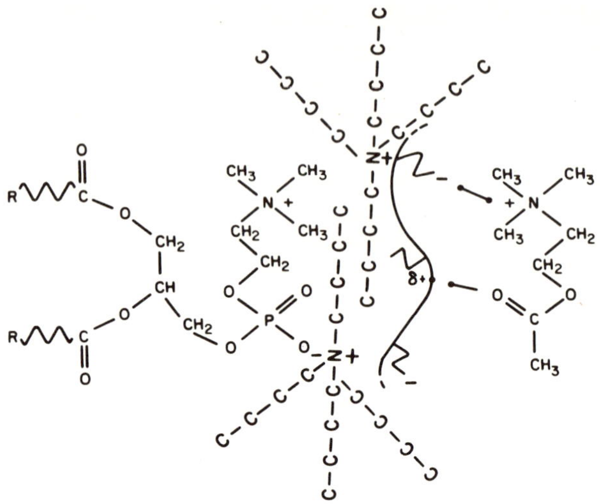

Fig. 1.11. Binding of tetrabutylammonium to a receptor site with intramolecular hydrophobic bonds stabilizing the protein-lecithin complex against dissociation by ACh.

a maximum in butyltrimethylammonium and decreased rapidly with increasing chain length (*227*), whereas in isolated preparations agonist activity increases progressively up to about the hexyl derivative (*158*, *227*, *229*). On the other hand, in some series there is a fairly rapid drop-off in activity with the butyl derivatives (*158*), even when an isolated tissue is used. Finally, as the chain length increases above about six carbon atoms, the type of activity invariably changes from agonist to antagonist (*158*).

It is fairly evident that with increasing chain length there is an increase in the ability to interact with many different types of macromolecules. The long-chain quaternary ammonium compounds* (see Figure 1.5) react strongly with acidic polysaccharides, nucleic acids, and a variety of proteins (*132*, *136*, *149*, *150*), whereas the parent compounds (ACh and 2-PAM) are both very weakly bound. When compounds in these series are injected into an animal, they progressively tend to combine with serum proteins as their chain lengths become longer. This may be the reason why diminishing potency at fairly short chain length is observed in whole animal experiments. However, it is still necessary to explain the reason for the change from agonist to antagonist, which occurs when the compounds are applied to isolated systems.

An increasing affinity with increasing chain length can be demonstrated with ChE (*6*) and lecithin (*133*). On this basis it is suggested that, as the carbon

* For example: *N*-(β-acetoxyethyl)-*N*,*N*-dimethyl-*N*-*n*-dodecylammonium; *N*,*N*-dimethyl-*N*-*n*-dodecyl-*N*-(β-hydroxyethyl)ammonium; and 2-PAD.

chain becomes longer, the affinity for the two anionic groups on the active site of the receptor increases. Interaction at these points results in stabilization of the active site against the dissociating action of ACh, because the larger alkyl chain has the tendency to become involved in many kinds of interaction: It could form cross-links between the phosphate group and the enzyme surface or between the anionic site and a fatty acid group on the lecithin, or intramolecular bonding between the chains of two molecules which are fixed simultaneously would be promoted (Figure 1.12). It is well known that with increasing alkyl chain length there is an increasing tendency to form micelles through association of hydrophobic groups. Simultaneous fixation to two adjacent sites would greatly facilitate such an association (Figure 1.12). The net effect of these kinds of interaction would be to stabilize the active site rather than promote its dissociation; that is, the compound would become an inhibitor rather than an agonist. However, at low concentrations these secondary interactions would be minimized, and hence the compound could act as an agonist. As the concentration increased, the reactions leading to stabilization would also increase, and the compound would inhibit the dissociation of the active-site complex. This partial agonist type of behavior has been observed with various members of different series of compounds, such as dioxolanes and unbranched alkyltrimethylammonium compounds (*158*).

As the alkyl chain increases above 9 or 10 carbons, the tendency to form hydrophobic bonds is so great that only the stabilization phase is observed, resulting in a pure anti-ACh action (*112, 158*). If the reactions were confined entirely to the active receptor site, then the compound would act as a competitive antagonist of ACh. However, owing to a wider spectrum of binding in conjunction with increasing lipid solubility these compounds could well react with macromolecules other than the receptor, such as those present in nerve endings, conducting membranes, and in the postsynaptic membrane;

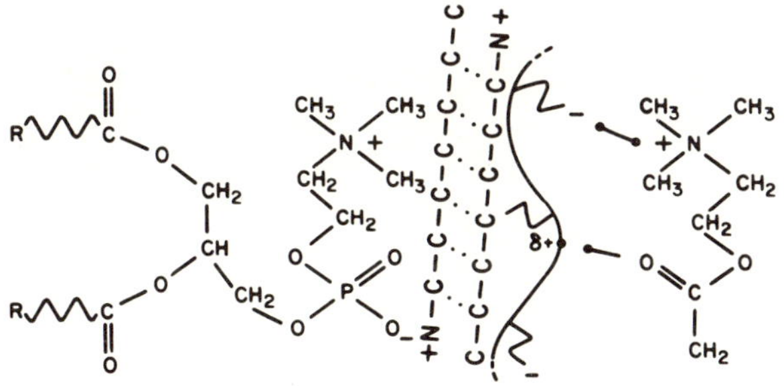

Fig. 1.12. Binding of heptyltrimethylammonium to a receptor site with intramolecular hydrophobic bonds stabilizing the protein-lecithin complex against dissociation by ACh.

these reactions might contribute to the anti-ACh action. The inhibitory effect would probably be mostly of the noncompetitive type, because ACh would not be able to displace the molecule from a site other than the receptor. This type of more or less nonspecific activity actually has been observed with long-chain (C_{12}) ammonium compounds on isolated aortic strip preparations (*112*). Not only are the compounds potent antagonists of ACh, but they also inhibit responses to norepinephrine, serotonin, histamine, and potassium chloride. The same compounds without the long chain are virtually inactive as inhibitors of contractions.

2. COMPETITIVE BLOCKING AGENTS: *d*-TUBOCURARINE AND GALLAMINE TRIETHIODIDE

d-Tubocurarine and TRIEG are visualized as combining exclusively by a two-point attachment, that is, as attaching simultaneously to the phosphate group of lecithin and to the protein anionic subsite (Figure 1.13), thereby creating a strong crosslinking of the lecithin–protein complex. Both compounds can react with lecithin (*133*), most likely by attaching to the phosphate group. *d*-Tubocurarine has been shown experimentally to combine with some macromolecules by a two-point attachment (*148*). Moreover, in the model the distance between the two anionic groups is probably close to 7 A, which would enable the active site to accommodate both charges on the *d*-tubocurarine molecule. This type of combination would produce complete stabilization of the receptor site and prevent ACh from causing dissociation. Since these compounds are highly lipid-insoluble, their effects would be confined exclusively to the junctional regions; the complications arising from presynaptic reactions would not be a factor in their competitive blocking of externally applied ACh.

Any compound that could combine with the phosphate group or the anionic site would cause a displacement of *d*-tubocurarine, because two-point attach-

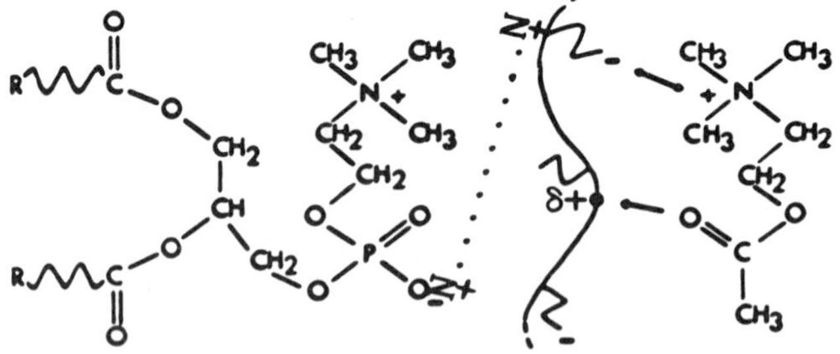

Fig. 1.13. Binding of curare or other diquaternary ammonium compounds to a receptor site. Crosslinking stabilizes the protein-lecithin complex against dissociation by ACh.

ment is required for its strong binding (*177*). This, then, may be why simple quaternary ammonium compounds are quite potent decurarizing agents.

3. DUAL-ACTING COMPOUNDS

Dual-acting compounds in general are fairly simple quaternary ammonium compounds and thus have an inherent ability to dissociate the receptor site and cause depolarization. Unlike *d*-tubocurarine, the decamethonium type of compound is weakly bound and so does not remain attached to the receptor site for long. However, as the concentration builds up due to the accumulation of C_{10} by the muscle, a two-point attachment might occur (Figure 1.13). This would have the effect of reassociating the active site, which could explain the change-over to a competitive type of blockade. In other words, once a two-point attachment occurred, repolarization could take place. It has been shown, in line with this concept, that *d*-tubocurarine can cause the repolarization of depolarized electroplax (*75*), although on this tissue decamethonium only causes depolarization.

On the basis of the picture of the receptor site structure–activity relationships among flexible bisquaternary ammonium compounds may be explained, particularly when it is considered that the active-site complex is in a somewhat mobile state and therefore can accommodate molecules of varying interquaternary distances; this flexibility had been proposed previously by Ehrenpreis (*132*) and Canepa (*230*). Bisquaternary compounds separated by small numbers of carbon atoms have difficulty in stretching between the two negative sites and hence are less potent in crosslinking the complex. As the number of carbons increases to ten, the optimal size for crosslinking is approached. Above ten carbon atoms the ability to react at both vicinal points diminishes, because a single receptor site is limited with respect to the distance by which the two negative sites may be distorted. In fact, with greatly increased interquaternary distances the fit would be poorer and the potency less; this is precisely what has been observed with many series of compounds (*231*).

A complication in the above mechanism is the fact that highly potent bisquaternary compounds are known in which the nitrogen atoms are separated by as many as twenty carbon atoms (*223*). In these instances, binding with negative groups occurs on two different receptor sites, not within a single site. The maximal distance between cationic groups in such a molecule is about 30 A; the length of a ChE molecule, which has a molecular weight of 250,000 (*232*), has not been determined but could be about 300 A.*

* This value was arrived at by comparing ChE with fibrinogen, both proteins being assumed to have a fairly elongated shape. It has been estimated that the length of the fibrinogen (molecular weight, 330,000) is about 475 A (*233*).

Assuming that there are ten uniformly distributed active sites per ChE molecule, the distance between adjacent sites would be about 30 A.

4. CHOLINESTERASE INHIBITORS

The compounds whose mechanism of action is the most difficult to analyze within the framework of the present hypothesis are, perhaps, the potent ChE inhibitors. Current concepts appear to explain their mode of action so convincingly as to discourage almost any alternative ones. Nevertheless, a number of important observations (some of which have been mentioned in Section 1.4) must be considered paradoxical if it is held that these compounds do not react with the receptor itself, in other words with that component which is directly concerned in events mediated by ACh and other agonists. A few of these findings will now be indicated.

(1) It is quite evident that the ChE inhibitors can have "direct" actions (*165*, *234*); i.e., they produce stimulation as a result of an interaction with the receptor rather than from inhibition of the enzyme as it is ordinarily understood. The interpretation usually given is that the receptor involved is not ChE, but this is considered to be somewhat unreasonable since these compounds would almost certainly combine selectively with the enzyme in preference to any other tissue component. An example of a direct action is the contraction of smooth muscle (e.g., of stomach) caused by physostigmine or neostigmine, which occurs very rapidly (within seconds) and without any evidence of build-up of endogenous ACh (*236*).

(2) The ChE inhibitors can potentiate nonhydrolyzable cholinotropic compounds (*235*).

(3) High concentrations of the inhibitors of ChE exert an anti-ACh effect (*70–73*), which has been attributed to reaction with the cholinergic receptor.

(4) The potentiation of ACh by inhibitors of ChE on isolated atria (*24*, *24a*), stomach smooth muscle (*236*), intestinal smooth muscle (*158*), and electroplax (*220*) requires scrutiny. As has been indicated, it is unlikely that at the concentrations used ACh is broken down by the enzyme of these tissues (except electroplax), and so there is no significant decrease in the bulk concentration of the ester. Yet, paradoxically, in each instance the ChE inhibitors strongly potentiate the ester. Further, this potentiation may occur when the extent of enzyme inhibition is extremely small or almost undetectable (*24*). Moreover, the potentiation may occur very rapidly, whereas the inhibition of ChE with physostigmine, neostigmine and, in particular, DFP is comparatively slow (*237*).

On the isolated electroplax physostigmine potentiates ACh 1000-fold (*220*), at a time when enzyme inhibition is only about 50% (*221*).

On the basis of this and much additional evidence, it is concluded that the generally accepted mechanism of action of the potent inhibitors of ChE, (particularly physostigmine and neostigmine) must be modified. The evidence suggests that potentiation of ACh does not entail inactivation of the bulk of the enzyme. Rather, these compounds appear to combine with the active site of the small fraction of ChE molecules that are involved in receptor function. This combination results in hydrolysis of the inhibitor (*211*, *218*) and subsequent occupancy of only part of the esteratic site, as previously discussed. Thus, it is considered that these kinds of ChE inhibitors "sensitize" the active receptor site: leaving a group on the site causes the lecithin–ChE complex to be placed in a more unstable, or partially dissociated, state, such that the subsequent interaction with ACh is magnified. Even non-hydrolyzed agonists would be potentiated. In some instances the ChE inhibitors produce so great an instability as to cause a direct action of their own as, for example, the rapid contraction of stomach smooth muscle.

It may be noted that the new concept is more in harmony with many important findings, including the degree of enzyme inhibition required for potentiation of ACh. According to Nachmansohn, who is strongly in favor of the nonidentity of enzyme and receptor, the amount of enzyme in a given tissue is far in excess of what is ordinarily needed to regulate ACh action, particularly in view of the presumed rapidity with which the enzyme inactivates ACh. Thus, he considers that the bulk of the enzyme, perhaps as much as 80% (*238*), must be inhibited if there is to be any effect on liberated ACh at various sites, such as at junctions of electroplax. In fact, he goes so far as to state that the depolarizing block of electroplax by neostigmine, occurring at an enzyme activity that is about 50% of initial, "must definitely be attributed to its action on the receptor rather than that on the enzyme" (*234*). Yet, as has been pointed out, marked potentiation of exogenously applied ACh may occur with even less inhibition of enzyme. This constitutes a direct contradiction of the current concepts of the function of ChE. In the case of electroplax it is undoubtedly true that at least part of the effect of physostigmine is the inhibition of nonreceptor enzyme, because the concentration of ACh required to depolarize the electroplax, 2×10^{-6} to 4×10^{-6} M (*220*), is high enough for the enzyme to hydrolyze the ester at a fairly rapid rate and thus reduce the concentration to below the threshold value.* This evidently is not the case when ACh acts at much lower concentrations, such as in atria, smooth muscle of the stomach, and intestinal smooth muscle.

There is little doubt that the major effects produced by the ChE inhibitors

* That this could not be the only factor in potentiation of ACh is indicated by the fact that the concentration of physostigmine used diminished the rate of hydrolysis of ACh by only 50% in studies with intact electroplax (*221*). This means that, at most, ACh should have been potentiated about 2-fold under these conditions. The fact that the potentiation was 1000-fold makes it apparent that inhibition of ChE could not be the primary factor.

are undoubtedly due to a reaction with tissue ChE. This conclusion derives from the fact that the duration of potentiation of ACh agrees qualitatively with the known duration of inhibition of ChE. On the atria, for example, the potentiating effects of neostigmine and physostigmine may last for 30 min. to an hour, whereas those of DFP are essentially irreversible. It must be stressed, however, that potentiation is now considered to be produced by reaction with only a limited number of enzyme-receptor molecules, since this effect may be unaccompanied by a significant inhibition of ChE.

In many instances the effectiveness of neostigmine in potentiating ACh is far greater than that of physostigmine (*24*, *216*), contrary to the relative potencies in inhibiting ChE in solution (*217*). This finding may be explained in one of the several following ways. The enzyme may have different properties, in terms of reactions with various compounds in situ, from those of the purified enzyme in solution; a number of such differences have been observed and are discussed by Barnard and Ostrowski (*16*). The enzyme may react faster with neostigmine than with physostigmine, resulting in a greater number of activated sites in a given period of time and a greater potentiation of ACh. Finally, the carbamoyl group that remains behind may influence the subsequent attachment of ACh in different ways: for some reason the dimethylcarbamate group of neostigmine might cause greater disruption of the complex than does the monomethylcarbamate of physostigmine.

The question arises why ACh should be far more strongly potentiated than other quaternary ammonium compounds. This is certainly true of isolated atria, in which ACh is potentiated about 8-fold, while carbamoylcholine is potentiated only about 2-fold by the same concentration of ChE inhibitor. The difference may be explained partly by the fact that the reaction of an ACh molecule at the active site is accompanied by hydrolysis, once the initial effect is achieved. However, this alone probably does not account for the profound degree of potentiation that sometimes occurs. For example, after the application of DFP (1 to 2 μg/ml) the threshold concentration for the effect of ACh on rabbit atria may be reduced several hundred times. Although the present proposed mechanism cannot fully account for this phenomenon, it cannot be explained simply on the basis of a reduction of enzyme activity in the usual sense, if for no other reason than that the ester is not hydrolyzed to a detectable extent while it is in the organ bath.

B. Some Limitations of the Proposed Mechanism

Among the facts that cannot be explained on the basis of the new proposal or, indeed, on any other basis are the following: the much greater sensitivity to ACh (by two or three orders of magnitude) of muscarinic receptors than of nicotinic receptors, the great potency of atropine and related compounds at muscarinic sites* and the ineffectuality of *d*-tubocurarine at such sites and the very weak action of certain bisquaternary ammonium compounds, such as hexamethonium, at muscarinic sites as compared with their great potency at cholinergic sites in ganglia.

The affinities of compounds to the particular ChE of the tissue upon which they act may answer some of the questions raised by these facts. Because the makeup of the "biophase" in which the enzyme-receptor is located may differ greatly from tissue to tissue, drug reactivities may be altered in a more or less unpredictable way. Use of tissue enzyme in situ will, perhaps, help to elucidate some of these factors.

I.7. SUMMARY

It is apparent from the preceding discussion that much progress has been made toward a greater understanding of cholinergic mechanisms at the molecular level. Some of the most important new results have been obtained through such sophisticated techniques as the electrophoretic jet, autoradiography, histochemistry with electron microscopy, together with methods for extracting and isolating in purified form physiologically active macromolecules. The advances made have strengthened the argument that ACh is the transmitter of information at most junctions; this is fundamental to formulating any molecular mechanism of action of cholinergic compounds. But it is now evident that neurohumoral theory as first enunciated grossly oversimplifies the facts, since ACh and other cholinergic compounds may have prominent actions at sites other than in the postsynaptic membrane, such as those in nerve terminals and in conducting membranes of nerve and muscle. These ancillary actions may at times be so pronounced as to suggest the presence of a functional cholinergic system within conducting membranes, although the evidence appears to be very much against such a hypothesis. It is possible that membrane components with which cholinergic drugs combine (the acceptors) can be isolated from nerve tissue; in vitro studies of the reactions between drugs and such components could afford insight into the molecular basis of bioelectric phenomena. All attempts at isolating the cholinergic receptor substance as a unique drug-binding tissue component have ended in failure.

Arguments favoring ChE as the cholinergic receptor continue to mount although, as stressed in this article, it may not be valid to use the purified enzyme for determining the binding of cholinergic compounds and comparing the results with their in vivo potency. Perhaps the most satisfactory approach is to study the interacting properties of the enzyme in situ and correlate such data with some physiological response of the tissue. When this is done many seemingly established properties of the enzyme may require revision: the rate

* But see footnote, p. 34.

at which it hydrolyzes ACh, the rate of reaction with inhibitors, the potency of inhibitors, etc. On the basis of such studies and the findings of other workers it is concluded herein that the primary function of tissue ChE may not be to limit ACh action in the usual sense. It has become evident that the enzyme may have some other function in the postsynaptic membrane; ChE is now considered to act as part of the receptor for ACh and other cholinergic compounds. Our picture of a hypothetical receptor site suggests how the reaction of ACh can produce depolarization and may be used as a basis for understanding the possible mechanism of action of some select cholinergic stimulants and blocking agents on the molecular level. Certainly, the model falls short of explaining all but a few aspects of receptor reactions and may well require revision as additional data are obtained. However, regardless of the precise manner in which it occurs, undoubtedly the evidence does seem to suggest that ChE could participate directly in the actions of cholinergic agonists and antagonists. If this is correct, there is eliminated the need of postulating a side-by-side existence of two distinctly different macromolecular entities, receptor and enzyme, which must be very closely related to each other with regard to their reaction with cholinergic compounds.

REFERENCES

1. A. O. Župančič, *Acta Physiol. Scand.*, **29**, 64 (1953).
2. A. O. Župančič, *Biochim. Biophys. Acta*, **81**, 411 (1964).
3. M. Wurzel, *Experientia*, **15**, 430 (1959).
4. M. Wurzel and N. Sapeika, *S. African J. Lab. Clin. Med.*, **4**, 229 (1958).
5. M. Wurzel, *Bull. Res. Council Israel*, **A9**, 5 (1960).
6. B. Belleau, *J. Med. Chem.*, **7**, 776 (1964).
7. J. Del Castillo and B. Katz, *J. Physiol.* (*London*), **128**, 157 (1955).
8. J. Del Castillo and B. Katz, *Proc. Roy. Soc.* (*London*), **B146**, 339, 362 (1957).
9. S. Ehrenpreis, unpublished results.
10. M. A. Gerebtzoff, *Cholinesterases*, Pergamon, London, 1959.
G. B. Koelle and J. S. Friedenwald, *Proc. Soc. Exptl. Biol. Med.*, **70**, 617 (1949).
G. M. Lehrer and L. Ornstein, *J. Biophys. Biochem. Cytol.*, **6**, 399 (1959).
11. R. J. Barrnett, *J. Cell. Biol.*, **12**, 247 (1962).
12. G. Rodriguez de Lores Arnaiz and E. D. P. De Robertis, *J. Neurochem.*, **9**, 503 (1962).
13. E. D. P. De Robertis, G. Rodriguez de Lores Arnaiz, L. Salganicoff, A. Pellegrino de Iraldi, and L. M. Zieher, *J. Neurochem.*, **10**, 225 (1963).
14. V. P. Whittaker, I. A. Michaelson, and R. J. Kirkland, *Biochem. J.*, **90**, 293 (1964).
15. K. Ostrowski and E. A. Barnard, *Exptl. Cell Res.*, **25**, 465 (1961).
16. E. A. Barnard and K. Ostrowski, *Exptl. Cell Res.*, **36**, 28 (1964).
17. D. Nachmansohn, *Chemical and Molecular Basis of Nerve Activity*, Academic Press, New York, 1959.
18. G. B. Koelle, *Nature*, **190**, 208 (1961).
19. F. A. Denz, *Brit. J. Exptl. Pathol.*, **34**, 329 (1953).
20. A. Silver, *J. Physiol.*, **169**, 386 (1963).
21. B. Klinar and A. O. Župančič, *Arch. Intern. Pharmacodyn.*, **136**, 47 (1962).

22. H. C. Lawler, *Biochim. Biophys. Acta*, **81**, 280 (1964).
23. S. Ehrenpreis, H. R. Munson, Jr., M. Bigo-Gullino, and M. A. Avery, *Life Sciences*, **3**, 809 (1965).
24. S. Ehrenpreis, D. MacFarlane, and M. Platthy-Lang, *Federation Proc.*, **24**, 610 (1965).
24a. S. Ehrenpreis, M. Platthy-Lang, and M. Bigo-Gullino, *Pharmacologist*, **7**, 138 (1965).
25. S. Ehrenpreis and M. Platthy-Lang, unpublished experiments.
26. D. Nachmansohn, *Chemical and Molecular Basis of Nerve Activity*, Academic Press, New York, 1959, pp. 37–38.
27. A. Rothenberg and D. Nachmansohn, *J. Biol. Chem.*, **168**, 223 (1947).
28. M. Dixon and E. C. Webb, *The Enzymes*, Academic Press, New York, 1958, pp. 15–18.
29. H. C. Lawler, *J. Biol. Chem.*, **236**, 2296 (1961).
30. H. O. Michel and S. Krop, *J. Biol. Chem.*, **190**, 119 (1951).
31. I. B. Wilson and M. A. Harrison, *J. Biol. Chem.*, **236**, 2292 (1961).
32. R. M. Krupka, *Can. J. Biochem. Physiol.*, **42**, 677 (1964).
33. K.-B. Augustinsson, *Acta Physiol. Scand.*, **15**, 1 (1948).
34. D. Nachmansohn, *Chemical and Molecular Basis of Nerve Activity*, Academic Press, New York, 1959, Chap. 3.
35. J. Jensen-Holm, *Acta Pharmacol. Toxicol.*, **18**, 379 (1961).
36. M. Dzoljic, *Arch. Intern. Pharmacodyn.*, **151**, 352 (1964).
37. G. H. Acheson, *Federation Proc.*, **7**, 447 (1948).
38. N. G. Emmelin and F. G. MacIntosh, *Acta Physiol. Scand. Suppl.*, **53**, 17 (1948); *J. Physiol.*, **131**, 447 (1956).
39. P. G. Waser, *J. Pharm. Pharmacol.*, **12**, 677 (1960).
40. E. D. P. De Robertis and H. S. Bennett, *J. Biophys. Biochem. Cytol.*, **1**, 47 (1955); E. D. P. De Robertis, *Exptl. Cell Res. Suppl.*, **5**, 347 (1958).
41. S. L. Palay, *J. Biophys. Biochem. Cytol.*, **2**, 193 (1956).
42. R. W. Ryall, *J. Neurochem.*, **11**, 131 (1964).
43. R. M. Burton, R. E. Howard, S. Baer, and Y. M. Balfour, *Biochim. Biophys. Acta*, **84**, 441 (1964).
44. R. M. Burton, *Intern. J. Neuropharmacol.*, **3**, 13 (1964).
45. G. A. Horrideg, D. M. Chapman, and B. MacKay, *Nature*, **193**, 899 (1962).
46. F. G. Canepa, *Nature*, **201**, 184 (1964).
47. K. Krnjevic and R. Miledi, *Nature*, **182**, 805 (1958).
48. J. I. Hubbard and W. D. Willis, *Nature*, **193**, 1294 (1962).
49. J. I. Hubbard and W. D. Willis, *Nature*, **193**, 174 (1962).
50. E. D. P. De Robertis, L. Salganicoff, L. M. Zieher, and G. Rodriguez de Lores Arnaiz, *Science*, **140**, 300 (1963).
51. V. P. Whittaker, I. A. Michealson, and R. J. Kirkland, *Biochem. Pharmacol.*, **12**, 301 (1963).
52. C. O. Hebb and A. Silver, *Nature*, **189**, 123 (1961).
53. R. Birks, B. Katz, and R. Miledi, *J. Physiol. (London)*, **150**, 145 (1960).
54. D. Nachmansohn, *Chemical and Molecular Basis of Nerve Activity*, Academic Press, New York, 1959, p. 18.
55. D. Nachmansohn, *Chemical and Molecular Basis of Nerve Activity*, Academic Press, New York, 1959, Chap. 6.
56. P. Karlson, *Introduction to Modern Biochemistry*, Academic Press, New York, 1963, p. 393.
57. S. Ehrenpreis, *Nature*, **201**, 887 (1964).
58. T. H. Bullock, H. Grundfest, D. Nachmansohn, and M. A. Rothenberg, *J. Neurophysiol.*, **10**, 11, 63 (1947).

59. D. Nachmansohn, *Chemical and Molecular Basis of Nerve Activity*, Academic Press, New York, pp. 55–60.
60. J. E. P. Toman, J. W. Woodbury, and L. A. Woodbury, *J. Neurophysiol.*, **10**, 429 (1947).
61. E. R. Whitcomb, S. L. Friess, and J. S. Moore, *J. Cellular Comp. Physiol.*, **52**, 275 (1958).
62. C. J. Armett and J. M. Ritchie, *J. Physiol.* (*London*), **152**, 141 (1960).
63. C. J. Armett and J. M. Ritchie, *J. Physiol.* (*London*), **155**, 372 (1961).
64. T. H. Bullock, D. Nachmansohn, and M. A. Rothenberg, *J. Neurophysiol.*, **9**, 9 (1946).
65. W.-D. Dettbarn and F. A. Davis, *Biochim. Biophys. Acta*, **66**, 397 (1963).
66. W.-D. Dettbarn, P. Rosenberg, and D. Nachmansohn, *Life Sciences*, **3**, 55 (1964).
67. E. Schoffeniels and D. Nachmansohn, *Biochim. Biophys. Acta*, **26**, 1 (1957).
68. D. Nachmansohn, *Chemical and Molecular Basis of Nerve Activity*, Academic Press, New York, 1959, p. 152.
69. M. Altamirano, C. W. Coates, H. Grundfest, and D. Nachmansohn, *Biochim. Biophys. Acta*, **16**, 449 (1955).
70. J. C. Eccles and M. V. MacFarlane, *J. Neurophysiol.*, **12**, 59 (1949).
71. M. Kimura, *Chem. Pharm. Bull.* (*Tokyo*), **11**, 40 (1963).
72. M. Kimura, T. Igarashi, and S. Iwashita, *Chem. Pharm. Bull.* (*Tokyo*), **11**, 51 (1963).
73. M. Kimura, *Chem. Pharm. Bull.* (*Tokyo*), **12**, 150 (1964).
74. P. Rosenberg and T. R. Podleski, *Biochim. Biophys. Acta*, **75**, 104 (1963).
75. H. B. Higman and E. Bartels, *Biochim. Biophys. Acta*, **54**, 543 (1962).
76. W.-D. Dettbarn, *Biochim. Biophys. Acta*, **32**, 381 (1959).
77. D. Nachmansohn, *Chemical and Molecular Basis of Nerve Activity*, Academic Press, New York, 1959, p. 167.
78. D. Nachmansohn, *Chemical and Molecular Basis of Nerve Activity*, Academic Press, New York, 1959, pp. 64–65.
79. M. A. Rothenberg, D. B. Sprinson, and D. Nachmansohn, *J. Neurophysiol.*, **11**, 111 (1948).
80. D. Nachmansohn, *Chemical and Molecular Basis of Nerve Activity*, Academic Press, New York, 1959, p. 183.
81. H. Grundfest, D. Nachmansohn, C. Y. Kao, and R. Chambers, *Nature*, **169**, 190 (1952).
82. A. L. Hodgkin and R. D. Keynes, *J. Physiol.* (*London*), **131**, 592 (1956).
83. C. S. Spyropoulos, discussion of paper by D. Nachmansohn, *Proc. 4th Intern. Cong. Biochem. Vienna 1958*, **3**, 26 (1959).
84. R. O. Brady, C. S. Spyropoulos, and I. Tasaki, *Am. J. Physiol.*, **194**, 207 (1958).
85. D. Nachmansohn, *Chemical and Molecular Basis of Nerve Activity*, Academic Press, New York, 1959, p. 65.
86. W.-D. Dettbarn, *Biochim. Biophys. Acta*, **41**, 377 (1960).
87. P. Rosenberg and S. Ehrenpreis, *Biochem. Pharmacol.*, **8**, 192 (1961).
88. D. Nachmansohn, *Chemical and Molecular Basis of Nerve Activity*, Academic Press, New York, 1959, p. 63.
89. I. B. Wilson and M. Cohen, *Biochim. Biophys. Acta*, **11**, 147 (1953).
90. T. R. Podleski and E. Bartels, *Biochim. Biophys. Acta*, **75**, 387 (1963).
91. M. N. Jindal and V. R. Deshpande, *Arch. Intern. Pharmacodyn.*, **130**, 322 (1961).
92. M. D. MacFarlane and T. Koppanyi, *Federation Proc.*, **24**, 710 (1965).
93. R. R. Walsh and S. E. Deal, *Am. J. Physiol.*, **197**, 547 (1959).
94. G. D. Webb and R. R. Walsh, *Federation Proc.*, **20**, 346 (1961).
95. R. R. Walsh and J. P. R. Lee, *Am. J. Physiol.*, **202**, 1241 (1962).
96. P. Rosenberg and S. Ehrenpreis, *Nature*, **190**, 728 (1961).
97. W. B. Cannon and A. Rosenblueth, *Supersensitivity of Denervated Structures*, Macmillan, New York, 1949.

98. S. Thesleff, *Physiol. Rev.*, **40**, 734 (1960).
99. L. Hinterbuchner and D. Nachmansohn, *Biochim. Biophys. Acta*, **44**, 554 (1960).
99a. A. D. Bergner and P. F. Wagley, *Proc. Soc. Exptl. Biol. Med.*, **97**, 90 (1958).
100. D. K. Myers and A. Kemp, *Nature*, **173**, 33 (1954).
101. K.-B. Augustinsson, T. Fredriksson, A. Sundwall, and G. Jonsson, *Biochem. Pharmacol.*, **3**, 68 (1959).
102. I. B. Wilson, in *Ciba Found. Symp. Enzymes Drug Action*, **1962**, p. 4.
103. W.-D. Dettbarn and P. Rosenberg, *Biochem. Pharmacol.*, **11**, 1025 (1962).
104. L. Lubinska, S. Niemierko, B. Oderfeld, and L. Szwarc, *J. Neurochem.*, **10**, 25 (1963).
105. J. Bernsohn, K. D. Barron, and A. R. Hess, *Nature*, **195**, 285 (1962).
106. E. Schoffeniels, I. B. Wilson, and D. Nachmansohn, *Biochim. Biophys. Acta*, **27**, 629 (1958).
107. P. Rosenberg and H. Higman, *Biochim. Biophys. Acta*, **45**, 348 (1960).
108. W.-D. Dettbarn, I. B. Wilson, and D. Nachmansohn, *Science*, **128**, 1275 (1958).
109. W.-D. Dettbarn, *Nature*, **186**, 891 (1960).
110. L. P. Hinterbuchner and I. B. Wilson, *Biochim. Biophys. Acta*, **32**, 375 (1959).
111. D. Nachmansohn, *Chemical and Molecular Basis of Nerve Activity*, Academic Press, New York, 1959, p. 166.
112. S. Ehrenpreis, M. Bigo-Gullino, and M. A. Avery, *Federation Proc.*, **23**, 383 (1964); *Arch. Intern. Pharmacodyn.*, **156**, 1, (1965).
113. D. Nachmansohn, *Chemical and Molecular Basis of Nerve Activity*, Academic Press, New York, 1959, Chap. 14.
114. R. Mitchell, A. P. Truant, and B. B. Clark, *Proc. Soc. Exptl. Biol. Med.*, **81**, 5 (1952).
115. B. B. Clark, in Conference on Neuromuscular Blocking Action of Anticholinesterase Compounds, Army Chemical Center, Edgewood, Md., 1952, p. 22.
116. P. Rosenberg and W.-D. Dettbarn, *Biochem. Pharmacol.*, **13**, 1157 (1964).
117. W.-D. Dettbarn, *Life Sci.*, **2**, 910 (1963).
118. W.-D. Dettbarn, *Nature*, **186**, 891 (1960).
119. W.-D. Dettbarn, personal communication.
120. F. E. Bloom, personal communication.
121. W.-D. Dettbarn, in *Bioelectrogenesis* (C. Chagas and A. P. de Carvalho, eds.), Elsevier, Amsterdam, 1961, p. 262.
122. E. R. Whitcomb and S. L. Friess, *Arch. Biochem. Biophys.*, **90**, 260 (1960).
123. F. E. Bloom and G. M. Schoepfle, *Am. J. Physiol.*, **204**, 73 (1963).
124. D. Nachmansohn, *Chemical and Molecular Basis of Nerve Activity*, Academic Press, New York, 1959, p. 168.
125. P. Mueller, *J. Gen. Physiol.*, **42**, 163 (1958).
126. A. M. Shanes, *J. Pharmacol. Exptl. Therap.*, **105**, 216 (1952).
127. F. A. Davis and W.-D. Dettbarn, *Biochim. Biophys. Acta*, **63**, 349 (1962).
128. A. Sandow and G. Kiebel, *Am. J. Physiol.*, **169**, 649 (1952).
129. M. G. Larrabee, J. D. Klingman, and W. S. Leicht, *J. Neurochem.*, **10**, 549 (1963.)
130. K. E. Neet and S. L. Friess, *Arch. Biochem. Biophys.*, *99*, 484 (1962).
131. S. Ehrenpreis, M. Platthy-Lang, and H. R. Munson, Jr., *Pharmacologist*, **5**, 254 (1963).
132. S. Ehrenpreis, *Biochim. Biophys. Acta*, **44**, 561 (1960).
133. S. Ehrenpreis, M. Platthy-Lang, and P. Patrick, unpublished work.
134. S. Ehrenpreis, *Intern. J. Neuropharm.*, **1**, 273 (1962).
135. S. Ehrenpreis, J. R. Munson, Jr., M. Bigo-Gullino, and H. L. Cooper, *Federation Proc.*, **22**, 215 (1963).
136. S. Ehrenpreis, *Proc. 1st Intern. Pharm. Meet. Stockholm*, **7**, 119 (1963).

136a. S. Ehrenpreis, in *Conference on Physical and Mathematical Approaches to the Study of the Electrical Behaviour of Excitable Membranes*, Woods Hole, Mass., July 1965; *J. Cell. Comp. Biol.*, **66**, 159, (1965).
137. E. Koenig and G. B. Koelle, *J. Neurochem.*, **8**, 169 (1961).
138. J. W. Clitherow, M. Mitchard, and N. J. Harper, *Nature*, **199**, 1000 (1963).
139. R. Miledi, *J. Physiol.* (*London*), **151**, 24 (1960).
140. J. Axelsson and S. Thesleff, *J. Physiol.* (*London*), **147**, 178 (1959).
141. S. Kuffler, *J. Neurophysiol.*, **6**, 99 (1943).
142. R. Miledi, in *Ciba Found. Symp. Enzymes Drug Action*, **1962**, p. 220.
143. W. C. Bowman and C. Raper, *Nature*, **201**, 160 (1964).
144. P. G. Waser, *J. Pharm. Pharmacol.*, **12**, 577 (1960).
145. P. G. Waser, in *Bioelectrogenesis* (C. Chagas and A. P. de Carvalho, eds.), Elsevier, Amsterdam, 1961, p. 353.
146. P. G. Waser, in *Ciba Found. Symp. Enzymes Drug Action*, **1962**, p. 206.
147. P. G. Waser, *Proc. 1st Intern. Pharm. Meet. Stockholm*, **7**, 101 (1963).
148. S. Ehrenpreis and M. M. Fishman, *Biochim. Biophys. Acta*, **44**, 576 (1960).
149. S. Ehrenpreis, 138th Meeting Am. Chem. Soc., New York, 1960, p. 15T.
150. S. Ehrenpreis, *Georgetown Med. Bull.*, **16**, 148 (1963).
151. S. Ehrenpreis, H. R. Munson, Jr., M. Bigo-Gullino, and H. L. Cooper, *Federation Proc.*, **22**, 215 (1963).
152. D. B. Taylor, *Anesthesiology*, **20**, 439 (1959).
153. R. Creese, D. B. Taylor, and B. Tilton, *J. Pharmacol. Exptl. Therap.*, **139**, 8 (1963).
154. W. L. Nastuk, *Ann. N.Y. Acad. Sci.*, **81**, 317 (1959).
155. W. D. M. Paton and E. J. Zaimis, *Pharmacol. Rev.*, **4**, 219 (1952).
156. W. D. M. Paton, *Proc. Roy. Soc.* (*London*), **B154**, 21 (1961).
157. W. D. M. Paton, in *Pharmacology of Smooth Muscle* (E. Buelbring, ed.), Macmillan, New York, 1964.
158. E. J. Ariëns, A. M. Simonis, and J. M. van Rossum, in *Molecular Pharmacology* (E. J. Ariëns, ed.), Vol. 1, Academic Press, New York, 1964, pp. 119ff., 287ff.
159. A. Hasson and L. L. Liepin, *Biochim. Biophys. Acta*, **75**, 397 (1963).
160. B. Witkop, R. C. Durant, and S. L. Friess, *Experientia*, **15**, 300 (1959).
161. W. F. Riker, Jr., J. Roberts, F. G. Standaert, and H. Fujimori, *J. Pharmacol. Exptl. Therap.*, **121**, 286 (1957).
162. W. F. Riker, Jr., G. Werner, J. Roberts, and A. Kuperman, *J. Pharmacol. Exptl. Therap.*, **125**, 150 (1959).
163. W. F. Riker, Jr., G. Werner, J. Roberts, and A. Kuperman, *Ann. N.Y. Acad. Sci.*, **81**, 328 (1959).
164. F. G. Standaert, *J. Pharmacol. Exptl. Therap.*, **143**, 181 (1964).
165. W. F. Riker, Jr., *Pharmacol. Rev.*, **5**, 1 (1953).
166. R. S. Masland and R. S. Wigton, *J. Neurophysiol.*, **3**, 269 (1940).
167. W. D. M. Paton and H. P. Rang, *Proc. Roy. Soc.* (*London*), **B163**, 1 (1965).
168. S. I. Oroszlan and G. D. Maengwyn-Davies, *Biochem. Pharmacol.*, **11**, 1213 (1962).
168a. S. Ehrenpreis and M. Bigo-Gullino, *Federation Proc.*, **25**, 472 (1966).
168b. P. B. Marshall, *Brit. J. Pharmacol.*, **10**, 354 (1955).
168c. S. Ehrenpreis, in *Cholinergic Mechanisms*, *Ann. N.Y. Acad. Sci.*, 1967, in press.
168d. E. J. Ariëns in *Cholinergic Mechanisms*, *Ann. N.Y. Acad. Sci.*, 1967, in press.
169. F. W. Schueler, *Chemobiodynamics and Drug Design*, McGraw-Hill, New York, 1960, p. 139.
170. D. W. Woolley, *Proc. Natl. Acad. Sci. U.S.*, **44**, 1201 (1958).

171. C. Chagas, E. Penna-Franca, K. Nishie, C. Crocker, and M. Miranda, *Compt. rend.*, **242**, 2671 (1956).
172. C. Chagas, E. Penna-Franca, K. Nishie, and E. J. Garcia, *Arch. Biochem. Biophys.*, **75**, 251 (1958).
173. A. Hasson and C. Chagas, *Biochim. Biophys. Acta*, **36**, 301 (1959).
174. C. Chagas, *Ann. N.Y. Acad. Sci.*, **81**, 345 (1959).
175. C. Chagas, in *Bioelectrogenesis* (C. Chagas and A. P. de Carvalho, eds.), Elsevier, Amsterdam, 1961, p. 341.
176. A. Hasson and C. Chagas, in *Bioelectrogenesis* (C. Chagas and A. P. de Carvalho, eds.), Elsevier, Amsterdam, 1961, p. 362.
177. S. Ehrenpreis and M. G. Kellock, *Biochim. Biophys. Acta*, **45**, 525 (1960).
178. S. Loewe and S. C. Harvey, *Arch. Exptl. Pathol. Pharmakol.*, **214**, 214 (1952).
179. C. J. Cavallito, A. P. Gray, and T. B. O'Dell, *Arch. Intern. Pharmacodyn.*, **101**, 38 (1955).
180. A. P. Gray, W. L. Archer, E. E. Spinner, and C. J. Cavallito, *J. Am. Chem. Soc.*, **79**, 3805 (1957).
181. T. B. O'Dell and M. D. Napoli, *J. Pharmacol. Exptl. Therap.*, **120**, 438 (1957).
182. E. W. Gill, *Proc. Roy. Soc.* (*London*), **B150**, 381 (1959).
183. S. Ehrenpreis and H. R. Munson, Jr., *Intern. J. Neuropharm.*, submitted.
184. J. P. Quilliam and D. B. Taylor, *Nature*, **160**, 603 (1947).
185. T. P. Feng, *Chinese J. Physiol.* **13**, 119 (1938).
186. W. Kalow, *J. Pharmacol. Exptl. Therap.*, **110**, 433 (1954).
187. D. H. Jenkinson, *J. Physiol.* (*London*), **152**, 309 (1960).
188. S. Ehrenpreis, *Nature*, **194**, 586 (1962).
189. S. Ehrenpreis, in *Ultrastructure and Metabolism of Nervous System*, *Res. Pub. ARNMD*, **40**, 368 (1962).
190. S. Ehrenpreis, in *Bioelectrogenesis* (C. Chagas and A. P. de Carvalho, eds.), Elsevier, Amsterdam, 1961, p. 379.
191. E. Trams, R. L. Irwin, C. J. Lauter, and M. M. Hein, *Biochim. Biophys. Acta*, **58**, 602 (1962).
192. E. G. Trams, *Biochim. Biophys. Acta*, **79**, 521 (1964).
193. D. W. Woolley, *Federation Proc.*, **18**, 461 (1959).
194. D. W. Woolley and N. K. Campbell, *Biochim. Biophys. Acta*, **40**, 543 (1960).
195. R. S. Dombra, L. S. Bradham, N. K. Campbell, and D. W. Woolley, *Biochim. Biophys. Acta*, **54**, 516 (1961).
196. D. W. Woolley and N. K. Campbell, *Biochim. Biophys. Acta*, **57**, 384 (1962).
197. D. W. Woolley, in *The Transfer of Calcium and Strontium Across Biological Membranes*, (R. H. Wasserman, ed.), Academic Press, New York, 1963, p. 375.
198. W. Vogt, *Z. Physiol. Chem.*, **331**, 239 (1963).
199. C. P. Bianchi and A. M. Shanes, *J. Gen. Physiol.*, **42**, 803 (1959).
200. D. Grob, T. Namba, N. A. Solomon, and D. S. Feldman, *J. Clin. Invest.*, **41**, 1363 (1962).
201. D. Grob and T. Namba, *Federation Proc.*, **22**, 215 (1963).
202. D. Grob, H. Himei, and T. Namba, *J. Clin. Invest.*, **43**, 1273 (1964).
203. T. Namba and D. Grob, in *Cholinergic Mechanisms*, *Ann. N.Y. Acad. Sci.*, 1967, in press.
204. D. Grob and T. Namba, *Federation Proc.*, **23**, 310 (1964).
205. I. B. Wilson and E. Cabib, *J. Am. Chem. Soc.*, **78**, 202 (1956).
206. L. A. Mounter, *Enzymologia*, **21**, 5 (1959).
207. I. B. Wilson, *J. Biol. Chem.*, **197**, 215 (1952).
208. A. H. Beckett, N. J. Harper, and J. W. Clitherow, *J. Pharm. Pharmacol.*, **15**, 362 (1963).

209. A. Inouye and Y. Shinagawa, *Bull. Chem. Soc. Japan*, **35**, 701 (1962).
210. L. A. Mounter and R. M. Cheatham, *Enzymologia*, **25**, 215 (1963).
211. I. B. Wilson, in *Ciba Found. Symp. Enzymes Drug Action*, **1962**, p. 408.
212. H. O. Schild, *Ciba Found. Symp. Enzymes Drug Action*, **1962**, p. 437.
213. T. Koppanyi and A. G. Karczmar, *J. Pharmacol. Exptl. Therap.*, **101**, 327 (1951).
214. T. Koppanyi, A. G. Karczmar, and G. C. Sheatz, *J. Pharmacol. Exptl. Therap.*, **107**, 482 (1953).
215. A. G. Karczmar, K. C. Kim, and K. Koketsu, *J. Pharmacol. Exptl. Therap.*, **134**, 199 (1961).
216. E. Xavier and J. R. Valle, *Acta Physiol. Latoam.*, **13**, 282 (1963).
217. D. Nachmansohn, *Chemical and Molecular Basis of Nerve Activity*, Academic Press, New York, 1959, pp. 47–49.
218. P. T. Nowell, C. A. Scott, and A. Wilson, *Brit. J. Pharmacol.*, **19**, 498 (1962).
219. I. B. Wilson, Chapter 7, this volume.
220. P. Rosenberg, H. Higman, and D. Nachmansohn, *Biochim. Biophys. Acta*, **44**, 151 (1960).
221. P. Rosenberg and W.-D. Dettbarn, *Biochim. Biophys. Acta*, **69**, 103 (1963).
221a. J. C. Watkins, *J. Theoret. Biol.*, **9**, 37 (1965).
222. C. J. Cavallito and A. P. Gray, *Progr. Drug Res.*, **2**, 135 (1960).
223. J. B. Stenlake, *Progr. Med. Chem.*, **3**, 1 (1963).
224. A. Goldstein, *Pharmacol. Rev.*, **1**, 102 (1949).
225. B. Collier and K. A. Exley, *J. Pharm. Pharmacol.*, **15**, 131T (1963).
226. K. Koketsu, *Am. J. Physiol.*, **193**, 213 (1958).
227. M. J. Dallemagne and E. Philipott, *Arch. Intern. Pharmacodyn.*, **87**, 127 (1951).
228. J. Thomas and G. A. Starmer, *J. Pharm. Pharmacol.*, **13**, 752 (1961).
229. F. M. Carey, D. Edwards, J. J. Lewis, and J. B. Stenlake, *J. Pharm. Pharmacol.*, **11**, 70T (1959).
230. F. G. Canepa, *Nature*, **195**, 573 (1962).
231. D. Bovet, in *Curare and Curare-Like Agents* (D. Bovet, F. Bovet-Nitti, and G. B. Marini-Battolo, eds.), Elsevier, Amsterdam, 1959, p. 230.
232. L. T. Kremzner, *Federation Proc.*, **23**, 177 (1964).
233. C. E. Hall and H. S. Slayter, *J. Biophys. Biochem. Cytol.*, **5**, 11 (1959).
234. D. Nachmansohn, *Chemical and Molecular Basis of Nerve Activity*, Academic Press, New York, 1959, p. 147.
235. B. Holmstedt, *Pharmacol. Rev.*, **11**, 567 (1959).
236. S. Ehrenpreis and J. Fleisch, unpublished experiments.
237. D. Nachmansohn, M. A. Rothenberg, and E. A. Feld, *J. Biol. Chem.*, **174**, 247 (1948).
238. D. Nachmansohn, *Chemical and Molecular Basis of Nerve Activity*, Academic Press, New York, 1959, p. 54.

CHAPTER 2

POSTGANGLIONIC PARASYMPATHETIC STIMULANTS (Muscarinic Drugs)

HARRIS L. FRIEDMAN

LAKESIDE LABORATORIES
DIVISION OF COLGATE–PALMOLIVE COMPANY
MILWAUKEE, WISCONSIN

2.1. MUSCARINIC ACTION

Relationships between the structure and the activity of compounds have intrigued chemists and pharmacologists ever since it was recognized that many compounds can elicit the same pharmacodynamic action. The synthesis of new molecules and the evaluation of their potency lead to speculation on the required structural features, which in turn leads to the synthesis of modified structures and to a more comprehensive pharmacological evaluation—a feedback mechanism, producing continuous advance in knowledge.

This chapter is concerned with structure–activity relations of compounds that are agonists for muscarinic neuroeffector sites. Because adequate background information concerning muscarinic action is available in standard textbooks, only phases pertinent to the subject will be mentioned. Descriptive information, discussion, and interpretation of data are given from the structure–activity point of view. Statements concerning the pertinency of data are the author's evaluation. Limited reviews of the subject have appeared in several books (*1–4*).

The presentation is as follows. Section 2.1 gives selected background information, methods of measurement, and the expression of activity. Section 2.2 contains tabulations of the activities of compounds reported in the literature as compared with acetylcholine, whose activity is given as 1. Section 2.3 reports the theories correlating structure and activity and some speculations on active conformation at the receptor site.

A. Definition and Morphology of Muscarinic Action

It has been known since 1870 that muscarine mimics the actions produced by stimulation of the cranial and sacral divisions of the autonomic nervous system, and later this was found to be true of acetylcholine (ACh) and many of its congeners. Speculations were made that a compound with similar action, perhaps muscarine itself, would ultimately be found in organisms belonging to the vertebrate kingdom. Following Hunt's (*5*) discovery in 1906, of the unusually high potency of ACh, Sir Henry Dale (*6*) in 1914 speculated on its possible occurrence and role in nerve function. These were established as facts after Loewi's epoch-making proof of humoral transmission in 1921.

The fact that ingested muscarine produces actions identical with those caused by nervous stimulation of the parasympathetic fibers indicates that many postganglionic neurohormone effector sites are exposed to compounds in the vascular fluid. One may wonder at the evolution of a nervous system vulnerable to dietary factors.

Dale in 1914 (*6*) defined muscarinic action as a "peripheral action broadly reproducing the effects of cranial and sacral involuntary nerves and readily paralyzed by atropine." In addition to the postganglionic parasympathetic neuroeffector sites (primarily smooth muscle and secretory glands) various brain neurons have recently been demonstrated to possess muscarinic sites: for example, pyramidal cells in the cerebral cortex (inhibitory) (*7*), and certain neurons in the brain stem (excitatory) (*8*) and in the cerebellum (excitatory) (*9*). Such sites probably exist also in certain autonomic ganglia, such as the inferior mesenteric ganglion of the cat (*10*). The term *muscarinic* will be used in this text, as it is well entrenched in nomenclature and still adequately characterizes the action of the compounds.

The ganglion cells of the parasympathetic system are situated close to or within the organs innervated; thus, their axons are quite short. The morphological details of the junction of the axon fibers and smooth muscle are only partially known. They have recently been reviewed by Burnstock and Holman (*11*) and by Daniel (*12*).

The axons branch and form a fine-meshed plexus of nonmyelinated fibers, which are usually enveloped (Schwann syncytium). There is no continuity between smooth muscle and nerve fiber, nor is there a specific area comparable to the end plate of the skeletal neuromuscular junction. In some smooth muscles each cell appears to possess axon terminals, but in other muscles only certain cells do (*11*). Electron microscopy shows the terminals of the nerve fibers to be packed with vesicles and mitochondria. The vesicles presumably are the storage place of ACh (*13*). The size of the synaptic gap is comparable to that at other synapses, about 200 to 300 A. Burnstock and Holman (*11*) postulated that the neurohormone transmitter, ACh, is released at many points close to the muscle cells and that those cells not directly stimulated by the transmitter are stimulated by electrical spread of excitation from neighboring cells.

It is unknown whether an identical amount of transmitter is released at all endings or whether different amounts are released by the same ending at different times. Del Castillo and Katz (*14*) demonstrated that at the skeletal neuromuscular junction the nerve impulse releases quantal amounts of ACh (one quantum containing probably a few thousand molecules). Data on muscarinic sites are lacking, although Burnstock and Holman consider a quantal mechanism possible at some sites (*11*). Koelle (*15*) postulated that at certain preganglionic sites the nerve-action potential liberates ACh, which in turn liberates additional amounts of ACh, and it is the latter, secondarily released and in increased amount, which effects the stimulus. He believes this likely also at postganglionic cholinergic sites (*16*). It is assumed that the postganglionic parasympathetic junctions at glands are similar to those at smooth muscle.

B. ACh, the Muscarinic Neurohormone

ACh occurs in both the plant and animal kingdoms (*17*); in the latter, from the lowest to the highest phyla. It has been isolated from protozoa and from nervous tissue of mollusca, annelida, arthropoda, insecta, etc. (*18*). The role of ACh in invertebrates and in vertebrates involves primarily modification of membrane permeability (*15*). Koelle (*15*) thought it likely that in the course of evolution ACh was introduced originally into nonneural tissues and developed eventually to a higher degree of specialization at the synapse (sympathetic and parasympathetic ganglia and the cholinergic neuroeffector sites of both smooth and striated muscle). As the craniosacral system is phylogenetically older than the thoracolumbar (*19*), it may well be that ACh was the earliest available compound that could be adapted to perform a neurotransmitter function. It is conceivable that a simple molecule (ethanolamine or a closely related amino acid) was available for adaptation to life processes at the dawn of evolution. It is of interest that the adrenergic neurohormones, epinephrine and norepinephrine, are ethanolamine derivatives.

Besides ACh several choline esters (propionyl, butyryl, acrylyl) have been isolated from various animal tissues (*20*), and this fact naturally stimulated speculation that one or more of these was involved in transmission at some muscarinic sites. There is, however, no evidence that this is so, and as it has not been proved otherwise, the assumption is made that ACh is the only muscarinic neurohormone.

C. Quantitation of Muscarinic Action

The ideal test is one that gives a reproducible quantitative measure of the response at the muscarinic neuroeffector site only, uninfluenced by action at other effector sites.

No single test for the evaluation of muscarinic agents exists, and each pharmacologist develops his own techniques, which vary in slight (and sometimes major) details from others. Luduena (*21*) has stressed the care required for significant results with smooth-muscle tissue. In the following are discussed factors that have produced nonuniform evaluations of muscarinic compounds in many published reports. It is fortunate that recent evaluations have given more significant data for structure–activity comparisons.

1. THE TISSUE CHOSEN

Early in this century most measurements were made in whole animals by measuring blood pressure depression. A large number of compounds were often run in one animal, and the action of later ones may have been affected by their predecessors. Although such experiments indicate muscarinic activity and can be "quantitated," the comparative value of the data remains uncertain, because factors of diffusion, metabolism, and excretion would produce various results, which may have been dependent also on the order in which the compounds were given. Isolated tissues will give more reproducible results, but there is no consensus as to which tissues are best. Thus, van Rossum and Ariëns (*22*) used rat jejunum on the basis that this gives feeble response to nicotinic agents, whereas others believe rabbit ileum is better in this respect. Isolated heart papillary muscle undoubtedly will give more significant results than blood pressure in whole animals, since the latter action may be caused both by dilatation of peripheral arterioles and by direct effect on the heart. Unfortunately, these data too often differ from those from intestinal tissue.

2. EQUIPMENT

Even in a simple test like the Magnus technique with isolated intestinal tissue certain mechanical factors, such as the type of lever and the working load, can affect the results. Of course, one hopes to eliminate the differences in absolute values by expressing potency relative to ACh, but there is no assurance that this is achieved (*21*).

3. TIME FACTORS

The rate of original addition of the drug, the time to wait before a second addition, the period for wash-out, and other time factors may give different absolute values, but these may be compensated for by comparisons with a standard.

4. HYDROLYSIS FACTOR

If the compound under study is an ester hydrolyzable by acetylcholinesterase (AChE), the effect measured in the presence of an AChE inhibitor may be different from that in its absence. By measuring the rate of hydrolysis it may be possible to correct for this effect (*23*). Poisoning AChE is preferable for comparing various esters.

5. ACTION AT OTHER EFFECTOR SITES

Small molecules, such as the simple alkyl quaternary ammonium ions, can interact with a variety of effector sites. To insure that the only stimulus being measured is that produced at the muscarinic receptor it may be necessary to block other receptor sites by adding specific antagonists. Thus, Ing et al. (*24*) added hexamethonium to block nicotinic sites, and Stephenson (*25*) added also an antihistamine to counteract the action of histamine liberation due to the hexamethonium.

6. STANDARD AS REFERENCE

There is no agreement on an ideal standard for comparison. Most workers prefer ACh because it is the natural neurohormone. Because of susceptibility to AChE some investigators prefer nonester types, such as muscarine, furtrethonium, or one of the Fourneau acetals (*26*). When Fourneau acetals are used, they should be carefully compared with ACh, to establish a ratio

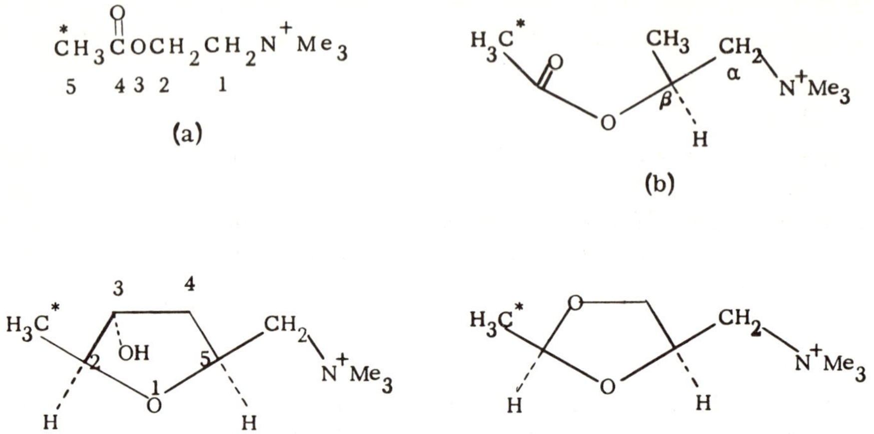

Fig. 2.1. Structures of selected muscarinic compounds to illustrate numbering of atoms. Asterisks denote the so-called "fifth atom." (a) Acetylcholine; (b) *dextro*-β-methyl-ACh; (c) L(+)-muscarine; (d) Belleau's acetal; L-(+)-*cis*.

necessary for conversion to values for comparison with published data. It is conceivable that Belleau's acetal (Figure 2.1) (*27*) will make an ideal standard, because it is stable and of known conformation and ultimately should be inexpensive.

7. DOSE–RESPONSE CURVES

The author believes one of the commonest deficiencies in the literature has been the lack of dose–response curves. Although a three-point determination may be adequate for comparison with a standard (provided the two lines are parallel), it is important to know whether an agonist can produce the maximal effect of ACh; otherwise, a value significant to a full understanding of the drug action is lost.

D. Quantitative Delineation of Action

For a quantitative comparison of muscarinic agents two values are required: effectiveness and potency. For a complete description the tissue used and the rate of response should be specified.

Effectiveness is that unknown quality which enables the drug to interact with the effector site in such manner as to trigger the response being measured. This quality has been termed "intrinsic activity" by Ariëns (*28*) and "efficacy" by Stephenson (*25*). To possess an effectiveness equal to that of ACh a drug must produce a maximal response equal to the maximal response produced by ACh. At present there is no way of expressing this value in absolute terms. Following Ariëns, it is usually presented as the ratio of the maximal response produced by the drug under study to the maximal response produced by ACh. The effectiveness of any muscarinic agent appears to be a function both of the structure of the compound and of the tissue being studied. Those drugs that in any dose would not produce maximal action equal to ACh were called by Stephenson "partial agonists." They have an activity intermediate between that of the antagonists and that of ACh, and because they will act as antagonists in the presence of compounds having greater intrinsic activity, they are also classified as "partial antagonists."

Potency, theoretically an expression of the number of molecules interacting with the effector site which is required to produce a particular stimulus, is commonly expressed in terms of concentration (dilution) or of weight. In Ariëns' terminology it is the measure of the affinity of the agonist for the receptor. Potency is also a function of both drug and tissue. The term is more often used in the relative sense: the ratio of the number of molecules of the drug to the number of molecules of ACh that will produce identical responses.

The rate of response comprehends many factors: time of onset of action, time to reach peak action, duration of effect, fade, etc. With the same drug the time factors vary with technique and tissue; with the same tissue, with the technique and drug. For example, Schueler and Keasling (*29*), using isolated guinea pig ileum, noted that an amount of "reversed ACh" required a period 250% longer than that required by an equal amount of ACh to produce the same final contraction, and they wondered whether the rate of response or the final effect was the more reliable measure of drug effector conformability or whether the slower rate was a reflection of access to the site of action. Rate factors being seldom quantitated and compared, they will be ignored in the following discussion.

2.2. STRUCTURAL TYPES AND ACTIVITIES

For a delineation of the activity of a muscarinic drug both the effectiveness and the potency must be expressed; these are independent of each other and vary with the tissue or organ used in the test.

The tables in this section contain data from the literature, selected to illustrate variation of structure with activity in terms of these three parameters. Most of the values are obtained from studies of isolated organs. Effectiveness is expressed in terms of Ariëns' intrinsic activity; potency, in terms of the reciprocal of the molecular ratio to ACh as unity. Thus, an intrinsic activity of 1 signifies that the drug produced an effect equal to the maximum effect produced by ACh, and a potency of 5 signifies that a concentration five times that of ACh was required to produce the same stimuli (that is, the potency is one-fifth that of ACh).

When informative, the results of several tests with the same compound are given in the tables in this section. As biological tests are not precise, the values have often been rounded. Organic structures can be printed only in two dimensions, but they must be thought of in their three-dimensional aspects. The tables must be read with some mental image of the chief polar regions and the force fields surrounding each molecule.

A. Variations in the ACh Molecule

1. VARIATIONS IN THE ONIUM HEAD

Table 2.1 illustrates the effect of replacing the onium N of ACh with other elements. It is evident that a positively charged atom is essential for activity. The carbon isostere (No. 4 in the table) is quite weak (*155*); however, it is a substrate for cholinesterase and appears to have some nicotinic action (*30*). The carbon isosteres of other potent compounds (such as muscarine) should be prepared and tested, before it can be concluded that this replacement always produces low activity. Ing noted that the potencies of ACh analogues containing other onium atoms (S, P, As) are in inverse order to the volumes occupied by these atoms (*31*).

As is evident from Table 2.2, maximal activity occurs with the trimethylammonium group; substitution of a methyl by any other group diminishes potency. Exchange of one methyl for ethyl (No. 5) lowers the potency only a little, but replacement of a second methyl with ethyl (No. 6) lowers it radically. A third ethyl (No. 11) does not markedly change the activity of its predecessor when the effect on isolated intestinal tissue is measured, but it abolishes activity when dog blood pressure is the criterion. Replacement of one methyl with

TABLE 2.1

Variations in Onium Atom; $Me_nXCH_2CH_2OAc$

No.	Me_nX	Potency	Test	Ref.
1	Me_3P^+	12	rab. ileum	*31*
2	Me_3As^+	90	rab. ileum	*31*
3	Me_2S^+	30	g. pig ileum	*24*
4	Me_3C	neglig.	g. pig ileum	*30*
		3200	g. pig ileum	*155*

groups higher than ethyl (Nos. 8 and 9) markedly reduces potency, and further substitution of such groups produces compounds with negligible activity (*32*). The successive omission of methyl to produce the tertiary (No. 3), secondary (No. 2), and primary (No. 1) amines diminishes, but does not entirely abolish, activity. It is presumed that these compounds possess a charged nitrogen at physiological pH.

It is to be noted that the preceding pertains to the ACh molecule. In most other structures the effect of replacement of an onium methyl with ethyl is more marked, and the triethyl analog is usually essentially inactive.

Thus, in amyl-N^+Me_3 replacement of one onium CH_3 with Et lowers the potency 250-fold (rat jejunum), whereas a replacement of two methyl groups with ethyls results in an inactive compound; similar results are noted in

TABLE 2.2

Variations in Onium Group; $R^2—N^+(R^1)(R^3)—CH_2CH_2OAc$

No.	R^1	R^2	R^3	Intrinsic activity	Potency	Test[a]	Ref.
1	H	H	H		20,000	rab. ileum	*31*
2	H	H	Me		1,000	rab. ileum	*31*
3	H	Me	Me		40	rab. ileum	*31*
	H	Me	Me	1	300	rab. ileum	*34*
4	H	Et	Et		60	rab. ileum	*35*
5	Me	Me	Et	1	4	rat jejun.	*36*
	Me	Me	Et		3	g. pig ileum	*37*
6	Me	Et	Et	1	300	rat jejun.	*36*
	Me	Et	Et		400	g. pig ileum	*37*
	Me	Et	Et		700	g. pig ileum	*31*
	Me	Et	Et		16	rab. ileum	*38*
7	Me	Me	NH_2		8	g. pig ileum	*39*
8	Me	Me	nPr		300	rab. ileum	*40*
9	Me	Me	nBu		weak	g. pig ileum	*24*
10	Me	Me	CH_2CH_2COOMe		100	g. pig ileum	*29*
11	Et	Et	Et	1	400	rat jejun.	*36*
	Et	Et	Et		300	g. pig ileum	*37*
	Et	Et	Et		1,700	g. pig ileum	*31*
	Et	Et	Et		inact.	dog b. press.	*41*
12	Me	Me	OCH_3		2	g. pig ileum	*33*
13	CD_3	CD_3	CD_3		1	dog b. press.	*156*

[a] Blood-pressure: lowering.

Table 2.10 (No. 5), Table 2.11 (No. 5), and Table 2.20 (No. 7), where the —N^+Et_2Me derivative is inactive (the inactive —N^+Et_3 analogue is not listed).

TABLE 2.3

Variations in Alkylene Chain; R_3N^+-Alkylene-OAc

No.	N^+R_3	Alkylene	Config.	Intrinsic activity	Potency	Test[a]	Ref.
1	N^+Me_3	absent			50	g. pig ileum	*45*
2	N^+Me_3	CH_2			5000	g. pig ileum	*45*
					1200	cat b. press.	*46*
3	N^+Me_3	$CH(CH_3)CH_2$	rac.		20	cat b. press.	*47*
			rac.		50	g. pig ileum	*42*
			(−)		230	g. pig ileum	*42*
			(+)		30	g. pig ileum	*42*
4	N^+Me_3	$CH_2CH(CH_3)$	rac.		1	cat b. press.	*47*
			rac.	1	1.5	rat jejun.	*34*
			rac.		1.6	g. pig ileum	*42*
			(−)		240	g. pig ileum	*42*
			(−)	1	400	rat jejun.	*43*
			(+)		1	g. pig ileum	*42*
			(+)	1	1.3	rat jejun.	*43*
5	N^+Me_2H	$CH_2CH(CH_3)$	rac.	0.9	1300	rat jejun.	*34*
6	N^+Me_2Et	$CH_2CH(CH_3)$	rac.		6	rab. ileum	*40*
7	N^+Me_3	$CH_2CH(Et)$			200	cat b. press.	*44*
	N^+Me_3	$CH_2CH(Et)$			20	rab. ileum	*40*
8	N^+Me_3	$(CH_2)_3$			900	rab. ileum	*48*
9	N^+Me_3	$(CH_2)_4$			740	rab. ileum	*48*
					100	rab. ileum	*49*
10	N^+Me_3	$CH_2CH{=}CHCH_2$	*cis*		50	dog heart	*50*
			trans		3	dog heart	*50*
11	N^+Me_3	$CH_2C{\equiv}CCH_2$			2	rab. ileum	*49*
12	N^+Me_3	$CH_2C{\equiv}CCH_2CH_2$			10	rab. ileum	*49*
13	N^+Me_3	$CH_2C{\equiv}CCH(CH_3)$			4	rab. ileum	*49*

[a] Blood pressure: lowering. Heart: inhibition.

An enigmatic substitution is that of OCH_3 for an onium CH_3, In ACh (Table 2.2, No. 12) the potency was halved, whereas in β-methyl-ACh the potency was diminished 11-fold (guinea pig ileum) and 120-fold (dog blood pressure); the same substitution in bethanechol increased the potency approximately 20-fold (guinea pig ileum or dog blood pressure), but in carbachol it increased it for guinea pig ileum but diminished it for dog blood pressure (*33*).

2. VARIATIONS IN THE ALKYLENE CHAIN

Complete absence of the connecting ethylene chain (Table 2.3, No. 1) surprisingly leaves not only an active compound but one more potent than the intermediate homolog (No. 2). In a saturated alkylene chain any departure from ethylene lowers the potency, with the exception of the *dextro* isomer of β-methyl-ACh (No. 4), which is at least as potent as ACh. This compound has been shown by Beckett and co-workers (*42*) and by Ellenbroeck and van Rossum (*43*) to have a configuration identical with that of the natural L(+) muscarine (Figure 2.1). Like muscarine it has little nicotinic activity. The *levo* isomer has approximately 1/300 the potency of the *dextro* isomer but can still produce maximal effect (intrinsic activity, 1). Beta groups larger than methyl (No. 7) lower the potency (*44*).

The *dextro* and *levo* isomers of α-methyl-ACh are both less potent than their corresponding beta analogs, and their potency ratio is only 8 (*42*).

The presence of a double bond (No. 10) enhances activity over the corresponding saturated analog, and a triple bond (No. 11) has a greater effect. Unfortunately, the true (two-carbon) analogs with ACh are unknown in the unsaturated series, so comparisons must be made with the butylene chain. The *trans* isomer of the butene analog (No. 10) is 16 times as potent as the *cis* isomer.

3. VARIATIONS IN THE ESTER GROUP

Alteration of the acyl methyl or any substitution in it produces compounds that are less potent than ACh (Table 2.4). Replacement of the three hydrogens with deuterium (No. 7) diminishes the potency slightly, and replacement of one hydrogen with fluorine (No. 3) does so substantially. Polar groups, such as OH (No. 4) and NH_2 (No. 5), markedly decrease potency. Alkyl groups higher than ethyl (Nos. 13 and 17) produce compounds having diminished intrinsic activity and leading ultimately to compounds that are competitive antagonists of ACh. The most active replacements for methyl are NH_2 (No. 2), $CH_2{=}CH{—}$ (No. 9), and $CH_3CO{—}$ (No. 12). The unsaturated compound (No. 9) is of interest, because this compound has been isolated from gastropods (*20*).

TABLE 2.4

Variations in Ester Group; $R\overset{\overset{O}{\|}}{C}OCH_2CH_2N^{+}Me_3$

No.	R	Config.	Intrinsic activity	Potency	Test[a]	Ref.
1	H		1	250	rat jejun.	*36*
	H			10	rab. ileum	*1*
2	H_2N		1	3	rat jejun.	*22*
3	FCH_2			15	g. pig ileum	*51*
4	$HOCH_2$			400	g. pig ileum	*52*
5	H_2NCH_2			450	rab. ileum	*1*
6	$EtOCH_2$			inact.	rab. ileum	*1*
7	D_3C			1.3	cat b. press.	*53*
8	CH_3CH_2			33	rab. ileum	*52*
	CH_3CH_2			15	g. pig ileum	*54*
	CH_3CH_2		0.9	400	rat jejun.	*36*
9	$CH_2{=}CH{-}$			5	g. pig ileum	*54*
10	CH_3CHOH	rac.		1400	g. pig ileum	*55*
	CH_3CHOH	(−)		900	g. pig ileum	*55*
	CH_3CHOH	(+)		5000	g. pig ileum	*55*
11	$CH_2OHCHOH$	rac.		2500	g. pig ileum	*55*
12	CH_3CO			7	rab. ileum	*52*
13	$CH_3CH_2CH_2$			400	rab. ileum	*52*
14	$CH_3\underset{\underset{CH_3}{\vert}}{C}H$		0.4	3000	rat jejun.	*36*
15	$H_2NCH_2CH_2CH_2$			2000	g. pig ileum	*54*
16	$CH_3CHOHCH_2$	rac.		1700	g. pig ileum	*55*
17	$CH_3CH_2CH_2CH_2$		0.3	6000	rat jejun.	*36*
	$CH_3CH_2CH_2CH_2$			500	rab. ileum	*52*
18	$\begin{matrix}H_3C\\H_3C\end{matrix}\!>\!C{=}CH$			1000	g. pig ileum	*54*

[a] Blood pressure: lowering.

TABLE 2.5

Variations in Ester Group; "Ether" Oxygen; $AcXCH_2CH_2N^{+}Me_3$

No.	X	Intrinsic activity	Potency	Test	Ref.
1	S	1	320	g. pig ileum	*56*
2	Se	1	220	g. pig ileum	*56*
3	NH	1	10,000	rat jejun.	*22*

Exchange of the "ether" O for S, Se, or NH (Table 2.5) markedly diminishes potency, but each of these compounds can produce maximal effect.

B. R-Alkylene-N^+R_3(R= H, Alkyl, Aryl)

The series alkyl-N^+Me_3 (Table 2.6) is one that has been studied by many investigators. The fact that maximal activity occurs at the normal amyl chain length was observed by Raventós (*57*) and became one of the bases of the five-atom rule (Section 2.3, C, 2) noted by Alles and Knoefel in 1939 (*58*) and proposed independently by Ing in 1948 (*31*). Although potency measurements vary, most pharmacologists have found that between methyl- and amyltrimethylammonium a minimum occurs at the ethyl or propyl group and that above heptyl the compounds become not only inactive as agonists but antagonistic to ACh.

When the compounds contain an unsaturated alkylene chain (Table 2.7), potency varies with the position of the unsaturation and with the number of carbons in the chain. Among compounds with either a double or triple bond those with a five-membered chain possess maximal potency. When a double

TABLE 2.6

Alkyl-N^+Me_3

No.	Alkyl	Intrinsic activity	Potency	Test[a]	Ref.
1	Me	1	4,000	rat jejun.	*22*
	Me		25,000	g. pig ileum	*45*
	Me		2,000	rab. ileum	*48*
2	Et	1	6,000	rat jejun.	*22*
3	Pr	1	8,000	rat jejun.	*22*
	Pr		700	rab. ileum	*48*
4	Bu	1	200	rat jejun.	*22*
	Bu		220	rab. ileum	*48*
5	Am	1	125	rat jejun.	*22*
	Am		110	rab. ileum	*48*
	Am		8	g. pig ileum	*24*
	Am		7	dog heart	*59*
6	Cyclopentyl		5,000	rab. ileum	*48*
7	Hexyl	0.9	300	rat jejun.	*22*
8	Heptyl	0.1	800	rat jejun.	*22*
9	Octyl		inact.	rat jejun.	*22*

[a] Heart: inhibition.

TABLE 2.7

Unsaturated Alkyl-N^+Me_3

No.	Unsaturated alkyl	Config.	Intrinsic activity	Potency	Test[a]	Ref.
1	$CH_2{=}CHCH_2$		1	2000	rat jejun.	*22*
2	$HC{\equiv}CCH_2$		1	2000	rat jejun.	*22*
	$HC{\equiv}CCH_2$			200	dog heart	*59*
3	$CH_3C{\equiv}CCH_2$			1	dog heart	*59*
4	$CH_3CH_2C{\equiv}CCH_2$			0.5	dog heart	*59*
5	$CH_3CH_2CH_2C{\equiv}CCH_2$			2	dog heart	*59*
6	$HC{\equiv}CCH_2CH_2$			5	dog heart	*60*
7	$CH_3C{\equiv}CCH_2CH_2$			0.5	dog heart	*60*
8	$CH_3CH{=}CHCH_2$	*cis*		30	dog heart	*50*
		trans		5	dog heart	*50*
9	$CH_3CH_2CH{=}CHCH_2$	*cis*		10	dog heart	*50*
		trans		2	dog heart	*50*
10	$CH_3CH{=}CHCH_2CH_2$	*cis*		2	dog heart	*50*
		trans		2	dog heart	*50*
11	$CH_3CH_2CH{=}CHCH_2CH_2$	*cis*		10	dog heart	*50*
		trans		10	dog heart	*50*

[a] Heart: inhibition.

TABLE 2.8

Aralkyl-N^+Me_3

No.	Aralkyl	Potency	Test	Ref.
1	C_6H_5	750	rab. ileum	*61*
2	$C_6H_5CH_2$	100	rab. ileum	*61*
3	$C_6H_5CH_2CH_2$	150	rab. ileum	*61*

bond is present, the *trans* compounds are usually more potent than the *cis*, but not necessarily.

In the aromatic series the compounds possess negligible activity, except those given in Table 2.8, in which, it will be noted, maximal potency is at the benzyl group (No. 2).

C. R—CHOH-Alkylene-N^+R_3

The presence of an OH group invariably decreases potency, and the same is true of its isosteres SH and SeH. Hunt found ACh to be 100,000 times more

TABLE 2.9

Hydroxy Compounds HX-Alkylene-N^+R_3

No.	HX	Alkylene	N^+R_3	Intrinsic activity	Potency	Test[a]	Ref.
1	HO	CH_2CH_2	N^+Me_3		1,300	rab. ileum	*52*
	HO	CH_2CH_2	N^+Me_3		100,000	cat b. press	*5*
	HO	CH_2CH_2	N^+Me_3	1	20,000	rat jejun.	*22*
	HO	CH_2CH_2	N^+Me_3		5,000	g. pig ileum	*56*
	HO	CH_2CH_2	N^+Me_3		200	dog heart	*62*
2	HO	CH_2CH_2	N^+Me_2Et	0.5	12,000	rat jejun.	*22*
3	HO	CH_2CH_2	N^+MeEt_2	0.2	25,000	rat jejun.	*22*
4	HO	$(CH_2)_3$	N^+Me_3		100,000	cat b. press	*32*
5	HO	$(CH_2)_4$	N^+Me_3		400	rab. ileum	*49*
6	HO	$(CH_2)_5$	N^+Me_3		100	rab. ileum	*49*
7	HO	$CH_2CH{=}CHCH_2$	N^+Me_3		1,000	rab. ileum	*49*
8	HO	$CH_2CH_2CH{=}CHCH_2$	N^+Me_3		300	rab. ileum	*49*
9	HO	$CH_2C{\equiv}CCH_2$	N^+Me_3		50	rab. ileum	*49*
10	HO	$CH_2CH_2C{\equiv}CCH_2$	N^+Me_3		20	rab. ileum	*49*
11	HS	CH_2CH_2	N^+Me_3		300	g. pig ileum	*56*
12	HSe	CH_2CH_2	N^+Me_3		180	g. pig ileum	*56*

[a] Blood pressure: lowering. Heart: inhibition.

potent than choline, as evidenced by blood-pressure lowering in cats, but on other organs (Table 2.9) the effect is not as great. The effect of acetylation of formo- and homo-cholines (next lower and higher homologs) is not as marked; for the former the potency produced by the Ac group is 10 and for the latter 10,000 (cat blood pressure) (*1*). It will be noted that the exchange of one (No. 2) or two (No. 3) methyls for ethyl in the onium head of choline has a much greater effect in diminishing intrinsic activity than an identical change in ACh.

D. R—O-Alkylene-N^+R_3 (Ethers)

Ethers are listed in Table 2.10; their sulfur isosteres, in Table 2.11. It is evident that most ethers are significantly less potent than ACh and that maximal activity occurs with the ethyl ether of choline. In the series of ethers possessing five atoms in the chain maximal activity is also found for the choline ethyl ether. The β-methylene derivative of choline methyl ether, Esmodil (No. 12), is an interesting variation, but the next lowest unknown homolog, which is the methylene isostere of reversed ACh, would be a more significant compound (Figure 2.2, a). The same is true of its reversed analog (Figure 2.2, b).

TABLE 2.10

Ethers; RO-Alkylene-N^+R_3

No.	R	Alkylene	N^+R_3	Intrinsic activity	Potency	Test[a]	Ref
1	Me	CH_2	N^+Me_3		60	g. pig ileum	*24*
2	Me	CH_2CH_2	N^+Me_3		10	g. pig ileum	*37*
3	Et	CH_2CH_2	N^+Me_3		15	rab. ileum	*65*
	Et	CH_2CH_2	N^+Me_3		10	g. pig ileum	*24*
	Et	CH_2CH_2	N^+Me_3	1	8	rat jejun.	*36*
	Et	CH_2CH_2	N^+Me_3		30	cat b. press.	*44*
4	Et	CH_2CH_2	N^+Me_2Et	1	25	rat jejun.	*36*
	Et	CH_2CH_2	N^+Me_2Et		40	g. pig ileum	*37*
5	Et	CH_2CH_2	N^+MeEt_2		inact.	rat jejun.	*36*
	Et	CH_2CH_2	N^+MeEt_2		3,000	g. pig ileum	*37*
6	i-Pr	CH_2CH_2	N^+Me_3		155	rab. ileum	*64*
7	Me	$(CH_2)_3$	N^+Me_3		100	g. pig ileum	*24*
	Me	$(CH_2)_3$	N^+Me_3		130	g. pig ileum	*37*
8	Me	$(CH_2)_3$	N^+Me_2Et		1,200	g. pig ileum	*37*
9	Me	$CH(CH_3)CH_2$	N^+Me_3		100	cat b. press.	*44*
10	Et	$CH(CH_3)CH_2$	N^+Me_3		55	rab. ileum	*64*
	Et	$CH(CH_3)CH_2$	N^+Me_3		20	cat b. press.	*44*
11	Me	$C(=CH_2)CH_2$	N^+Me_3	1	30	rat jejun.	*22*
12	$HOCH_2CH(CH_3)$	CH_2CH_2	N^+Me_3		930	rab. ileum	*64*
13	$HOCH_2CH(CH_3)$	$CH(CH_3)CH_2$	N^+Me_3		12,000	rab. ileum	*64*

[a] Blood pressure: lowering.

TABLE 2.11

Thioethers; RS-Alkylene-N^+R_3

No.	R	Alkylene	N^+R_3	Potency	Test[a]	Ref.
1	Me	CH_2	N^+Me_3	slight	cat b. press.	*66*
2	Et	CH_2CH_2	N^+Me_3	1200	rab. ileum	*48*
3	Me	$(CH_2)_3$	N^+Me_3	60	rab. ileum	*48*
4	Me	$(CH_2)_3$	N^+Me_2Et	900	rab. ileum	*48*
5	Me	$(CH_2)_3$	N^+MeEt_2	neglig.	rab. ileum	*48*
6	Et	$(CH_2)_3$	N^+Me_3	600	rab. ileum	*48*
7	Pr	$(CH_2)_3$	N^+Me_3	2800	rab. ileum	*48*

[a] Blood pressure: lowering.

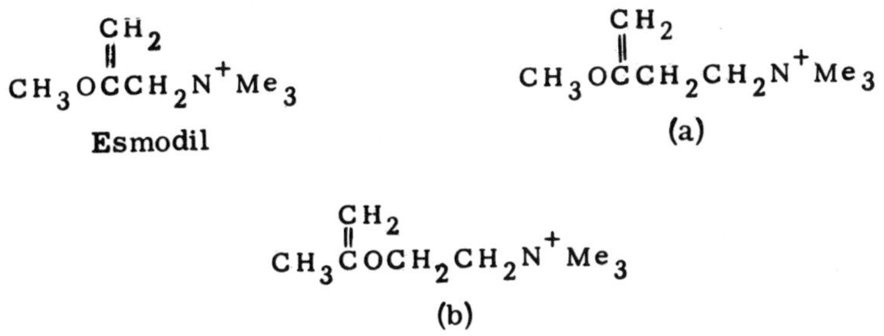

Fig. 2.2. Esmodil (top) and related compounds.

Aromatic ethers, such as phenylcholine, are inert as muscarinic agents but have pronounced nicotinic activity (*63*). The last two compounds in Table 2.10 together with choline isopropyl ether (No. 6) were studied by Gyermek (*64*) as "opened" muscarines. Their low activity is quite surprising, but may be due to the fact that they are complicated mixtures of optical isomers.

Thioethers are less active than the corresponding oxygen compounds.

E. R—C(=X)-Alkylene-N⁺Me₃ (Ketones)

In general the ketones are weaker than their corresponding hydrocarbon analogs, and the thioketones are still weaker (see Table 2.12). These com-

TABLE 2.12

Ketones; RC(=X)-Alkylene-N^+Me_3

No.	R	X	Alkylene	Potency	Test[a]	Ref.
1	H	O	CH_2	35	cat. b. press.	*1*
2	Pr	O	CH_2	1000	g. pig ileum	*24*
3	Me	O	CH_2CH_2	500	g. pig ileum	*24*
4	Et	O	CH_2CH_2	2000	g. pig ileum	*24*
	Et	O	CH_2CH_2	150	rab. jejun.	*65*
5	Et	O	$CH(CH_3)CH_2$	2000	g. pig ileum	*24*
6	Me	O	$(CH_2)_3$	250	g. pig ileum	*24*
	Me	O	$(CH_2)_3$	75	rab. jejun.	*65*
	Me	O	$(CH_2)_3$	900	rab. ileum	*48*
7	Me	S	$(CH_2)_3$	1400	rab. ileum	*48*
8	Et	S	$(CH_2)_3$	neglig.	rab. ileum	*48*

[a] Blood pressure: lowering.

pounds have a more predominantly nicotinic than muscarinic action, and evaluation of potency is complicated because of this (*24*).

F. Polyhydroxy and Hydroxy Ketone Analogues

Before the structure of muscarine was correctly ascertained, it was thought to be a choline type containing both a hydroxyl and an aldehyde group (*67*). Several compounds were synthesized following this erroneous model (see Figure 2.3, a, b) but were exceedingly weakly active. ACh containing a β-acetoxymethyl substituent (Figure 2.3, c) is little more potent than choline itself.

G. "Inorganic" Esters and Halides

The nitrate and nitrite esters (Table 2.13, Nos. 1 and 2) are quite active and of historic interest. One of the earliest structures considered for muscarine was the aldehyde corresponding to choline (Figure 2.3, d). Ewins (*68*) showed that the muscarinic compound formed from nitric acid oxidation of choline and thought to be the aldehyde was actually the nitrite ester (No. 2). Dale (*6*) demonstrated that it differed pharmacologically from natural muscarine. In the series of halogen-substituted compounds little difference is found between Cl, Br, and I; when there is a difference, the iodo compound is the most potent. The sulfate (No. 15) and phosphate (No. 14) esters are very weakly active or inactive.

H. Betaines

Betaine itself is practically inert (*73*) but becomes active when esterified with lower alkyl groups. The next higher homolog (Table 2.14, No. 2), named

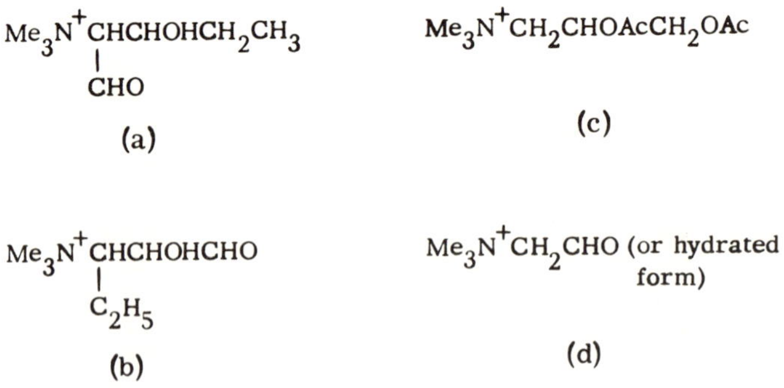

Fig. 2.3. Old formulas for muscarine.

TABLE 2.13

"Inorganic" Esters and Halides; X-Alkylene-N^+Me_3

No.	X	Alkylene	Intrinsic activity	Potency	Test[a]	Ref.
1	O_2NO	CH_2CH_2		1	cat b. press.	*1*
	O_2NO	CH_2CH_2		4	g. pig ileum	*69*
2	ONO	CH_2CH_2		100	cat b. press.	*1*
3	Cl	CH_2CH_2		100	rab. ileum	*70*
4	Br	CH_2CH_2		100	rab. ileum	*70*
	Br	CH_2CH_2	1	200	rat jejun.	*22*
5	I	CH_2CH_2		100	rab. ileum	*70*
6	Br	$CH_2CH(CH_3)$		100	rab. ileum	*70*
7	Br	$CH(CH_3)CH_2$		1000	rab. ileum	*70*
8	Cl	$(CH_2)_3$		50	rab. ileum	*70*
9	Br	$(CH_2)_3$		10	rab. ileum	*70*
	Br	$(CH_2)_3$	1	50	rat jejun.	*22*
10	I	$(CH_2)_3$		10	rab. ileum	*70*
11	Cl	$CH{=}CHCH_2$		20	rab. ileum	*70*
12	Br	$CH{=}CHCH_2$		10	rab. ileum	*70*
13	^-O_3SO	CH_2CH_2		inact.	cat. b. press.	*71*
14	$(MeO)_2POO$	CH_2CH_2		weak	cat b. press.	*71*
15	$MeSO_2O$	CH_2CH_2		3000	g. pig ileum	*72*

[a] Blood pressure: lowering.

TABLE 2.14

Betaines; R_3N^+-Alkylene-COOR′

No.	R_3N^+	Alkylene	R′	Intrinsic activity	Potency	Test[a]	Ref.
1	Me_3N	CH_2	Et		200	cat b. press.	*41*
2	Me_3N	CH_2CH_2	Me	1	1	g. pig ileum	*74*
	Me_3N	CH_2CH_2	Me		3	frog heart	*75*
3	Me_3N	CH_2CH_2	Et		10	g. pig ileum	*29*
	Me_3N	CH_2CH_2	Et	1	160	rat jejun.	*3*
4	$EtMe_2N$	CH_2CH_2	Me		10	g. pig ileum	*29*
5	$EtMe_2N$	CH_2CH_2	Et	0.6	1,200	rat jejun.	*3*
6	Et_2MeN	CH_2CH_2	Me		500	g. pig ileum	*29*
7	NH_2Me_2N	CH_2CH_2	Me		30	g. pig ileum	*39*
8	Me_3N	$CH_2CH(CH_3)$	Me		10,000	g. pig ileum	*29*
9	Me_3N	$CH(CH_3)CH_2$	Me		neglig.	g. pig ileum	*29*
10	Me_3N	$CH_2CH_2CH_2$	Me		12	frog heart	*75*
11	Me_3N	$CH_2CH{=}CH$	Me		2	g. pig ileum	*76*
	Me_3N	$CH_2CH{=}CH$	Me		17	frog heart	*75*

[a] Blood pressure: lowering. Heart: inhibition.

by Schueler "reversed ACh," and ACh are equipotent (*74*). The homolog containing a link of three carbons (No. 10) is also very potent, particularly when a double bond (No. 11) is present. Variations in the onium head and in the alkylene chain of the reversed ACh molecule produce compounds whose potencies generally are similar to those of the congeners of ACh with the same modifications. An exception is the β-methyl derivative (No. 8), which is surprisingly weak.

I. Cyclic Derivatives

1. NITROGEN IN THE RING

In general, putting the nitrogen of ACh into a ring markedly lowers potency. An exception is the naturally occurring compound arecoline (Table 2.15, No. 6). This compound is unusual in that it is a tertiary amine which, when further methylated to the onium derivative (No. 7), results in a compound

TABLE 2.15

Onium N in Ring

No.	Compound	Intrinsic activity	Potency	Test[a]	Ref.
1	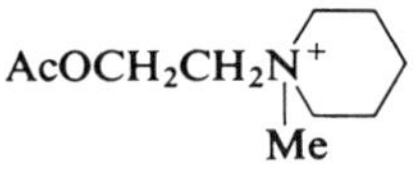		1000	cat b. press.	*78*
2	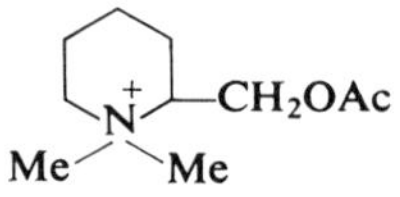		30	cat b. press.	*79*
3	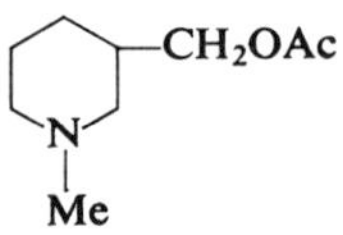		100	rab. ileum	*35*
4	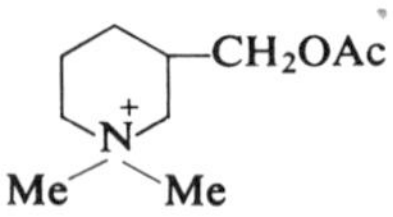		10	cat b. press.	*79*
			2000	rab. ileum	*38*
5	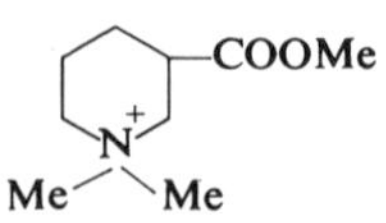		4000	rab. ileum	*38*

TABLE 2.15—*continued*

No.	Compound	Intrinsic activity	Potency	Test[a]	Ref.
6	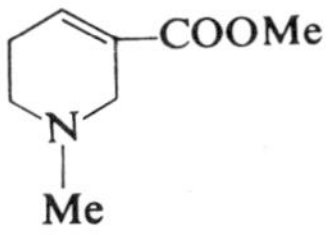	1	75	cat b. press.	*78*
			5	rab. jejun.	*34*
			1	g. pig ileum	*80*
7	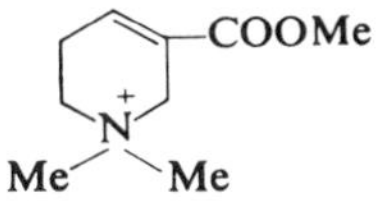	0.9	160	rat jejun.	*34*
			40	g. pig ileum	*80*
8	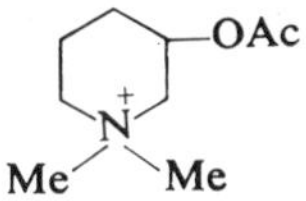		1000	rab. ileum	*40*
9	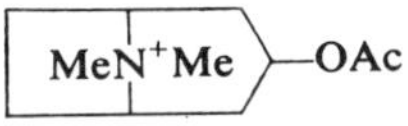		100	rab. ileum	*81*
10	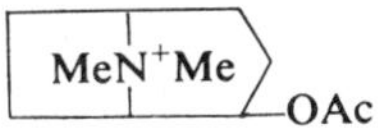 *trans*-oid		100	rat colon	*82*
	cis-oid		neglig.	rat colon	*82*

[a] Blood pressure: lowering.

with lower potency. The acetyl derivative of 3-hydroxyquinuclidine is claimed to be a potent muscarinic agent, which also becomes less potent when methylated (*77*).

Schueler (*40*) tested 3-acetoxydimethylpiperidinium (No. 8) as a cyclized ACh (or a cyclized β-methyl-ACh) and found it to be weak.

2. ONE OXYGEN IN THE RING

This class comprises many compounds of interest: furans (Tables 2.16 and 2.17), muscarines (Table 2.18), and muscarones (Table 2.19). As Table 2.16 shows, high potency is found for some of the furans. Ing (*24*), as an extension of his five-atom rule, investigated the 2-methyl derivative (No. 3) of the previously known parent furan compound (No. 1) and showed it to have the greater potency anticipated. Other variations diminish activity, and saturation of the ring also produces compounds which are less active. The saturated analog (Table 2.17, No. 9) of Ing's active compound has not been purified;

TABLE 2.16

One Oxygen in Ring Furans

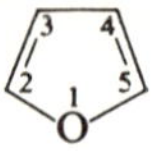

(hydrogens not designated)

No.	Position 2	4	5	Intrinsic activity	Potency	Test[a]	Ref.
1			$CH_2N^+Me_3$		20	rab. jejun.	*90*
			$CH_2N^+Me_3$		12	g. pig ileum	*24*
			$CH_2N^+Me_3$	1	13	rat jejun.	*34*
2			$CH_2N^+Me_2H$	0.9	800	rat jejun.	*34*
3	CH_3		$CH_2N^+Me_3$	1	0.8	rat jejun.	*34*
	CH_3		$CH_2N^+Me_3$		⩾1	g. pig ileum	*24*
4	CH_3		$CH_2N^+Me_2H$	0.8	500	rat jejun.	*34*
5	CH_3CH_2		$CH_2N^+Me_3$		35	g. pig ileum	*91*
6			$CH_2CH_2N^+Me_3$		100	g. pig ileum	*91*
7	CH_3	N^+Me_3	CH_3		5000	cat b. press.	*86*

[a] Blood pressure: lowering.

the mixture reported (*23*) is stated to be mainly of the *cis* form. The ketone derivative (lactone) (Table 2.17, No. 2) is surprisingly weak, considering the fact that it is a cyclized β-methyl-ACh.

TABLE 2.17

One Oxygen in Ring-Saturated Furans

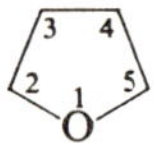

(hydrogens not designated)

No.	Position 2	3	4	5	Potency	Test	Ref.
1				$CH_2N^+Me_3$	200	rab. jejun.	*90*
2	O=			$CH_2N^+Me_3$	1000	rab. ileum	*92*
3	$HOCH_2$			$CH_2N^+Me_3$	>1000	rab. ileum	*93*
4		N^+Me_3	OH	CH_2CH_3	>1000	rab. ileum	*93*
5			N^+Me_3		3000	cat. b. press.	*86*
6	CH_3CH_2		N^+Me_3		150	cat b. press.	*86*
7	CH_3CHOH		N^+Me_3		1000	cat b. press.	*86*
8	$Me_3N^+CH_2$			$CH_2N^+Me_3$	1000	cat b. press.	*86*
9	CH_3			$CH_2N^+Me_3$	20	g. pig ileum	*23*

TABLE 2.18

Muscarines

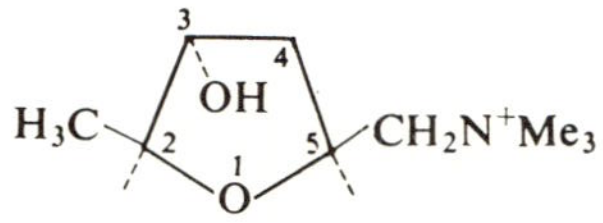

No.		Position[a] 2	3	5	Config.	Rab. ileum, poten. (88)	Rat jejun. (34, 89) Intr. act.	Poten.	Frog heart[b] (34, 89) Intr. act.	Poten.	Cat b. press.,[c] poten. (86)	Frog heart, poten. (86)
					Muscarines							
1		S	R	S	*dl*	1	1	2	1	6		
		S	R	S	L(+)	0.4	1	0.8			0.2	5
		S	R	S	D(−)	160						
2	acetyl	S	R=OAc	S	L(+)						0.8	
3	nor	S	R	$S{=}NMe_2$	L(+)		0.9	1600			600	2,500
4	epi	S	S	S	*dl*	280	1	1500	0.1	weak	330	100,000
5	allo	S	R	R	*dl*	190	1	500	0.4	weak	200	7,500
6	epiallo	S	S	R	*dl*	260	1	125	1	500	125	6,000
					Analogs							
7			R	S	*dl*						125	14,000
8			S	S	*dl*						1,000	200,000
9		R=H, S=Pr	R	S	*dl*						60	25,000
10		R=H, S=Pr	S	S	*dl*						10,000	500,000
11		R=Me, S=Me	R	S	*dl*						1,100	2,000
12		S	$R{=}OH, S{=}C_6H_5$	S	*dl*						0.8	
					4,5-Dehydro muscarines							
13		S	R		*dl*						1.3	100
14		S	S		*dl*						2.5	200

[a] S: group above plane of ring. R: group below plane of ring.
[b] Heart: inhibition.
[c] Blood pressure: lowering.

The incorrect designation of the muscarine structure by Kögl et al. in 1931 (*67*) caused confusion and for many years held up progress in structure–activity relationships. Several workers recognized that the structure proposed (Figure 2.3, a) could not be correct and proposed an alternative formula: Fourneau and co-workers (*26*), an acetal type, and Rogers (*83*), an *N*-alkoxy type. Reinvestigation of muscarine by Kögl et al. (*84*) and by Eugster and Waser (*85*) resolved this perplexing problem in 1957, and muscarine (Figure 2.1) fell into line with known potent muscarinic agents.

Waser (*86*) has tabulated the pharmacological studies made with muscarine up to the year 1961. With few exceptions muscarine is more potent on smooth muscle than ACh. Its action is slower in onset and more persistent. It is highly selective in action, being without effect on skeletal muscle and possessing nicotinic activity only in large doses. Waser (*86*) found it without effect on erythrocyte AChE; however, Witkop et al. (*87*) found it active on AChE from electric eel tissue.

Gyermek and Unna (*88*) first published potency data for the optical isomers of muscarine and showed the remarkable stereospecificity of the natural compound (Table 2.18). Van Rossum (*89*) found that the epi, allo, and epi-allo isomers, although of low potency, have an intrinsic activity of 1 when tested

TABLE 2.19

Muscarones

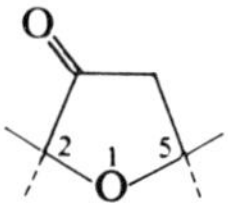

No.	Position 2	Position 5	Config.	Rab. ileum, poten. (*88*)	Cat b. press.,[a] poten. (*86*)	Frog heart,[b] poten. (*86*)
1	$S=CH_3$	$S=CH_2N^+Me_3$	*dl*	0.16		
			(+)	0.18	0.37	
			(−)	0.08	0.13	4
2	$S=CH_3$	$R=CH_2N^+Me_3$	*dl*	0.3	0.37	10
3		$S=CH_2N^+Me_3$	*dl*		8	4000
4	$S=CH_3$	$S=CH_2N^+Me_2H$	*dl*		125	
5	$S=CH_3$, $R=CH_3$	$S=CH_2N^+Me_3$	*dl*		6	8000
		4,5-Dehydro muscarone				
6	$S=CH_3$	$CH_2N^+Me_3$	*dl*	0.6	0.19	5

[a] Blood pressure: lowering.
[b] Heart: inhibition.

on rat jejunum, but the epi and the allo forms are only partial agonists on the frog heart. In general, variation from the natural muscarine structure (in the saturated muscarine series) produces compounds of lesser activity, with the exception of the 3-phenyl derivative (Table 2.18, No. 12). This compound has unusually high potency in the presence of the large intruding planar phenyl group. Introduction of a double bond in the 4,5 position (Nos. 13 and 14) enhances potency, and oxidation of the hydroxyl to carbonyl not only produces a more potent muscarinic compound (Tables 2.18 and 2.19) but one with high nicotinic activity. The more potent isomer of muscarone, according to Waser (*86*), has the *dextro* configuration, not the *levo* as has muscarine. Others (*23*) have questioned Waser's steric designation, but the matter is not significant, because both the *dextro* and *levo* forms of muscarone are highly potent, and the low ratio, 3, of the activity of the two forms is in marked contrast to that of the corresponding muscarines, in which the potency of the *levo* isomer is 400 to 1000 times that of the *dextro*.

Replacement of the ring oxygen with sulfur in muscarine and muscarone leads to the thio derivatives, which are 1500 and 26 times less potent (*86*) (see Table 2.17, cat blood pressure).

3. TWO OXYGENS IN THE RING

Fourneau in 1944 (*26*) published a series of cyclic acetal derivatives which, in contrast to previously known variations of ACh, had unusually high potency, and he speculated that natural muscarine might bear some structural relation to those compounds. Later work justified the speculation. The compounds originally prepared by Fourneau were mixtures of *cis* and *trans* isomers, and not until Triggle and Belleau's studies in 1962 (*94*) was their stereochemistry elucidated. Triggle and Belleau proved that the compound designated F-2268 (Figure 2.4, a) was a 60:40 mixture of the *cis* and *trans* forms and that the most potent isomer, the *cis* L(+), had a configuration identical with the natural L(+) muscarine. They further showed that variations from this configuration resulted in compounds with markedly lower potency. Unfortunately,

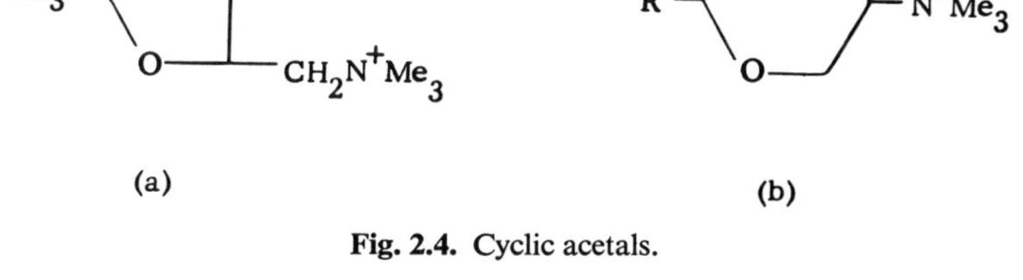

Fig. 2.4. Cyclic acetals.

TABLE 2.20

Two Oxygens in Ring

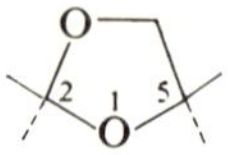

No.	Position 2	Position 5	Config. Stereo.	Config. Opt.	Rat jejun. (*22*) Intr. act.	Rat jejun. (*22*) Poten.	G. pig ileum, poten. (*94, 96*)	Other ref.
1		$CH_2N^+Me_3$		*dl*	1	160	1000	
2	Me	$CH_2N^+Me_3$	*cis*	*dl*			1	
	Me	$CH_2N^+Me_3$	*cis*	D(−)			16	
	Me	$CH_2N^+Me_3$	*cis*	L(+)			0.16	
	Me	$CH_2N^+Me_3$	*trans*	*dl*			5	
	Me	$CH_2N^+Me_3$	mix.	*dl*	1	1		
3	Et	$CH_2N^+Me_3$	mix.	*dl*	1	125		
4	Pr	$CH_2N^+Me_3$	mix.	*dl*	0.5	400		
5	Cl_3C	$CH_2N^+Me_3$	*cis*	*dl*			100	
	Cl_3C	$CH_2N^+Me_3$	*trans*	*dl*			1000	
6	Me	$CH_2N^+Me_2Et$	mix.	*dl*	1	2.5		
7	Me	$CH_2N^+MeEt_2$	mix.	*dl*	0.3	500		
8	Me	$CH_2N^+Et_3$	mix.	*dl*	0	inact.		
			cis	*dl*			200	
9	Me	$CH_2N^+Me_2H$	mix.	*dl*	1	600		
10	$CH_2N^+Me_3$		mix.	*dl*				100 rat ileum, (*26*)
11	$CH_2N^+Me_3$	Me	mix.	*dl*				50 rat ileum, (*26*)
12	$CH_2N^+Me_2H$	Me	mix.	*dl*				50 g. pig ileum, (*97*)

their acetal (Figure 2.1) has not been adequately studied pharmacologically. Its action on tissues other than guinea pig ileum will be awaited with great interest. Ariëns and co-workers (*22*) showed that structural variations in the Fourneau acetal series of compounds of mixed *cis* and *trans* isomers decrease the intrinsic activity and potency as much as in ACh, except that the triethylammonium derivative is inactive (Nos. 6, 7, and 8). Similar studies should be made with the pure *cis* isomers. In the homologous six-membered acetal ring (Figure 2.4, b), where R is H or CH_3, the potency is one-tenth that of ACh (Table 2.20, No. 3), but when R is phenyl the compound is inactive (*95*).

4. OXYGEN AND NITROGEN IN THE RING

In general, those compounds which resemble cyclized ACh are much less active than the parent substance (Table 2.21). The nitrogen isostere of F-2268 (Table 2.21, No. 8) and ACh are equipotent.

TABLE 2.21

O and N in Ring

No.	Compound	Potency	Test[a]	Ref.
1	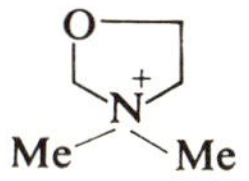	inact.	cat b. press.	*6*
2	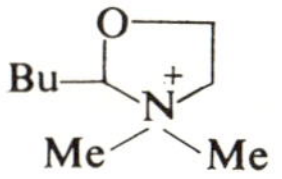	100	cat b. press.	*86*
3	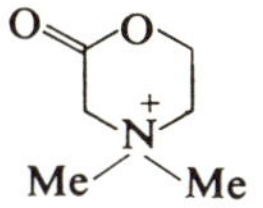	400	g. pig ileum	*98*
4	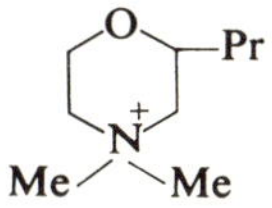	300	cat b. press.	*86*
5	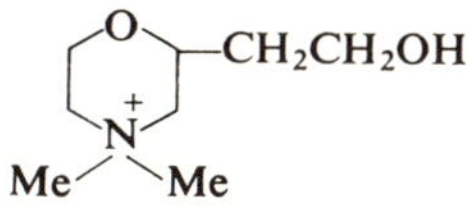	1400	cat b. press.	*86*
6	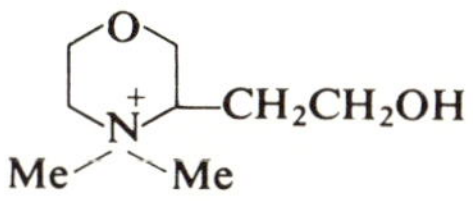	4000	cat b. press.	*86*
7	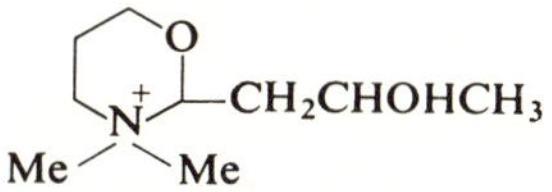	neglig.	cat b. press.	*86*
8	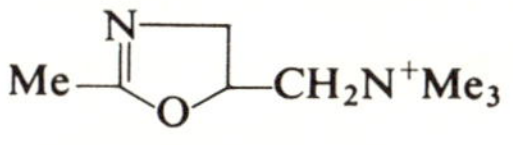	1	g. pig ileum	*94*

[a] Blood pressure: lowering.

J. Bisonium Compounds

Although the presence of two onium groups does not abolish activity, in practically all instances the resulting compounds are much less potent than ACh. The one exception seems to be compounds containing double or triple bonds in the alkylene chain (Nos. 11 and 12) (Table 2.22) but, until data are

TABLE 2.22

Bisonium Compounds; Me_3N^+-X-N^+Me_3

No.	Connecting group, X	Potency	Test[a]	Ref.
1	$CH_2CH(OAc)CH_2$	6,000	cat b. press.	*32*
2	$CH_2CH_2OCH_2CH_2$	100,000	cat b. press.	*6*
3	$CH_2COOCH_2CH_2$	1,000	g. pig heart	*100*
4	$CH_2COOCH_2CH_2CH_2$	1,000	g. pig heart	*100*
5	$CH_2CH_2COOCH_2CH_2$	10	g. pig heart	*100*
	$CH_2CH_2COOCH_2CH_2$	500	g. pig ileum	*29*
6	$(CH_2)_8$	10,000	g. pig ileum	*99*
7	$(CH_2)_9$	8,000	g. pig ileum	*99*
8	$(CH_2)_{10}$	3,200	g. pig ileum	*99*
9	$(CH_2)_{11}$	1,300	g. pig ileum	*99*
10	$(CH_2)_{12}$	1,300	g. pig ileum	*99*
11	$CH_2C{\equiv}CCH_2$	12	cat heart	*101*
12	$CH_2C{\equiv}CCH_2CH_2$	2	cat heart	*101*
13	$CH_2C{\equiv}CCH_2CH_2CH_2$	2	cat heart	*101*
14	$CH_2CH_2C{\equiv}CCH_2CH_2$	110	cat heart	*101*
15	$CH_2CH{=}CHCH_2$	500	cat heart	*101*
16	$CH_2CH{=}CHCH_2CH_2$	weak	cat heart	*101*
17	$CH_2CH{=}CHCH_2CH_2CH_2$	30	cat heart	*101*

[a] Blood pressure: lowering. Heart: inhibition.

available on tissues other than the more sensitive cat auricle, definite conclusions must be withheld. Paton (*99*) noted that compounds in the saturated series showed activity in guinea pig or rabbit ileum but were without effect on cat blood pressure. He concluded these might not be true muscarinic agents.

K. Miscellaneous Compounds

A number of compounds, whose structures do not readily fit into simple classifications, possess substantial muscarinic activity. Pilocarpine (Figure 2.5) has been known for many years to be such a compound. Van Rossum (*34*) recently clarified the action of pilocarpine. It has an intrinsic activity of 0.8 and

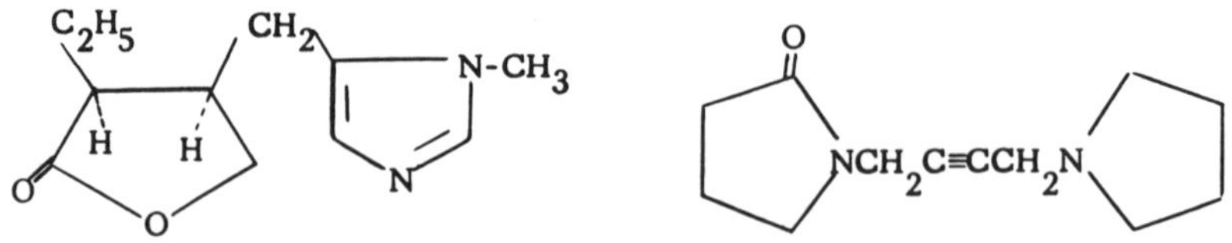

(a) (b)

Fig. 2.5. (a) Pilocarpine and (b) oxotremorine.

is therefore a partial agonist, becoming lytic in higher doses. At still higher doses it becomes a noncompetitive antagonist, probably through binding to sites other than muscarinic.

Variations in the pilocarpine structure, such as are caused by opening of the lactone ring or removal of the methyl group, produce weak or inert compounds (*1*). Schild et al. (*102*) noted that the effect of pilocarpine on guinea pig ileum was much more diminished at pH 9 than at pH 7.

A compound reported to be of the same potency as ACh was first isolated as a metabolite of Tremorine and shown to be the mono-oxo derivative (Figure 2.5) (*103*). The activity was unanticipated in view of the lack of muscarinic activity of both the parent compound (Tremorine) and its monomethyl derivative (*104*).

Many compounds with a wide variety of structure have been reported to possess weak muscarinic activity but are not deemed important enough to be considered herein.

2.3. THEORIES RELATING STRUCTURE AND ACTIVITY

The activity data of the previous section have two major applications: in deducing those structural features of agonists which correlate with intrinsic activity and those which correlate with potency and in deducing the topological features of the cellular site where these agonists produce their effect (the muscarinic receptor).

The prime structural features to be resolved are those which cause some compounds to be pure agonists of either high or low potency, some to be partial agonists, and some to be antagonists. In discussion of the hypotheses here the assumption is made that no chemical change occurs in the agonist during production of the muscarinic stimulus, even in instances in which chemically reactive groups are present; that is, ACh produces its measured effect independent of its later disposition (by hydrolysis). A change in the effector site (the receptor) is not excluded. As this site is a biochemical structure, its features cannot be deduced from activity data alone, but hypotheses can be eliminated, refined, or newly formulated with such data.

Over the years proposals and theories have varied with the information available. The following discussions present them in substantially chronological order.

A. Site of Muscarinic Action

1. RECEPTORS

Clark (*105*) demonstrated that ACh inside a smooth muscle cell produced no stimulus, and he calculated that the amount required to produce a stimulus could cover only a small fraction of the involved cell surface. This and other evidence indicate that ACh acts at certain restricted cell sites and, according to the terminology of Langley (*106*), who called these "receptive sites," they are termed receptors. Receptors may be pictured as local areas on a large macromolecule such as a protein. More broadly, following Schueler (*107*), a receptor may be defined as a pattern of diverse forces forming a part of some biological system and having roughly the same dimensions as the pattern of forces presented by the drug molecule under discussion, such that a relationship of complementarity for interaction exists.

2. VARIOUS ACh RECEPTORS

Because ACh is a neurotransmitter at many different sites, the obvious question arises whether the receptors at the ganglionic and postganglionic synapses and at the skeletal neuroeffector junction are identical or, if not, in what way they differ. Adequate data indicate that the ganglionic (nicotinic) and the striated neuromuscular receptors do differ from the muscarinic, as evidenced by the dissimilar structural requirements of drugs that stimulate these sites (see Chapters 3 and 5).

A more important question is whether the various muscarinic receptors are identical for, if they are not, data from tests involving different sites should not be used for quantitative comparisons. There is evidence both for and against identity; atropine, for example, abolishes ACh action at all muscarinic sites and in a way quantitatively similar to that of different muscarinic agents (*22*). Gyermek and Unna (*108*) concluded from a study of ACh and of muscarinic agents on rabbit and rat intestine and uterus, on frog and dog heart, and on dog bladder, that the constancy of potency ratios for all the compounds and the similar ranks in potency revealed a single type of receptor. On the other hand, Gyermek (*109*) obtained results according to which he proposed different functional sites for the bladder and for other organs. Lee and Shideman (*110*) found that higher homologs of amyltrimethylammonium have a muscarinic effect on the heart-lung preparation of the dog but not on isolated cat papillary muscle. Van Rossum (*89*) demonstrated a difference in receptors of rat intestine and frog heart.

Although it appears that all muscarinic receptors are not identical, they certainly possess remarkable similarities. Whether the differences result from transport through the surrounding area (the biosphere or biophase) or from the receptor itself is unknown. Certainly, caution must be exercised in comparing values obtained from one tissue with those from another. For this reason the tables of data contain tests from more than one tissue.

3. RECEPTOR SPECIFICITY

Whether drug receptors are essentially "active sites" on proteins, such as exist in enzymes, is not known, but the comparison is often made (*111*). Even if they are, there is no a priori reason why a drug receptor should be as structurally specific for agonists as some enzymes are for substrates. However, as seen in the previous section, there is a limited structural range of high potency, and minor changes can have major effects in decreasing potency. Thus, it appears that the muscarine receptor is rigidly built (*112*). The question whether the receptor pre-exists in whole or in part or whether the proximity of the agonist induces it (in whole or in part) is one for which an answer is as yet unavailable but most desirable.

4. ACTION VIA DISPLACEMENT OF ACh

It is conceivable that a compound would be inactive if attached to the muscarinic receptor but would mimic muscarinic action as a result of the displacement of ACh from storage sites near the receptor. Renshaw et al. (*113*) explained the brief duration of the action of ethoxycholine by postulating that the action was really due to ACh liberation from storage sites via exchange adsorption. Cavallito (*114*) proposed the same for amyltrimethylammonium.

If such were, in whole or in part, the mode of action of some compounds, then comparisons often would be misleading, as they might be comparisons of structural requirements for displacement from silent, or storage, binding sites rather than of muscarinic receptors.

5. ACTION AT THE RECEPTOR

a. Qualitative Aspects

Since the action of ACh at the muscarinic receptor produces a stimulus, there must be some specific union between ACh and the receptor. As ACh is easily washed off most tissues, this binding is readily reversed. The ACh molecule can form a limited number of bonds with other molecules: polar or coulombic (onium N, oxygens), hydrogen (oxygens), van der Waals (hydrocarbon moieties), and hydrophobic.* Clark (*105*) and Renshaw (*73*) pictured the initial process of binding as a selective adsorption mainly of a saltlike type; Croxatto (*116*) as a "crystallization" into the receptor; and Riker (*117*), as ionic attraction plus additional forces of chemical binding. Belleau (*96*) has stressed the concept that van der Waals forces are significant only where there is a true lock and key fit of drug and receptor. Wilson (*118*) stressed the role of hydrophobic bonds in the attachment of Me_4N^+ to receptors, and Belleau (*96*) extended this concept to the muscarinic receptor. Whether hydrogen bonds play a role in receptor–ACh interaction is not known, but the role of this bond in the ring oxygen of muscarine has been emphasized by Waser (*86*).

* Hydrophobic bonding was originally defined as involving nonpolar groups of proteins (*115*) but is now conceived of as involving small molecules too.

Whatever the manner of attraction and interaction, the presence of ACh at the receptor site leads to increased cell permeability followed by rapid influx and efflux of biophase ions. Most important appear to be increased sodium influx and potassium efflux (or, according to Daniel (*12*), increased calcium influx). The flow of ions is followed by an energy change that results in either excitation or inhibition of the innervated tissue. In the case of smooth muscle an excited cell can produce action in neighboring cells by electric stimulation. How one common action can produce both excitation and inhibition is not known. Eccles (*119*) pictures the action of ACh as an opening of fine channels or pores in the membrane structure through displacement of naturally occurring plugs; the opening of large channels, permitting ingress of sodium ions, causes excitation, and the opening of small channels, allowing escape of potassium ions but hindering entrance of the larger hydrated sodium ions, causes inhibition.

Clark (*105*) had postulated that for maximal activity all receptors were occupied and that submaximal action was proportional to the number of receptors occupied. Schild et al. (*102*) calculated that only about one in ten thousand receptors needs to be occupied by ACh to produce a maximal stimulus. This would indicate a receptor reserve, or spare receptors, as an insurance factor. Paton (*120*) pictures the degree of excitation as proportional not to the occupation of receptors but to the rate of receptor combination with ACh. Thus, he pictures ACh as rapidly "dancing on and off" the receptor. Belleau (*121*), postulating the receptor as part of a proteinlike macromolecule that has conformational adaptability to certain compounds, visualizes agonists as producing an effective conformational perturbation and inert compounds as producing an ineffective or nonspecific one. Which picture is correct is unknown, and probably every experimenter has a different one in his own mind.

b. Quantitative Aspects

On the basis of their theories of drug receptor action various authors have developed thermodynamic or kinetic equations to portray the variation of effect with concentration of agonist. Expressions developed by Clark (*105, 122*), Ariëns (*28*), and Stephenson (*25*) are well documented and thoroughly discussed by Ariëns and collaborators (*3*). Essentially, these are mass-action law equations or Langmuir adsorption isotherms, which relate the concentration of drug to that of the drug receptor complex, which latter in turn is related to the stimulus. Both Ariëns (*3*) and Furchgott (*123*) have stressed that the mathematical expressions are similar no matter what the theory of receptor action and that the equations derived offer no experimental method of differentiation. As thermodynamic calculations are independent of mechanism, this is not strange. At present little aid to comprehending *structural* relationships is offered by the mathematical equations relating concentration and stimulus. Utilizing Ariëns' equations (*3*) one can predict the type of curve resulting from dose–response studies with single drugs or with combinations of drugs and make some forecast of the change in a homologous series.

B. AChE and the Muscarinic Receptor

Nachmansohn (*124*) stressed the inseparability throughout the animal kingdom, of AChE and electric activity of all conducting tissue and postulated a primary role of ACh in nerve conduction. His postulates concerning the role of ACh in the nervous system are not generally accepted (*125*, *126*).

ACh ultimately is hydrolyzed by AChE to choline, a compound of such low potency as to be inactive at the final concentration. Whether the action of ACh is always terminated by hydrolysis of the enzyme or by diffusion from the site is unknown. Speculations have been made from both viewpoints (*14*). The fate of the ACh or choline formed also is unknown; possibly, some choline is returned to storage sites, where cholineacetylase converts it to ACh for future use (*14*).

Roepke (*127*), Gyermek (*128*), and Witkop (*87*) noted common structural features of compounds that interact with both the muscarinic receptor and with AChE. From his studies Schild (*129*) proposed two reactive sites for the ACh receptor of guinea pig ileum that he considered similar, if not identical, with the two reactive sites of AChE.

Župančič (*130*) on the assumption that Nature was too economical to utilize two proteins when one would do, postulated that the muscarinic receptor is identical with the site of hydrolysis of ACh on AChE. Waser (*131*) also regarded this as one possibility, others being two entirely different protein structures or two separate functional units in the same protein. He felt the last possibility was the most likely for the cholinergic skeletal muscle receptor. Both Beckett (*132*) and Belleau and Lacasse (*96*) noted the similar absolute and relative stereospecificities displayed for AChE and the muscarinic receptor by various series of compounds. Belleau et al. (*133*) drew an analogy between the energies of binding on AChE of the members of the homologous series alkyl-N^+Me_3 (alkyl = methyl to *n*-dodecyl) and the known effect of these compounds on the muscarinic receptor. A plot of free energy of binding versus length of alkyl group showed breaks at the amyl and nonyl derivatives, which correlated with muscarinic intrinsic activities (1 and 0, respectively). Further, a transition from negative to positive entropy of complex formation occurred at the nonyl compound, which was characterized as a change from an ordering to a disordering effect on the enzyme; on the assumption that the same changes would occur at the muscarinic receptor, Belleau (*133*) explained the change of agonist via partial agonist to antagonist in this series (see Table 2.6).

Thus the data indicate a close relationship between compounds acting at the muscarinic receptor and at AChE. Whether the receptors are similar sites (on different proteins or on the same protein) or whether they are dissimilar sites with some features in common will remain for future study to elucidate.

C. Spatial and Electronic Correlations

1. GENERAL DIMENSIONAL THEORIES

Hunt and Taveau (*32*) noted that those compounds which depart least from the choline structure produce the greatest effects. They postulated that the role of this group was to carry compounds to definite cell structures or to make them fit in a "certain mosaic." Dale (*6*), differentiating between muscarinic and nicotinic actions, noted that these varied independently with molecular modification and that active compounds possess some of each action. Renshaw (*73*) also believed that a special spatial configuration was required for the selective adsorption of these compounds, but after the synthesis and pharmacological evaluation of hundreds of onium compounds he was not able to characterize the structural features essential for muscarinic action (*134*).

By contrast, Barnes and Beutner (*135*) denied the importance of structure either in the compound acting or in the site of action; adequate electric potential at cell boundaries was considered the only necessary factor. Although the electric potential of a boundary is certainly of importance, theories based on the nonnecessity of specific structural features for muscarinic action have turned out to be fruitless.

A small or a highly flexible compound should be able to fit more effector sites in a cell structure than a larger or more rigid molecule. Such a compound should possess a wide spectrum of action. Schueler (*40*) felt that flexibility was advantageous and that it should be possible by statistical calculations to determine optimal configurations. An inspection of potent, naturally occurring compounds shows that they are often characterized, not by flexibility of structure, but by rigidity (e.g., steroids). It appears unlikely that a statistical calculation of the probability that a molecule will be in one conformation rather than in another would permit conclusions as to which conformation would be the most active. Information gleaned from highly flexible molecules must be tempered with data from fixed structures.

Ing et al. (*24*), by analogy with the furans, concluded that the carbons of the ACh appendage lie in a plane, but the determination of the correct structure of muscarine showed that this is not a necessary condition of activity; the ACh structure can be fitted almost perfectly to that of muscarine. 4,5-Dehydromuscarine and muscarone fit in between the two ring systems in both structure and potency.

Archer and co-workers (*82*), basing their ideas on rigid-ring tropane compounds (Table 2.15, No. 10), postulated a *trans* configuration of the nitrogen and ether oxygen of ACh as essential for muscarinic action. The spatial relationship of the tropane *trans* isomer is similar to that of 3-acetoxyquinuclidine, but neither is one of the most potent muscarinic types.

2. THE FIVE-ATOM RULE

Raventós (*57*) and Alles and Knoefel (*58*) had both noted that maximal muscarinic activity of compounds of the type $R\text{-}N^{+}Me_3$ resulted when the

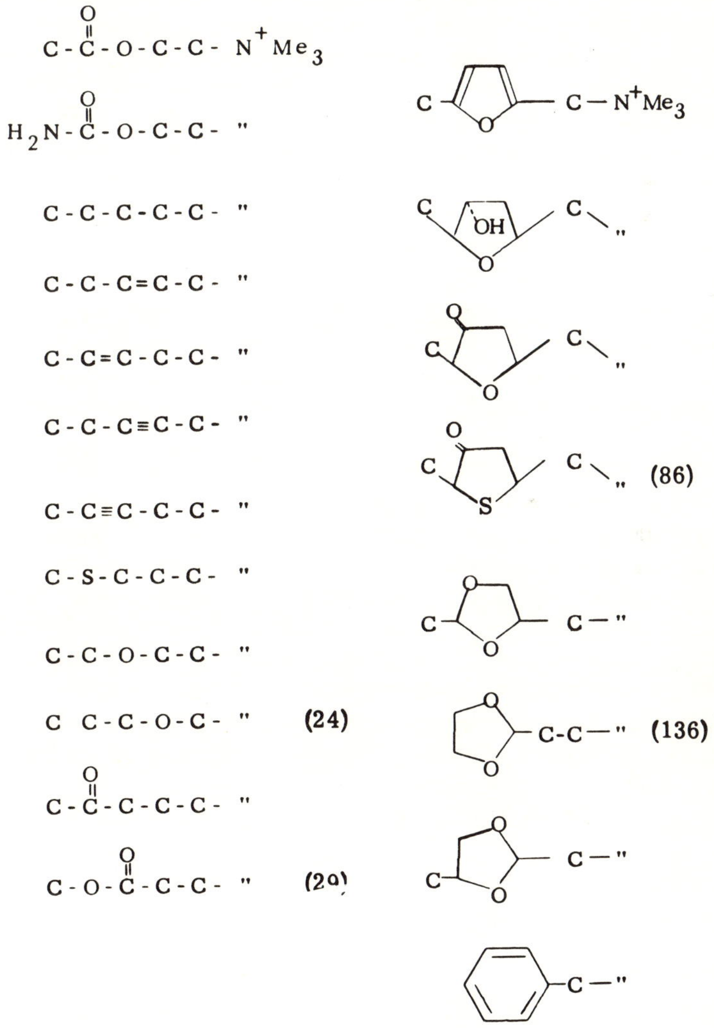

Fig. 2.6. Structures conforming to the five-atom rule. New references in parentheses.

substituent R contained a chain of five atoms exclusive of the hydrogens. It was Ing in 1949 (*31*) who formalized this into his well-known rule and who utilized it to prepare compounds of greater potency. The unusual scope of this simple rule is evidenced by the variety of structures that reach peak potency at

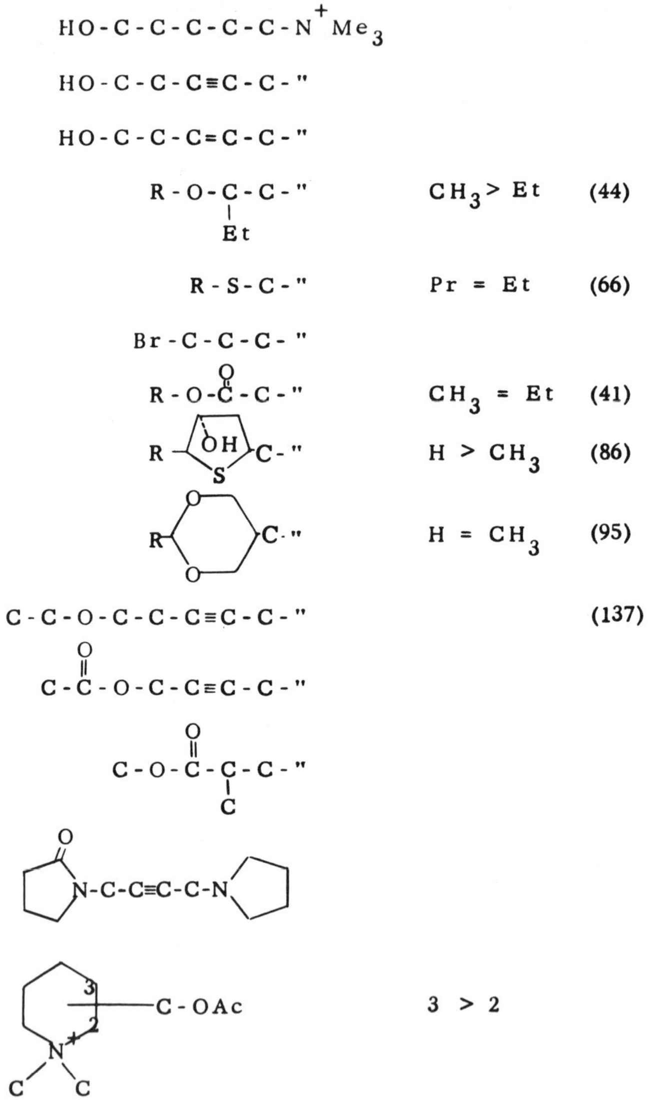

Fig. 2.7. Exceptions to the five-atom rule. New references in parentheses.

this chain length (Figure 2.6). Polar groups (S, O) or unsaturation can vary in position in the chain. In the ethylenic compounds both *cis* and *trans* forms reach maximal potency at five atoms.

Exceptions to the rule are listed in Figure 2.7. The fact that 2-trimethylammoniumethylfuran is less potent than its lower homologue led Ing to modify his rule (*91*) so as to specify maximal potency for the unit: oxygen function–$(C)_2$—N^+Me_3, but β-ethylcholine ethers do not fit this modification. The most glaring misfits in Figure 2.7 are those compounds containing a C≡C group. If it is assumed that larger atoms, such as Br and S, occupy the space of two CH_2— groups, then bromopropyltrimethylammonium and thiomuscarine are not true exceptions.

The fifth-atom group is most often methyl, and the effect of such an inert small moiety in producing extra potency has stimulated many to offer explanations. Ing (*31*) postulated that a precise fit between drug and some macromolecular cell structure was required for high activity. Waser (*86*) felt that van der Waals forces binding this otherwise inert group might be the explanation and, that in the case of muscarine, an inductive effect of the CH_3 on the ether oxygen might additionally play a role. Beckett et al. (*23*) likewise proposed that the fifth atom might increase electron availability for those compounds in which the ether oxygen was present. Belleau and Lacasse (*96*) also stressed the role of van der Waals forces for certain preferred configurations. They further felt (*121*) that Ing's rule of five was relevant where the phenomena of hydrophobic interactions were significant.

It is of interest that in the series of alkyl-N^+Me_3 (Table 2.6), where alkyl varies from methyl to amyl, minimal potency is found when alkyl is ethyl or propyl. This has never been explained satisfactorily, but it appears that here, as in the five-atom rule, spatial factors are of prime significance.

3. INTERPROSTHETIC DISTANCES

Alles and Knoepel (*58*), after noting that amyltrimethylammonium was the compound of maximal potency in the alkyl-N^+Me_3 series, calculated the length of this ion as 11.4 A and postulated a head-on fit to the receptor. Pfeiffer (*138*) measured on atomic models the distances between what he termed prosthetic groups. He proposed that muscarinic action depended on prosthetic oxygen atoms at a distance of approximately 5 and 7 A, respectively, from one or more methyl groups attached to the onium nitrogen. Ing (*31*) immediately criticized this concept, pointing out that many active compounds did not fit these measurements and many inactive ones did. Lands and Cavallito (*48*) calculated from measurements on models an appendage length of 7.5 A for a five-atom chain on the onium head and postulated that this size was associated with maximal potency. Hanna (*139*) modified this to maximal activity for onium ions at a distance of 5 to 7 A from a polarized group containing an electrophilic atom bound to a nucleophilic heteroatom to which are attached small substituents. From the structure of muscarine and the activity of all its isomers Gyermek and Unna (*140*) showed that the concept of distances between pharmacophore groups was not of itself a sufficient criterion, for the isomers they studied often had identical intergroup distances but markedly different potencies. Waser (*86*) found it necessary to postulate different configurations for muscarine and muscarone in an endeavour to account for the high activity of the wrong isomer in the muscarone series. He believed that in muscarone the C═O was responsible for hydrogen bonding (in place of the ether O of muscarine) and postulated that a distance of 4.2 A from nitrogen to ketone oxygen in muscarone corresponded to a 3.8 A distance (N to ether O) in muscarine. Synthesis of a few muscarone variants (keto group in place of ring O and C═O and O interchanged) might help to clarify the situation. Unfortunately, the onium group in these tetrahydrofuran compounds can rotate on the alpha carbon and, therefore, the actual O—N distances for the active conformation are not known. It may be that in the muscarine and muscarone series the five-atom rule plays a greater role than do specific distances between nitrogen and oxygens.

4. EFFECT OF SPECIFIC GROUPS

a. Cationic Head

The cationic head appears to be the only essential structural requirement for muscarinic activity; in Ariëns' terminology it confers intrinsic activity. It need not contain nitrogen, as other ionizable atoms are effective. The smallest cationic head, the trimethylammonium group, invariably confers the highest potency. Ing (*141*) postulated that two methyls are required for high activity and that these must fit into some component molecule of the receptor; thus, replacement of two methyls with larger groups, such as ethyl, would statistically reduce the correctness of fit and cause a large drop in activity. Van Rossum and Ariëns (*142*) pointed out that larger groups replacing methyl resulted in a decrease of the positive charge on the nitrogen, and they considered both this and the spatial factor of importance. Cavallito (*114*) also felt that the reduction in concentration of charge on the onium head weakened the binding of the electrostatic bond with an anionic group in the receptor, thus decreasing effectiveness.

In the change from N-diethylmethyl to N-triethyl-ACh the appreciable lowering of potency anticipated does not occur and, further, the compound has an intrinsic activity of 1 (on intestinal tissue). In other molecules the triethyl analog is either a partial agonist or an antagonist. Wilson (*143*) demonstrated that for ACh attachment to AChE the third methyl group on the nitrogen interacted with a marked decrease in the entropy of the complex without affecting affinity. Belleau and Lacasse (*96*) applied this same explanation to the lack of effect on replacement of the third onium methyl of ACh at the muscarinic receptor. On the assumption that hydrophobic forces were involved they predicted that groups bulkier than methyl would induce nonspecific perturbations leading to less active or inactive compounds.

When the onium nitrogen is in a ring system anomalies may result. Arecoline, which is a tertiary base, is about 30 times as potent as its corresponding methiodide (*80*, *112*). No good explanation of the decreased potency of this onium derivative has been offered. In some piperidine derivatives the N-methyl compounds are less potent than the N-dimethyl (onium) derivatives (*144*), and in others they are more potent. In 3-acetoxyquinuclidine methylation lowers activity 200-fold (*112*). Burgen (*80*) thought that the decrease in certain instances could be explained by an increased separation of the positive N from its opposite group in the muscarinic receptor. Whatever the cause, it does not appear predictable from present data.

b. Oxygens

Edwards and Marsh (*65*) concluded from a study of related ethers and ketones that the ether oxygen of ACh was more essential than the keto oxygen to muscarinic activity. Sekul and Holland (*145*) postulated that the fractional positive charge on the ether oxygen determined the degree of muscarinic potency and showed that in a series of ethers ($R—O—CH_2CH_2N^+Me_3$) the potency diminished with decrease in the electron-attracting effect of R. Both Barlow et al. (*37*) and Beckett et al. (*23*) attributed to the ether oxygen in the 3 position a function in production of intrinsic activity, characterizing it as a primary binding group effected via hydrogen bonding.

A keto group alone appears to be of negative value in an open chain, yet it greatly enhances potency in muscarone. When a keto group replaces a methylene adjacent to an ether oxygen, activity is potentiated (as in ACh and reversed ACh). In the case of muscarine and muscarone the keto and hydroxyl groups appear to be equivalent. If they are bound to identical sites by electronic forces, then it is difficult to picture a common bonding.

In general, introduction of a hydroxyl group lowers the potency of the parent compound. Both Lands (*38*) and Riker (*117*) felt that the OH group actually hindered attachment to the muscarinic receptor. However, in muscarine the hydroxyl is an exception, as it enhances potency 20-fold over the parent compound (Table 2.17, No. 9), and this potency is not increased by acetylation (Table 2.18, No. 2).

c. Effect of Unsaturation

Introduction of a C═C bond usually reduces activity in open-chain compounds, whether the bond is one or two —CH_2's removed from the onium ion, and this holds for both the *cis* and *trans* isomers. The same decrease in activity is found for the C≡C bond when it is one CH_2 removed, but marked enhancement is found when it is two CH_2's from the onium group. Many potent compounds containing the triple bond appear to violate Ing's five-atom rule. It does not appear that spatial factors are involved in enhancement of activity; indeed, the additional linear structure would be expected to decrease potency. Jacob et al. (*49*) attributed the enhancing effect to electronic influence exerted or transmitted (or both) by the triple bond. If this is so, it is difficult to account for the low potency of $AcOCH_2CH{=}CHCH_2N^+Me_3$, this being a vinylog of ACh.

5. POLARIZING FORCES

To account for differences in potency in molecules with similar interatomic distances Schueler (*146*) calculated what he termed the polarizing forces of atoms and of groups of atoms situated at the extremities of the ACh molecule and its congeners. An example is the series $Me_3N^+CH_2CH_2X$, where X can be OAc, I, Br, Cl, or OH. His calculations indicated a numerical trend, but one independent of sign. He therefore postulated that for any series of related groups the potency decreased as the absolute value of the polarizing force varied from that for ACh. Inspection of Schueler's data does show a trend, but the correlation is not adequate for prediction of quantitative potency. Certainly, a quantitation of the polar character of the onium head would be valuable, and it is hoped that Schueler's concept will be refined and become a more fruitful one.

6. ISOSTERIC REPLACEMENT

The determination of which groups are bioisosteric (*147*) can give an indication of those parts of the molecule which have a "space-filling" effect. It has already been noted that onium ions, where sulfur or phosphorus replace nitrogen, produce active compounds, whereas a quaternary carbon, which is not charged, causes loss of muscarinic activity. In Table 2.5 it is seen that replacement of the ACh ether oxygen with sulfur, selenium, or nitrogen gives compounds having an intrinsic activity of 1, although their potency is markedly decreased. In amyltrimethylammonium the exchange of an ether oxygen for CH_2 in position 3 ($Me_3N^+CH_2CH_2OCH_2CH_3$) gives a compound with retention of substantially equal potency; in other positions the replacement of the CH_2 by an ether oxygen markedly decreases potency. It appears that in these other positions the oxygen repels the compound from its receptor. There are inadequate data for determining whether one of the common bioisosteric pairs, CH_3 and Cl, produces equipotent compounds in the muscarinic series, but it appears that they do not. Thioketones are markedly less potent than their corresponding ketones. In the one instance known the replacement of keto with methylene (Table 2.10) produces a highly active compound. Replacement of the carbonyl of ACh with the SO_2 group markedly diminishes potency. Reversal of the ester group produces bioisosteric compounds, as has been shown in several other series (*147*).

More compounds need to be prepared and evaluated; for example, the hydroxyl group of muscarine should be replaced with the methyl group, and the ring oxygen should be replaced with CH_2. Where methyl occurs as the fifth-atom group, replacement with CF_3 should produce compounds of theoretical interest.

7. ROLE OF ANTAGONISTS

Clark (*122*) showed that atropine, acting as an antagonist to muscarinic agents, presumably acts at the same site as the agonists, as could be demonstrated by the equivalency of mass-action law constants. Ariëns (*3*) has also shown that in most instances this must be so, but he pointed out that the antagonist need not be attached at exactly the same site but could be bound on an adjacent point and thus block access of ACh. Fastier (*148*) showed schematically how structurally unrelated antagonists might block ACh. He pointed out that an antagonist need not present the same pattern of forces to the acceptor as ACh but, if the binding force were adequate, blockade could occur by means of a drug with an affinity for part of the receptor. There is a definite three-dimensional structural resemblance between atropine and ACh, but antagonist molecules require structural features not found in ACh. The fact that an antagonist need not possess a positive onium group (*3*) additionally points up the differences in binding. This is not to deny the great value of the study of muscarinic antagonists, but it does not appear that the data so obtained will lead to a better comprehension of structural relationship among the muscarinic agonists, nor is it definite that they will lead to a fuller comprehension of the specific mode of binding of ACh.

Antagonists are the subject matter of Chapter 3, and their structure–activity relationships will not be discussed here. However, as a general rule, substitution of increasingly large hydrocarbon groups on either terminus of ACh (the onium head or the ester CH_3) leads first to muscarinically inactive compounds and then to antagonists.

8. HYDROPHOBIC INTERACTIONS

Belleau has endeavored to account for the variable intrinsic activity of muscarinic agents and to establish a predictive rule (*121*) based on the induced-fit theory of enzyme action. He postulated that drugs could produce two types of perturbation in the protein component of the muscarinic receptor: a specific conformational perturbation, which would result in a muscarinic stimulus, and a nonspecific conformational perturbation, which would not. Belleau used the extended conformation of ACh as a reference structure and postulated that hydrophobic interactions in excess of those produced by ACh would determine whether a molecule would act as an agonist, a partial agonist, or an antagonist. With fifty-three selected compounds he showed that an almost perfect correlation existed between his calculation of excess hydrophobic interactions and the known intrinsic activity of these compounds. There are, however, exceptions. It is possible to replace two or even three of the *N*-methyl groups of ACh and still retain a compound with intrinsic activity equal to 1. As noted in Table 2.18, it is possible to introduce the phenyl group in the 3 position of muscarine with practically no loss of activity. According to Belleau's theory, this compound should be completely inactive, probably a potent antagonist. It is further noted in Table 2.18 that epimuscarine, which has an intrinsic activity of 1 when tested on the rat jejunum, has an intrinsic activity of only 0.1 when tested on frog heart; therefore, Belleau's hypothesis would probably have to be restricted to intestinal muscle. The intrinsic activity of the trichloromethyl analog of Belleau's acetal (Table 2.20) will be awaited with interest, as indicating how well it fits in his theory. It is difficult to see how potent compounds, such as oxotremorine and the acetylenic compounds of Jacob et al. (*49*, *59*, *60*), would fit into this system.

Until the intrinsic activity of many more compounds is measured, one must question whether Belleau's hypothesis is much more than a reflection of Ing's rule of five or, more logically (if we count the nitrogen and one of its methyls), a rule of seven over-all atoms. Linear extension at either end may produce compounds that have an intrinsic activity of less than 1, whereas substitution in the middle is subject to other, at present unknown, rules. It must be remembered that here no correlation with potency was attempted or implied.

9. OVERALL CONFIGURATION

Pfeiffer in 1948 (*138*) was the first to characterize the essential structural requirements for muscarinic activity. The limited number of compounds that had been studied and the erroneous designation of the structure of muscarine obviously hampered a correct solving of the problem. Exceptions to Pfeiffer's postulates were quickly pointed out. After studying a larger series of compounds Lands (*38*) recognized that oxygen was not a required atom, that the most potent compounds have at least one methyl group in the ionic head and another terminal methyl group at a distance of about 7 A units from the nitrogen, and that hydroxyl groups or large groups, such as aromatic or heterocyclic rings, were detrimental to muscarinic activity. Lands and Cavallito

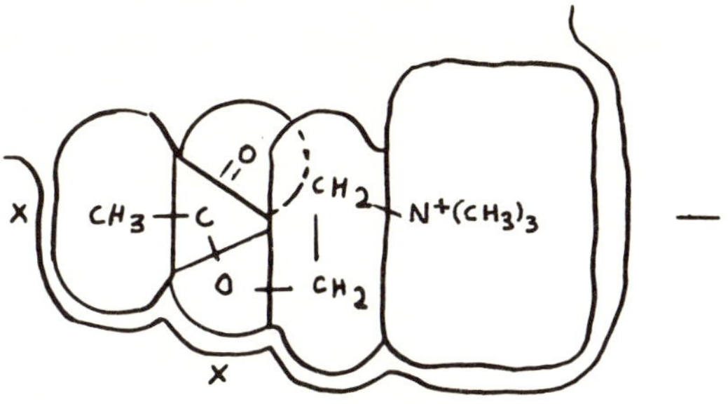

Fig. 2.8. The muscarinic conformation of ACh according to Marsh (*149*).

(*48*) further refined these concepts by including a cationic head of minimal size with an appendage of optimal length of approximately 7.5 A, the appendage being mainly linear and not containing strongly polar constituents. Marsh (*149*) was the first to delineate a spatial arrangement of the atoms of ACh that might account for its muscarinic (and also nicotinic) activity (Figure 2.8).

With the determination of the correct structure of muscarine and the synthesis of all its isomers and with the determination of the stereoconfiguration of β-methyl-ACh it became possible to see the structural similarity of a large number of the most potent muscarinic agents and to account for the low potency of many other compounds. Figure 2.9 depicts the similarity in stereochemistry of a substantial number of muscarinic compounds. It shows the flat furan ring with planar bonds and the tetrahydrofuran with nonplanar substituent bonds. High muscarinic potency is characterized by structural features, as follows.

In position 5 a methylene carrying a trimethylammonium group must be either in the plane of the ring or above it (in terms of the projection shown); in position 3 there must be a hydroxyl group below the ring or a ketone oxygen in the same plane; in position 2 the methyl group must either be in the plane of the ring or above it. It must further be assumed that position 4 is a neutral

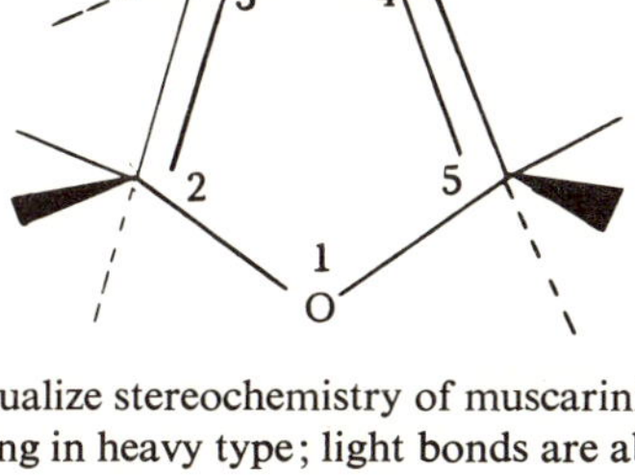

Fig. 2.9. Diagram to visualize stereochemistry of muscarinic compounds. Heavy bonds are in plane of ring in heavy type; light bonds are above and below ring.

position, as is also a substituent (other than a polar group) above the ring in positions 3 and 4. The carbon at position 4 may be absent; in place of one of the ring carbons in positions 3 or 4 there can be an ether oxygen, the 3—4 bond can be lacking, and the 3 or the 4 atom, or both, can be omitted.

With the exception of the acetylenic compounds and, perhaps, pilocarpine and some of the betaines, a vast number of muscarinic compounds fit into this limited structure. There are exceptions, such as the more active form of muscarone (Table 2.19) and the unexpectedly potent 4,5-dehydroepimuscarine (Table 2.18, No. 14).

Waser (*86*) explained the anomalous high potency of D(−) muscarone by assuming a conformation of the molecule in which the carbonyl group was located at the same portion of the receptor as was the ether oxygen of muscarine; the muscarone ether oxygen then took the place of the muscarine hydroxyl group. This offers an explanation, in the sense that the carbons and the onium group of muscarone are now superimposable on the muscarine structure. However, the high potency of the (+) isomer of muscarone is not thereby explained, nor does Waser's postulate accord with the low potency of open-chain ketones (Table 2.12). The author believes it more likely that the ether oxygen of muscarone plays the same role at the same site as does that of muscarine and that serious consideration should be given to the possibility that the ketone group of muscarone has a warping effect on the area adjacent to the receptor site, such that groups are accommodated below the plane of the ring. Thus, there is a sequence from muscarone to 5-methylfurtrethonium to muscarine, maintaining the same position for the locus of the ether oxygen.

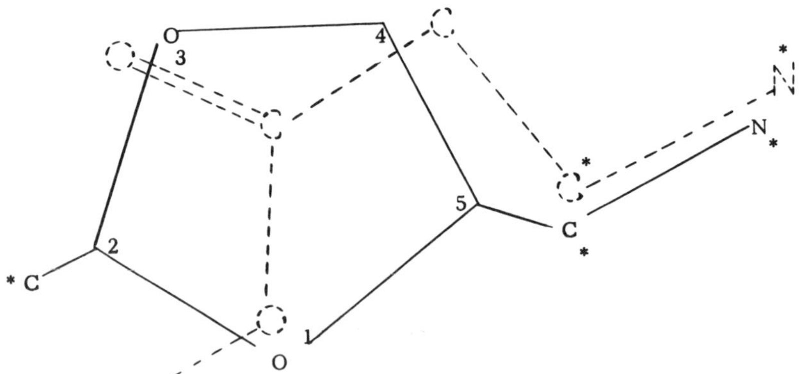

Fig. 2.10. Relation of reversed ACh to Belleau's acetal. Dreiding molecule projection, looking down on plane of ring. Starred atoms are above the plane of the ring, the carbonyl oxygen slightly below.

It is possible to find a conformation of reversed ACh (Figure 2.10) that has its atoms located almost exactly spatially, as in muscarine or Belleau's acetal. In this instance the beta carbon of the reversed ACh corresponds to the 4-ring carbon of the acetal, and this may be the reason why a β-methyl substituent in reversed ACh markedly lowers potency. Arecoline can fit into this pattern in a similar fashion; this is different from the active conformation suggested by van Rossum (*112*).

There are many compounds of low potency that fit the scheme given above. It does not appear at present possible to find one structure that will account for both potency and intrinsic activity. Further measurements of compounds known and yet to be made may make this goal attainable.

10. COMPOUNDS WITH MUSCARINIC SPECIFICITY

Whereas ACh is a multiple agonist, it was early recognized that muscarine possesses highly specific muscarinic activity; that is, it has negligible nicotinic or curaremimetic effects under usual experimental conditions. The same is true of the acetyl ester and the ethyl ether of β-methylcholine, pilocarpine, and oxotremorine. Numerous other compounds have been found to be more or less specifically muscarinic. This specificity appears to result from a poor fit of the nicotinic and curare receptors rather than from any special structural feature of these compounds.

D. Delineation of the Muscarinic Receptor

At the moment that a muscarinic agent triggers an impulse there must be a specific, active conformation of the receptor, whether the receptor is fixed or is induced. It is an interesting mental exercise to delineate a receptor structure that will explain the potency and intrinsic activity of muscarinic agents.

The major characteristic of all muscarinic agents is the onium head, and it has already been noted that this alone is adequate for activity. The main binding must therefore be made via this group and, logically, with a group of opposite charge in the receptor. Clark (*122*) postulated that the onium group probably reacted with a carboxyl group. He adduced as support the fact that on frog heart the concentration of ACh required to produce a given action increased with increasing pH. On the other hand, Ariëns (*150*) found that in rat intestine there was no change of the compounds furtrethonium and butyltrimethylammonium with pH, and he concluded that the anionic site on the receptor was a strong acid group. Schild (*129*) observed that raising the pH to 9 for guinea pig ileum abolished the effects of a weak base, such as pilocarpine, but had no effect on a strong base, such as ACh. Segre (*151*) studied the effect of pH (5.5 to 9.0) on guinea pig ileum, utilizing ACh, and found the affinity of the drug to the receptor to be a minimum at pH 6.7. Thus, the published results are inconclusive and require further experimentation to characterize the negatively charged group of the receptor. Speculation has been made that the onium binding might be effected with a sulfonic or phosphoric acid moiety, but there is at present no consensus, nor are there adequate data to designate what group is involved (*123*).

It is generally agreed that the ether oxygen or the keto oxygen can be bound either by hydrogen bonds or by coulombic bonds and that the methyl group, when in Ing's fifth position, must be held by van der Waals bonds. It is also generally held that the receptor itself is probably part of a protein molecule similar to an enzyme, although this still requires experimental proof.

Marsh (*149*), from evaluation of the available data, portrayed the muscarinic receptor as shown in Figure 2.8. He did not define stereochemical aspects and, had he known the correct structure of muscarine, he undoubtedly would have modified his representation. Lands and co-workers (*48*, *82*, *152*) conceived of the receptor as having the characteristics of a crevice or troughlike structure, in which the active drug is held at one end by electrostatic attraction to an anionic area by a small cationic head and by a second point of attachment to a polar oxygen at a distance of 4 to 7 A from the cationic head, the over-all length of the receptor surface being 7 to 8 A, measured from the anionic site, and being so structured as to accommodate the onium group *trans* to the ether oxygen.

Cavallito (*2*) further emphasized the limited accessibility of the onium head which, he felt, needed to be attached to a methylene "neck" so it could accommodate the onium head in the trough. Because α,α-dimethyl-ACh is approximately one twenty-fifth as active as ACh (dog blood pressure) (*153*, *154*), further studies are required to clarify the actual effect of substituents on the α-methylene group.

From his comprehensive studies of the muscarine and muscarone series Waser (*86*) felt that muscarine must have a close fit to the receptor and that it should be possible to elucidate the major aspects of the receptor from this series of compounds. He postulated ionic binding of the quaternary nitrogen and hydrogen bonding to the ether oxygen atom at a distance from the nitrogen of 3.8 A, slight binding of the hydroxyl group, and strong binding of the methyl group by van der Waals forces. Thus, Waser felt there were three strong binding groups in the receptor. He postulated that the ketone group, to accommodate the active form of muscarone, took the place of the ether oxygen, as previously discussed. Gyermek and Unna (*140*) felt that the receptor bound four groups of muscarine and that in addition to the ether oxygen of the ring the other three substituents of the tetrahydrofuran ring were bound. If one confines the data to muscarine, the receptor of Gyermek and Unna would appear to be identical with that postulated by Waser.

The most complete portrayals of the total muscarinic receptor are those presented by Beckett et al. (*23*) (Figure 2.11) and by Belleau and Puranen (*27*) (Figure 2.12). Barlow (*4*) has similarly shown the relation of natural muscarine to its surrounding receptor configuration; his picture appears a refinement of Beckett's. Beckett pictured the primary sites of association as the onium nitrogen and the ether oxygen (of muscarine or ACh) and considered the OH of muscarine (or the ketone of ACh) as secondary. Belleaú portrayed the same three sites but postulated a special role for the carbonyl of D(−)-muscarone (Figure 2.12, a) and ACh (Figure 2.12, b), which contributes additional binding energy. Belleau (*121*), by an alternate and more schematic picture, illustrated the specific conformational change produced by an agonist (Figure 2.12, c); this change should obviously be conceived in terms of the structure of Figure 2.12, b.

Eccles (*119*) has portrayed in a schematic, visualizable form how the receptor might look and how ACh could act on the one hand as a stimulant and on the other hand as a depressant. His picture of the action at the receptor shows a molecule that acts by pivoting another molecule to uncover a pore. For a molecule to act in this fashion it would have to be attached at two points and, although ACh and many other compounds might fit this picture, it is most difficult to see how tetramethylammonium could so act (except via ACh itself).

The receptor, being part of a living organism, presumably is characterized by mobility and adaptability. Yet, as structural requirements for potent muscarinic activity are limited, it is obvious that the receptor affords limited accommodation.

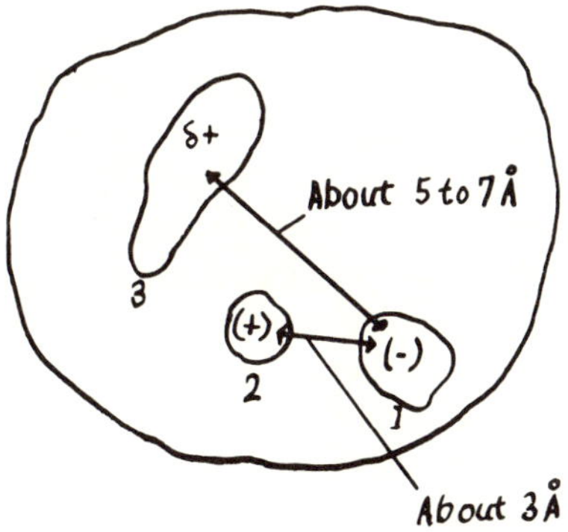

Fig. 2.11. The muscarinic receptor according to Beckett (*23*). 1, Anionic cavity to accommodate N^+; 2, positive point to accommodate ether O; 3, positive area for OH of muscarine, =O of ACh, =CH of furan. Quaternary N and ether O of muscarine lie in one plane and the lower portion of this plane (that with the OH) is the surface presented to the receptor.

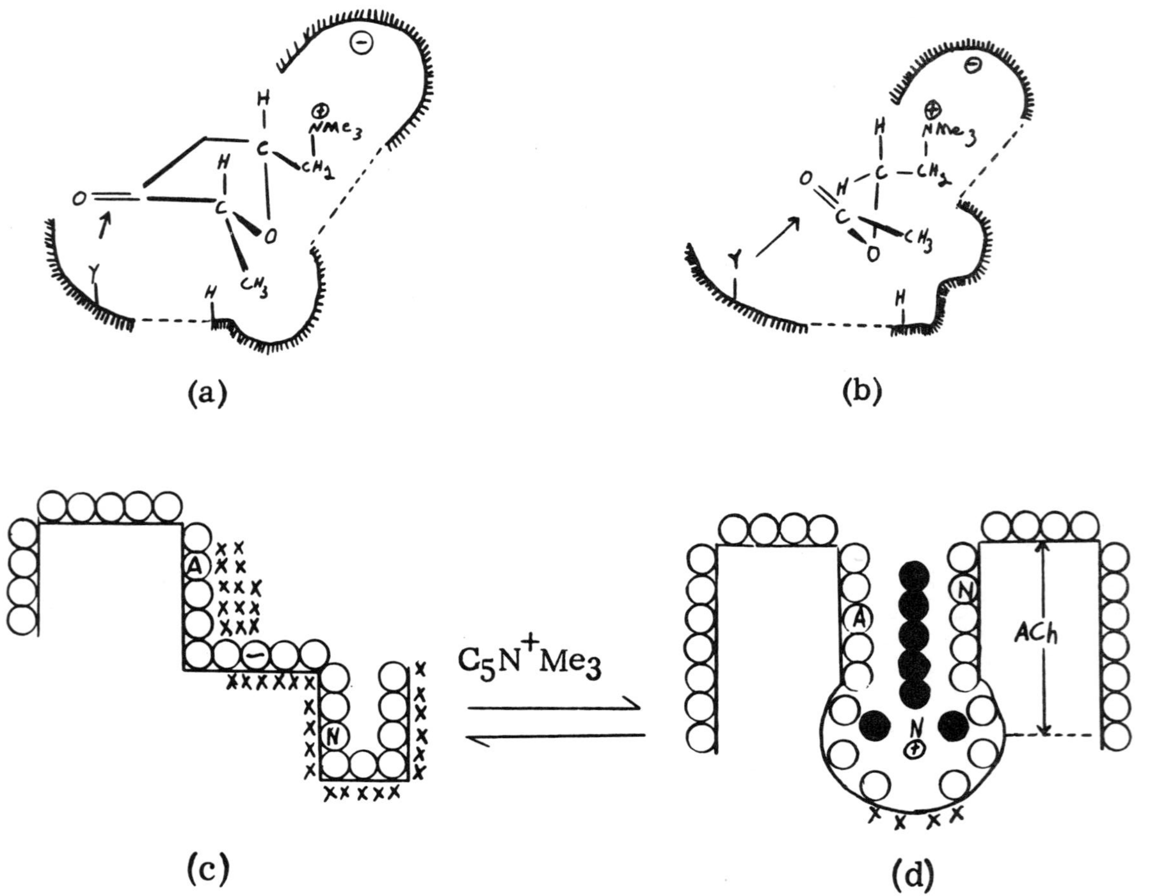

Fig. 2.12. The muscarinic receptor according to Belleau (*27*, *121*). (a) D(−)-Muscarone, (b) ACh, (c) $X = H_2O$, (d) $^{-}nH_2O$.

The author believes that the ACh receptor portrayed by Belleau (Figure 2.12, b) can be modified to give a fuller explanation of the molecules with high intrinsic activity and potency, if the following assumptions are made.

The muscarinic receptor is composed of two distinctly different areas: a small primary site containing a negative charge and a larger, more diffuse, secondary area.

The primary anionic site is limited in size and access of the onium group to it is somewhat restricted by the adjacent area. Small organic cations, if they approach closely enough, induce an interaction that triggers the muscarinic stimulus; this site alone is adequate to be termed the muscarinic receptor.

The occluding areas are adjacent to, and extend on, one side of the anionic site. These contain in a definite pattern an area of hydrogen bonding (the site of the ether O of ACh or muscarine), a limited area of van der Waals attraction (the "fifth-atom" site), and a coulombic area (the site of the C=O of ACh or muscarone). The function of these sites is to so orient the ACh molecule (or other related molecules) that the cationic head can reach the receptor anionic site. The first two of these sites are attractive forces. The third is postulated to be a repulsive force, one which has a special function in causing a warping action, which permits greater access of the whole molecule. Thus, although OH and C=O groups in general are repelling or disorienting and normally decrease the potency of compounds, their presence in one particular locus, that of the oxygen in the OH of muscarine or in the C=O of muscarone, is beneficial. It is likely that this same role is played by the C=O in oxotremorine and the C≡C in various compounds (Tables 2.2, 2.7).

The fit of the tetramethylammonium must be somewhat restricted, or else it would be as potent as ACh. A correct appendage is necessary for high potency. The effect of a proper appendage and, particularly, the effect of the "repulsing oxygen" can be seen in compounds containing the onium head —N^+Me_2Et (Tables 2.2, 2.3, 2.10, 2.14, 2.20); for, where the appendage lacks this group these compounds have an intrinsic activity of less than 1, and where it possesses this, the intrinsic activity is equal to 1. The greater effect of the muscarone ketone than of the muscarine hydroxyl is reflected in the potencies of the 2,2-dimethyl derivatives, the muscarone derivatives being the more potent (Table 2.18, No. 11, and Table 2.19, No. 5). It is acknowledged that more examples are required to prove this point, but it appears a logical one from the present data. It is to be noted that this "warping effect" is not adequate to overcome Ing's five-atom rule.

REFERENCES

1. D. Bovet and F. Bovet-Nitti, *Médicaments du Système Nerveux Végétatif*, S. Karger S. A., Basel, 1948.

2. C. J. Cavallito and A. P. Gray, *Progr. Drug Res.*, **2**, 136 (1960).

3. E. J. Ariëns, ed., *Molecular Pharmacology*, Academic Press, New York, 1964.
4. R. B. Barlow, *Introduction to Chemical Pharmacology*, 2nd ed., Wiley, New York, 1964.
5. R. Hunt and R. de M. Taveau, *Brit. Med. J.*, **2**, 1788 (1906).
6. H. H. Dale, *J. Pharmacol. Exptl. Therap.*, **6**, 147 (1914).
7. K. Krnjević and J. W. Phillis, *J. Physiol.*, **166**, 328 (1963).
8. P. B. Bradley and J. H. Wolstencroft, *Brit. Med. Bull.*, **21**, 15 (1965).
9. J. W. Phillis, *Brit. Med. Bull.*, **21**, 26 (1965).
10. L. Gyermek, E. B. Sigg, and E. Bindler, *Am. J. Physiol.*, **204**, 68 (1963).
11. G. Burnstock and M. E. Holman, *Ann. Rev. Physiol.*, **25**, 61 (1963).
12. E. E. Daniel, *Ann. Rev. Pharmacol.*, **4**, 189 (1964).
13. E. de Robertis, A. P. de Iraldi, G. R. de Lores Arniaz, and L. Salganicoff, *J. Neurochem.*, **9**, 23 (1962).
14. J. del Castillo and B. Katz, *Progr. Biophys. Biophys. Chem.*, **6**, 121 (1956).
15. G. B. Koelle, *J. Pharm. Pharmacol.*, **14**, 65 (1962).
16. G. Koelle, personal communication, 1965.
17. J. H. Welsh, *Bull. Johns Hopkins Hosp.*, **83**, 568 (1948).
18. E. Florey, in *Neurochemistry* (K. Elliott, I. Page, and J. Quastel, eds.), Charles C. Thomas, Springfield, Ill., 1962, p. 673.
19. W. C. Wescoe, in *Pharmacology in Medicine*, 2nd ed. (V. A. Drill, ed.), McGraw-Hill, New York, 1958, Chap. 25.
20. V. P. Whittaker, *Ann. N.Y. Acad. Sci.*, **90**, 695 (1960).
21. F. P. Luduena, in *Methods of Medical Research*, Vol. 8 (H. D. Bruner, ed.), Yearbook Publishers, Chicago, 1960, p. 142.
22. J. M. van Rossum and E. J. Ariëns, *Arch. Intern. Pharmacodyn.*, **118**, 418 (1959).
23. A. H. Beckett, N. J. Harper, and J. W. Clitherow, *J. Pharm. Pharmacol.*, **15**, 362 (1963).
24. H. R. Ing, P. Kordik, and D. P. H. Tudor Williams, *Brit. J. Pharmacol.*, **7**, 103 (1952).
25. R. P. Stephenson, *Brit. J. Pharmacol.*, **11**, 379 (1956).
26. E. Fourneau, D. Bovet, F. Bovet, and G. Montezin, *Bull. Soc. Chim. Biol.*, **26**, 516 (1944).
27. B. Belleau and J. Puranen, *J. Med. Chem.*, **6**, 325 (1963).
28. E. J. Ariëns, *Arch. Intern. Pharmacodyn.*, **99**, 32 (1954).
29. F. W. Schueler and H. H. Keasling, *J. Pharmacol. Exptl. Therap.*, **103**, 222 (1951).
30. J. Banister and V. P. Whittaker, *Nature*, **167**, 605 (1951).
31. H. R. Ing, *Science*, **109**, 264 (1949).
32. R. Hunt and R. de M. Taveau, *Hygienic Laboratory*, **Bull. 73**, 11 (1911).
33. T. F. Burks, J. P. Long, L. L. Darko, and J. G. Cannon, *Federation Proc.*, **24**, 611 (1965).
34. J. M. van Rossum, *Arch. Intern. Pharmacodyn.*, **140**, 592 (1962).
35. F. C. Nachod and A. M. Lands, *Trans. N.Y. Acad. Sci.*, **16**, 2 (1953).
36. E. J. Ariëns and A. M. Simonis, *J. Pharm. Pharmacol.*, **16**, 137 (1964).
37. R. B. Barlow, K. A. Scott, and R. P. Stephenson, *Brit. J. Pharmacol.*, **21**, 509 (1963).
38. A. M. Lands, *J. Pharmacol. Exptl. Therap.*, **102**, 219 (1951).
39. F. W. Schueler and C. Hanna, *Arch. Intern. Pharmacodyn.*, **88**, 351 (1951).
40. F. W. Schueler, *Arch. Intern. Pharmacodyn.*, **93**, 417 (1953).
41. R. R. Renshaw and R. Hunt, *J. Pharmacol. Exptl. Therap.*, **37**, 309 (1929).
42. A. H. Beckett, N. J. Harper, J. W. Clitherow, and E. Lesser, *Nature*, **189**, 671 (1961).
43. B. W. J. Ellenbroek and J. M. van Rossum, *Arch. Intern. Pharmacodyn.*, **125**, 216 (1960).
44. A. Simonart, *Arch. Intern. Pharmacodyn.*, **48**, 328 (1934).
45. W. B. Geiger and H. Alpers, *Arch. Intern. Pharmacodyn.*, **148**, 352 (1964).
46. R. Hunt and R. R. Renshaw, *J. Pharmacol.*, **25**, 315 (1925).
47. A. Simonart, *J. Pharmacol. Exptl. Therap.*, **46**, 157 (1932).

48. A. M. Lands and C. J. Cavallito, *J. Pharmacol. Exptl. Therap.*, **110**, 369 (1954).
49. J. Jacob, I. Marszak, L. Bardisa, A. Marszak-Fleury, and R. Epsztein, *Arch. Intern. Pharmacodyn.*, **91**, 303 (1952).
50. I. Marszak, M. Olomucki, R. Epsztein, and J. Jacob, *Compt. Rend.*, **238**, 166 (1954).
51. J. Salle, *Arch. Intern. Pharmacodyn.*, **91**, 339 (1952).
52. H. C. Chang and J. H. Gaddum, *J. Physiol.*, **79**, 255 (1933).
53. H. Erlenmeyer and H. Lobeck, *Helv. Chim. Acta*, **20**, 142 (1937).
54. V. P. Whittaker, in *Hefter's Handbuch der Experimentellen Pharmakologie*, Vol. 15, Springer, Berlin, 1963.
55. B. V. R. Sastry, C. C. Pfeiffer, and A. Lasslo, *J. Pharmacol. Exptl. Therap.*, **130**, 346 (1960).
56. K. A. Scott and H. G. Mautner, *Biochem. Pharmacol.*, **13**, 907 (1964).
57. J. Raventós, *Quart. J. Exptl. Physiol.*, **26**, 361 (1936).
58. G. A. Alles and P. K. Knoefel, *Univ. Calif. (Berkeley) Publ. Pharmacol.*, **1**, 200 (1939).
59. I. Marszak, J. Guermont, R. Epsztein, and J. Jacob, *Compt. Rend.*, **233**, 530 (1951).
60. J. Jacob, I. Marszak, R. Epsztein, and J. Guermont, *Compt. Rend.*, **234**, 1230 (1952).
61. G. A. Alles, *Univ. Calif. (Berkeley) Publ. Pharmacol.*, **2**, 161 (1944).
62. I. Marszak, R. Epsztein, and J. Jacob, *Compt. Rend.*, **231**, 1578 (1950).
63. P. Hey, *Brit. J. Pharmacol.*, **7**, 117 (1952).
64. L. Gyermek, personal communication, 1964.
65. J. E. Edwards and D. F. Marsh, *J. Pharmacol. Exptl. Therap.*, **103**, 196 (1951).
66. R. Hunt and R. R. Renshaw, *J. Pharmacol. Exptl. Therap.*, **44**, 151 (1932).
67. F. Kögl, H. Duisberg, and H. Erxleben, *Ann. Chem.*, **489**, 156 (1931).
68. A. J. Ewins, *Biochem. J.*, **8**, 209 (1914).
69. K. Credner, *Arzneimittel-Forsch.*, **6**, 31 (1956).
70. E. Fourneau, D. Bovet, and F. Bovet, *Ann. Pharm. Franc.*, **4**, 166 (1946).
71. R. Hunt and R. R. Renshaw, *J. Pharmacol.*, **35**, 99 (1929).
72. E. T. Eckhardt and F. W. Schueler, *J. Pharmacol. Exptl. Therap.*, **141**, 343 (1963).
73. R. R. Renshaw, *Science*, **62**, 384 (1925).
74. W. B. Bass, F. W. Schueler, R. M. Featherstone, and E. G. Gross, *J. Pharmacol. Exptl. Therap.*, **100**, 465 (1950).
75. E. Strack and K. Försterling, *Z. Physiol. Chem.*, **285**, 207 (1950).
76. A. S. V. Burgen and F. Hobbiger, *Brit. J. Pharmacol.*, **4**, 229 (1949).
77. M. D. Mashkovsky, *Intern. J. Neuropharmacol.*, **1**, 227 (1962).
78. R. Hunt and R. R. Renshaw, *J. Pharmacol.*, **35**, 75 (1929).
79. R. R. Renshaw, M. Ziff, B. Brodie, and N. Kornblum, *J. Am. Chem. Soc.*, **61**, 638 (1939).
80. A. S. V. Burgen, *J. Pharm. Pharmacol.*, **16**, 638 (1964).
81. L. Gyermek and K. Nador, *J. Pharm. Pharmacol.*, **9**, 209 (1957).
82. S. Archer, A. M. Lands, and T. R. Lewis, *J. Med. Pharm. Chem.*, **5**, 423 (1962).
83. E. F. Rogers, D. Bovet, V. G. Longo, and G. B. Marini-Bettolo, *Experientia*, **9**, 260 (1953).
84. F. Kögl, C. A. Salemink, H. Schouten, and F. Jelinek, *Rec. Trav. Chim.*, **76**, 109 (1957).
85. C. H. Eugster and P. G. Waser, *Helv. Chim. Acta*, **40**, 888 (1957).
86. P. G. Waser, *Pharmacol. Rev.*, **13**, 465 (1961).
87. B. Witkop, R. C. Durant, and S. L. Friess, *Experientia*, **15**, 300 (1959).
88. L. Gyermek and K. R. Unna, *Proc. Soc. Exptl. Biol. Med.*, **98**, 882 (1958).
89. J. M. van Rossum, *Science*, **132**, 954 (1960).
90. E. J. Fellows and A. E. Livingston, *J. Pharmacol. Exptl. Therap.*, **68**, 231 (1940).
91. A. K. Armitage and H. R. Ing, *Brit. J. Pharmacol.*, **9**, 376 (1954).

92. A. Enders and U. Schmidt, *Arzneimittel-Forsch.*, **4**, 331 (1954).
93. K. Bowden and G. A. Mogey, *J. Pharm. Pharmacol.*, **10**, 145 (1958).
94. D. J. Triggle and B. Belleau, *Can. J. Chem.*, **40**, 1201 (1962).
95. G. Tsatsas, *Ann. Pharm. Franc.*, **8**, 273 (1950).
96. B. Belleau and G. Lacasse, *J. Med. Chem.*, **7**, 768 (1964).
97. J. P. Fourneau, C. Menin, and A. Beauvillain, *Ann. Pharm. Franc.*, **16**, 630 (1958).
98. F. W. Schueler, *J. Am. Pharm. Assoc., Sci. Ed.*, **45**, 197 (1956).
99. W. D. M. Paton and E. J. Zaimis, *Brit. J. Pharmacol.*, **4**, 381 (1949).
100. S. Katsh and G. Keighley, *Am. J. Physiol.*, **174**, 431 (1953).
101. H. G. Schoepke and F. E. Shideman, *J. Pharmacol. Exptl. Therap.*, **129**, 322 (1960).
102. H. O. Schild, in *Enzymes and Drug Action* (J. L. Mongar and A. V. S. Reuck, eds.), Little, Brown, Boston, 1962, p. 435.
103. A. K. Cho, W. L. Haslett, and D. J. Jenden, *J. Pharmacol. Exptl. Therap.*, **138**, 249 (1962).
104. D. J. Jenden, data presented at Federation Meeting, Atlantic City, N.J., April, 1965.
105. A. J. Clark, *The Mode of Action of Drugs on Cells*, Edward Arnold, London, 1933.
106. J. N. Langley, *J. Physiol.* (*London*), **33**, 374 (1905).
107. F. W. Schueler, *Chemobiodynamics and Drug Design*, McGraw-Hill, New York, 1960.
108. L. Gyermek and K. R. Unna, *J. Pharmacol. Exptl. Therap.*, **128**, 30 (1960).
109. L. Gyermek, *Am. J. Physiol.*, **201**, 325 (1961).
110. W. C. Lee and F. E. Shideman, *J. Pharmacol. Exptl. Therap.*, **127**, 219 (1959).
111. J. L. Mongar and A. V. S. Reuck, eds., *Enzymes and Drug Action*, Little, Brown, Boston, 1962.
112. J. M. van Rossum, *J. Pharm. Pharmacol.*, **15**, 285 (1963).
113. R. R. Renshaw, D. Green, and M. Ziff, *J. Pharmacol. Exptl. Therap.*, **62**, 430 (1938).
114. C. J. Cavallito, in *Curare and Curare-Like Agents*, Little, Brown, Boston, 1962, p. 55.
115. W. Kauzmann, in *Advances in Protein Chemistry*, Vol. 14 (M. L. Anson and J. T. Edsall, eds.), Academic Press, New York, 1959, p. 37.
116. R. Croxatto and F. Huidobro, *Arch. Intern. Pharmacodyn.*, **106**, 207 (1956).
117. W. F. Riker, Jr., in *Pharmacology in Medicine*, 2nd ed. (V. A. Drill, ed.), McGraw-Hill, New York, 1958, Chap. 26.
118. I. B. Wilson, in *Enzymes and Drug Action* (J. L. Mongar and A. V. S. Reuck, eds.), Little, Brown, Boston, 1962, p. 460.
119. J. C. Eccles, *Science*, **145**, 1140 (1964).
120. W. D. M. Paton, *Proc. Roy. Soc. Med.*, **53**, 815 (1960).
121. B. Belleau, *J. Med. Chem.*, **7**, 776 (1964).
122. A. J. Clark, *Handbuch der Experimentellen Pharmakologie*, Vol. 4, Springer, Berlin, 1937.
123. R. F. Furchgott, *Ann. Rev. Pharmacol.*, **4**, 21 (1964).
124. D. Nachmansohn, *J. Am. Med. Assoc.*, **179**, 639 (1962).
125. S. Ehrenpreis, *Nature*, **201**, 887 (1964).
126. G. B. Koelle, in *Handbuch der Experimentellen Pharmakologie*, Springer, Berlin, 1963, p. 268.
127. M. H. Roepke, *J. Pharmacol. Exptl. Therap.*, **59**, 264 (1937).
128. L. Gyermek, *Acta Physiol. Acad. Sci. Hung.*, **8**, 43 (1955).
129. H. O. Schild, *J. Physiol.* (*London*), **153**, 26 (1960).
130. A. O. Župančič, *Acta Physiol. Scand.*, **29**, 63 (1953).
131. P. G. Waser, in *Enzymes and Drug Action* (J. L. Mongar and A. V. S. Reuck, eds.), Little, Brown, Boston, 1962, p. 206.

132. A. H. Beckett, *Proceedings First International Pharmacology Meeting*, Vol. 7, Macmillan, New York, 1963, p. 30.
133. B. Belleau, H. Tani, and F. Lie, *J. Am. Chem. Soc.*, **87**, 2283 (1965).
134. R. R. Renshaw, personal communication, 1937.
135. T. C. Barnes and R. Beutner, *Nature*, **164**, 109 (1949).
136. K. Balenović, N. Bregant, T. Galijan, Z. Štefanac, and V. Škarić, *J. Org. Chem.*, **21**, 115 (1956).
137. J. Jacob, I. Marszak, S. Cruck, and J. P. Guermont, *Compt. Rend.*, **239**, 1551 (1954).
138. C. C. Pfeiffer, *Science*, **107**, 94 (1948).
139. C. Hanna, *Proc. Iowa Acad. Sci.*, **58**, 245 (1951).
140. L. Gyermek and K. R. Unna, *J. Pharmacol. Exptl. Therap.*, **128**, 37 (1960).
141. H. R. Ing, *Chem. Ind.* (*London*), **(1951)**, 926.
142. J. M. van Rossum and E. J. Ariëns, *Experientia*, **13**, 161 (1957).
143. I. B. Wilson, *J. Biochem.*, **197**, 215 (1952).
144. J. Jaramillo, M.S. Thesis, Tulane University, New Orleans, La., 1962.
145. A. A. Sekul and W. C. Holland, *Arch. Intern. Pharmacodyn.*, **144**, 347 (1963).
146. F. W. Schueler, *Science*, **115**, 548 (1952).
147. H. L. Friedman, *Natl. Acad. Sci.-Natl. Res. Council Publ.*, *206*, Washington, D.C. 1951.
148. F. N. Fastier, in *Annual Review of Pharmacology*, Vol. 4 (W. C. Cutting, ed.), Annual Reviews, Inc., Palo Alto, Calif., 1964, p. 51.
149. D. F. Marsh, *Outline of Fundamental Pharmacology*, Charles C Thomas, Springfield, Ill., 1951.
150. E. J. Ariëns, in *Curare and Curare-Like Agents*, Little, Brown, Boston, 1962, p. 73.
151. G. Segre, *Arch. Intern. Pharmacodyn.*, **124**, 53 (1960).
152. A. M. Lands and F. P. Luduena, *J. Pharmacol. Exptl. Therap.*, **116**, 177 (1956).
153. W. B. Wheatley, *J. Am. Chem. Soc.*, **76**, 2832 (1954).
154. W. B. Wheatley, personal communication, 1965.
155. A. S. V. Burgen, *Brit. J. Pharmacol.*, **25**, 4 (1965).
156. B. Belleau, *Isotopes in Pharmacology* (L. Roth, ed.), Univ. Chicago Press, Chicago, 1965, p. 469.

CHAPTER 3

POSTGANGLIONIC PARASYMPATHETIC DEPRESSANTS (CHOLINOLYTIC OR ATROPINELIKE AGENTS)*

JOSEPH G. CANNON and J. P. LONG

STATE UNIVERSITY OF IOWA
IOWA CITY, IOWA

Although postganglionic parasympathetic depressants are specific antagonists of acetylcholine at the muscarinic receptor, in high concentration they may demonstrate many pharmacological properties (antihistaminic, adrenolytic, ganglionic, and neuromuscular, or skeletal, inhibition, and also direct musculotropic depressant action); the tertiary derivatives demonstrate varying actions on the central nervous system. This discussion of the relationships of structure to activity will be limited to the inhibitory action at the muscarinic receptor.

3.1. HISTORICAL

An accurate study of the actions of belladonna dates from the isolation of its alkaloids in pure form. Atropine was isolated by Mein in 1831, but it was not until the early part of the present century that samples of pure scopolamine became available. Bezold and Bloebaum in 1867 demonstrated the blocking of cardiac effects of vagal stimulation by atropine; various other inhibitory actions of atropine on the parasympathetic nervous system were noted during the next decade. Because of the availability of the pure alkaloid atropine was used by Crum-Brown and Frazier in their classic work on the increase in pharmacological properties (usually neuromuscular inhibitory actions) due to the quaternization of various naturally occurring alkaloids. It is only

* This investigation was supported in part by Research Grants M-10753 and NB-1396 from the Public Health Service, Bethesda, Maryland.

reasonable that early workers in this field devoted their attention to altering the structure of atropine or scopolamine, hoping to find a compound more selective in its actions or of significantly different duration of action. The standard of biological activity during this period was the compound's ability to produce mydriasis in rabbits. Results of these earlier studies have already been reviewed (*1–3*). Synthesis and evaluation of compounds containing neither the tropane ring nor tropic acid were reported in the late nineteen-thirties; since then most research has centered on synthetic compounds. References to these important contributions will be cited during the discussion of the influence of specific substitutions on activity.

3.2. STRUCTURAL FEATURES OF ANTICHOLINERGIC AGENTS

Certain structural features appear repeatedly in the many anticholinergic agents that have been synthesized and evaluated biologically. Pfeiffer (*4*) has pointed out steric influences involved in antagonizing acetylcholine; Lands (*5*) has outlined maximal and minimal spatial requirements for various substituents of the molecule.

A. Constituent Groups

The following molecular skeleton defines the structural features that appear in virtually every series of active compounds:

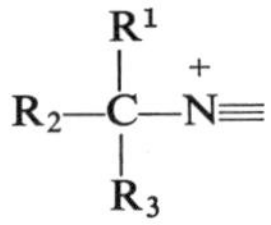

where R_1 is a planar ring, such as phenyl, thienyl, or furan, R_2 is a secondary substitution, which may be alkyl, aryl, or hydrogen, and R_3 is a hydrogen bonding group, such as hydroxyl or amide. The triple bond is a cationic head, which is quaternary ammonium or a tertiary amine with a pK_a such that a high percentage of the compound is protonated at biological pH; the carbon-to-nitrogen portion of the molecule may or may not contain an ester linkage.

B. Molecular Volume

The over-all molecular volume of the molccule and the charge distribution appear to be important factors:

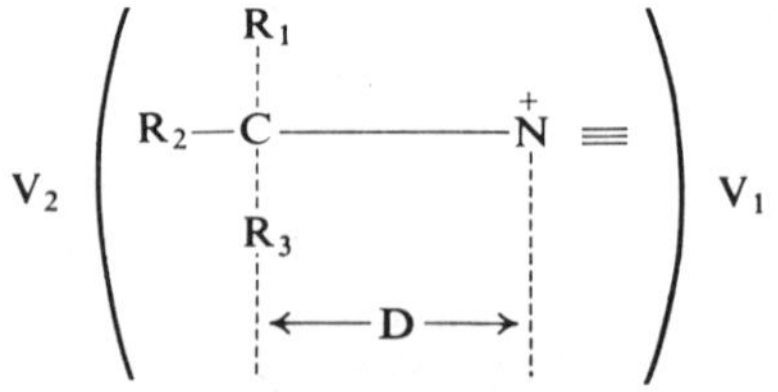

The various volume factors involved in inhibition at the postganglionic parasympathetic nerves (muscarinic receptors) do not appear to be as structurally specific as they are in stimulation of these receptors. The size of substitutions on the cationic head (V_1), the lipid-soluble portion of the molecule (V_2), and the over-all length of the molecule can be varied simultaneously and still retain significant blocking activity. The lipophobic portion of the molecule (V_1) may have widely varying substituents without loss of blocking activity, in contrast to the rather limited substitution permissible for cholinergic stimulating action. The steric factor shows a reverse effect from the blocking agents to the stimulating agents. Holton and Ing (*6*) demonstrated that progressive replacement of the *N*-methyl groups of acetylcholine with ethyl groups produces a progressive reduction in muscarinic activity. This may, perhaps, be expected if the cationic group in muscarinic agents serves to anchor the molecule to the receptor. Ing et al. (*7*) obtained maximal blocking activity by replacing the *N*-methyl groups of β-dimethylaminoethyl benzilate methyl chloride with ethyl groups. However, further increases in size to butyl or larger groups reduces or abolishes activity (*7–12*). The phosphonium and arsonium analogues of acetylcholine are clearly less active blockers than nitrogen analogues; this indicates further the maximal size restriction for the cationic head. The *N*-oxide derivatives appear to be less active than their parent compounds (*19*). These results make it tempting to speculate that for muscarinic or stimulating activity the small cationic head must fit into a definite space and must aid the neutralization of charge on the corresponding portion of the receptor surface. The inhibitory action is obtained when large enough groups are substituted on the cationic portion to prevent close contact with the receptor and, hence, a neutralization of charge (*13*, *14*). The cationic portion of the blocking agents provides the electrostatic forces necessary to orient the molecules toward the receptor and to hold them in place.

The lipophilic portion of the molecule (V_2) can also vary widely, as long as certain specific requirements are met. One of the substitutions must be a planar ring which is equal to or less than a phenyl group in volume. Compounds containing a substituted phenyl ring show a decrease in anticholinergic activity (*8*). It is improbable that inductive effects on the ring system cause this, considering that the decrease in activity is observed with both electron-attracting and electron-repelling substituents. The phenyl ring itself is not essential for activity (*5*). Moffett and Neil (*15*) reported high activity with various esters of Δ-α-cyclohexenyl, and Moffett et al. (*16*) reported high activity for Δ^2-cyclopentenyl-substituted and cyclopentyl-substituted acetic acids. Replacement of the phenyl group with α-thienyl does not interfere with the high activity (*17*, *18*). The secondary substitution (R_2) may be an alkyl group up to normal hexyl or an aryl group (*17*) equal to or less than phenyl in volume. It is interesting to note that an asymmetric quaternary carbon atom often increases the activity (*8*, *14*, *19*). A group capable of hydrogen-bond formation (R_3) attached to the quaternary carbon is a further requirement. Of course, the most likely group is a hydroxyl group, and it has been demonstrated many times that this substitution increases the activities of various homologous series (*5*, *9*, *20*, *21*). The inductive effects of an aryl group adjacent to or, at most, one carbon removed from, the hydroxyl or amide undoubtedly increases the tendency to hydrogen-bond formation. Many examples in organic chemistry substantiate this suggestion. The substitution for the hydroxy by sterically comparable groups, such as nitrile, leads to a sharp reduction in activity. R_1 and R_2 may be incorporated in the same substituents, as in fluorene and phenothiazine.

The structure between the substituted terminal carbon and the quaternary nitrogen, D, may be varied considerably without altering markedly the inhibitory action. The interatomic distance can vary from 5 to 9 A and still maintain high activity. Fromherz (*24*) obtained many potent esters with 3-diethylamino-2,2-dimethyl-1-propanol. Similarly, Schaumann (*25*) obtained significant atropinelike action with esters of 1-methyl-4-phenylpiperidine-4-carboxylic acid. However, the ester linkage is not essential for anticholinergic action and may serve only as a "spacing" group between the cationic head and the quaternary carbon. Winder et al. (*22*) observed significant atropinelike action with various quaternary salts of dimethylaminoethyl benzhydryl ether (diphenhydramine). Becker et al. (*23*) and Cunningham et al. (*20*) reported strong atropinelike activity with various substituted α-piperidinopropanes, and Lands et al. (*18*) described potent anticholinergic action with 2-diphenylaminoalkyl cyanides. Lands (*5*) obtained derivatives of 1-methylpiperidine approximately equal to atropine in activity. From this he concluded that the methylpiperidine ring was the important structure in the tropane ring and that relatively little additional activity is contributed by the second ring.

3.3. SUMMARY OF BASIC STRUCTURAL REQUIREMENTS

(1) The cationic site is essential for the binding of either muscarinic agents or their inhibitors. The steric factors appear less critical for inhibition than for stimulation. Optimal inhibitory activity usually appears with substitutions larger than methyl. Substitution with alkyl groups larger than isopropyl result in reduction in activity. Heterocyclic rings also appear to yield high activity.

(2) Cyclic substitution: at least one planar ring not larger than phenyl is needed for high activity, and the other substitution on the quaternary carbon may be an aryl, alicyclic, or alkyl group; thus far, substitution with groups larger than phenyl (e.g., *p*-bromophenyl) have resulted in a sharp reduction in activity, but whether this reduction is due to steric or inductive effects has not been established.

(3) The introduction of a hydroxyl group at an optimal distance from the nitrogen leads to significant increase in anticholinergic activity. The function of the hydroxyl group is probably to serve as a point of attachment on the receptor surface through hydrogen bonding.

(4) The "esteratic," or ester, linkages found in many anticholinergic agents may contribute to optimal activity, but their absence in a number of series of compounds clearly indicates that they are not essential for activity.

3.4. STEREOCHEMISTRY

Asymmetric substitution on the terminal carbon atom may produce an increase in anticholinergic activity (*8*, *14*, *19*). Whether this increased activity is due to a peculiar property of asymmetry, to a decreased free rotation of the quaternary carbon, or to some other factor has not been established. Since enantiomorphs possess the same chemical properties, the most obvious explanation of differences in activity would be a multipoint interaction with an optically active receptor. Much work has been done with the optical isomers of anticholinergic agents, and a discussion of stereoisomerism as related to this fundamental biological phenomenon is rightfully included in this chapter.

A. Nomenclature

From the beginning workers in the field of stereoisomerism and optical isomerism, in particular, have been plagued by difficulties in terminology. Emil Fischer could not determine the absolute configuration of an asymmetric carbon atom but, feeling an urgent need of some point of reference, he adopted the C-5 of glucose. He degraded the sugar to glyceraldehyde, in which a single asymmetric carbon remained, and arbitrarily assigned the following names and structures:

(+)-glyceraldehyde (−)-glyceraldehyde

All structures whose configuration correlated with (+)-glyceraldehyde were assigned by Fischer to this series; by the same token, those which correlated with the L-glyceraldehyde were placed in that series. Serine was adopted as the reference standard for α-amino acids, and its configuration was related to the glyceraldehydes.

Many different concepts for expressing configurations have been used. For a discussion of this aspect one should refer to a modern text of biochemistry. The Fischer method of notation has been used quite consistently through the years and is the most familiar, but other methods have been devised. One of them will be discussed (*26*, *27*). It depends on the three following steps. (1) Each of the four groups attached to the asymmetric carbon atom is assigned a priority sequence. This priority sequence is a function of the atomic number of the substituent. (2) From the priority sequence a clockwise or counter-clockwise pattern is determined; once this pattern is established a configurational label is assigned to the asymmetric pattern. R is used for the right-handed pattern and S for the left-handed pattern. The application of priority in a sequence may be illustrated by a compound CABCD, in which the substituents in decreasing atomic number are ABCD; the molecule is viewed from a direction remote from the smallest, or D, as in **(I)**.

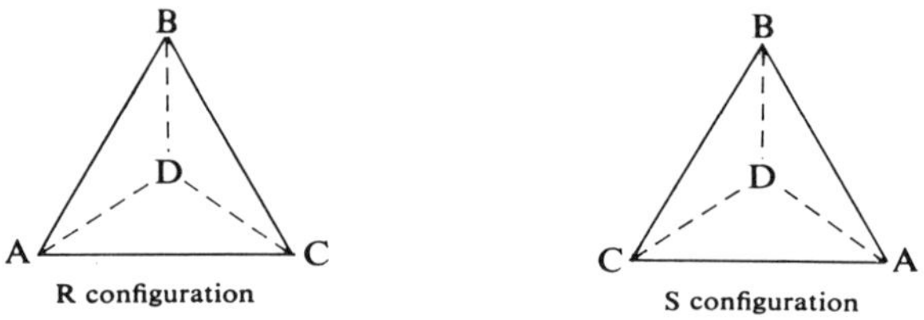

(I)

If the plane defined by A, B, and C shows these in clockwise sequence, the center is assigned the R configuration. If counterclockwise, it is assigned the S configuration. Obviously, this method must overcome certain problems before it will be readily accepted. First, most workers are acquainted with Fischer's terminology and, second, substitutions with the same atomic number must arbitrarily be assigned priority sequence. Nevertheless, the system appears to possess advantages and is being used more widely.

B. Stereochemical Configurations

Assigning correct absolute configurations to enantiomorphs is difficult. Fischer made an arbitrary assignation to (+)-glyceraldehyde. This stood until 1951, when X-ray analysis confirmed the absolute configuration. There is no correlation between the absolute configuration and the rotation of polarized light; on occasion the direction of rotation may even be inverted by changing the solvent. The usual methods of assigning stereochemical configurations (*28*) are conversion to D- or L-glyceraldehyde or to a compound already correlated, shifts in rotation dependent on temperature, dilution, addition of neutral salts, etc., application of optical rotatory dispersion, especially for polycyclic steroids, selective reactivity of an enzyme system, and selective adsorption of one isomer on an active surface.

The separation of stereoisomers is discussed in detail by Eliel (*29*). The formation of diastereoisomers has proved to be the most satisfactory method of separating rotamers.

C. Role of Stereoisomers in Biology

Pasteur's discovery that *Penicillium* preferentially attacks D tartrates marked the beginning of the importance of stereoisomerism in biology. Many examples have been cited during the past century that substantiate the influence of stereoisomers on biological activity. That various enzymes attack selectively one of a pair of enantiomorphs has been recognized for many years. Specific activity of a single enantiomorph has been observed repeatedly in autonomic pharmacology. However, after a century of observations and speculations biologists still have not explained the marked differences in activity usually observed with stereoisomers; for example, a D amino acid will taste sweet and the L isomer sour (*30*), and the various analgetic series, such as racemorphan (Dromoran) (*31*), and analgetic agents in general (*32*) demonstrate marked spatial selectivity with regard to their analgetic activity. The relatively inactive isomer usually has the same qualitative action as its epimer, but examples of antagonism of the active isomer by the weaker agent have been reported (*33*). The question of why this difference in biological activity exists has not been resolved. The usual explanation points to the possibility of multipoint attachment of a chemical to a receptor surface. This is shown for the anticholinergic agent trihexyphenidyl **(II)**; similar illustrations have been presented for atropine (*34*).

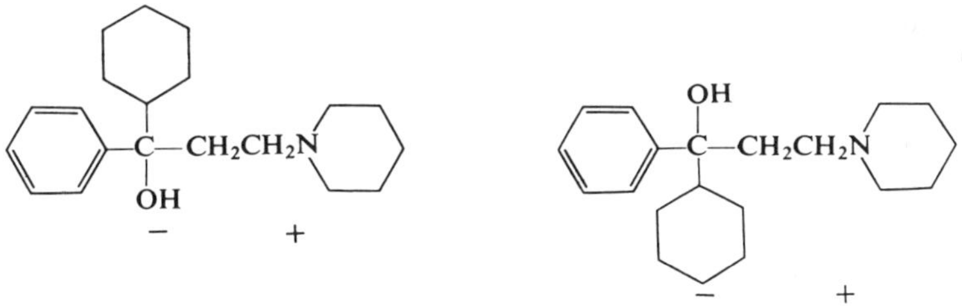

correct configuration — incorrect configuration

(II)

Other possible reasons for differences in biological activity may be related to selective absorption, distribution, or excretion of the isomers. The usual concept of drug–receptor interaction, in which a drug is adsorbed on the surface of an enzyme or an enzymelike material, is undoubtedly an oversimplification of the complex forces involved in attracting, arranging, and holding a molecule to the surface. Drug–receptor interactions, often overlooked as possible explanations of differences in biological activity, include charge-transfer complexes and alteration in the matrix of the receptor. Upon association with the receptor surface there is no longer a single isomer, but diastereoisomers. The number of possible combinations and interactions increases tremendously. Some of these possibilities are outlined in an excellent review by Hartung and Andrako (*28*). The elucidation of reaction mechanisms is further complicated by difficulties in obtaining pure isomers. Even with the most refined techniques it is often quite impossible to effect an absolute separation. The small activity of the relatively inactive species may be due entirely to contamination by the active one.

Therefore, whatever systems are used to explain the great biological differences in stereoisomers, whether they be merely a matter of orientation in space or in kinetics or of the energy requirements of interactions and binding forces between isomer and receptor, much additional study is needed to elucidate the mechanisms. This, as it did in the days of Pasteur and Cushny, probably offers one of the greatest challenges to biology.

3.5. SOME PHYSICOCHEMICAL ASPECTS

The cationic head of acetylcholine, its ester oxygens, and their distances from the cationic head are factors involved in the union of acetylcholine with its receptor cell protein and, thus, with its ultimate activity. An anticholinergic drug must have sufficient similarity to acetylcholine to displace it from its receptor sites. Since it is generally agreed that the functional group of prime importance in the acetylcholine molecule is the quaternary nitrogen head, and since all common anticholinergic agents are amino compounds (tertiary, quaternary, or tertiary amine oxides), and since it is likely (*35*) that non-quaternary amines exist in cellular fluids in the protonated form, it seems profitable to cite certain properties of organic nitrogen-containing cations. In an aqueous medium a nitrogen-containing cation is hydrated by a shell of electrostatically held water molecules. If appropriate structural features are present in the molecule, the water molecules will be held even more tightly by hydrogen bonds. The process of binding of a cationic drug molecule to an anionic receptor site must involve the loss of much of this water of hydration; furthermore, in bonding with a receptor site the cation must assume a fixed, or a relatively fixed, orientation, which results in a loss of entropy (*36*). These over-all losses in free energy must be compensated for by gains from bond formation. The chief stabilizing force is the electrostatic bond formed between the cationic head and the anionic receptor. This electrostatic bond is not a directed bond, and hence it does not impose the strict steric requirements of a covalent bond. Secondary contributions to bonding are derived from hydrogen bonding and from other covalent attractions, dipole interactions, and van der Waals attractions, which involve other portions of the molecule (*37*). The secondary attracting forces involve effects over a relatively short distance; thus, they will be greatly influenced by the shape of the molecule and by its ability to complement the shape of the site to which it is bonding. Conversely, to a greater or lesser extent the receptor site can apparently modify its stereochemical nature to accommodate the drug molecule.

From a purely physicochemical viewpoint the nature of the substituents on a cationic head derived from nitrogen is of the utmost importance and can be expected to determine the activity and the site of action of the molecule. Structure **(III)** represents a quaternary tetraalkylammonium ion; **(IV)**, a salt of a tertiary amine; **(V)**, the unprotonated form of a tertiary amine; **(VI)**, an amine oxide; and **(VII)**, the protonated form (salt) of a tertiary amine oxide. In solution, **(IV)** and **(VII)** are in equilibrium with their conjugate free base, whereas **(III)** exists completely in the ionic form shown. Because of this, **(III)** will exhibit a markedly different and more restricted distribution between cells than will **(IV)** and **(VII)**; it will be less able to penetrate membranes for which some degree of lipophilicity is necessary (*36*). The tertiary amine and the amine oxide can form stable hydrogen bonds with water in both the protonated forms [**(IV)**, **(VII)**] and the free-base forms [**(V)**, **(VI)**], whereas the quaternary **(III)** can be surrounded only by a loosely held shell of water bound by electrostatic attraction (*36*). No conclusion can be drawn about the net effect of these hydration phenomena at receptor sites; although the electrostatically held shell of water surrounding the quaternary **(III)** will be more readily displaced during the receptor bonding process, **(IV)** can hydrogen-bond with the receptor as well as with water. Moreover, **(IV)** may be expected to approach more closely the receptor and thus be held more firmly, by virtue of the diminished steric hindrance about the nitrogen atom (*36*). Klages et al. (*38*) have cited the slight basicity of tertiary amine oxides, which is further reduced

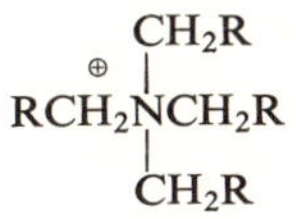

(III)

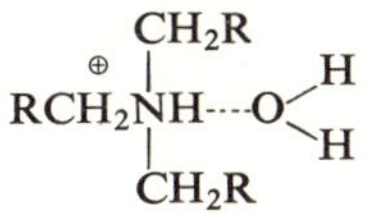

(IV)

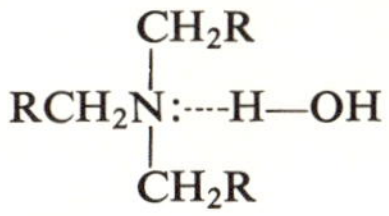

(V)

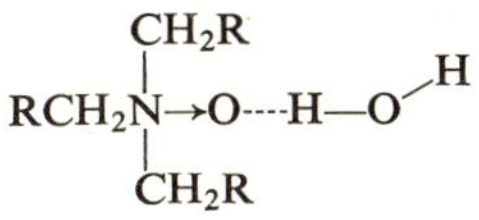

(VI)

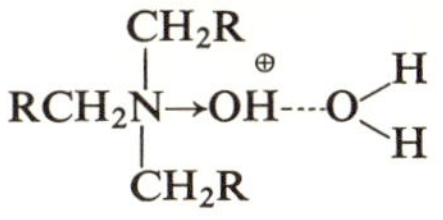

(VII)

by mesomeric or inductive effects. Despite their ability to form "onium" compounds with hydrogen chloride and with antimony pentachloride (*38*) it seems likely that an amine oxide will react with an in vivo receptor in the nonprotonated form **(VI)**. It should not be assumed, however, that a bond between a receptor and an amine oxide is necessarily weaker than one between a receptor and a quaternary ammonium moiety or an amine salt.

The proposals of Cavallito and Gray (*36*) regarding the role of hydration in the activity of amine cations seem eminently tenable and may have wide application in chemical pharmacology. Pempidine, **(VIII)**, and mecamylamine, **(IX)**, are ganglionic blocking agents, as is the primary amine analogue of **(IX)** (*39*). Bennett et al. (*40*) have suggested that the mode of action of mecamylamine differs from that of the quaternary ganglionic blocking agents. However, the ganglionic blocking potency of **(VIII)** and **(IX)** and of quaternary ammonium compounds may be related (inversely) to the extent to which their cations are hydrated in solution. Hall (*41*) has suggested that, although tertiary amine salts can bond covalently with only one water molecule, larger numbers of water molecules may hydrate primary and secondary amine salts through covalent linkages. Increasing the degree of steric hindrance about a primary or

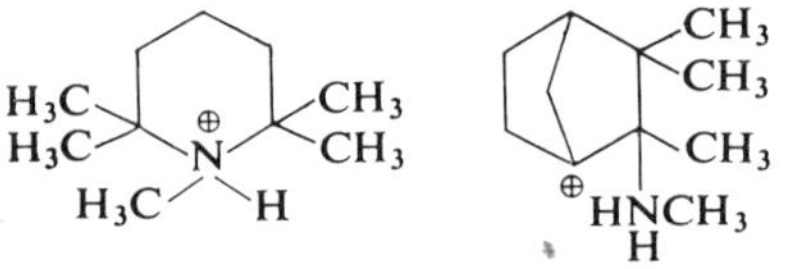

(VIII) **(IX)**

secondary ammonium ion apparently reduces greatly the ability to bond covalently with water, and thus the ion becomes more similar to a quaternary ammonium ion. It would follow that poorly hydrated cations are more capable of gaining access to, and bonding with, a muscarinic receptor site. Both mecamylamine and pempidine represent structures in which the amino group is highly shielded by adjacent groups. It is pertinent to note that Pierce (*35*) lists no primary or secondary amines as active cholinolytic agents.

The charge distribution on a quaternary ion can be modified by the groups surrounding the nitrogen. Tetramethylammonium ion exhibits maximal positive charge on the nitrogen (*36*). Substitution by larger alkyl groups will result in displacement of electrons toward the nitrogen, thus spreading the cationic charge. This process might be viewed as analogous to hyperconjugation in olefins (*42*); see structure **(X)**.

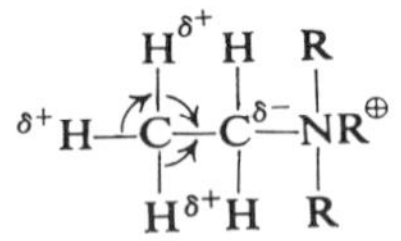

(X)

Cavallito and Gray (*36*) stated that the higher the concentration of charge on the nitrogen, the greater the stabilization derived from an electrostatic bond with an anionic site and the greater the strength of the stabilization. They further stated that substituents with loosely held, readily polarized π electrons will contribute effectively to the self-stabilization of the ion, as in **(XI)**. Thus, there is less energy to be gained from bonding with an external ionic group. If the quaternary group is further removed from the source of electrons, the interaction will be less. Ingold (*43*) has proposed that the trimethylammonium group attached to a benzene ring withdraws electrons from the ring by a negative *inductive effect* (the "−I mechanism"). The intensity of this effect at the aromatic nucleus is diminished by relay through a chain of saturated carbon atoms, becoming barely appreciable after relay through three intervening carbon atoms, as in **(XII)**. Unusually great charge delocalization occurs

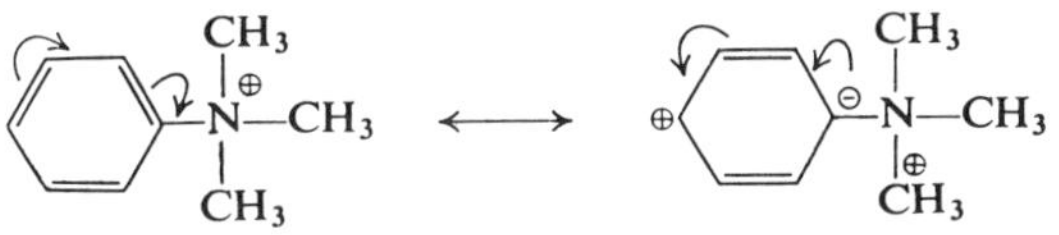

(XI)

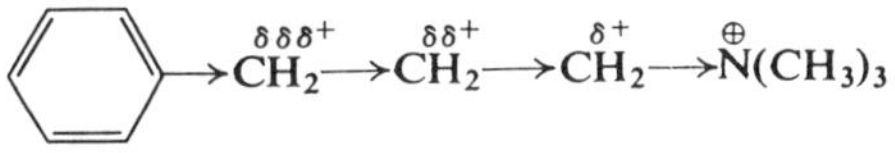

(XII)

in quaternary ions derived from aromatic nitrogen heterocycles, such as **(XIII)**. In addition to the form illustrated extreme resonance forms of **(XIII)** can be drawn, in which the unit positive charge resides on carbon 2, 4, or 6.

Cavallito and Gray (*36*) have cited the well-documented equilibrium between a quaternary such as **(XIII)** and an un-ionized *pseudo base*, **(XIV)**, and they have indicated that the concentration of the un-ionized form **(XIV)** increases with increasing pH. The ability of a quaternary compound to assume a form such as **(XIV)** in a reversible manner could facilitate passage of the molecule through a lipophilic barrier. Cavallito and Gray's statement that the proportionate amount of pseudo base increases with each aromatic ring that is fused to the heterocyclic system agrees with the findings of Hantzsch and Kalb (*44*) that the contribution of the pseudo base form is greater in quinolinium, isoquinolinium, and acridinium systems than in the pyridinium system. However, it must be borne in mind that the pseudo base equilibrium exists only under conditions of extreme alkalinity (*45*), such as are not attainable in vivo. Furthermore, Aston and Lasselle (*46*) have shown that even in strongly basic media the equilibrium in the quinoline system is far in the direction of the quaternary form. Thus, it would seem that caution should be exercised in attempting to ascribe physiological significance to the equilibrium between a quaternary and a pseudo base.

It should not be inferred that a tendency to delocalization of the positive charge on the cationic head of a cholinolytic molecule is necessarily undesirable; a partial dissipation of the positive charge may serve to give the molecule a greater degree of specificity of biological effect. There is a multiplicity of anionic receptors in the body, all of which have some degree of affinity for the cationic head of the drug, and with which the drug will interact. Some of these interactions will give rise to side effects, and others will merely bind the cation to an inactive site and prevent its reaching and attaching to an active center. A cationic head, especially a quaternary, with a somewhat dispersed charge would not be expected to bind to many weaker anionic sites and so provide a more potent and more specific action. It is of some interest

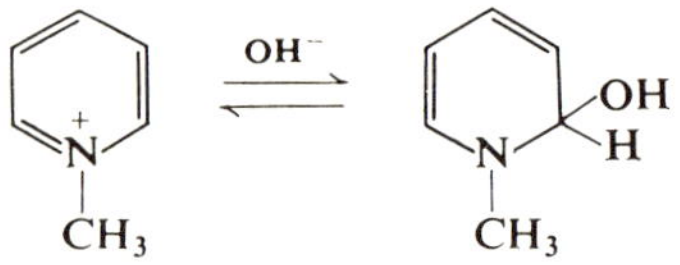

(XIII) **(XIV)**

that the hydrazinium analogue **(XV)** of acetylcholine was reported by Schueler and Hanna (*47*) to be much less potent than acetylcholine, whereas the methoxylamine analogue **(XVI)** has been shown to be at least one half as potent as acetylcholine (*48*). Both **(XV)** and **(XVI)** represent structures in which an electron-rich atom attached to the quaternary head would be expected to diminish the positive-charge concentration. It is difficult to rationalize the difference in activity between the two acetylcholine congeners according to charge distribution phenomena or steric effects. It must be concluded that with the present knowledge it is not possible to predict with any accuracy the biological effect resulting from either charge dissipation or charge concentration on the cationic form of a cholinergic or cholinolytic molecule.

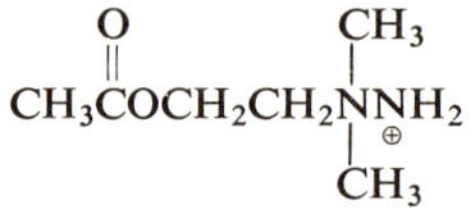

(XV)

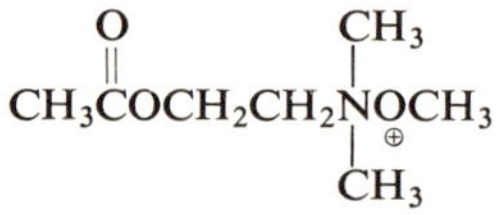

(XVI)

Thomas and Marlow (*49, 50*) have reached some conclusions concerning charge distribution effects in a series of quaternary acetylcholinesterase inhibitors, which may also be pertinent to quaternary cholinolytic structure. On the basis of Pauling's (*51*) representation of the electrical nature of the ammonium ion, NH_4^+, these workers proposed that the unit positive charge of a tetraalkylammonium ion is more or less uniformly distributed among the one nitrogen and four carbon atoms attached to it. These α carbon atoms have partial carbonium ion character and bear approximately 0.2 unit positive charge each. Thus, the unit positive charge on a quaternary molecule is dispersed over a five-atom system. See structure **(XVII)**. If this concept is true, it is incorrect to consider that a quaternary cation (and perhaps a primary, secondary, or tertiary amine salt) possesses a discrete, concentrated center of electropositivity. Even in the simplest system there would be a considerable dissipation of the charge. The affinity of the quaternary compound for the receptor is postulated (*49, 50*) to be due to the attraction between the anionic site and the partial positive charges on three of the α carbons, with a smaller contribution from the more distant partial charge on the nitrogen atom which, because of its tetrahedral nature, cannot approach the receptor as closely as

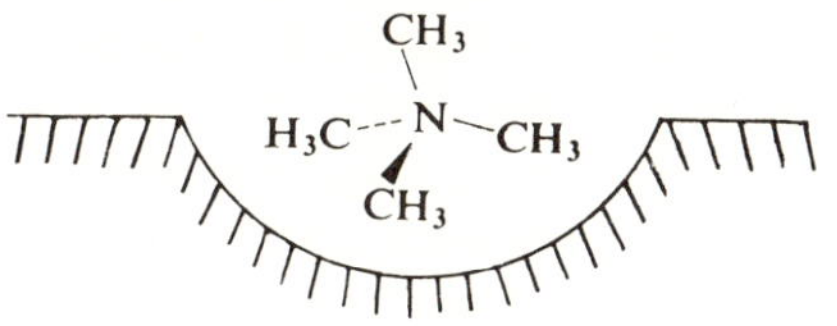

(XVII)

can the α carbons. In such a representation of the cation-receptor complex the stereochemistry of the quaternary head assumes even more importance.

Although the useful cholinolytic agents discovered up to the present time have been nitrogen compounds, it must be borne in mind that other members of the nitrogen family of elements (phosphorus, arsenic, antimony) may be incorporated into organic molecules, and cationic heads containing these elements have been prepared. Similarly, organic divalent sulfur compounds may be converted into trivalent "onium" structures. The literature has revealed that little consideration has been given to cholinolytic agents derived from sulfur, phosphorus, arsenic, or antimony rather than from nitrogen. However, Hunt and Renshaw (*52*) have reported studies on the cholinergic activities of a series of "onium" salts (*18–21*), which show the effect of replacement of the nitrogen in an organic cation with another atom. The sulfonium **(XVIII)** and phosphonium **(XIX)** analogues of tetramethylammonium had muscarinic effects analogous to, but somewhat less than, the parent nitrogen structure; the arsonium **(XX)** and stibonium **(XXI)** structures were of a very low order of activity. This same pattern of activity was followed in the nicotinic effects of the four compounds. Ing and Wright (*53*) concluded that the activity in this series is a function of the *total volume* of the cation (Table 3.1).

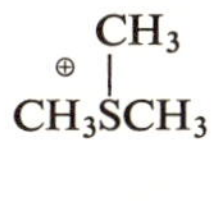

(XVIII)

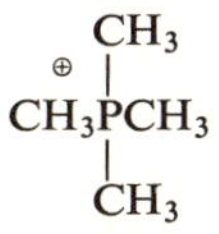

(XIX)

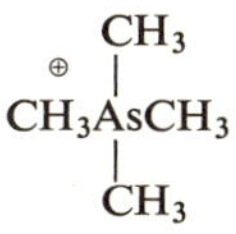

(XX)

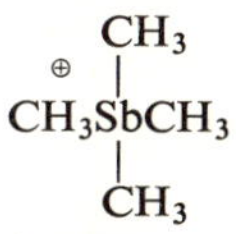

(XXI)

TABLE 3.1

Element	Covalent radius, A (*54*)	Volume, A³
N	0.75	1.77
S	1.04	4.7
P	1.10	5.6
As	1.18	6.9
Sb	1.36	10.5

Since the volume of a sphere varies with the cube of the radius ($V=4/3\pi r^3$), moderate changes in radius produce sizable changes in volume. The addition of methyl groups to the larger atoms further extends the size of the cation and may make the "onium" head too large to penetrate membranes or attach properly to a receptor. It appears that useful cholinolytic agents may be limited to the nitrogen series of compounds.

Among the most important structural moieties in the family of cholinolytic agents is the tropane system **(XXII)**. A vast literature exists on the relationship of the stereochemistry of tropane derivatives to biological activity (*55*). It is presumed by most organic chemists that in the ground state the piperidine ring of tropane exists in the chair form **(XXIII)** and not in the boat form **(XXIV)**. Considerations of dynamic equilibria favor the chair form (*55*). However, Hardegger and Ott (*56*) and Fodor and Nador (*57*) have presented chemical data indicating that in certain reactions in vitro the tropane alcohols exist in the boat conformation **(XXIV)**. The possibility exists that a biological receptor site can enforce a less favored conformation, such as **(XXIV)**, on the molecule

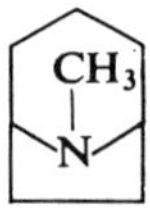

(XXII)

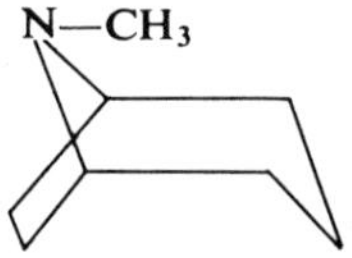

(XXIII)

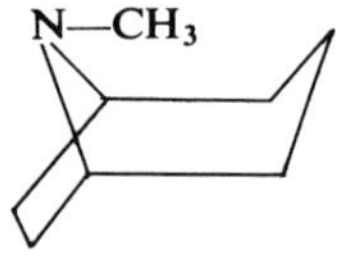

(XXIV)

of a tropane-derived cholinolytic agent. If the piperidine ring can indeed be converted from the chair to the boat, any ring substituents at position 3 or 4 (whether axial or equatorial) will have undergone a marked change of position in space relative to the nitrogen of the molecule. Such spatial changes may alter the ability of the molecule to attach to the receptor. The possibility of conformational interchanges in the tropane-derived series of cholinolytic agents greatly complicates considerations of interatomic distances and other stereochemical phenomena.

REFERENCES

1. A. R. Cushny, *Biological Relations of Optically Isomeric Substances*, Williams and Wilkins, Baltimore, 1926.
2. W. F. v. Oettingen, *The Therapeutic Agents of the Pyridine Group Including the Tropinol, Scopoline, Ecgonine and Granatoline Derivatives. The Relation between Their Chemical Constitution and Pharmacological Action*, Edward Bros., Ann Arbor, Mich., 1936.
3. E. Nyman, *Acta Physiol. Scand.*, **3**, 1 (1942).
4. C. C. Pfeiffer, *Science*, **107**, 94 (1948).
5. A. M. Lands, *J. Pharmacol. Exptl. Therap.*, **102**, 219 (1951).
6. P. Holton and H. R. Ing, *Brit. J. Pharmacol.*, **4**, 190 (1949).
7. H. R. Ing, G. S. Daws, and I. Wajda, *J. Pharmacol. Exptl. Therap.*, **85**, 85 (1945).
8. V. R. Meier and K. Hoffmann, *Helv. Med. Acta, Suppl. 6*, **7**, 106 (1941).
9. A. M. Lands, V. L. Nash, and K. Z. Hooper, *J. Pharmacol. Exptl. Therap.*, **86**, 129 (1946).
10. R. R. Burtner and J. W. Cusic, *J. Am. Chem. Soc.*, **65**, 262 (1943).
11. D. K. de Jongh, E. G. Van Proosdij-Hartzema, and P. Janssen, *Arch. Intern. Pharmacodyn.*, **103**, 141 (1952).
12. M. H. Ehrenberg, J. A. Ramp, E. W. Blanchard, and G. R. Treves, *J. Pharmacol. Exptl. Therap.*, **102**, 141 (1952).
13. A. M. Lands and G. J. Cavallito, *J. Pharmacol. Exptl. Therap.*, **110**, 369 (1954).
14. A. M. Lands and F. P. Luduena, *J. Pharmacol. Exptl. Therap.*, **116**, 177 (1956).
15. R. B. Moffett and J. Neil, *J. Org. Chem.*, **15**, 354 (1950).
16. R. B. Moffett, C. A. Hart, and J. Neil, *J. Org. Chem.*, **15**, 343 (1950).
17. A. M. Lands and V. L. Nash, *Proc. Soc. Exptl. Biol. Med.*, **57**, 55 (1944).
18. A. M. Lands, E. Ananenko, G. Jones, J. O. Hoppe, and T. J. Becker, *J. Pharmacol. Exptl. Therap.*, **96**, 1 (1949).
19. J. P. Long and A. M. Lands, *J. Pharmacol. Exptl. Therap.*, **120**, 46 (1957).
20. R. W. Cunningham, B. K. Harned, M. Clark, R. R. Cosgrove, N. S. Daugherty, C. Hine, R. E. Vessey, and N. N. Yuda, *J. Pharmacol. Exptl. Therap.*, **95**, 151 (1949).
21. J. P. Long and H. H. Keasling, *J. Am. Pharm. Assoc., Sci. Ed.*, **43**, 616 (1954).
22. C. V. Winder, M. E. Kaiser, M. M. Anderson, and E. M. Glassco, *J. Pharmacol. Exptl. Therap.*, **87**, 212 (1946).
23. T. J. Becker, E. Ananenko, G. Glenwoods, and L. C. Miller, *Federation Proc.*, **5**, 163 (1946).
24. K. Fromherz, *Arch. Exptl. Pathol. Pharmakol.*, **173**, 86 (1933).
25. O. Schaumann, *Arch. Exptl. Pathol. Pharmakol.*, **196**, 109 (1940).
26. R. S. Cahn and C. K. Ingold, *J. Chem. Soc.*, **1951**, 612.
27. R. S. Cahn, C. K. Ingold, and V. Prelog, *Experientia*, **12**, 81 (1956).
28. W. H. Hartung and J. Andrako, *J. Pharm. Sci.*, **50**, 805 (1961).
29. E. L. Eliel, *Stereochemistry of Carbon Compounds*, McGraw-Hill, New York, 1962.
30. C. P. Berg, *Physiol. Rev.*, **33**, 145 (1953).
31. E. L. May, in *Medicinal Chemistry*, 2nd ed. (A. Burger, ed.), Wiley-Interscience, New York, 1960, p. 327.
32. A. H. Beckett, *Progr. Drug Res.*, **1**, 455 (1959).
33. M. L. Tainter and M. A. Seidenfeld, *J. Pharmacol. Exptl. Therap.*, **40**, 23 (1930).
34. J. P. Long, F. P. Luduena, B. F. Tullar, and A. M. Lands, *J. Pharmacol. Exptl. Therap.*, **117**, 29 (1956).
35. J. S. Pierce, in *Medicinal Chemistry*, 2nd ed. (A. Burger, ed.), Wiley-Interscience, New York, 1960, p. 470.
36. C. J. Cavallito and A. P. Gray, *Progs. Drug. Res.*, **2**, 141 (1960).

37. J. H. DeBoer, *Advan. Colloid. Sci.*, **3**, 1 (1950).
38. F. Klages, E. Muhlbauer, and W. Uhl, *Angew. Chemie*, **68**, 704 (1956).
39. G. A. Stein, M. Sletzinger, H. Arnold, D. Reinhold, W. Gaines, and K. Pfister, *J. Am. Chem. Soc.*, **78**, 1514 (1956).
40. G. Bennett, C. Tyler, and E. Zaimis, *Lancet*, **II**, 218 (1957).
41. H. K. Hall, *J. Am. Chem. Soc.*, **79**, 5441, 5444 (1957).
42. L. F. Fieser, and M. Fieser, *Advanced Organic Chemistry*, Reinhold, New York, 1961, p. 141.
43. C. K. Ingold, *Structure and Mechanism in Organic Chemistry*, Cornell Univ. Press, Ithaca, N.Y., 1953, p. 232.
44. A. Hantzsch and M. Kalb, *Ber.*, **32**, 3109 (1899).
45. R. C. Elderfield, in *Heterocyclic Compounds*, Vol. 4 (R. C. Elderfield, ed.), Wiley, New York, 1952, p. 231.
46. J. G. Aston and P. A. Lasselle, *J. Am. Chem. Soc.*, **56**, 426 (1934).
47. F. W. Schueler and C. Hanna, *Arch. Intern. Pharmacodyn.*, **88**, 351 (1951).
48. T. F. Burks, J. P. Long, L. L. Darko, and J. G. Cannon, *J. Med. Chem.*, **8**, 841 (1965).
49. J. Thomas, *J. Med. Pharm. Chem.*, **3**, 309 (1961).
50. J. Thomas and W. Marlow, *J. Med. Chem.*, **6**, 107 (1963).
51. L. Pauling, *The Nature of the Chemical Bond*, 2nd ed., Cornell Univ. Press, Ithaca, N.Y., 1940, p. 71.
52. R. Hunt and R. R. Renshaw, *J. Pharmacol. Exptl. Therap.*, **25**, 315 (1925).
53. H. R. Ing and W. M. Wright, *Proc. Roy. Soc.* (*London*), **B114**, 48 (1933).
54. T. Moeller, *Inorganic Chemistry*, Wiley, New York, 1952, p. 134.
55. L. Gyermek and K. Nador, *J. Pharm. Pharmacol.*, **9**, 209 (1957).
56. E. Hardegger and H. Ott, *Helv. Chim. Acta*, **36**, 1186 (1953).
57. G. Fodor and K. Nador, *J. Chem. Soc.*, **1953**, 721.

CHAPTER 4

GANGLIONIC STIMULANT AND DEPRESSANT AGENTS

*LASZLO GYERMEK**

SYNTEX RESEARCH CENTER
AND
DEPARTMENT OF PHARMACOLOGY
SCHOOL OF MEDICINE, STANFORD UNIVERSITY
PALO ALTO, CALIFORNIA

4.1. INTRODUCTION

Since the physiologic functioning of autonomic ganglia involves acetylcholine (ACh) as the synaptic transmitter substance, stimulation and blockade

* Present address: Department of Anesthesia, School of Medicine, Stanford University, Palo Alto, California.

of the ganglia caused by other chemical agents must also involve ACh. Accordingly, ganglionic stimulants and blocking agents may function by influencing the formation, binding, transport, release, or metabolism of ACh. The action of the majority of ganglionic drugs may consist of either substituting ACh at a certain ganglionic receptor site or influencing enzymatic or other chemical factors (such as ionic ones) involved in the stimulating and blocking processes. The autonomic ganglion cells are in a unique position with respect to other neural synapses, where either the cholinergic nature of neurotransmission has not been established or the existence of additional "noncholinergic" transmission phenomena has been strongly suggested (*1*). Whether the relationship between the ganglionic stimulant and blocking agents and the synaptic transmission is restricted to cholinergic mechanisms or not is still a basic question. A comprehensive evaluation of all these topics would cover the relationships of ganglionically active drugs to all facets of ACh-mediated and other neurotransmission phenomena. This seems to be an almost impossible task at present, and therefore attention in this review will be directed primarily to areas of research where adequate information is available. Information is fairly full regarding the chemical structures of the substances in relation to biological actions that are accessible to quantitative evaluation. In many studies of the relationship between structure and activity in ganglia the drugs employed are considered to be substitutes for the neurotransmitter substance itself. The exact site of interaction, however, is not well defined, and it must be stressed that the effects of known ganglionic stimulant and blocking agents on the basic physiologic phenomena of neurotransmission are largely unexplored.

4.2. PHYSIOLOGIC AND PHARMACOLOGIC ASPECTS OF GANGLIONIC STIMULATION AND BLOCKADE

A. Reviews

Most of the reviews of the physiology and pharmacology of ganglionic synapses appearing in the last two decades were the results of an increasing interest in ganglionic blocking drugs following a detailed pharmacologic reevaluation of TEA about 20 years ago (*2*).

Neurophysiologic analysis of autonomic synapses was independent of the practical efforts of medicinal chemistry and pharmacology. It was started in the thirties and was continuously pursued. Outstanding reviews by Rosenbluth (*3*) and Eccles (*1*) concerned the transmission of nerve impulses at neuroeffector junctions and peripheral synapses. The recent, most comprehensive review of Eccles (*1*) on synaptic physiology offers a detailed discussion of important anatomic aspects and predominantly neurophysiologic explorations of autonomic ganglia. Eccles and his associates have published a long series of fundamental papers on these subjects in the last three decades. The results of recent neuropharmacologic studies (*4–8*) indicate the existence and functional complexity of different receptors within the substrate of sympathetic ganglia. Other important reviews of the physiology of synapses are those of Paton (*9*) and Perry (*10*), which deal with problems of chemical transmission at cerebral and autonomic synapses, give comprehensive descriptions of methods (including microelectrode techniques), and discuss the problem of acetylcholine release. Evaluating changes of ionic compositions of perfusing fluids in ganglia resulted in the suggestion that blockade of the transmission at the autonomic ganglia is not necessarily a competitive blocking of receptors of ACh but may be a direct action on the nerve cell metabolism (*10*). The reviews of Konzett and Rothlin (*11*) and of Trendelenburg (*12*) reflect the approach of the pharmacologists to problems involving the autonomic ganglia by outlining the characteristics of different stimulant and blocking agents with attempts to classify them pharmacologically as accurately as possible. Nicotinic and non-nicotinic receptors are discussed in detail by Trendelenburg (*12*, *13*). The similarities and differences between ganglionic and adrenal medullary receptor sites and chemoreceptors have been thoroughly described by Konzett and Rothlin (*11*). The reviews cited also give comprehensive descriptions of earlier work and of such physiologic aspects as the role of different receptive sites, possible transmitter agents, biogenic amines, the development of tolerance to blockade, and differences between sympathetic and parasympathetic ganglia. The physicochemical nature and the molecular structures of receptors in the ganglion cells may be analyzed by applying the techniques of drug–receptor interaction; these have been summarized and evaluated by Ariëns and Simonis (*14*) and include a critical appraisal, not only of the incompletely known structural features of receptors, but also of the still unexplored correlations between chemical structure and physicochemical properties of different classes of drugs, including the quaternary ammonium* type of neural stimulant and blocking agents. Whereas their review was concerned with the search for suitable means of expressing drug–receptor combinations, Barlow (*15*) embarked on other crucial aspects of drug–receptor mechanisms, the steric relationships. These are represented by three major facets: the arrangement in space of the pharmacodynamic groups of drugs, the arrangement in space of the receptor groups in the receptor unit, and the arrangement in space (on the biological surface) of the receptor units themselves. Specifically, the stereochemical criteria of nicotinic actions were analyzed by utilizing the structure of nicotine isomers and bisquaternary ganglionic blocking agents. The suspicion, raised earlier by Perry (*10*), concerning the existence of a mechanism other than competition for a receptor

* In this text many quaternary ammonium compounds and amines are listed in the cationic or free-amine form instead of the salt form.

site emerges also in Barlow's work. The suggestion is made that in the action of ACh a primary protein structure alteration takes place and leads to permeability changes before enzymatic mechanisms can come into play.

Two major reviews appearing in recent years summarize structure–activity relationships in a comprehensive fashion: that of Nador (*16*) on ganglionic drugs and that of Cavallito and Gray (*17*) on quaternary ammonium compounds. The latter deals extensively with such problems as the role of structural variations in the binding of blocking agents to specific and nonspecific sites and the distribution of the agents between sites of action and loss. It also offers an excellent compilation of data on curarelike agents. Because both reviews have several aspects in common with the present one, references will be made to them throughout the text.

An abundance of chemical and also qualitative pharmacological data is found in the detailed monographs of Guggenheim (*18*), Bovet and Bovet Nitti (*19*) and, especially, Craig (*20*). Comprehensive but shorter reviews have appeared on quaternary ammonium compounds (*21–24*), hypotensive drugs (*25*), and clinical aspects (*26*). Researches on selected classes of ganglionic drugs were the subject of a few major papers. Moe and Freyburger (*27*) described tetraethylammonium and other early ganglionic blocking agents. Ambache (*28*) summarized the pharmacological effects of atropine on the autonomic ganglia. Gyermek (*29*) and Gyermek and Nador (*30*) reviewed the ganglionic, atropinelike, and curarelike properties of a large class of tropane derivatives. Spinks et al. (*31*) presented a summary of the extensive work done in England on pempidine analogues. Guyonneau (*32*) summarized the autonomic pharmacology of diphenylaminoalkanes, amino ethers, and ester derivatives. Trendelenburg (*13*) described the pharmacological differences between the noncholinergic ganglionic stimulant and blocking agents and the "classical" cholinergic type of agent, and Gyermek (*33*) reviewed the ganglionic actions of 5-HT, related indoles, and their antagonists.

B. Pharmacologic Considerations of Transmission of Nerve Impulses in Autonomic Ganglia

A simplified scheme of the processes involved in ganglionic neurotransmission is depicted in Figure 4.1, where seven phases of transmission are indicated: (1) conduction of impulses in the myelinated presynaptic fibre, (2) conduction in the presynaptic terminals that are nonmyelinated, (3) release of ACh at the presynaptic terminals, (4) crossing of ACh at the synaptic gap, its occupation of receptors of the cell membrane, and its hydrolysis, (5) local response of postganglionic neuron to ACh, (6) initiation of propagated action potential, and (7) conduction in the postsynaptic axon.

Although these seven phases, outlined by Perry (*34*) in 1957, generally hold

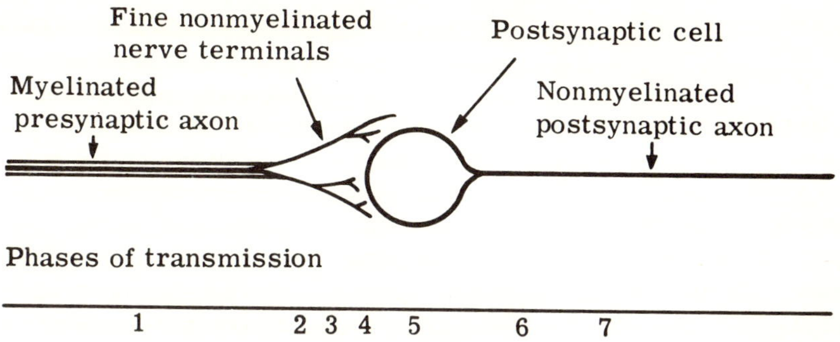

Fig. 4.1. Diagram of ganglionic synapse. Line at bottom shows transmission phases according to Perry (*10*).

today, some additions and modifications concerning phases 3 to 5 are indicated. It has been shown (*5*) that when ACh is liberated at the presynaptic terminal, besides passing to the postsynaptic receptor sites it acts on the presynaptic endings. Further, a positive feedback action of ACh in ganglionic transmission has been proposed on the assumption that the neurotransmitter substance may act at several receptor sites (that is, preganglionic and ganglionic sites). Regarding the nature of the receptor sites, recent studies indicate that the situation is far from being as simple as had been thought even a few years ago, when ACh was considered to act only on a single ganglionic receptor type. Pharmacologic studies made fairly long ago called attention to the possible existence of different cholinergic and noncholinergic receptor types. Lundberg (*35*) described the inhibitory action of epinephrine on ganglionic transmission, an action which is probably brought about through its hyperpolarizing effect on the ganglionic cell membrane. Since ACh can liberate epinephrine in the ganglionic chromaffin tissue, this device may provide a negative feedback circuit for regulating ganglionic transmission. A theory of ganglionic inhibitory action of physiologically occurring norepinephrine has recently been proposed by Costa et al. (*36*). The results of Muscholl and Vogt (*37*), in which the ganglionic norepinephrine content is depleted, does not, however, support this theory. The observations of Reinert (*38*) indicate that the bulk of epinephrine present in the ganglion originates from postganglionic adrenergic neurones and that under physiologic conditions epinephrine does not alter cholinergic neurotransmission. These results make it difficult to interpret the existence of ganglionic P waves, which were proposed by Eccles and Libet (*4*) to be of adrenergic origin.

Trendelenburg (*13*) first summarized the information on nonnicotinic types of ganglionic stimulants, among which histamine and 5-HT may have physiologic importance. Although these amines are not known to be liberated by stimulation of the preganglionic nerves their changing blood levels may influence ganglionic transmission.

Additional indication for the existence of different ganglionic receptors derives from older (*39*) and recent neurophysiologic studies (*4*, *40*, *41*) in which a series of pharmacological agents were extensively utilized as useful tools of exploration. Eccles and Libet (*4*) analyzed and evaluated the significance of three different types of postganglionic potentials elicited by preganglionic volleys. The first postganglionic spike potential (N) is the one which can be suppressed by typical ganglionic blocking agents (i.e., hexamethonium and *d*-TC). It is followed by a small second (P) wave and a later negative (LN) wave. The following behavior is characteristic of the last two components of the evoked action potential complex, as distinguished from that of the spike potential and from each other: (a) repetitive stimulation enhances the LN wave; (b) ganglionic blocking agents which block the spike potential do not influence the latter two; (c) anticholinesterases selectively depress the LN wave; (d) reserpine and to a lesser extent Dibenamine selectively depress the P wave; (e) atropine depresses P as well as LN; finally, (f) botulinum toxin which interferes with the release of ACh from presynaptic terminals depresses all these components. Based on these significant findings Eccles and Libet (*4*) proposed a scheme for illustrating the nature of chemical mediation at a sympathetic ganglion; the preganglionically liberated ACh may act at two receptor sites of the ganglion cell surface, those producing the spike potential (N-receptors) and those producing the delayed potential (LN-receptors), shown to be independent of the spike potential. It is possible that at least one bypass of monosynaptic cholinergic transmission exists which, through stimulation of chromaffin cells, liberates epinephrine by acting on another ganglionic receptor type. Although there is no evidence yet, it may be that other amines (for example, 5-HT) are involved in a similar bypass circuit. The triggering stimulus in such case also could be the presynaptically liberated ACh. Volle (*42*, *43*) showed that, besides ACh, agents like carbachol and tetramethylammonium (TMA) can act on the presynaptic terminals and may release ACh. These effects are blocked by atropine and procaine but remain unaltered by hexamethonium. On the basis of recent observations it is proposed that there are three different acetylcholinergic receptor sites in the ganglia (*42*, *43*): the *E-1* type, which is sensitive to ACh, TMA, nicotine, and 1,1-dimethyl-4-phenylpiperazinium bromide (DMPP) and is vulnerable to hexamethonium, the *E-2* type, which reacts to ACh, muscarine, methacholine, and anticholinesterases (this type can be inhibited by atropine), and the *I* type, on which ACh and methacholine act through hyperpolarization (this type also is sensitive to atropine). See Table 4.1.

This information clearly indicates that in autonomic ganglionic neurotransmission only one transmitter substance, ACh, is of major importance,

TABLE 4.1

Different Types of Ganglionic Stimulant Agents and Receptor Sites

Type of agent	Type of receptor *a*	*b*	*c*	Stimulant agent	Blocking agent
Cholinergic					
Nicotinic	N	E-1		ACh, DMPP, TMA, nicotine	Competitive: TEA, hexamethonium, nicotine Depolarizing: nicotine, TMA
Nonnicotinic	LN	E-2[d]		ACh, muscarine, methacholine, pilocarpine, McN-A-343, AHR-620	Atropine (cocaine, morphine), nicotine (depolarizing), TMA (depolarizing)
	P[e]			ACh	
Noncholinergic			M, B	Histamine, 5-HT, guanidines	Cocaine, morphine[f] (against all three), pyrilamine (against histamine), indoleacetamides, quaternary indolealkylamines, guanidines (against 5-HT and guanidines)

[a] Classification based on differences in action of different agents eliciting or modifying different components of evoked ganglionic potentials (*4*).

[b] Classification based on characteristics obtained in cat ganglion experiments with evoked ganglionic potentials and spontaneous postganglionic nerve activity (*42*).

[c] M and B receptors are distinguished from the muscular (D) or A receptors (*33*, *455*).

[d] ACh and methacholine act by a hyperpolarizing action on this receptor; atropine blocks.

[e] Through mobilization of epinephrine, producing inhibition.

[f] Cocaine and morphine blockade was reported for McN-A343 (*180*).

but this substance may act on three different receptor sites by different types of action. Although the proof of this might have been obtained through the purely neurophysiologic approach, the pharmacologic application of different ganglionic stimulants and blocking agents provided more decisive, although still not final, conclusions. In addition to the role of ACh the minor and modulating roles of other agents, such as the catecholamines, 5-HT, histamine, and inorganic ions, must be considered. The findings also show that in discussing structure–activity relationships of ganglionic agents a great deal of caution should be exercised, not only because of the possible heterogeneity of the chemical moieties that influence the type of action, but also because of the major differences attributable to the different conditions of known and generally used pharmacologic preparations. Therefore, comparisons are preferably made only concerning a series of a few closely related members of a certain chemical class, and the test objects. The experimental criteria for testing the compounds to be compared should be identical or at least very similar.

C. Receptor Sites and Ganglionic Agents

At present we are still far from being able to pinpoint the exact sites of action of ganglionic blocking agents. This problem can be approached through refined electrophysiologic methods and through biochemical model systems of interaction of drug and protein receptor. The results of electrophysiologic studies available so far are discussed in Section 4.2, B. The use of biochemical model systems is in its early stage, and knowledge is very limited. Certain protein fractions were found to react vigorously with some quaternary ammonium compounds but not necessarily with those which produce ganglionic blockade. A specific protein complex was obtained through precipitation with *d*-tubocurarine from the electric organ of the eel, and it showed high affinity to several quaternary ammonium compounds. This study suggested to Ehrenpreis (*44*) that interaction of tubocurarine involves hydrogen bonding with the protein and that phosphate protein groups may also be involved in the binding interactions.

The problem of ganglionic drug–receptor interaction is an important one. Because of the existence of structurally different classes of highly active ganglionic agents and a heterogeneity of the receptor sites the theories concerning optimal structural features and possible ways of interacting can differ considerably. The majority of investigators accept the concept that the basis of the interaction between ganglionic receptors and stimulant agents is a physicochemical bond formation operating mainly through the attachment of a cation to an anionic surface. It is generally thought that in ganglionic blockade the fundamental step is a replacement reaction between two cationic compounds which are exchangeable at the receptor surface and operate through a single or a multiple point of attachment. Ariëns and Simonis (*14*) postulate that the chief action of different antagonists occurs not at the receptor site of the agonist but in an adjacent, more indifferent, receptor area. The observation that many agonists show little or no chemical relation to the corresponding antagonists is also in favor of this hypothesis. The theory that blocking agents of highly polarized amine and ammonium types of stimulants (histamine, epinephrine, ACh) have less to do with the anionic sites of the receptors of the amines than with adjacent "supporting" sites calls for careful consideration and critical evaluation. In the case of the antagonism to ACh the theory may be valid with respect to the muscarinic receptor sites. Some stimulants of receptors strictly require an onium cation of limited size and, consequently, at least two methyl groups at the cationic portion of the molecule; by contrast, the antagonists of muscarinic sites are characterized by bulky acidic moieties or fused and usually three-membered ring systems, e.g., phenothiazines. Here the nature of the cationic portion seems to be of less importance. These structural requirements indicate that the assumption of Ariëns and Simonis (*14*) probably is valid for antimuscarinic, cholinolytic agents.

The different structural requirements of ganglionic blockade, as distinguished from blockade of the postganglionic parasympathetic receptor sites, has been widely discussed and will not be mentioned in detail here. In reviews such as that of Bergel (*45*) these differences are outlined with the conclusion that a change in the ester group of ACh reflects the combination and subsequent events at the muscarinic receptors rather than at the corresponding "nicotinic receptors."

The presently available data on the structure–activity relationships of ganglionic stimulant and blocking drugs indicate that, in contrast to the muscarinic receptor sites, ganglionic receptors are activated by a simple monoquaternary ammonium cation (for example, TMA) and are blocked to a considerable extent by a similarly simple ethyl-substituted congener (for example, TEA). It is true that additional functional groups can enhance ganglionic stimulant and blocking potencies either by increasing the affinity of the modified molecules or by increasing their selectivity through reducing their chances of being taken up by nonspecific receptors. However, most of the data indicate that ganglionic stimulant and blocking agents act by attachment to a single anionic site on the surface of the synaptic cell body. Chemical (primarily ionic and steric) factors may markedly influence this attachment to the receptor, but there seems no need to assume a multifocal type of attachment at the surface of ganglionic sites.

Regarding the nature of the onium cation, a high charge concentration is generally considered to be favorable to both stimulant and blocking actions at the ganglia (*17*). However, in the action of certain monoquaternary cations the redistribution of electric charge due to the polarization of electrons around a quaternary nitrogen seems to be important (*46*). This shift of charge is dependent on the electronegativity of the substituents on the nitrogen atom. Holmes et al. (*47*) reached the conclusion that in case of curarelike action a certain accumulation of charge on the nitrogen atom is necessary. However, in a series of alkyl and aralkyl monoquaternary ammonium compounds the relationships between the ganglionic activities and the structures of the compounds suggested that in ganglionic actions the electronic charge density of the nitrogen should be within a certain limit. Reciprocal correlations between curarelike and ganglionic effects in series of ammonium compounds with the general structure **(1)*** seemed to justify this assumption.

* Boldface numerals in parentheses refer to List of Chemical Formulas, pp. 309–315.

The problem of the combination of different bisquaternary ammonium ganglionic blocking agents and the receptor in a large number of different asymmetric and symmetric bisammonium compounds has been extensively studied. Contrary to earlier studies, which proposed a two-point attachment of these agents to anionic sites, Fakstorp et al. (*48*, *49*) concluded that one ammonium group attaches to the receptor while the rest of the molecule, including the second quaternary ammonium group, serves as a diffuse screen on the other adjacent parts of the receptor. Gill and Ing (*50*) suggested that the spatial configuration of the bisquaternary cation appears to be more important in ganglionic blocking action than the interquaternary distance, a consideration also in favor of a one-point attachment. Based on crystallographic measurements of pentamethonium iodide, Canepa (*51*) also questioned the validity of the two-point-attachment theory concerning configurational entropy, and he advanced the idea of an attachment to a single area of the membrane surface. It was also suggested that during synaptic transmission the ACh molecule is oriented with the quaternary cationic group toward the receptor membrane and with the esteratic site toward the emitting membrane. It appears that the solid state of the molecule does not support the hypothesis of a two-point attachment. Whereas the ganglionic blocking activity of less bulky quaternary groups is a function of the chain length, the more bulky quaternary cations (the triethylammonium groups) do not allow the solid-state forces to act, and they block by their bulky character, regardless of the chain length involved.

An important structural characteristic of bisquaternary ammonium compounds is that shortening the chain length between two cationic nitrogens results in an increased probability of interaction between them. Two closely situated onium groups would thus become less independent as separated ions and may resemble in physicochemical characteristics single divalent cations in a single solvent cage. Besides the quaternary ammonium groups, attention has to be given to the role of other structural elements found in several ganglionic blocking agents. The nonionic bulk of large ring substituents can, for example, influence activity by different means: favoring distribution to sites of action, stabilizing adsorption at receptors by preventing access to them for displacing ions, contributing to bonding energy by Van der Waals forces, and reducing affinity of water for the ionic groups (*17*).

It was emphasized that structural variations may exert a greater effect on membrane penetration than on binding characteristics with the receptors. Thus, the problem of exploring the accessibility of compounds to receptor sites through localization studies seems to be imperative.

The shortcomings of the available studies derive from the well-recognized limitations of our knowledge not only of the action, but also of the structure, of the agents (*14*). Thus, it should be realized that not only the planar formula of compounds, but even molecular models, without supportive physicochemical data, are sometimes inadequate, because chemical structure and physicochemical properties are often unrelated. Future studies, therefore, must satisfy certain clearly recognized criteria with respect to structure and action. A clear separation should be made between the pharmacological actions of isolated systems, in which the potency of an agent must be determined first, and those of more complex systems, in which additional factors, such as metabolism, distribution, and elimination, must be studied, before a conclusion regarding the action of the agent in question can be reached.

For a better understanding of the mode of action of ganglionic drugs, a more complete knowledge of receptor sites is also of prime importance. Very little is known about them. According to the concepts presently favored, the ganglionic receptor surface involves a lattice of anionic groups distributed in patterns roughly analogous to that of a crystal surface. The mosaiclike surface of fairly closely spaced anionic groups could permit a variety of compounds, including bisquaternaries of various intercationic distances, to bond in preferred sequences or patterns to these receptor surfaces (*17*).

Only a complex approach involving neurophysiologic, biochemical, stereochemical, and physicochemical experimentation with the proper biological substrates and adequate pharmacological agents will raise our knowledge to the level required for solving the problems of mechanism.

D. Methods

Confronted with problems of exploring the biological activities of different classes of agents, the pharmacologist tries to analyze drug action in simple but still adequate test preparations. For studying the effects of drugs on autonomic ganglia the preparations of mammals are preferred. Any studies that analyze ganglionic agents exclusively in the whole animal and observe phenomena of such complexity as blood-pressure rise or fall without further pharmacological characterization should be looked upon with a certain caution. The often used practical approach of structure–activity studies, in which ganglionic blocking action is sought on the basis of hypotensive effects, offers some possibility of finding an effective ganglionic blocking drug, but it deprives the investigator of the benefit of correlating chemical structure with a specific biological activity and defeats its most important purposes, that of exploring the selectivities, potencies, and pharmacologic types of the agents. Such biological parameters obtained in suitable test objects support our knowledge not only of the drugs but also of the receptors they act upon. Thus, properly analyzed stimulant and blocking drugs become very useful tools in the exploration of the nature of biological receptors. The significance of this is obvious.

The two basic types of methods of analyzing ganglionic drugs are the measurement of the change in an end-organ response by assuming that its response is largely or entirely due to the change in neurotransmission at the ganglia, which are stimulated electrically or chemically, and the recording of changes in postganglionic nerve potentials, either spontaneous or evoked, that follow drug administration. The variations in the different stimuli (electric or chemical), the different degrees of isolation of the responding organs (in vivo, in situ, and in vitro), the species and the various types of administration of the blocking drug, all yield a confusingly large number of methods which can be, and have been, used. Some of the methods have achieved general recognition and are of obvious theoretical and practical importance. Their merits and limitations may be evaluated relatively easily. Reliance on a few well-explored procedures is justified, and even with the development of newer and more accurate or sensitive methods these workhorses of autonomic pharmacology would be difficult to replace. A short description of the most frequently used methods is found in Table 4.2.

TABLE 4.2

Some Common Methods of Studying Ganglionic Agents

Test object	Ganglionic pharmacologic response		Ref.
	Stimulation	Blocking	
Cat nictitating membrane (superior cervical ganglion)	Contractions of membrane by stimulant agent; can be prevented by ganglionic blocking drugs (different classes) or removal of the ganglion	Relaxation of membrane or inhibition of contractions produced by electrical stimulation or ganglionic stimulants[a]	*2*, *13*, *53*, *54*, *247*
Cat and dog blood pressure	Blood pressure rise or biphasic response in normal animals; can be prevented by ganglionic blocking agents in atropinized or spinal animals	Blood pressure drop, during which ganglionic stimulants or stimulation of splanchnic nerve and carotid occlusion are ineffective[b]	*92*, *163*, *247*, *320*, *345*, *355*, *471*
Dog pelvic nerve bladder preparation	Rapid contraction of the bladder on intra-arterial injection; prevented by ganglionic blocking agents	Inhibition of bladder contraction produced by electrical stimulation of pelvic nerves or ganglionic stimulants given intra-arterially[c]	*71*, *74*, *154*, *189*, *277*, *302*

TABLE 4.2—*continued*

Test object	Ganglionic pharmacologic response: Stimulation	Ganglionic pharmacologic response: Blocking	Ref.
Isolated rabbit and guinea pig ileum	Contractions; prevented by ganglionic blocking agents[d]	Inhibition of contractions produced by ganglionic stimulants; without influence on effect of muscarine or methacholine[d]	*28*, *158*, *311*, *431*
Stimulation and blockade of chemoreceptors (cat, dog)	Various respiratory and cardiovascular reflex actions sensitive to ganglionic blockade or denervation of chemoreceptor zones (carotid, aortic bodies)[e]	Prevention of respiratory and cardiovascular reflex actions of ganglionic stimulants by local injections into the chemoreceptor areas[e]	*2*, *11*, *239*
Changes in spontaneous postganglionic nerve activity related to different ganglia in cat (superior cervical,[f] inferior mesenteric, stellate, ciliary)	Increase in spontaneous nerve activity on intra-arterial administration; blocked by ganglionic blocking agents	Decrease in spontaneous nerve activity or inhibition of stimulant action of ganglionic stimulants[g]	*40*, *58*, *169*, *177*, *185*
Changes in evoked potentials of postganglionic nerve related to different ganglia of the cat (superior cervical, stellate,[h] ciliary)		Inhibition	*58*, *60*, *61*, *84*, *85*, *241*

[a] Compounds should be ineffective against postganglionic stimulation (electric or epinephrine). Differentiation between cholinergic and noncholinergic blocking agents (potency against 5-HT) is possible. For modifications, see text.

[b] Pressor response to catecholamines is enhanced; depressor response to ACh is either unchanged or only slightly reduced.

[c] No inhibition of contraction produced by "muscarinic" agents (muscarine, methacholine). Differentiation between cholinergic and noncholinergic blocking agents (potency against 5-HT) is possible.

[d] Several classes of stimulants of the intramural nerve plexuses exist.

[e] Cholinergic and noncholinergic stimulant and blocking agents exist.

[f] Also in the rat and rabbit.

[g] Different classes of agents are known.

[h] Also in the rat.

Use of the nictitating membrane has undergone several modifications. Instead of administering the blocking drugs intravenously, which produces marked systemic changes, the investigator injects them into the common carotid artery via a suitable branch (usually the thyroid or lingual artery), so that the drug is channelled primarily to the ganglionic area (*13*). For prevention of possible effects of the drug on the end organ (nictitating membrane) a complete isolation and perfusion of the superior cervical ganglion may be required. Kibjakow (*52*) described the perfused cat superior cervical ganglion preparation, which was successfully applied to the study of ganglionic neurotransmission and drug effects (*53–57*). Volle (*58*) used the nonperfused ganglion preparation, recording postganglionic nerve activity for the analysis of the mechanism of action of a few typical ganglionic drugs.

Considering the complexity of the nervous and humoral mechanisms regulating blood pressure and the different groups of ganglia participating in the over-all response, the measurement of blood pressure, although still used quite frequently, should be considered a preliminary, exploratory approach necessitating further analysis and more refined techniques.

In several studies isolated excised ganglia were studied, and a change of nerve conduction across the ganglion by drugs was determined. Thus, the superior cervical ganglion of the rat has been isolated and tested with pentobarbital (*59*) and with many other drugs of the tranquilizing, local anesthetic, and sympathomimetic type (*60*). The superior cervical ganglion (*61*) and the stellate ganglion of the rat (*62*) have also been employed for studying drugs on isolated ganglia.

Several other sympathetic-ganglion preparations have been used sporadically in the study of ganglionic blocking agents. The role of the stellate ganglion in the vasomotor reaction of the rabbit ear has been explored with unilaterally denervated ears. Compounds that produce vasodilation only on the innervated ear were believed to act by blocking the stellate ganglion. Hexamethonium and pentamethonium have been tested (*63*). A preparation of isolated sympathetic ganglion and pulmonary artery of the rabbit has recently been developed (*64*), on which TEA has been shown to be fairly effective. Studies of a nerve muscle preparation, in which the guinea pig vas deferens with different ganglionic blocking and postganglionic sympatholytic drugs was used, indicated that there are sympathetic ganglia in the "postganglionic" section of the hypogastric nerve. Typical ganglionic blocking drugs interfered with the nerve stimulation but not with the direct muscular stimulation, whereas agents with a postganglionic type of action, such as hemicholinium, guanethidine, bretylium, and procaine, usually were effective against both types of electric stimulation (*65*). A differentiation between ganglionic and postganglionic sympathetic nerve blockade was made possible by using a cat preparation and recording spontaneous nerve activity in the sympathetic fibers to the kidney. Compounds that selectively depress ganglia in addition to the spontaneous nerve activity block the action of asphyxia-induced increased nerve activity; azamethonium belongs to this group of drugs. On the other hand, drugs that act centrally depress spontaneous nerve activity but are not effective against the stimulation produced reflexly through asphyxia; narcotine belongs to this group (*66*). Neural after-discharges in the postganglionic portion of the sympathetic nerves originating from the cat stellate ganglion were studied with different ganglionic blocking agents. The agents decreased the amplitude of action potentials but did not produce complete block of ganglionic transmission in the dose range used (*67*).

1. PARASYMPATHETIC GANGLIA

There are two major problems in analyzing pharmacologically the functions of the parasympathetic ganglia: the anatomic situation of a very short postganglionic fiber portion, which hardly permits direct recording from the postganglionic nerve, and the nature of chemical neurotransmission at this division of the autonomic nervous system, which is cholinergic at both the ganglionic and the postganglionic receptor sites. This is in contrast to the case of sympathetic ganglia, in which a drug with an ACh-blocking property can easily be employed without interfering with the function of the adrenergically innervated end organ; drugs possessing this property may influence both ganglionic and postganglionic cholinergic sites, thereby complicating evaluation. Several preparations have been tested and almost all are handicapped by one of these methodological difficulties. In certain studies and particularly when a selective blocking action on the parasympathetic ganglionic division is claimed, it is mandatory to clarify the type of action. Unfortunately, this is impossible with many preparations. Therefore, as in the case of sodium citrate, which was supposed to act at parasympathetic but not at sympathetic ganglia, the ganglionic site of action cannot be established beyond doubt by measuring pupillary and heart-frequency changes of the turtle (*68*). Two methods using end-organ responses and still circumventing the problem of interference between the ganglionic and postganglionic cholinergic receptor sites are a modified mouse pupil method (*69*) and the dog bladder preparation (*70–72*). In the mouse pupil method, a differentiation between the mydriatic responses produced by ganglionic blocking agents (which paralyze the ciliary ganglion) and those produced by atropinelike agents (which affect the parasympathetic nerve endings) is possible by using pretreatment with carbamoylcholine. Suitable doses of this cholinomimetic agent prevent the dilatation of the pupil elicited by ganglionic blocking drugs (hexamethonium, mecamylamine) but do not alter the pupil response to atropine and atropinelike agents (scopolamine, benactyzine). The mydriatic response of agents producing both ganglionic and postganglionic parasympathetic blockade is reduced to a variable degree by the pretreatment. Although no quantitative assessment of the individual mydriatic components could be made concerning the action of the latter type of agent, it was demonstrated that in the action of certain quaternary tropane derivatives the ganglionic blockade takes a measurable part, whereas such compounds as butylscopolaminium bromide and metantheline bromide produce mydriasis only through postganglionic parasympathetic blockade.

The use of the dog bladder preparation, which gives measurements of the pressure changes in the bladder of anesthetized dogs stimulated either by the parasympathetic pelvic nerves or by ganglionic stimulants, and the administration of the drugs to be studied, which is made through a suitable arterial branch into the abdominal aorta, are based on the presence of a somewhat unique receptor system of this organ. Studies with cholinomimetic and cholinergic blocking agents indicated that a substantial portion of parasympathetic bladder ganglia are not connected functionally to typical parasympathetic nerve endings, because even after blockade of the typical parasympathetic nerve endings (by eliminating the action of muscarinic stimulants by atropine) stimulation of the pelvic nerve remains effective, and ganglionic stimulant agents produce excitation of almost unchanged intensity. Compounds that have blocking properties at sympathetic ganglia are highly effective in this stage of the preparation. The parallelism between the blockade of the pelvic ganglia through use of the bladder preparation and that of the superior cervical ganglion in the dog and cat has been demonstrated (*73*). The dog preparation has been used with very satisfactory results in testing several noncholinergic ganglionic stimulant and blocking agents (*74–76*).

Several nerve muscle preparations of the gastrointestinal tract have been used for studying ganglionic blocking agents. In the case of the isolated vagus stomach preparation of the cat the ganglionic blocking action has been distinguished from a postganglionic action by separately testing the same compounds on an isolated piece of stomach strip. The sensitivity of the electrically stimulated nerve muscle preparation to blocking agents was compared with that of the ACh-stimulated isolated stomach preparation in an attempt to separate ganglionic and postganglionic actions (*77*). The isolated guinea pig esophagus was used for studying atropinelike and ganglionic blocking agents (*78*). Different types of the isolated guinea pig ileum preparation have been used in several studies of the physiologic role of intramural nerve plexuses and the influence of blocking agents acting at the ganglionic receptor sites in the plexuses. Cholinergic blocking agents (hexamethonium) and noncholinergic blocking agents (morphine) have been studied (*79–82*). The guinea pig ileum stimulated by ganglionic stimulants (nicotine, DMPP, or TMA) is suitable for testing ganglionic blocking activity, but a separation of this action from a cholinolytic atropinelike property is possible only by checking the compound also against ACh or muscarine. An analysis of ganglionic stimulant and blocking agents in the isolated rat duodenum indicated the existence both of a preganglionic stimulant action on the eserinized preparation and of a depolarizing effect producing spasm, which is peculiarly reversed by atropine (*83*).

These nerve-end organ preparations are most frequently used for studying agents acting on parasympathetic ganglia; a more adequate means of evaluation, however, is the recording of postganglionic nerve activity. Because of methodological difficulties this approach is restricted practically to the ciliary ganglion of the cat, where nerve activity at the branches of the small ciliary nerves can be recorded (*84*, *85*), but even this method is much too demanding for routine investigational purposes.

Several studies were devoted to solving the problem of the differential sensitivity of different ganglia by using various species and various organs of the same species with different ganglionic blocking agents. Often the main effort was directed to a more thorough evaluation of a certain compound with several different methods and different ganglia. These studies are summarized in Table 4.3.

TABLE 4.3

Comparative Tests with Ganglionic Blocking Agents

Test method[a]	Blocking agent	Notes	Ref.
Cat nictitating membrane (CNM). Isolated guinea pig ileum	Methonium compounds	No difference in potencies between sympathetic and parasympathetic ganglion preparations	*221*
CNM. Dog: vagus blockade, ACh pressor response after atropine, splanchnic nerve stimulation, carotid occlusion	Azamethonium		*354*
Different species: hypotensive action, carotid occlusion, ACh pressor response after atropine, nicotine and lobeline pressor responses, epinephrine pressor response potentiation, protective action against nicotine toxicity, vagus blockade	Plegarol		*385b*

TABLE 4.3—*continued*

Test method[a]	Blocking agent	Notes	Ref.
Rabbit, mouse: hypotensive action, mydriatic response, SCG preparation with constant perfusion	Piperidine compounds	Comparison of hypotensive action with ganglionic blockade	*469*
Mouse: nicotine tremor, mydriasis after sympathetic denervation. Cat: CNM, nicotine pressor response, vagus stimulation	Pempidine, bisquaternary ammonium compounds	Action on nicotine tremor: peripheral	*315*
CNM. Isolated guinea pig ileum	Pempidine		*431*
Isolated guinea pig ileum. Cat: SCG-evoked action potentials, ACh pressor response, carotid occlusion, splanchnic nerve stimulation, bladder contractions in situ	Pempidine and analogues		*220*
Cat: CNM, stellate ganglion, vagus stimulation	TEA		*2*
Dog: carotid occlusion, ACh pressor response after atropine, vagus stimulation, epinephrine-induced reflex bradycardia	Different blocking agents		*345*
Carotid occlusion, central vagus stimulation	1,1-Diethyl-2,6-dimethylpiperidinium		*471*
Rabbit: isolated nerve-bladder strip, isolated ileum, isolated atria. Steer: isolated iris sphincter	ACh, atropine		*472*
CNM, splanchnic nerve stimulation, preparation of vagus nerve and heart, nicotine pressor response, submaxillary gland stimulation	Magnolia and cocculus alkaloids	Ganglia to the submaxillary gland most sensitive to ganglionic blockade, adrenal medulla least sensitive	*470*

TABLE 4.3—*continued*

Test method[a]	Blocking agent	Notes	Ref.
CNM. Dog: DMPP pressor response, nicotine pressor response, vagus stimulation, carotid occlusion, bladder stimulation by DMPP	Phenylalkylamines		
CNM. Mouse: nicotine convulsions, mydriasis	Mecamylamine	Parallelism between tests only within a series of compounds	*419*
CNM. Dog: vagus stimulation, carotid occlusion, chorda tympani stimulation Rabbit: nicotine pressor response CNM. Isolated guinea pig ileum. Rat, rabbit: gut propulsion	Mecamylamine		*420*
Cat: CNM, nicotine pressor response, splanchnic nerve stimulation. Dog: vagus stimulation. Mouse: mydriatic response	Bisquaternary ammonium compounds and aliphatic polyamines	Mouse mydriasis is extremely sensitive to pentolinium type of agent	*327*
Cat: CNM, stellate ganglion	Different well-known ganglionic drugs	Short duration of action on stellate ganglion	*241*
SCG. Cat: ciliary ganglion	Methonium compounds, TEA, chlorisondamine, catecholamines, pentolinium	Comparison, sympathetic and parasympathetic ganglion	*84*, *85*, *473*, *474*
Cat: CNM, changes in pupil diameter	Methyl ethyl isooctenylamine	Comparison, sympathetic and parasympathetic ganglion	*242*
CNM, dog bladder, mouse pupil, isolated rabbit ileum	Quaternary tropines	Comparison, sympathetic and parasympathetic ganglion	*297*, *29*, *291*
Dog: nictitating membrane, preparation of pelvic nerve and bladder	TEA, methonium compounds, quaternary tropines	Comparison, sympathetic and parasympathetic ganglion	*73*
Cat heart: sympathetic and parasympathetic nerve stimulation	Methonium compounds	Comparison, sympathetic and parasympathetic ganglion	*94*

[a] CNM, cat nictitating membrane; SCG, superior cervical ganglion.

4.3. GANGLIONIC STIMULANT AGENTS

A. Definition of Ganglionic Stimulants

Ganglionic stimulant agents are molecules that produce or increase post-ganglionic nerve activity through a selective action on autonomic ganglion cells. They may be classified as follows:

(1) Directly acting ganglionic stimulants that influence either the same receptor sites at which acts ACh, the only neurotransmitter substance known, or ganglionic receptors other than those sensitive to ACh.

(2) Indirectly acting stimulants that either (a) increase the formation or the release (or both) of ACh at the preganglionic terminals or (b) promote its passage to the receptor sites of the ganglionic cell body or interfere with its inactivation (or both).

Unfortunately, at present it is impossible to classify clearly the ganglionic stimulant agents according to these criteria. A few agents, especially DMPP, satisfy the first alternative under (1), but with others the situation is not nearly so simple.

An important consideration is that there must be a clear distinction between conditions applying to agents that selectively stimulate ganglia and conditions applying to the neurotransmitter substance. ACh, the neurotransmitter substance, is not a typical ganglionic stimulant by the definition of ganglionic stimulants outlined above, because it does not selectively stimulate ganglion cells when injected. Physiologically it still fulfils its role as a transmitter substance, because its release and degradation close to the site of action assures selectivity. This implies that the molecular structure of ACh is not optimal for a certain cholinergic receptor site. Therefore, in attempts at synthesizing new, highly potent, and selective ganglionic stimulants structural features other than those of ACh should be considered.

B. Optimal Structural Requirements for Ganglionic Stimulant Action

In view of recent physiologic and pharmacologic studies of autonomic ganglia it is obvious that the problem of the optimal structural requirements for ganglionic stimulant action is not as simple as it was in the past, when a single receptor site was thought to be the target of ganglionic stimulant drugs. The following factors must be considered: (a) the existence of at least two ACh-sensitive receptor sites in autonomic ganglia and the possibility of physiologically significant noncholinergic receptors, (b) the probably different distributions of the receptor sites at different "typical" ganglia, and (c) the existence of other neural elements in the organism, which are morphologically and physiologically similar to, but not identical with ganglia, but which are pharmacologically reactive to ganglionic agents. The use of adequate testing methods and the correct interpretation of the data restricted to the biological sites may help somewhat in overcoming these problems. Among the molecular factors necessary for nicotinic ganglionic stimulation an onium cation or the adequate ionization of a suitable tertiary base is important. Of the two tertiary nitrogen atoms of nicotine the pyrrolidine nitrogen exists at physiologic pH in the form of an *N*-pyrrolidinium ion, and this seems to be the cause of the stimulant action. The degree of ionization of ditertiary bases, however, cannot be accurately determined on the basis of the dissociation constants of the individual basic groups. There are several factors involved; one is the mutual interactions between the differently ionizable groups. Ionization may also change during the process of attachment of the molecule to ionic receptors and in the case of close proximity by Van der Waals forces. Thus, to consider the dissociation constant a crucial factor in the action of ganglionic stimulant drugs resembling nicotine has limitations and requires caution. In view of this a suggestion for producing compounds with one dissociating tertiary nitrogen atom and one quaternary group has been made; Barlow (*15*) and Gyermek and Nador (*86*) have described monoquaternary and bisquaternary derivatives of nicotine.

On the basis of observations with phenacyl and phenylalkyltrimethylammonium compounds, Wong and Long (*87*) claimed that the structural requirements for nicotinic activity are less rigid than those for muscarinic activity. Compounds in this series which had approximately a three-carbon atomic distance between the phenyl group and the quaternary nitrogen were the most effective, and ganglionic stimulant activity was enhanced when the atom adjacent to the phenyl ring carried a negative charge. The nicotinic potency in the phenacyl derivatives decreased as the electron density around the carbonyl oxygen decreased. Hey (*88*) described the ganglionic stimulant potencies of a series of substituted choline phenyl ethers which surpassed that of nicotine by a factor of 6 to 8. At that time the compounds were the most potent agents known, and the following structural features were suggested as being optimal for ganglionic stimulant action: a trimethylammonium cationic group, an ethylene chain between the onium group and the aromatic nucleus, and an ether oxygen whose electron density has to be influenced by the inductive effect of the substituents of the phenyl ring. 3,5-Dibromo-substituted and *m*-bromo-substituted phenyl ethers showed the optimal effect. In accord with the theory methyl substitution, unlike halogen substitution, decreased the potency relative to the parent compound (choline phenyl ether); similarly, substitution with any group at the *p* position markedly diminished potency (Table 4.4). Because the study of Hey (*88*) was based not only on a limited number of substituted choline phenyl ethers but also on extensive work on the structure–activity relationships of large series of choline ether and aliphatic ammonium-type ganglionic stimulants, it seemed that the structural features

TABLE 4.4

Ganglionic Stimulant Activity of Some Ethers and Esters of Choline and Related Alkyl Ammonium Compounds (Pressor Response on Cats)[a]

$RO(CH_2)_2N^+(CH_3)_3 \cdot Br$

R	Potency, molar[b]	Potency, molar[c]
Ethyl		0.07
Butyl		0.13
3,5-$Br_2C_6H_3$	7.1	
m-BrC_6H_4	7.8	40.00
m-ClC_6H_4	4.6	
C_6H_5	2.1	10.4
m-Tolyl	0.27	
p-ClC_6H_4	0.22	0.91
3,5-Xylyl	0.11	
p-Tolyl	0.008	
ACh	0.046	0.12
Carbamolycholine	0.15	
Propionylcholine	0.071	0.19
n-Butyrylcholine		0.25
Isobutrylcholine	0.18	0.47
n-Valerylcholine		0.29
Trimethyl-ACh	0.44	1.25
Benzoylcholine	0.052	
Phenacetylcholine	0.15	
4-Ketoamyltrimethylammonium iodide		3.04
n-Amyltrimethylammonium bromide		1.1

[a] Molar potency relative of nicotine 1.0.
[b] Data of Hey (*88*).
[c] Data of Wiley (*121*).

described represented the ideal molecular configuration for ganglionic stimulant action. More recent studies of tropane derivatives, however, indicated that compounds with entirely different structural features yield markedly higher stimulant potencies. In a series of alkyltrimethylammonium compounds the ketoamyltrimethylammonium analogue showed the optimal potency on the isolated heart of *Venus mercenaria*.

Although the action of ACh and of alkylammonium compounds on this preparation is designated "nicotinic," this test organ seems to be not equivalent to mammalian ganglionic preparations, because *d*-tubocurarine shows no blocking action and because the potencies of several compounds related to ACh were similar to those obtained on "muscarinic" preparations. Thus, the structural requirements for optimal actions described by Welsh and Taub (*89*) probably do not hold for mammalian ganglia. Using a series of benzoylcholine derivatives with substitutions in the aromatic nucleus, Ormerod (*89a*) described the correlations between the ganglionic stimulant potency and mesomeric effects of the substituents in the benzene ring. In this series the potency decreased with the electron-attracting power of substituents. By contrast, choline phenyl ethers gain in potency when the electron-attracting power of substituents increases. The explanation was offered that with esters the inactive surface of the ganglion appears to act as an electrophilic reagent and, with ethers, as a nucleophilic reagent. Assuming a functional methyl group at the receptor surface, the mechanism of attachment of an ester type **(2)** of agent may be through the carbonyl oxygen to the nucleophilic receptor. In the case of an ester type of agent the binding is established through a hydrogen bond between the electrophilic surface group and the ether oxygen **(3)**. According to Ing (*90*), the relations between structure and nicotinelike actions of the choline group are much more obscure than those involving the "muscarinic" actions. A study of the requirements concerning the size of the cationic group necessary for ganglionic stimulation indicates that replacement of the ammonium group with any other onium group in ACh (that is, with P or As) decreases activity (*90*).

C. Selectivity of Ganglionic Stimulants

The problem of selectivity of ganglionic stimulant agents concerning receptors of the autonomic ganglia is of basic pharmacologic importance. One of the first pertinent observations was that of Dale in 1914 (*91*), who used atropine to differentiate between the "nicotinic" and "muscarinic" actions of ACh and related choline derivatives. Nicotinic properties were described as insensitive to atropine and sensitive to blocking doses of nicotine, whereas muscarinic action was vulnerable to atropine. Among structural features the trimethylammonium group was early recognized as important in nicotinic and muscarinic action (*92*). ACh for a long time was claimed to produce exclusively nicotinic effects at the ganglia, and almost fifty years passed before it was recognized that there are also muscarinic sites at the autonomic ganglia. ACh possibly acts on both (*4*, *41*, *243*).

Many studies of structure–activity relationships have dealt with the characterization of the optimal nicotinic and muscarinic structural moieties; they will be discussed only as far as they pertain to ganglionic stimulants. It should suffice to mention that the structural requirements for obtaining stimulation of these different receptor sites differ considerably. Nevertheless, many compounds structurally satisfy more than one cholinergic receptor site. The motor end plates in some respects are pharmacologically similar to autonomic ganglia. Thus, ACh, nicotine, and several other ganglionic stimulants are also stimulants of the motor end plates. Besides the classic peripheral cholinergic receptor sites, however, there exist other neural receptor elements (adrenal medulla, chemoreceptors, certain sensory nerve endings) that are pharmacologically very similar to autonomic synapses (*11*, *93*). Only a few studies have delineated the properties of ganglionic stimulant agents at these different ganglionlike receptor sites. The review of Konzett and Rothlin (*11*) leaves little doubt that chemoreceptors are very similar to ganglia in structural requirements and it might be expected that only quantitative rather than qualitative differences exist. However, examples of the relative selectivities of certain agents that stimulate ganglia, chemoreceptors, and the adrenal medulla also have been reported (*11*, *94–97*). There is a difference in the relative potencies of ganglionic stimulants when determined at typical ganglionic sites, chemoreceptors, and the adrenal medulla. Lobeline chiefly stimulates the aortic bodies, DMPP the adrenal medulla, and McN-A-343 the ganglionic receptor sites (*96*).

A separation of activity of different stimulant agents for these sites is also noted (*98*). Whereas lactylcholine produces predominantly stimulation of the adrenal medulla, pyruvylcholine acts mainly by stimulating the sympathetic ganglia. Large doses of TEA produce stimulation of the adrenal medulla, which cannot be inhibited by hexamethonium (*99*). Certain sensory receptors were described by Gray and Diamond (*93*) as being ACh-sensitive; there this substance acts as a nicotinic agent. Effective doses of ACh and the types of blocking agent (excess nicotine, curare, hexamethonium) were the same at these receptors as at autonomic ganglia. As to whether ACh is indeed a neurotransmitter substance at a variety of sensory receptors remains to be proved and seems not to be likely at such sites as the mechanoreceptors.

The possibilities of a selective blockade at one division of autonomic ganglia or at a particular ganglion have been rather well explored, but little work has been done with selectively acting ganglionic stimulants. Although it has been shown that TMA produces more prolonged stimulation of sympathetic than of parasympathetic ganglia, the reverse may apply regarding the intensity of stimulation. The explanation, that the accessibility of different cells within the same organ or in different organs is different whereas the basic level of sensitivity to the agent may remain the same, might also be applicable to other stimulant agents. These considerations are important in evaluating claims for selective stimulant or blocking actions at different ganglia. The selectivity toward sympathetic ganglia of the choline cresyl ether type of stimulant (*100*) may be valid only for certain organ systems. The proposition of a general lack of efficacy at parasympathetic ganglia of these agents seems to be incorrect, because a definite stimulant action, sensitive to hexamethonium blockade, was demonstrated on the dog bladder with choline cresyl ether (*95*).

D. Actions of Ganglionic Stimulants at Sites Other Than Ganglionic

Nicotine, a tertiary amine, is well known to show stimulant action on the CNS, including a typical tremor in certain species, Data are now available that indicate that prototypes of ganglionic stimulants, such as nicotine and DMPP, exhibit peripheral pharmacologic effects other than their ganglionic action. Nicotine, for example, has a nonganglionic action on peripheral sympathetic nerves, which results in a pilomotor response, contraction of the isolated nictitating membrane of the cat, and vasoconstriction of peripheral vessels. It has been suggested that it liberates norepinephrine from peripheral stores through an action on chromaffin cell elements (*101*). DMPP, one of the most frequently utilized ganglionic stimulant agents, shows the following "atypical" effects: peripheral release of sympathetic transmitter substances independent of a ganglionic stimulant action, as described for nicotine (*102, 103*), blockade of ganglionic and neuromuscular transmission in certain preparations (*104*), and stimulation of visceral sensory nerve endings in the pulmonary area, producing bradycardia, hypotension, and apnea (*105*). Besides nicotine and DMPP, the 2,6-dichloro analogue of choline phenyl ether seems to have an effect on postganglionic adrenergic nerves and adrenals, where it inhibits release or storage of catecholamines (*106*). Some of the highly potent ganglionic-stimulant tropane compounds were also shown recently to have adrenergic neurone blocking effects similar to those of bretylium (*107*).

E. Classes of Ganglionic Stimulant Agents

1. SIMPLE MONOQUATERNARY ALKYL- AND ARALKYLAMMONIUM COMPOUNDS

In an early study Hunt and Renshaw (*108*, *109*) investigated tetraalkylammonium compounds and described their ganglionic stimulant action. More recently Wien (*110*) analyzed the role of the substitution of ethyl groups for methyl in tetramethylammonium and observed a transition of stimulant actions into blocking properties. Using a series of hydroxyalkyltrimethylammonium compounds, Dallemagne and Philippot (*111*) reported on the ganglionic stimulant actions of hydroxyethyldimethylethylammonium, hydroxyethyldimethylbutylammonium, and hydroxyethyldimethylhexylammonium.

A series of dimethylammonium compounds, in which the fourth substituent of the quaternary nitrogen was an aromatic group, has been recently studied by Levy et al. (*83*). None of these compounds, however, approached ACh or nicotine with respect to ganglionic stimulant actions. Other tetraalkyl and mixed alkyl–aralkyl quaternary derivatives with usually moderate ganglionic stimulant properties are listed in the summarizing work of Craig (*20*).

2. ALKYLAMMONIUM COMPOUNDS WITH UNSATURATED GROUPS

One class of alkyltrimethylammonium compounds, in which the alkyl chain of varying lengths contained one double or triple bond, was described by

TABLE 4.5

Comparison of the Ganglionic Stimulant Activities of Saturated and Unsaturated Alkylammonium Compounds[a]

n	$CH_3(CH_2)_nN^+Me_3\cdot I^-$	$CH_2{=}CH(CH_2)_nN^+Me_3\cdot I^-$	$CH_3C{\equiv}C(CH_2)_nN^+Me_3\cdot I^-$
1		0.4	0.5
2	0.2 to 0.4	1.5	1 to 2
3	1 to 6	3 to 10	6
4	3 to 10	5 to 10	3 to 4
5	5 to 10	2 to 4	1
6	2 to 3	0	
7	0		
8	0		

[a] Nicotinic activity of ACh on dog blood pressure, 1.0. From data of Jacob (*112*).

TABLE 4.6

Ganglionic Stimulant Activity of Some Saturated Ethylenic and Acetylenic Alkylammonium Compounds and Their Acetyl Ester Derivatives[a]

Compound	Nicotinic activity: Leech muscle	Nicotinic activity: Dog blood pressure (atropinized)
$HO(CH_2)_4N^+Me_3\cdot I^-$	0.5	0.5 to 1
$HO(CH_2)_5N^+Me_3\cdot I^-$	1	1
$CH_3CH(OH)(CH_2)_3N^+Me_3\cdot I^-$	2	3 to 5
$HOCH_2CH{=}CHCH_2N^+Me_3\cdot I^-$	0.5	0.5
$HO(CH_2)_2CH{=}CHCH_2N^+Me_3\cdot I^-$	0.5	1
$CH_3CH(OH)CH{=}CHCH_2N^+Me_3\cdot I^-$	2	1.5 to 2
$HOCH_2C{\equiv}CCH_2N^+Me_3\cdot I^-$	2	0.5 to 1
$HO(CH_2)_2C{\equiv}CCH_2N^+Me_3\cdot I^-$	1	1 to 1.5
$CH_3CH(OH)C{\equiv}CCH_2N^+Me_3\cdot I^-$	4 to 10	2 to 3
$CH_3COO(CH_2)_4N^+Me_3\cdot I^-$		0.5[b]
$CH_3COOCH{=}CHCH_2NMe_3\cdot I^-$		1 to 2[b]
$CH_3COOCH_2CH{=}CHC{\equiv}CCHNMe_3\cdot I^-$		0.3[b]
$CH_3COCH_2C{\equiv}CCH_2N^+Me_3\cdot I^-$	2 to 4	0.25 to 1
$CH_3CO(CH_2)_2C{\equiv}CCH_2N^+Me_3\cdot I^-$	0.8	0.5 to 1.0
$CH_3COCH(CH_3)C{\equiv}CCH_2N^+Me_3\cdot I^-$	2 to 4	0.5 to 1
$CH_3COOCH(CH{=}CHCH_3)C{-}C{\equiv}CCH_2NMe_3\cdot I^-$		0.17[b]

[a] Nicotinic activity of ACh, 1.0. From data of Jacob (*116*).
[b] From data of Marszak et al. (*123*).

Jacob et al. (*112–114*) and Marszak et al. (*115*); (see Table 4.5). It was concluded that in compounds with an alkyl chain of five carbon atoms introduction of one unsaturated group either slightly increases or does not change nicotinic activity. The same authors also investigated the ganglionic stimulant actions of oxyethyltrimethylammonium compounds with one unsaturated group. Hydroxyalkyltrimethylammonium compounds, their acetyl derivatives (for structures see Table 4.6), and the corresponding saturated analogues usually showed similar potencies. Some of the unsaturated compounds and derivatives of the five-carbon chain length were the most potent in this series (Table 4.6) (*116*).

In addition to variations of the chain length the influence of the position of hydroxyl and of unsaturated groups was also studied (*116*, *117*). No marked influence on ganglionic stimulant activity was observed with these changes. The most active compounds surpassed the potency of ACh by a factor of 5 to 10. The importance of both electronic and steric factors in nicotinic action was emphasized.

3. ESTERS AND ETHERS OF AMINO ALCOHOLS

a. Betaine Esters

Weak ganglionic stimulant activity has been reported with methyl-, propyl-, *n*-butyl-, and phenyl-substituted betaine ethyl esters by Hunt and Renshaw (*118*). A stimulant action on the cat blood pressure preparations has been found also with carbamoylmethyl trimethylammonium chloride and four *N*-alkylcarbamoyl derivatives. Most of these compounds showed only weak ganglionic stimulant action (*119*).

b. Choline Esters and Ethers

The choline esters and ethers constitute a large portion of those compounds which were tested for ganglionic stimulant actions.

In the early studies of Dale (*91*), besides ACh and choline, the nicotinic actions of choline nitrite ester, choline nitrate ester, and choline ethyl ether were analyzed in relation to their cholinomimetic muscarinic actions. Guggenheim (*18*) summarized the available information on choline esters and ethers, listing approximately thirty derivatives, of which α-methylcholine, butyrylcholine, and α-homocholine methyl ether were outstanding as stimulant agents.

Holton et al. (*120*) studied the role of alternations of substituents at the cationic head by gradually replacing the methyl groups with ethyl groups. The presence of more than one terminal ethyl group abolished ganglionic stimulant action in the atropinized cat blood pressure preparation. The ganglionic stimulant potency of ACh is surpassed by longer-chain acid esters of choline. Propionyl-, butyryl-, valeryl-, and isobutyrylcholine all showed higher ganglionic stimulant activity than ACh. Trimethylacetylcholine was ten times more potent (*121*). Lands and Cavallito (*122*) studied the ganglionic stimulant action of longer-chain choline derivatives as compared with amyltrimethylammonium, and Marszak et al. (*123*) reported on the acetyl esters of several longer-chain unsaturated amino alcohols. The activities of these compounds were usually lower than that of ACh on the atropinized dog blood pressure preparation.

Carbamoylcholine, an enzymatically nonhydrolyzable choline derivative, was first described by Kreitmair (*124*) and is known to possess marked ganglionic stimulant properties besides its predominantly cholinomimetic muscarinic characteristics. The *N*-methyl and *N,N*-dimethyl derivatives of carbamoylcholine are stronger stimulants of autonomic ganglia of the cat than is the parent compound. Their effective doses range between 20 and 100 μg/kg (*125*). The muscarinic actions of carbamoylcholine, however, are eliminated by alkyl substitution on the carbamoyl nitrogen (*126*).

A recent comparison of acetyl-, propionyl-, butyryl-, and benzoylcholine and their thiocholine analogues indicated varying degrees of ganglionic stimulant actions on blood pressure responses of cats, but the same agents depressed ganglionic transmission when tested on neostigmine-treated animals, the ganglionic transmission of which was measured with stimuli evoked at the superior cervical ganglion (*127*).

Butyryl-β-methylcholine and, to a lesser extent, benzoyl-β-methylcholine were stimulant at the superior cervical ganglion (*128*).

An indication of ganglionic stimulation was detected in the isolated guinea pig ileum and rabbit heart with butyrylcholine and propionylcholine. The higher homologues, pentanoylcholine and hexanoylcholine were less effective (*98*). Mesylcholine, a relatively new sulfonic acid analogue of ACh, showed considerably higher ganglionic stimulant potency than ACh, although its muscarinic action was merely a hundredth that of ACh (*129*, *130*). Valeroylcholine produces, besides ganglionic stimulation, autoinhibition at the ganglia of the guinea pig ileum (*131*). Senecioylcholine (β,β-dimethylacrylylcholine) is another recently described choline derivative, which predominantly shows ganglionic stimulant actions (*132*). A few interesting ACh derivatives were studied by Schueler et al. (*133*), in which the order of the oxygen atoms of the ester group had been changed ("reversed carboxy analogs of ACh"). Marked ganglionic stimulant pressor effects were observed with the reversed carboxy analogues of propionylcholine as compared with propionylcholine. However, by introducing this relatively minor change in the oxygen–nitrogen distances no difference in the ganglionic potency of ACh and its reversed carboxy analogue could be detected (*133*, *134*). The pharmacology of dicholine esters

TABLE 4.7

Effect of Branching-Chain Moieties on the Ganglionic Stimulant Activity of Choline Ethers and Acetylcholine[a]

	Nicotinic activity in cat blood pressure[b]				
	$R-CH_2CH_2N^+(Me)_3$	$R-CH(CH_3)CH_2N^+(Me)_3$	$R-CH(C_2H_5)CH_2N^+(Me)_3$	$R-CH(C_3H_7)CH_2N^+(Me)_3$	$R-CH(C_4H_9)CH_2N^+(Me)_3$
CH_3OR	+	−	−	−	++
C_2H_5OR	+	−	−	−	−
C_4H_9OR	++	−	−	−	−
CH_3OCOR	++	−	±	−	−

[a] Data of Simonart (*136*).

[b] − = no action, ± = extremely weak action, + = weak action, ++ = strong action.

was reviewed by Brücke (*135*). The following dicholine derivatives were reported to have ganglionic stimulant action (in order of increasing action): succinyl-, glutaryl-, adipyl-, pimelyl-, suberyl-, azelayl-, and sebacyldicholines.

c. Alkyl Ethers of Alkylammonium Compounds

One series of this class has been studied by Simonart (*136*) and is presented in Table 4.7. The *N*-propyloxymethyl-, *N*-butoxymethyl-, isobutoxymethyl-, and allyloxymethyltrimethylammonium iodides were described by Hunt and Renshaw (*137*, *138*). Alkyl ether compounds with longer aliphatic chains and unsaturated groups of the general structure $RO(CH_2)_{4-5}N^+(CH_3)_3X^-$, where R is methyl through butyl and X is halogen, were studied.

Some of the compounds contained an acetylenic group in the connecting chain between the ammonium group and the ether oxygen (*139*). Most of these compounds were weaker ganglionic stimulants than ACh on the blood pressure of the dog.

While β-methylcholine methyl and ethyl ethers do not exhibit nicotinic effects, the isopropyl ether of β-methylcholine produces slight ganglionic stimulation in the cat blood pressure preparation (*140*). Choline isopropyl ether and choline 1-hydroxy-2-propyl ether show considerable ganglionic stimulant actions in the pelvic ganglia of the dog. The corresponding β-methylcholine derivatives were practically devoid of such an action. All four compounds were practically ineffective as cholinomimetic agents (*141*).

d. Thioethers of Alkylammonium Compounds and Related Sulfur-Containing Derivatives

A fairly large number of thioethers of alkylammonium compounds and sulfur-containing derivatives were studied by Hunt and Renshaw (*137*) and by Lands and Cavallito (*122*). Some of the thioether compounds, such as the isopropyl thioether of homocholine, were quite potent on the atropinized dog blood pressure preparation.

e. Aromatic Choline Ester and Choline Ether Derivatives

The nicotinic properties of benzoyl-, phenylacetyl-, and β-phenylpropionylcholines were described more than fifty years ago (*142*), and a re-evaluation of benzoylcholine showed that it has various autonomic effects: depending on the dose, it produces muscarinic, hexamethonium-sensitive, and hexamethonium-resistant ganglionic effects (*143*).

The D(−)-phenylglycolate ester of trimethylammoniumethanol was claimed recently to have a predominantly ganglionic stimulant effect on sympathetic ganglia, less influence on the parasympathetic division, and no inhibiting action (*144*).

Some choline ester derivatives with heterocyclic rings possess significant ganglionic stimulant properties. The naturally occurring murexine **(4)** shows relatively moderate ganglionic stimulant action on the spinal cat (*146*). Dihydromurexine and its 2-pyridyl analogue, however, are quite potent ganglionic stimulants. Imidazoleacetylcholine and 2-pyridylacetylcholine also show ganglionic stimulant characteristics. Imidazoleacryloylcholine is less potent, and imidazolepropionylcholine significantly more potent, than the acetyl derivatives in the cat, producing nicotinic blood pressure rise (*147*, *148*).

A systematic study of different ganglionic preparations with dialkylaminoalkyl esters of cyclohexyl-1-cyclohexanecarboxylic acid and with similar ether and alkane derivatives has been reported. The role of the aromatic groups, the chain length, the presence or absence of ester and ether moieties, and the nature of the substituted amino groups were investigated. Only some of the trimethylammonium derivatives of the ether type exhibited ganglionic stimulant action exceeding that of choline phenyl ether. However, in vivo either they were weaker or no quantitative data were available on their efficacy. With the use of normal and eserinized rat duodenum preparations a distinction has been made between preganglionic (ACh-liberating) and depolarizing actions; the two different types of action seemed to require different structural characteristics (*32*).

The ganglionic stimulant actions of choline phenyl ether and its nuclear-substituted analogues have been recognized for a long time. Hunt and Renshaw (*138*) studied analogues of choline phenyl ethers with *p*-hydroxy, benzoyloxy, methoxy, and acetamido substituents in the phenyl ring. These substitutions resulted in considerably weaker ganglionic stimulants than the parent compound.

Choline phenyl ether itself was known to be one of the most effective ganglionic stimulants, being effective at 50 μg/kg in the cat. It produces a nicotinic blood pressure rise; the *o*-, *m*-, and *p*-tolyl ethers of choline were less effective.

The corresponding β-methylcholine compounds showed only ganglionic blocking effects (*140*).

In a series of amino- and ammonioalkyl phenyl and naphthyl ethers of the general structure $R_1R_2R_3N^+—CH_2CH_2OR_4$, where R_1R_2 are alkyl or cycloalkyl, R_3 is H or alkyl, and R_4 is phenyl, substituted phenyl, or naphthyl, a few showed moderate ganglionic stimulant action whereas the majority exhibited blocking properties (*145*).

Choline ethers of type **(5)** were potent ganglionic stimulants. The structure–activity relationships of nuclear substituents on ring I and alterations of the substituents of N also were studied. The claim (*100*) that this class shows marked selectivity for the ganglia of the sympathetic system could not be confirmed (*95*).

In another series of choline ether derivatives the peak potency appeared with the *m*-bromophenyl ether of choline, which was one of the most potent nicotinelike stimulant agents (*88*, *121*). The structure–activity relationships of this and related choline phenyl ethers were explored in detail by Hey (*99*); see Section 4.3, B. Potencies of these compounds are shown in Table 4.4.

4. ONIUM COMPOUNDS OTHER THAN AMMONIUM

Sulfonium, arsonium, phosphonium, and stibonium derivatives, which are analogues of tetramethylammonium with ganglionic stimulant activity, were described by Hunt and Renshaw (*109*). Except for the sulfonium analogue, they were considerably weaker than TMA. Few sulfonium derivatives were further studied, and of these β-phenoxyethyldimethylsulfonium nitrate, the sulfonium analogue of choline phenyl ether, was fairly potent.

5. NICOTINE AND AGENTS RESEMBLING NICOTINE

Compounds included in this class are chemically fairly heterogeneous. This presents a puzzle to anyone who is dealing with problems in structure–activity relationships. Instead of discussing at this point the different suggested optimal molecular configurations for nicotinelike ganglionic stimulant action it will be pertinent to discuss the problem of classifying these agents. A classification of nicotinelike agents cannot be accurate as long as it is not proved that all the compounds included in a certain group act identically. What is known at present is only that these agents stimulate autonomic ganglia, are fairly specific in that they do not markedly influence other autonomic receptor sites or receptor sites of ACh outside the ganglion, are readily blocked by a certain class of specific ganglionic blocking agents (the majority by hexamethonium), and produce electrophysiologic changes resembling that of nicotine in its stimulating phase. The last, however, is far from being adequately elucidated with respect to many of the compounds listed. Thus, suitable pharmacologic evidence that these compounds act by an identical mechanism at identical receptor sites is not yet available, and the present classification should be considered temporary and subject to future correction.

a. Nicotine

Since the classic studies of Langley, who applied it locally and first described in detail its marked effects on ganglionic transmission, nicotine has become the favorite prototype of a ganglionic stimulant agent in spite of the following disadvantages. Nicotine is a ditertiary base with very little, if anything, in common structurally with the neurotransmitter substance; it is not selective enough as a ganglionic stimulant, and it has blocking characteristics that are due both to its primary stimulant action (depolarization block) and to a competitive type of blockade, which is independent of the stimulating phase; when tested on the whole animal its effects at the carotid chemoreceptors, the adrenal medulla, and the CNS contribute to the over-all effect.

Modern re-evaluations of nicotine from the points of view of ionization of its N-containing groups (*149*) and its stereostructure (*15*) have improved our knowledge to such an extent that, at least within this class, the optimal molecular forms are recognized and are available for comparative studies with other molecular species. The ionization studies indicate that at physiologic pH nicotine exists mainly in the form of a mono-quaternary nicotinium ion whose proton is on the pyrrolidine nitrogen.

The absolute configuration of nicotine has been determined, and no difference in toxicity between its (L) and (D) forms was found. Similarly, no difference was observed between the ganglionic stimulant actions of the (D) and (L) forms of nornicotine (*15*).

Regarding the role of the pyrrolidine ring, it is interesting that the connection between the piperidine and pyrrolidine rings of nicotine need not necessarily be at the α carbon of the pyrrolidine system. *N*-(β-Pyridylmethyl) pyrrolidine is equiactive with nicotine, and substitution of the pyrrolidine group for a trimethylammonium group also yields a potent compound.

These considerations led Barlow and Hamilton (*150*) to investigate in great detail a large number of pyridine derivatives that had been developed from nicotine (*6*). The role of the attachment to the α, β, and γ carbon atoms of the piperidine ring of the groups pyrrolidine, piperidine, and trialkylammonium has been studied. The influence of the length of the connecting chain between the two *N*-containing groups was determined, and the role of the following factors was evaluated: the distribution of the electronic charge in the pyridine ring as influenced by different substituents (*150*) and the spatial constellation of the functional group as influenced by size of substituents and length of connecting chain. Some details of this comprehensive study are presented in Table 4.8. Barlow and Hamilton (*150*) conclude that optimal nicotinic potency is obtained within the class of nicotine-model compounds when a quaternary ammonium group, either trimethylammonium or *N*-methylpyrrolidinium, is attached to the pyridine ring at the β position. Several of the potent compounds had a relatively positive carbon atom in the pyridine ring at a distance from the onium group that was similar to that given by Hey (*88*) for the ganglionically potent choline phenyl ether derivatives. The same data concerning interprosthetic distances for nicotinic action suggest that even in ACh the partially positive carbonyl carbon atom is a more important component than the ether oxygen, which in ACh does not carry any positive charge.

TABLE 4.8

Ganglionic Stimulant Potencies of Analogues of Nicotine[a]

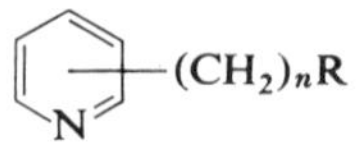

Point of attachment	n	R	Relative potency
3	1	Trimethylammonium	2.0
		Monomethylnicotinium	0.28
3	1	Ethyldimethylammonium	0.78
3	1	Dimethylamino	0.04
3	2	Piperidino	0.022
3	2	Pyrrolidino	0.03
2	2	Pyrrolidino	0.012
2	2	Dimethylamino	0.41
4	1	Dimethylamino	0.0025
4	2	Pyrrolidino	<0.0012
		Choline phenyl ether	5.5
		Nicotine	1.0

[a] Cat superior cervical ganglion. Data of Barlow and Hamilton (*308*).

b. Quaternary Derivatives of Nicotine

Some mono- and bisquaternary analogues of nicotine were studied by Barlow and Dobson (*151*), who reported on the three possible methyl quaternary forms of nicotine. Of these the *N*-pyrrolidinium methiodide proved to be about as potent as nicotine but to be without the secondary blocking action of the tertiary base. The other two compounds, the *N*-pyridinium methiodide and the dimethiodide of nicotine, were only very slightly potent. Gillis and Lewis (*152*) found discrepancies between the effects of nicotine monomethiodide and nicotine. The quaternary derivative was more potent on neuromuscular preparations but weaker on ganglia, and its action was more sensitive than that of nicotine to atropine blockade. They found the other two methyl quaternary derivatives also considerably less potent. Of several aralkyl quaternary derivatives of nicotine studied by Gyermek and Nador (*86*) the bisquaternary derivative of nicotine that carried a methyl quaternary group on the pyridyl nitrogen and a *p*-phenylbenzyl quaternary group on the piperidyl nitrogen showed marked nicotinic stimulant properties, whereas the other derivatives exhibited only ganglionic blocking effects (Table 4.9).

TABLE 4.9

Ganglionic Actions of Some Quaternary Salts of Nicotine[a]

Code no.	Salt	Ganglionic blocking potency[b]
A-103	Methyl(*N*-pyrrolidyl)nicotinium iodide	<0.2
A-100	Methyl(*N*-pyridyl)methyl(*N*-pyrrolidyl)nicotinium diiodide	<0.5
N-494	Methyl(*N*-pyridyl)benzyl(*N*-pyrrolidyl)nicotinium iodide bromide	2.2
N-495	Methyl(*N*-pyridyl)*p*-phenylbenzyl(*N*-pyrrolidyl)nicotinium iodide bromide	stimulant[c]
N-496	*p*-Phenylbenzyl(*N*-pyridyl)methyl(*N*-pyrrolidyl)nicotinium bromide iodide	15.0
A-95	Benzyl(*N*-pyridyl)benzyl(*N*-pyrrolidyl)nicotinium dibromide	0.5

[a] Data of Gyermek and Nador (*86*).
[b] Potency of tetraethylammonium on cat nictitating membrane preparation, 1.0.
[c] About five times less potent than nicotine.

c. 1,1-Dimethyl-4-phenylpiperazinium bromide

DMPP has been described (*153*, *154*) as having primarily ganglionic stimulant properties in the cat and dog. Because it did not show the disadvantages of nicotine (ganglionic blocking, central effects), it soon became one of the most widely used agents for eliciting and evaluating ganglionic stimulation. Its pharmacology was further explored by recording spontaneous and evoked postganglionic nerve activity in the cat (*6*, *155*, *156*). The actions of this agent also were analyzed in intestinal preparations (*28*, *81*), and in intact dogs (*157*), and its receptor interactions were studied (*158*). Although it is a very suitable pharmacologic test compound, recent studies indicate the presence of ganglionic blocking properties and actions other than at ganglia (*103*, *159*). However, as long as a much more selective ganglionic stimulant agent is not available, DMPP remains the ganglionic stimulant "reference standard" compound of choice. The piperazine ring of DMPP can be replaced with a piperidine ring without major loss of ganglionic stimulant potency (*160*, *161*). Further substitution, with an *N*-isopropyl instead of an *N*-methyl group, resulted in a ganglionic blocking agent (*160*).

6. TROPANE DERIVATIVES

In studies of ganglionic blocking tropane derivatives it was found that few showed ganglionic stimulation besides their blocking properties. The most

TABLE 4.10

Ganglionic Stimulant Tropane Derivatives[a]

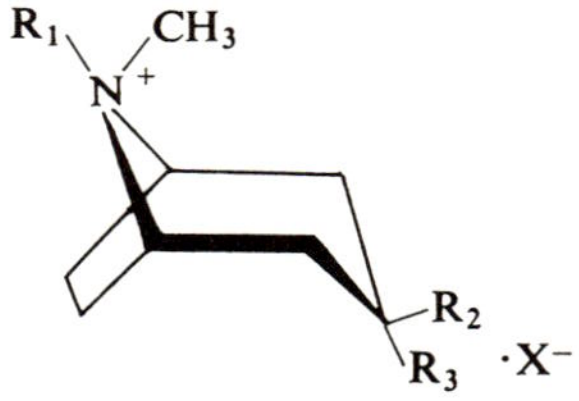

Compound	R_1	R_2	R_3	X	Ganglionic stimulant potency ([b])	([b])	Reflex respiratory stimulant potency in the cat
N-417	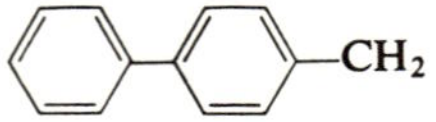	H	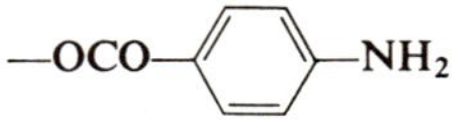	Br	60	15	13
N-361	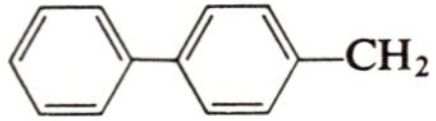	H	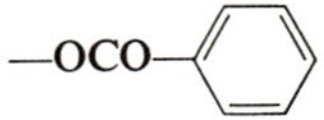	Br	2.5		0.3
N-406	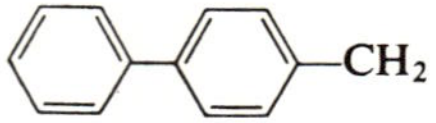	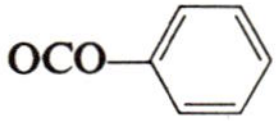	H	Br	0.5		0.2
N-293	CH_3	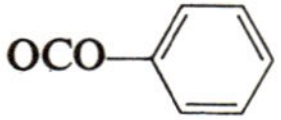	H	I	0.1		0.1

N-447	CH_3	H	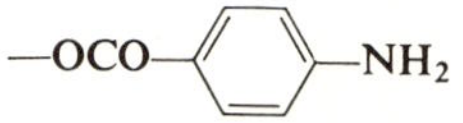	I			
N-451	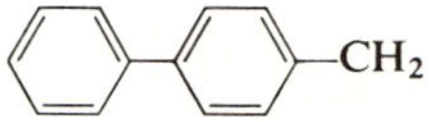	H	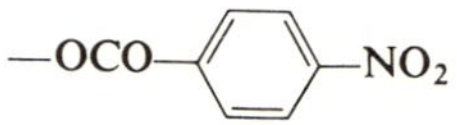	Br			
Na-88	CH_3	H	H	I	0.1		0.1
N-427	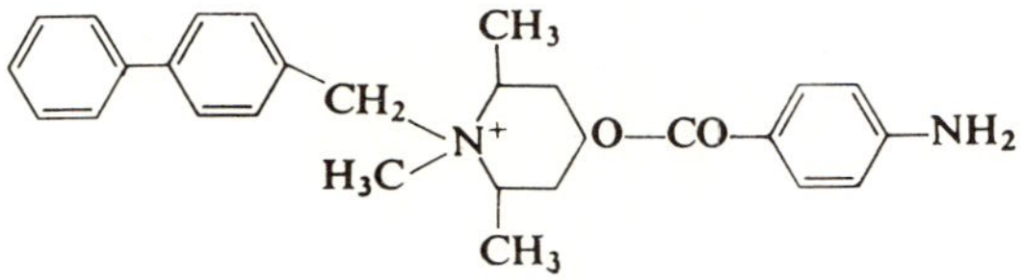			Br	6.0	2.0	5.0
N-284	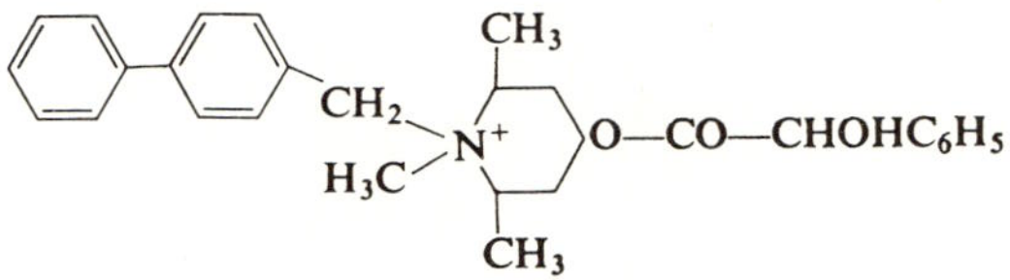			Br	0.2		0.2
N-412	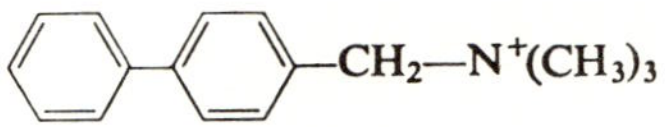			Br	0.2		0.1
Lobeline					0.1	0.2	0.2
Nicotine					1.0	1.0	1.0

[a] Data of Gyermek and Nador (*95*).
[b] Cat pressor response.
[c] Cat nictitating membrane.

potent compound in the series was *p*-phenylbenzyl(*p*-aminobenzoyl α-tropinium bromide), N-417, which in cat blood pressure experiments exhibited a ganglionic stimulant potency surpassing that of nicotine by a factor of 60 (*95*). In the cat nictitating membrane preparation it was 15 times more potent than nicotine, thus yielding the most potent ganglionic stimulant so far encountered (Table 4.10). It also elicited intensive stimulation of the respiration through the carotid chemoreceptors and produced stimulation on the isolated rabbit ileum. Like many other ganglionic stimulant agents it produced a secondary blocking phase. Repeated administration caused an increasingly lower degree of rise in blood pressure. As to its mechanism of action, norepinephrine mobilized from the adrenal medulla must play a definite role, for three reasons: because a fairly large difference in potency between the cat blood pressure and the nictitating membrane was shown, because after ligation of the adrenal gland N-417 acts considerably more weakly, and because, if given in the abdominal aorta through the superior mesenteric artery, it produces a significantly greater effect. After N-417 the blood pressure rise is followed by a definite fall, caused by a blockade of the sympathetic ganglia. This secondary block is not competitive but, rather, of the depolarizing type. Whereas a competitive type of agent (TEA) can be antagonized by cholinesterase blocking agents, such as diisopropyl fluorophosphate, the action of N-417 usually is enhanced by it.

N-417 and few similar agents represented an entirely new chemical class of ganglionic stimulant agents. The known compounds that stimulated autonomic ganglia belonged to simple monoquaternary ammonium derivatives (TMA, DMPP) or to quaternary ammonium compounds of the aliphatic ester and ether types (choline derivatives). Of the naturally occurring ganglionic stimulants nicotine, cytisine, and lobeline contain tertiary and secondary amino groups. The most active compounds in the tropine ester series were in many respects different from the known compounds. In studies dealing with the correlation of ganglionic stimulant action and chemical constitution Hey (*88*) claimed that to obtain an optimal ganglionic stimulant action structures containing the following moieties were needed: a cationic head with three methyl groups, an ether oxygen with a two-carbon connecting chain toward the cationic head, and an aromatic group containing electronegative substituents and capable of influencing the polarity of the ether oxygen by reducing its electron density. The observations of Hey were supported by earlier findings of Hunt and Renshaw (*138*) and of Loewe and Puttuck (*100*) with the choline ether type of molecules. Choline phenyl ethers, however, did not seem to represent the optimal nicotinic structure, because compounds that exhibit maximal potency belong to a chemical class entirely different from choline ethers. These compounds do not contain a trimethylammonium cationic group and are not of the ether, but of the ester, type. In contrast to the suggested role of the electronegative substituents, which in the *ortho* or *meta* position of the aromatic nucleus increase markedly the nicotinic action, potency can be markedly enhanced by introducing an amino substituent in the *para* position (Table 4.10). Although the results with this class of tropines and related structures were not adequate for establishing the optimal chemical requirements of ganglionic stimulant activity, it can be stated that in the most active ganglionic stimulants there is a *para* phenylbenzyl quaternary ammonium group, that the quaternary group is located on the nitrogen atom of a cyclic amine, which can be either tropane or 2,6-dimethylpiperidine, and that an aromatic ester group in which an amino group in the *para* position is optimal. Elimination of the first condition (that is, elimination of the *para* phenylbenzyl group by substitution and by using other groups, such as methyl, benzyl, or naphthylmethyl) results in a marked decrease or cessation of ganglionic stimulant action. Elimination of the second requirement (that is, the complete opening of the cyclic tropane ring into an aliphatic compound (N-443)) also leads to a complete elimination of ganglionic stimulant action. Elimination of the third structural condition (that is, the ester group) results in a compound (*N*-*p*-phenylbenzyltropanium bromide, N-421) which does not stimulate, but markedly blocks, the autonomic ganglia (Table 4.28). However, in the series of nicotine quaternaries the (*N*-*p*-phenylbenzyl$_{\text{pyrrolidyl}}$) (*N*-methyl$_{\text{pyridyl}}$) nicotinium derivative showed considerable stimulant potency.

Regarding the mechanism of action of ganglionic stimulant agents, the study with the tropane and piperidine types of agent mentioned above confirmed the general concept that every compound that stimulates the ganglia produces a secondary blocking effect. It must be realized that the competitive blocking capacity influences the stimulating action and that the competitive and depolarizing types of blockade are mingling and produce an over-all effect that can be extremely varied. It is worth while to mention that N-417, which produces an intensive stimulation of sympathetic ganglia, does not evoke stimulation of the guinea pig ileum and rat ileum. On the isolated rabbit ileum it produces a biphasic effect, and increasing the dose results in a predominantly blocking action. N-361, which is somewhat weaker in its ganglionic stimulant actions, does not produce stimulation on the isolated rabbit ileum at all. The different results obtained with compounds that produce a double effect (ganglionic stimulation and blocking actions) can offer an explanation of the findings of Loewe and Puttuck (*100*), that certain choline cresyl ether types of agent only stimulate the sympathetic ganglia. This claim was based on negative results obtained from the isolated guinea pig ileum, in which the parasympathetic ganglia were not stimulated by these agents.* The only other type of

* The reason for a virtual selectivity was that the methods used were not adequate to detect the qualitatively present, but not readily measurable, parasympathetic ganglion stimulation. As mentioned, the guinea pig ileum is a test organ that does not respond even

tropane derivative that exhibited nicotinic stimulant properties was 3β-phenyltropane, which is about as potent as nicotine. The structural requirements for its action were found to be quite specific: the 3α-phenyl analogue was much less active. Methyl quaternization did not increase the potency of the compounds, whereas the presence of the phenyl group was necessary for the nicotinic action (*161*).

A few derivatives containing the granatane ring system* were tested for ganglionic actions. Methyl quaternaries of acetyl α-granatane and β-granatane showed mild stimulant actions on the cat nictitating membrane and dog bladder preparations (*141*).

F. Nonnicotinic Cholinergic and Noncholinergic Ganglionic Stimulants

It was recognized a few years ago that several nontypical ganglionic agents, such as histamine, 5-HT, pilocarpine, and muscarine, can stimulate autonomic ganglia and that their actions on the ganglia are unlike that of ACh and nicotine. Trendelenburg (*13*), for example, found that on the cat superior cervical ganglion preparation the stimulation produced by histamine, pilocarpine, and 5-HT can be abolished only by depolarizing agents (TMA) but cannot be inhibited by hexamethonium.

Konzett and Rothlin (*11*) distinguished between direct and indirect ganglionic stimulants that act by sensitizing the receptors to ACh. ACh, choline, nicotine, ATP, KCl and several other compounds belong to the first type, whereas physostigmine and histamine belong to the second type. The different degrees of blocking of DMPP, nicotine, and TMA by hexamethonium on the nervous (ganglionic) receptors of guinea pig ileum suggested to Day and Vane (*81*) that the sites of action of these conventionally used ganglionic stimulant agents are not identical. TMA, for example, seems to act not only at cholinergic, but also at 5-HT-sensitive and histamine-sensitive, receptor sites. The stimulant action of 5-HT on the isolated gut is different from the other above-mentioned agents, in that it is blocked by morphine and hyoscine but not by methysergid, which blocks 5-HT at other muscular receptors. In the dog two different types of cholinergic ganglionic stimulant can be described (*162*). The

---

to the most active ganglionic stimulant compounds, although stimulation is obtained on other preparations, such as rabbit ileum. Because of these discrepancies choline cresyl ether was tested on the dog bladder, where it produced an obvious stimulating action susceptible to hexamethonium blockade. It seems that so far there is no indication of the existence of a selective ganglionic stimulation in the absolute sense, just as there is no completely selective ganglionic blocking agent that would act exclusively on a certain type of ganglion.

* Obtained through the courtesy of Prof. G. Fodor and Dr. B. Matkovics, Department of Organic Chemistry, University of Szeged, Hungary.

ganglionic stimulant characteristics of nicotine and DMPP could be distinguished from stimulant agents such as McN-A-343 and AHR-602 in the spinal cat. The effects of the latter agents could be blocked by cocaine, morphine, and methadone, but even these two agents are not alike in their over-all stimulant action (*163*). On the dog bladder ganglia a definite separation of the effects of nicotinic drugs (nicotine, DMPP, and ACh) and 5-HT could be demonstrated by using specific blocking of agents (*74*). On the guinea pig ileum the drugs nicotine, DMPP, and choline phenyl ether represent one group of stimulants that are sensitive to ganglionic blocking agents, and ACh, histamine, and 5-HT belong to a group not sensitive to these agents. Receptors of ACh, histamine, and 5-HT, however, seem not to be identical (*164*). A pharmacologic distinction between different ganglionic receptor sites of the guinea pig ileum has also been demonstrated by Harry (*82*) by means of selective desensitization to 5-HT and histamine and selective blocking against histamine by antihistaminic agents. The differential sensitivity of nicotine, histamine, and 5-HT to botulinium toxin blockade also indicates that probably three different sites are involved in the action of these agents.

From experiments with selective competitive antagonists Van Rossum (*158*) analyzed the correlations of affinity and intrinsic activity of different ganglionic drugs and concluded that DMPP and nicotine react with the same receptor type. On the basis of the results obtained from the isolated superior cervical ganglion of the cat by monoamine oxidase inhibition, Kalbermatten (*165*) proposed that 5-HT was involved in altering ganglionic transmission.

1. NONNICOTINIC CHOLINERGIC STIMULANTS OF GANGLIA

a. Anticholinesterase Drugs

Neostigmine and eserine produce a pressor response in the dog under ganglionic blockade with hexamethonium. The pressor response is blocked by small doses of atropine (*166*, *167*) or by TMA. This is suggestive of a nonnicotinic sympathetic ganglion stimulant action (*167*). A direct ganglionic stimulant effect of neostigmine was also found in the cat nictitating membrane preparation (*168*). Eserine similarly produced ganglionic stimulation in the superior cervical ganglion, which was insensitive to hexamethonium and *d*-tubocurarine (*40*). Neurophysiologic analysis showed that neostigmine acts at autonomic ganglia by mechanisms other than those connected to blockade of cholinesterase. It possibly influences both presynaptic and postsynaptic receptor sites and may combine with sites that are atropine-sensitive (*169*). It was also suggested that neostigmine acts by two distinct mechanisms in autonomic ganglia: first by a direct action and then by ACh release, as indicated with the moving-fluid electrode technique on isolated ganglion (*170*). Besides the direct ganglionic actions there is a restoring effect of neostigmine on ganglionic conduction following blocking agents (*171*, *172*). Atropine interferes with the conduction-restoring effect of neostigmine; thus, it seems that this effect is also manifested at the nonnicotinic type of ganglionic receptor. The antagonistic action of another anticholinesterase drug, diisopropyl fluorophosphate, to ganglionic blockade seems to parallel its inhibitory action on specific cholinesterase (*173*).

b. Muscarine

A study of natural muscarine chloride, made by Ambache and co-workers (*7*), first called attention to the possible ganglionic stimulant effect of muscarine, a prototype cholinomimetic drug considered earlier to be absolutely free from ganglionic action. On the perfused superior cervical ganglion preparation of the cat it was demonstrated that doses of muscarine as minute as 0.1 to 0.2 μg were capable of stimulating ganglion cells. Konzett and Waser (*174*) reported similar results on the perfused ganglion preparation. Ambache et al. (*7*) stated that the ganglionic stimulant action of muscarine can be abolished by atropine, nicotine, and hexamethonium, and only the denervated ganglion was insensitive to hexamethonium blockade. Recently Gyermek et al. (*175*) provided direct evidence that muscarine stimulates the inferior mesenteric and superior cervical ganglion of the cat by recording the electrical activity of the postganglionic nerve filaments. Muscarinic activity and ganglionic stimulant potency seem to be parallel within the chemical group of muscarine analogues because isomers of muscarine inactive at the postganglionic sites were also inactive at the ganglion.

An electrophysiologic analysis of the action of muscarine on the superior cervical ganglion indicated that the components of the action potential produced by muscarine and DMPP are different. A correlation between the muscarine-induced S_1 and S_2 components of the postganglionic neurograms and the contractions of the nictitating membrane has been found (*156*). These studies and that of Jones et al. (*163*) with the superior cervical ganglion indicated that the muscarine-induced ganglionic stimulation, although extremely sensitive to atropine blockade, is insensitive to hexamethonium. Correspondingly, earlier attempts to demonstrate the ganglionic stimulant action of crystalline and synthetic muscarine on atropinized preparations yielded negative results (*176*, *177*).

c. Pilocarpine

The cholinomimetic alkaloid pilocarpine exhibits some ganglionic stimulant properties that can be demonstrated in cat blood pressure response (*178*), in dog bladder (*141*), and in isolated intestine (*179*). Pappano and Volle (*180*) recently presented evidence of the ganglionic stimulant action by using electrophysiologic methods of analysis. The type of action of pilocarpine is similar to that of muscarine.

d. McN-A-343 and AHR-602

McN-A-343, [4-(*m*-chlorophenylcarbamoyloxy)-2-butynyl]-trimethylammonium chloride, is another of the better explored cholinergic but nonnicotinic types of ganglionic stimulant agents (*8*). It is resistant to hexamethonium but can be blocked readily by atropine. The muscarinic actions of this agent are relatively weak. This is interesting in view of the observations with muscarine isomers, in which the ganglionic stimulant action and the peripheral muscarinic actions seemed to parallel each other. The example of McN-A-343 suggests that the structural features required for stimulating the atropine-sensitive cholinergic nonnicotinic receptor sites are not identical with those required for stimulating the postganglionic muscarinic receptor. On the other hand, examples of the muscarine analogues indicate an identity of structural requirements at these two receptors. The ganglionic stimulant characteristics of McN-A-343 were further explored by Murayama and Unna (*181*) in a careful comparison with DMPP and pilocarpine. The findings of Roszkowski (*8*) regarding resistance to ganglionic blocking agents and sensitivity to atropine were confirmed, and blocking by cocaine and morphine was noted. A similarity to, but not a full identity with, pilocarpine action was claimed.

Results obtained with AHR-602, *N*-benzyl-3-pyrrolidylacetate methobromide, indicate that it also belongs to the class of cholinergic nonnicotinic types (*182*).

The study of Jones (*183*) showed that muscarine, McN-A-343, and AHR-602 resemble each other in their stimulant action on the ganglia. Since cocaine, morphine, and methadone also block the effect of these muscarinic substances, it seems possible that these agents act at ganglionic receptors similar to those at which 5-HT acts. Newly developed classes of selective antagonists to the neural activity of 5-HT, such as indoleacetamidines, guanidines, and indolealkylammonium compounds (*75*, *76*, *184*), thus would be expected to affect the ganglionic effects of muscarinic agents.

2. NONCHOLINERGIC GANGLIONIC STIMULANTS

a. 5-HT and Related Compounds

Indirect evidence obtained on the cat nictitating membrane preparation (*178*) and direct evidence obtained by recording spontaneous postganglionic nerve activity on the inferior mesenteric ganglion of the cat (*185*) are now available for the ganglionic stimulant action of 5-HT. Pharmacologic analysis with different blocking agents indicated that its action is different from cholinergic ganglionic stimulants and that the 5-HT receptors at the ganglion are also markedly different from the smooth-muscle receptors sensitive to this amine (*185*). Further studies (*186*) demonstrated that several *N*-methylated derivatives of 5-HT also stimulate ganglionic receptors. While the *N*-monomethyl derivative acts at the same receptors as 5-HT, the *N*,*N*-di- and *N*,*N*,*N*-trimethyl derivatives (bufotenin and bufotenidine) predominantly stimulate the cholinergic nicotine-sensitive receptor types (*187*). An indole type of blocking agent of 5-HT at the ganglion, 5-hydroxy-3-indoleacetamidine, also produces transient ganglionic stimulation affecting the 5-HT-sensitive ganglionic receptors (*186*). Comparison of a few indoles on the inferior mesenteric ganglion of the cat is given in Table 4.11.

5-HT-sensitive receptors can be found not only at autonomic ganglia but at chemoreceptors and in ganglionlike receptors of the intestines and the dog bladder. 5-HT produces stimulation at these sites and often also potentiates the effect of other neuronal stimuli (electric stimulation, DMPP, ACh, and potassium chloride), as demonstrated, for example, on the dog bladder (*74*). The receptors sensitive to 5-HT in these ganglia are also distinctly different pharmacologically from the nicotine type of ganglionic receptor. The receptors of 5-HT are susceptible to cocaine and morphine blockade and to 5-HT tachyphylaxis, but are not influenced by ganglionic blocking agents, such as hexamethonium (*33*).

TABLE 4.11

Effects of Indole Compounds on the Inferior Mesenteric Ganglion of the Cat[a]

Compound	Stimulant potency	Blocking potency
5-Hydroxytryptamine	++	++
N-Methyl-5-hydroxytryptamine	++	++
Bufotenine (*N*,*N*-dimethyl-5-hydroxytryptamine)	++[b]	++[b]
Bufotenidine, $^{-}$O-indolyl-$(CH_2)_2N^+(CH_3)_3$	++[c]	++[c]
5-Hydroxy-3-indoleacetamidine	++	++
5-Hydroxy-α-methyltryptamine		+
5-Benzyloxygramine		+
N,*N*-Dimethyltryptamine	+[b]	+
N,*N*,*N*-Trimethyltryptamine	++[c]	
Tryptamidine (3-indoleacetamidine)	+	+
7-Benzyloxygramine		+

[a] Very potent, ++; weakly potent, +. Data of Gyermek and Bindler (*186*).
[b] Partly cholinergic type.
[c] Mainly cholinergic type.

b. Guanidine Derivatives

Some of these, especially phenyldiguanide and 2-naphthylguanidine, stimulate autonomic ganglia; their site of action is similar to that of 5-HT (*75*). A few characteristics of guanidine derivatives are shown in Table 4.12.

c. Histamine

Histamine is known to stimulate certain autonomic ganglia. This is manifested, for example, in contractions of the cat nictitating membrane on close intraarterial injection and in an increase of the responses of the superior cervical ganglion to ACh. These effects are not influenced by hexamethonium, but are blocked by cocaine and morphine (*132*). Histamine was also shown to stimulate the paravertebral sympathetic ganglia, producing a rise in blood pressure in the cat (*178*). However, no significant increase of the spontaneous postganglionic nerve activity has been observed on injecting low doses (1 μg) of histamine into the cat inferior mesenteric ganglion preparation (*141*). When histamine stimulates the adrenal medulla it liberates norepinephrine in addition to epinephrine. This stimulant action is resistant to TEA but can be suppressed by antihistamines (*94*).

The first subgroup of ganglionic stimulants consists of the typical nicotinic type of agent, including DMPP, TMA, and nicotine itself, which are easily characterized pharmacologically by their hexamethonium-sensitive and atropine-resistant ganglionic effects. A major part of the ganglionic action of ACh is also attributable to this kind of mechanism.

TABLE 4.12

Stimulant and Blocking Potencies of Guanidine Derivatives on Autonomic Ganglia (Inferior Mesenteric Ganglion of the Cat)[a]

	Minimal effective stimulant dose, μg/kg	Minimal effective blocking dose against 5-HT, μg/kg	Minimal effective stimulant dose,[b] μg/kg
Phenyldiguanide	6.2	12.0	0.6
Benzylguanidine	14.0	55.0	14.0
2-Naphthylguanidine	0.7	5.0	0.5
2-Anthrylguanidine	2.5	1.6	
2-Anthrylbiguanide	20.0	15.0	
2-Acridylbiguanide	40.0	10.0	
5-Hydroxytryptamine	3.3		1.0

[a] Data of Gyermek (*75*).

[b] Dog pelvic nerve bladder preparation.

The second subgroup includes, besides the characteristic muscarinic agents (muscarine, pilocarpine, etc.), ACh which, besides having nicotinic ganglionic stimulant properties, acts on muscarinic receptor types of ganglion. The following evidence is available for this second action of ACh. Two temporally distinct effects of ACh on the superior cervical ganglion of the cat have been found. The first, an early effect that can be obtained after eserine treatment or tetanic stimulation, is sensitive to *d*-tubocurarine and hexamethonium; the second, later, effect is sensitive to atropine (*40*). The second seems to be connected with a lowered resting membrane potential; in this respect the superior cervical ganglion is very similar to the parasympathetic pelvic ganglion of the dog, in which the effect of ACh and electrical stimulation can also be divided into two phases: a hexamethonium-sensitive phase and an atropine-sensitive phase (*71*). The remarkable similarity between these two organs indicates that at the intramural pelvic ganglia of the dog bladder either the functioning of typical parasympathetic nerve endings is independent of a superimposed ganglionic element, or the pelvic ganglia possess two types of receptor, which also substitute for the end-organ receptors. Small doses of ACh produce a diphasic action obtained by recording from the surface of the ganglion cells of the superior cervical ganglion of the cat. The diphasic action consists of a low-amplitude hyperpolarization followed by a low-amplitude depolarization. Larger doses produce a triphasic response with an initial depolarization followed by a hyperpolarization and a second delayed depolarization. Very large doses produce a single phase of depolarization (*41*). In distinction to the first group, these sites are characterized pharmacologically by their sensitivity to atropine blockade and their resistance to hexamethonium.

The third group of compounds comprise those agents which act on probably noncholinergic receptor sites at the ganglion; 5-HT, phenylguanidine, and histamine belong to this group. Their action on the receptors, however, can be either direct or indirect through the possible participation of a cholinergic nonnicotinic synapse (for example, the E-2 type).

G. Miscellaneous Compounds with Ganglionic Stimulant Action

In contrast to muscarine, which is one of the typical representatives of nonnicotinic ganglionic stimulant agents, its keto derivatives, muscarone, and a few of its isomers are fairly potent ganglionic stimulants of the nicotinic type. Stimulation of atropinized dog and cat ganglia and isolated frog rectus muscle has been obtained that was sensitive to hexamethonium blockade (*71*, *176*, *188*, *189*); see Table 4.13. A stimulation of the atropinized inferior mesenteric ganglia of the cat has been shown for (±) muscarone in doses five to ten times larger than that of nicotine (*177*).

Certain aliphatic choline ether types of "model" substances of muscarine,

TABLE 4.13

Nicotinic Stimulant Effects of Muscarone Derivatives[a]

Compound	Minimal effective "nicotinic" stimulant dose, μg/kg: Dog nictitating membrane	Cat nictitating membrane	Cat respiration	Frog rectus muscle, activity ratio[b]
(−)Muscarone	150	50	50	2
(±)Muscarone	180	65	125	2
(+)Muscarone	120	100	160	2
(±)Allomuscarone	160	40	70	3
(±)4,5-Dehydromuscarone	60	50	40	2
(±)4,5-Dehydropropylmuscarone	150	120	180	$\frac{1}{4}$
L(+)-Muscarine	200	400	250	1/400
DMPP	10	8	8	
ACh	300	50	70	1

[a] Data of Gyermek and Unna (*188*).
[b] Activity of ACh, 1.0.

which contained several of its functional groups except the tetrahydrofuran ring moiety and showed only weak cholinomimetic actions, possessed fairly pronounced ganglionic stimulant action in the dog bladder (*141*).

Furfuryltrimethylammonium and its 5-methyl analogue are structurally related to muscarine. Their ganglionic stimulant actions on the cat blood pressure, on the superior cervical ganglion preparation, and on the dog bladder are moderate (*141*, *179*, *190*). δ-Trimethylammonium-γ-valerolactone, besides its muscarinic properties, shows predominantly nicotinic effects (*191*). Methylated derivatives of histamine, which carry two or three methyl groups on the terminal N atom of the side chain, show definite ganglionic stimulant action. N^1,*N*,*N*-Trimethylhistamine was found to be as potent as nicotine on the spinal cat blood pressure preparation and nictitating membrane (*192*, *193*). *N*,*N*-Dimethylhistamine showed only weak nicotinic action (*193*).

Leptodactyline [*N*,*N*,*N*-trimethyl-*N*-β-(*m*-hydroxyphenyl) ethylammonium], a naturally occurring ammonium ion, has very extensive ganglionic stimulant action in cat and dog blood pressure experiments (*194*).

Quaternary methyl derivatives of tyramine, dopamine, and norepinephrine were reported to be stimulant to autonomic ganglia of the cat (blood pressure and nictitating membrane). Dopamine methobromide showed a remarkable degree of potency, surpassing that of nicotine (*195*).

Some of the sympatholytic benzodioxane derivatives of Fourneau were studied by Bacq (*196*) for their action on autonomic ganglia of the cat. Ethylethanolaminomethyl-3-benzodioxane (F-997) and diethylaminomethyl-3-benzodioxane methiodide showed nicotinelike stimulant properties, whereas most of the other sympatholytic benzodioxanes had ganglionic blocking effects.

Of the group of coniine alkaloids, coniine itself is a weak ganglionic stimulant and γ-coniceine a more potent one on the cat superior cervical ganglion (*197*).

A tremor-producing agent, 1,4-dipyrrolidino-2-butyne (Tremorine), which also exhibits relatively marked parasympathetic effects, shows signs of ganglionic stimulation in the cat. The effect is blocked by atropine and by ganglionic blocking agents (*198*). An active metabolite of Tremorine, 1-(2-oxo-1-pyrrolidinyl)-4-(1-pyrrolidinyl)-2-butyne (oxotremorine), first claimed to be free from ganglionic action (*199*), was shown later to produce long-lasting postganglionic firing, which was similar to that of anticholinesterase agents and was also sensitive to atropine (*200*).

4.4. GANGLIONIC BLOCKING AGENTS

A. Modes and Types of Action of Ganglionic Blocking Agents

It is now recognized that drug-induced blockade of autonomic ganglia may develop through various mechanisms. From the pharmacologic point of view, criteria of ganglionic blockade can change considerably, depending on the types of drug and biological preparation used. Since a large number of ganglionic blocking agents belong to the methonium type, and because these agents also occupy an important position as being therapeutically useful, a description of the criteria of ganglionic blocking agents, outlined by Paton and Zaimis (*201*), for methonium compounds will be pertinent here. A ganglionic blocking compound must interfere only with ganglionic neurotransmissions and not any other. It should block the synapses without previous excitation, and it should not interfere with the release of ACh. Compounds belonging to the methonium type, represented by the prototype agent hexamethonium, satisfied these criteria. When tested on the spinal cat blood pressure and nictitating membrane preparation, hexamethonium did not influence the effect of epinephrine or that of postganglionic electric stimulation of the nictitating membrane. It did not produce signs of ganglionic stimulation; on the perfused superior cervical ganglion the output of ACh was the same before and after administration of methonium compounds, which exceeded the ganglionic blocking dose by a factor of 1000. This agent blocks the blood pressure responses produced by nicotine and TMA but not that of epinephrine. The studies of Paton and Zaimis (*201*), outlining the criteria of ganglionic blockade, actually only characterized the site of action for certain types of agent but made no reference to the mode or mechanism of action. Additional studies were made (*202*) to classify the most important ganglionic blocking agents according to their mode of action. Two major categories have been described: agents that produce initial stimulation followed by blockade through depolarization (called depolarizing blocking drugs) and agents that produce block in the absence of depolarization and stimulation (called competitive blocking compounds). Besides the classic agents of the methonium group, which belong to the competitive type of agent, certain compounds such as nicotine exhibit a dual action, having an initial depolarizing phase and a concomitant competitive blocking phase. Its possible mode of action, that of reversibly inhibiting ACh at the ganglionic sites, was suggested relatively early by Koppanyi et al. (*203*), who demonstrated an antagonistic action of physostigmine against the nicotine blockade. This resulted in the proposition that there is a competitive type of blockade produced by nicotine. The complicating details of nicotine action, however, were not recognized at that time. According to recent studies its action is quite complex. Takeshige et al. (*204*) studied ACh, methacholine, and nicotine, and the last one seems to be the most complicated in mode of action. The complexity of nicotine action is illustrated by observations of the perfused superior cervical ganglion, nicotine combining first with the free, later on with the activated, ganglionic receptors. Whereas its ganglionic stimulating action is produced on the free receptors, the blocking effect may be manifested mostly on the activated receptors (*205*). The influence on facilitation of ganglionic transmission has been evaluated by using nicotine. Facilitation by repetitive preganglionic volleys is unaffected by eserine or by anesthetics, but it is abolished by doses of nicotine below those that normally affect ganglionic transmission. Thus, besides the conventional blocking actions of nicotine and its direct stimulant action on ganglionic transmission, there is an inhibitory action against ganglionic facilitation, which is independent of the others. It is obvious from these considerations that in addition to, and in contrast to, hexamethonium blockade the ganglionic inhibition produced by nicotine, which outlasts the period of depolarization, is probably due to diminished release of acetylcholine from presynaptic terminals (*207*). Thus, it should be realized that different mechanisms of blockade of transmission come into play when different doses of nicotine are employed (*206*).

Decamethonium and eserine were found to produce a competitive type of blockade on the superior cervical ganglion. Thus, decamethonium seems to exhibit a unique feature, being a competitive blocking agent at one cholinergic synaptic receptor site and a depolarizing blocking agent at another. A recent study of the isolated guinea pig ileum indicated that, although hexamethonium is a surmountable competitive antagonist when tested against DMPP, newer ganglionic blocking agents, such as chlorisondamine and mecamylamine, show a noncompetitive type of antagonism. TEA showed a mixed type of action. These differences were detected in the shift or change in slope of dose–response curves in the presence of both ganglionic blocking agents and the stimulant (*208*). Similar dose–response correlations from studies of frog rectus muscle indicated the competitive nature of hexamethonium blockade and the noncompetitive nature of chlorisondamine and mecamylamine blockade (*209*).

By using neurophysiologic methods and analyzing correlations of stimulus frequency and blockade with the application of ganglionic blocking agents of different structures it was possible to distinguish between these agents. It was indicated that frequency-connected variations in ganglionic drug–receptor affinities or intrinsic activities are possible and that such differences cannot be found by using cruder methods of exploration. Several blocking agents displayed a positive linear relationship between the degree of block and stimulus frequency, but the slopes of these relationships were usually markedly variable among the different blocking agents (*210*). A similar study with mecamylamine and hexamethonium showed that their modes of action on ganglionic transmission were similar (*211*). However, other studies indicate that mecamylamine does not act by a competitive type of blockade against acetylcholine and that its type of action is completely different from that of hexamethonium and pentolinium. Mecamylamine is readily diffusable into cells and, when it acts on the whole animal, several other factors than ganglionic blockade are involved (*212*). Another indication of a difference in type of action between mecamylamine and methonium compounds is the observation that excess carbon dioxide antagonizes the action of hexamethonium while the action of mecamylamine is being enhanced (*23*). A discrepancy between the hypotensive and ganglionic doses of mecamylamine and those of methonium compounds has also been noted (*213*).

A separation of ganglionic depolarization from ganglionic block has been detected by using the sympathetic ganglion cells of frog (*214*). ACh, carbachol, nicotine, and TMA depolarize the ganglion cells and depress synaptic transmission. In the continued presence of any of these drugs the depolarization subsides, but the depression of synaptic transmission persists. Succinylcholine and decamethonium in high concentration depress transmission without causing initial depolarization. That the depolarization type of block is independent of the preceding stimulatory action at the ganglia is indicated by the observations of Gold and Reinert (*215*), who showed that amphetamine produced a ganglionic depolarization and block similar to those produced by nicotine and did not produce any stimulatory action in the ganglion. Neurophysiologic findings indicate that ACh produces ganglionic blockade that coincides with the ganglionic depolarization and postganglionic firing, whereas blockade by methacholine coincides with ganglionic hyperpolarization and electrical silence of the postganglionic nerve. Atropine antagonizes the blockade produced by both agents. Concerning the possibilities of ganglionic blockade with various depolarizing and hyperpolarizing types of agents, Takeshige and Volle (*41*) offer the following classification: depolarization antagonized by atropine (this is produced by ACh or tetramethylammonium), hyperpolarization antagonized by atropine (produced by ACh and methacholine), hyperpolarization not antagonized by atropine (produced by large doses of ACh), and late depolarization not antagonized by atropine (produced by large doses of tetramethylammonium). Concerning compounds with a complex type of action, Komalahiranya and Volle (*216*) described the different phases of the ganglionic action of *N*-ethylmaleimide. The first is an enhancement of the evoked postganglionic spike potential and a depression of the responses produced by ACh, KCl or TMA and, conversely, a later change that consists of an enhancement of the responses of the ganglia to ganglionic stimulants when the response to stimulation of the preganglionic nerve is depressed. Further, retrograde firing along the preganglionic nerve evoked by KCl is enhanced by *N*-ethylmaleimide, indicating the complexity of action.

This summary of data available on the modes and types of action of a few of the more significant blocking agents of autonomic ganglia merely illustrates that present knowledge is still quite superficial regarding them. The expression "mechanism of action" has been rather avoided, because it covers the total series of events, from an agent approaching a receptor to the final response through and beyond those stages outlined in Section 4.2, B. However, a summary of modes and types of action can be at least of some practical help in the critical assessment of new drugs, especially in selecting proper methods of evaluation and placing the compounds in a channel of techniques that may lead eventually through more refined techniques to an understanding of at least some of the "mechanisms" of ganglionic drug actions.

B. Sensitivities of Sympathetic and Parasympathetic Ganglia to Ganglionic Blockade

The theoretically and therapeutically important problem of the comparative sensitivities of sympathetic and parasympathetic ganglia to ganglionic blockade has been extensively explored. Several times it was claimed that certain agents blocked exclusively a division of autonomic ganglia or a certain ganglion, but the claims were usually not substantiated later. It was Shafer (*68*) who first found that sodium citrate blocked the parasympathetic pathways to the pupil and heart of the turtle, but the same doses of citrate did not paralyze sympathetic pathways, and so he concluded that calcium ions are more necessary to the functioning of the parasympathetic ganglia than to that of the sympathetic. Ganglionic blocking agents may be classified as outlined below.

1. COMPOUNDS OF HIGH SELECTIVITY

Cavallini et al. (*217*) reported that certain alkylammoniumstilbene and diphenyl derivatives blocked the vagal ganglia of the cat in preference to its cervical sympathetic ganglia. Similar observations were reported by Pardo et al. (*218*), who obtained selective blockade of vagal ganglia of the cat with ethylmethylisooctenylamine.

2. COMPOUNDS WITH MODERATE SELECTIVITY

In contrast to the few data given above, which report relatively high selectivity toward certain parasympathetic ganglia, there are several studies which have shown only a moderate degree of selectivity between different ganglia. A comparison of the various studies is fairly difficult, because each investigator has used different methods and species of animals.

Sometimes marked differences in sensitivity occur among different organs even in the same species, as in the nictitating membrane as compared with the salivary glands of the cat, but the latter is much too sensitive to any kind of blocking agent. An attempt was made to resolve these problems by using the cat heart stimulated through the vagus and through the sympathetic nerves, determining the blocking concentrations of several different types of blocking agent and expressing the ratio of sympathetic to parasympathetic blockade. Four out of five compounds showed approximately the same blocking ratios (about 1), but pentamethonium showed a ratio of 10, indicating a possible true selectivity toward a certain parasympathetic ganglion. The reason for such a selectivity may reside in the different accessibilities to the compound of different cells within the same organ.

3. COMPOUNDS WITH NO SELECTIVITY

In a third group of studies practically no difference between the sensitivities of the two divisions of the autonomic nervous system was reported. The following agents were used: ganglionic blocking agents of different classes (*85*); bisquaternary ammonium compounds (*219*); mecamylamine, pempidine, and their derivatives (*220*); and bisquaternary ammonium compounds and heterocyclic bisquaternary ammonium compounds (*221*, *222*). Of several ganglionic blocking compounds belonging to different chemical classes only one showed relatively selective depression of pelvic parasympathetic ganglia of the dog (*223*). Chandrasekhar et al. (*73*) studied structurally different ganglionic blocking agents. Although the ganglionic blocking potencies were approximately identical in the same species (dog), the same compounds tested in the mouse for pupillary dilatation showed markedly different degrees of relative potency. Thus, the variability in ganglionic blocking selectivity seems to reside in a species difference rather than in a difference between individual ganglia or divisions of ganglia of the same species.

The reason for a virtual selectivity in certain ganglion preparations was investigated by several groups. More detailed pharmacological analysis usually revealed that an effect other than ganglionic was involved in producing this difference. β-Triethylammonium (β'-triethylammoniumethyl) propionate dibromide, for example, was found to have, besides the ganglionic blocking capacity, a weak muscarinic action which, by an overlap with the ganglionic blockade, could well produce a picture indicating a selective inhibition of sympathetic ganglia (*224*). The interesting possibility that selectivity toward blockade in one division of the autonomic ganglia develops through a different degree of tolerance on repeated administration was discussed by Zaimis (*225*). Holtz and Schümann (*226*), in a careful study of the sympathetic and parasympathetic ganglion blockade with different types of blocking agent, offered an explanation of the possible differences between two divisions of ganglia when certain types of animal preparation were used. Their work emphasizes the nonidentity of receptors and even the difference in the responding organs when the whole animal is used. Thus, the possibility of drawing a proper conclusion from the whole animal concerning the blockade of a certain division or group of ganglia is quite difficult.

Several drugs reported earlier to be selective toward the parasympathetic ganglia were found to possess certain atropinelike side effects which mask ganglionic blockade at certain organs. A high blocking ratio at a particular ganglion of such an agent as compared to a standard blocking drug is therefore misleading. Furthermore, local anesthetic property can interfere with the function of certain postganglionic nerve elements where penetrability of an agent may selectively influence the membrane characteristics of a nerve fiber. The most conclusive evidence for a basically equal sensitivity of sympathetic and parasympathetic ganglia to conventional ganglionic blocking agents comes from electrophysiological studies performed on the superior cervical and ciliary ganglia of the cat (*84*, *85*, *94*, *227*). In these studies the responses of the sympathetic superior cervical ganglion of the cat was compared with the response of the parasympathetic ciliary ganglion by simultaneously recording postganglionic action potentials. By using structurally different ganglionic blocking agents, no difference between the sensitivity of these two ganglia has been found. With reference to earlier studies conducted in less suitable organ preparations, it was suggested that the observed differences were due not so much to variations in the nature of receptor sites or in receptor density at the different ganglia, but rather to unrecognized direct actions of the drugs at the effector organs or to differences in the access to ganglionic structures of the circulating drugs. Nonlinearity of the relations between effector response and ganglionic response or variations in the frequency-response of different ganglia to different electrical stimulations may contribute to the differences observed in certain studies. This was demonstrated by Schneider and Moore (*84*) by simultaneous comparison of the blockade of the superior cervical ganglion and ciliary ganglion of the cat and recording of postganglionic nerve activity. By changing the frequency of stimulation, a difference between the blocking potency of chlorisondamine and pentapyrrolidinium as compared to hexamethonium could be shown.

C. Relationships of Ganglionic Blockade to Other Pharmacologic Actions

The relationships between ganglionic blockade to inhibition of other cholinergic neurotransmission mechanisms is one of the basic problems, since curarelike and cholinolytic agents all revolve around one transmitter substance, ACh. The distinctly different structural characteristics of curarelike, atropinelike, and most ganglionic blocking agents, however, clearly indicate the major differences in structural requirements of different cholinergic receptor sites. Structural variations in the tropane group serve perhaps best to illustrate the usually reciprocal correlations between ganglionic blocking and cholinolytic actions and the more closely related, but still distinctly different, features that satisfy neuromuscular rather than ganglionic receptor sites (see Section 4.4, E, 5).

In a group of mono- and bisquaternary tropane derivatives the ganglionic blocking and curarelike actions parallelled the blocking potencies to AChE whereas blocking action at the parasympathetic nerve endings was related to the degree of blockade of pseudocholinesterase. These findings seem to indicate that the surface of receptors at various cholinergic sites is similar to the surface of cholinesterase dominant at that particular type of receptor (*228*). Several ganglionic blocking agents, such as nicotine, TMA, and mecamylamine, were tested to reveal correlations between ganglionic blocking potencies and actions on enzymes (such as specific and nonspecific cholinesterase, phosphomonoesterase, succinate dehydrogenase) and those on the SH content of the cat superior cervical ganglion (*229*). The relationship between anesthetic, nervous-system depressant actions and ganglionic transmission has been explored with the superior cervical ganglion of the cat. In a study conducted with many ganglionic blocking agents no hypnotic, sedative, or local anesthetic agent showed any correlation between anesthetic activity and ganglionic blockade (*230*, *231*). The relationship between oxygen consumption of the cervical sympathetic ganglion of the cat and ganglionic blockade was investigated by Vysotskaia et al. (*229*), but no correlation between the two could be established.

D. Actions of Ganglionic Blocking Agents Manifested at Other Than Ganglionic Receptor Sites

1. INHIBITION OF RELEASE AND SYNTHESIS OF ACh

The possibility of inhibiting the release of ACh from presynaptic nerve endings or storage sites was suggested recently. The reason is that newer ganglionic blocking agents, such as the pempidine and mecamylamine class of compounds, exhibited certain properties which were not explainable by the conventional theory of competitive antagonism at ganglionic sites with ACh. It was demonstrated that mecamylamine can inhibit synthesis of ACh (*232*), but in a later study Gardiner (*233*) could not demonstrate any such action of it or of pempidine, although hemicholinium (HC-3) effectively reduced the synthesis in the same concentration.

2. POTENTIATION OF CATECHOLAMINES AND OTHER VASOACTIVE AGENTS

In several species doses of ganglionic blocking agents, such as TEA, hexamethonium, and pentamethonium, too small to block ganglionic transmission, produce sensitization of the pressor effects of epinephrine and norepinephrine and of reflex vasoconstriction. It is probable that changes in the tissue stores are connected with this sensitization. The agents do not "seal the stores" of catecholamines as cocaine probably does, but increase the rate of uptake of norepinephrine and accelerate conversion into epinephrine. A possible blockade of O-methyl transferase might also be involved (*234*). Earlier observations of Lum and Rashleigh (*317*) indicate potentiating actions of TEA and mecamylamine. These agents enhance the actions of catecholamines and also that of angiotonin, 5-HT, histamine, and barium chloride on isolated arterial strips.

The studies of Zaimis (*225*) and Mantegazza et al. (*236*) indicate that the possible mechanism of development of tolerance to ganglionic blocking agents on continuous administration may reside in the phenomena of sensitization of vascular end-organ cells to epinephrine and norepinephrine. Sensitization of these sites can well produce effects that mask ganglionic blockade. It seems important to analyze these side effects while developing new ganglionic blocking agents, because it might be that a satisfactory degree of separation of catecholamine sensitization from ganglionic blocking action could be achieved. The rationale for this is based on findings that the receptor sites for these actions, although similar, are not identical. Furthermore, they are located apart from each other. Therefore, selective access to one site and not to any other can be envisioned.

3. BLOCKING ACTIONS OTHER THAN GANGLIONIC

Large doses of hexamethonium not only block the ganglia but also inhibit releasing of norepinephrine by sympathetic nerves (splenic nerve) of the cat

(*237*). Phenothiazines, besides blocking ganglia and chemoreceptors, block the ACh and K^+-induced activation of the potentials at the saphenous nerve. These results seem to show that the agents have a nonspecific nerve depressant effect that is similar to a local anesthetic action (*238*).

E. Classes of Ganglionic Blocking Agents

1. ALIPHATIC ALKYLAMMONIUM COMPOUNDS

Of the fair number of compounds that belong to the aliphatic alkylammonium group of ganglionic blocking agents TEA is the most important and has been investigated the most intensively. The first pharmacological study of it was made in 1915 by Burn and Dale. A more detailed pharmacological evaluation was undertaken by Achison and Moe (*2*) in 1946. In their study primary emphasis was placed on the cardiovascular effects of TEA, and it was concluded that its action is due mainly to a blockade of autonomic ganglia. This was demonstrated with the superior cervical ganglion, with the stellate ganglion, and at the cardioinhibitory ganglia of the vagus nerve. As regards structures functionally closely related to autonomic ganglia, TEA blocks the action of ganglionic stimulants on carotid body chemoreceptors, but it does not block stretch receptors and actions of stimulants on afferent vagal endings (*239*). A comprehensive review by Moe and Freyburger on the subject of TEA and related ganglionic blocking agents covers many aspects of the pharmacology of TEA (*27*). Several pharmacological studies have appeared since, a few of which will be quoted here. In most of the investigations TEA alone was used as reference standard in the study of new groups of ganglionic blocking agents. Investigations into TEA itself covered ganglia such as the celiac ganglion (*240*), the superior cervical, and stellate and ciliary ganglia in a comparative fashion (*241*, *242*), and the sympathetic and parasympathetic ganglia of the cat heart (*94*). The action of TEA on the stellate ganglion of the cat, which depresses the spontaneous after-discharges of the postganglionic nerve, has been studied by Karkevich (*67*). It was compared with other well-known ganglion blocking agents on the isolated superior cervical ganglion separation of the rat (*61*). Its actions against ganglionic stimuli of various frequencies, delivered to the preganglionic nerve of the superior cervical ganglion, has been studied, and a direct relationship between the intensity of ganglionic block and stimulus frequency has been established (*210*). On the isolated guinea pig ileum TEA, compared with other agents, did not show a very pure ganglionic blocking action when tested against DMPP (*208*). Dose–response relationships have been studied with the superior cervical ganglion of the dog, and complete blockade of the ganglionic transmission could be demonstrated with large doses. This was in contrast to other ganglionic blocking agents, such as chlorisondamine. The mode of action of

TEA has been investigated in conjunction with its antagonism to DFP. The reversal of the blockade produced by DFP was proportional to its inhibitory effect on specific cholinesterase (*173*). In contrast to DFP, eserine did not completely antagonize the blocking effects of TEA (*243*).

Several reports are available which, in addition to its typical ganglionic blocking properties, call attention to other actions of TEA that cannot be attributed to ganglionic blockade. In the isolated sympathetic ganglion pulmonary artery preparation of the rabbit TEA showed both postganglionic and preganglionic effects. A sensitization of the effect of *l*-norepinephrine occurs (*244*). TEA, like many other ganglionic blocking agents, stimulates the gastrointestinal tract; the mechanism probably involves excitation of parasympathetic spinal centers (*245*). TEA is almost completely ineffective against tonic nicotine convulsions in the mouse (*246*). Several ganglionic blocking agents of the methonium type antagonize these convulsions, but so far no satisfactory explanation of this phenomenon has been obtained. A central and also peripheral sympathetic inhibitory mechanism appears to be involved in the hypotension produced by TEA, which is missing with other ganglionic blocking agents (*247*). TEA and other ganglionic blocking agents cause a sensitization against the pressor effects of epinephrine, norepinephrine, and reflex vasoconstrictions. It also releases epinephrine from the adrenal medulla (*11*). Its action in the myoneural junction is illustrated by the finding that it produces blockade against ACh on the dorsal muscle of the leech (*248*). It was found to be effective against the arrhythmia induced in rabbit hearts by electrical stimulation or aconitine (*249*). Of the structure–activity studies conducted with analogues of TEA the work of Moe and Freyburger must be mentioned. They reported on approximately eighty compounds, but none of them surpassed TEA in potency. Subsequent studies of Winbury (*250*), Winbury et al. (*251*), and Cook et al. (*252*) described quite potent aliphatic ammonium compounds structurally related to TEA.

Of the series of aliphatic monoquaternary ammonium compounds synthesized by Robinson (*253*) and studied by Cook et al. (*252*) diethyldiisopropylammonium chloride (SC-3376) showed a peak potency; it was twelve times more potent than TEA (Table 4.14). Almost all compounds of this series that surpassed TEA in potency carried one or two α-branched aliphatic side chains. Winbury (*250*) concluded that the variation of molecular size was not so much required as the presence of an α-branched aliphatic chain, which restricts rotation around a quaternary nitrogen and offers a favorable configuration for a suitable attachment to ganglionic receptor sites. The same structural requirements for monoquaternary types of ganglionic blocking compound were found to be important with piperidinium compounds (*29*), with 2,6-disubstituted piperidine, and with 2,5-disubstituted pyrrolidine derivatives (*251*). The role of increasing the chain length of one aliphatic

TABLE 4.14

Aliphatic Monoquaternary Ammonium Compounds[a]

Code no.	Compound: Cation	Compound: Anion	Ganglionic blocking potency[b]: Sympathetic[c]	Ganglionic blocking potency[b]: Parasympathetic[d]
SC-1854	$(CH_3)_3(BrCH_2CH_2)N^+$	Br^-	0	0
SC-2552	$(CH_3)_3(HOOCCH_2CH_2)N^+$	Br^-	0	0
SC-2967	$(CH_3)_3(C_2H_5OCOCH_2)N^+$	Br^-	0	
SC-2677	$(CH_3)_3(C_2H_5OCOC_2H_4)N^+$	I^-	0	
SC-3563	$(C_2H_5)_2(CH_3)(HOC_2H_4)N^+$	Br^-	0	
SC-1953	$(C_2H_5)_2(HOC_2H_4)N^+$	Br	0.24	0.32
SC-1905	$(HOC_2H_4)_4N^+$	Br	0	0
SC-1920	$(C_2H_5)_2(C_3H_7)_2N^+$	Br	0.92	1.3
SC-1919	$(C_2H_5)_3(C_4H_9)N^+$	Br	1.1	1.9
SC-1921	$(C_2H_5)_2(C_4H_9)_2N^+$	Br	0.43	0.77
SC-3433	$(CH_3)_3[CH_3(CH_3)CH]N^+$	Br	0.24	
SC-3346	$(CH_3)(C_2H_5)_2[CH_3(CH_3)CH]N^+$	Br^-	0.84	
SC-3496	$(CH_3)(C_2H_5)[CH_3(CH_3)CH](HOC_2H_4)N^+$	Br^-	0.27	
SC-3378	$(C_2H_5)_3[CH_3(CH_3)CH]N^+$	Br^-	2.6	
SC-1885	$(CH_3)_2[CH_3(CH_3)CH]_2N^+$	Cl^-	1.9	1.9
SC-2108	$(CH_3)(C_2H_5)[CH_3(CH_3)CH]_2N^+$	Br^-	5.9	6.7
SC-3475	$(CH_3)[CH_3(CH_3)CH](HOC_2H_4)N^+$	Br^-	0.86	
SC-3376	$(C_2H_5)_2[CH_3(CH_3)CH]_2N^+$	Cl^-	12.6	
SC-2206	$(C_2H_5)[CH_3(CH_3)CH]_2(HOC_2H_4)N^+$	Cl^-	2.8	2.5
SC-2135	$(CH_3)(C_2H_5)[C_2H_5(CH_3)CH]_2N^+$	I^-	6.4	6.4
SC-2336	$(CH_3)(C_2H_5)[CH_3(CH_3 \cdot CH)CH_2]_2N^+$	I^-	1.1	3.1
SC-3513	$(CH_3)_2[C_2H_5(C_2H_5)CH]_2N^+$	I^-	3.0	
SC-3424	$(CH_3)(C_2H_5)[C_3H_7(CH_3)CH]_2N^+$	I^-	3.3	
SC-3377	$(CH_3)(C_2H_5)[CH_3(CH_3 \cdot CH)C_2H_4]_2N^+$			

[a] Data of Cook et al. (*252*).
[b] Potency of TEA, 1.0.
[c] Cat nictitating membrane preparation.
[d] Cat bladder preparation.

group in tetraalkylammonium compounds was summarized by Craig (*20*). However, no particularly potent compounds have been reported. A similar structural modification of amines of the general type $HOC_2H_4N^+(CH_3)_2R$, where R varied from ethyl to octadecyl, has been studied in the cat with an optimal blocking effect at a chain length of C_8 to C_{10} (*111*). The C_{12} compound of this series was more potent than the C_{10} derivative on the dog blood pressure preparation (*254*). In contrast to most of the ganglionic blocking agents of the aliphatic ammonium type, which block the sympathetic and parasympathetic ganglia about equally, ethylmethylisooctenylamine was reported to have considerable specificity to parasympathetic ganglia (*218*). This selective blockade, however, has not been substantiated (*85*).

2. ARALKYL ALIPHATIC MONOQUATERNARY AMMONIUM COMPOUNDS

Monoquaternary ammonium compounds containing one or two aromatic groups with ganglionic blocking potency have been known for a long time [for

TABLE 4.15

Arylalkyl Aliphatic Monoquaternary Ammonium Compounds[a]

Compound		
Cation	Anion	Ganglionic blocking potency[b]
$(C_2H_5)_3N^+CH_2C_6H_5$	I	0.5
$(CH_3)(C_2H_5)_2N^+CH_2C_6H_5$	I	<0.3
$(CH_3)_2N^+(CH_2C_6H_5)_2$	Br	1.0
$(C_2H_5)_2N^+(CH_2C_6H_5)_2$	Br	0.4
$(CH_3)_2N^+ \langle {CH_2C_6H_5 \atop CH_2CH_2C_6H_5}$	Br	<0.2
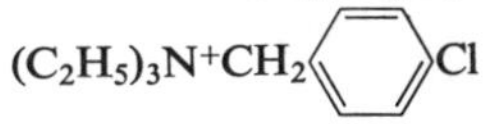	I	0.3
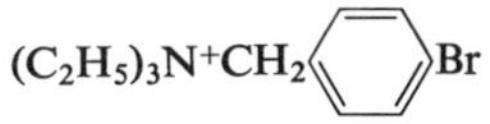	Br	0.3
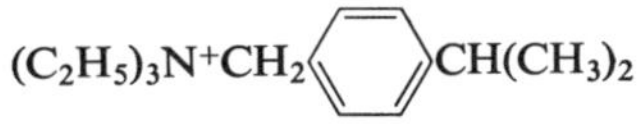	Br	1.9[c]
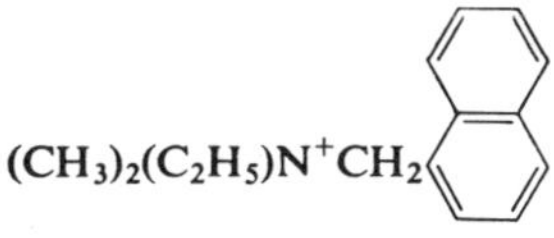	I	0.4
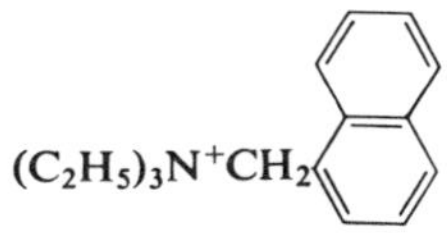	Cl	0.5
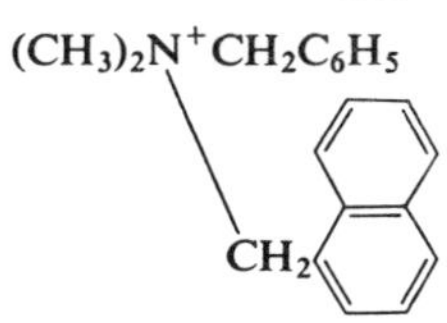	Br	0.8

[a] Data of Gyermek (*29*) and Gyermek and Nador (*358*).
[b] Potency of TEA, 1.0.
[c] Data of Winbury (*250*).

a summary see Craig (*20*)]. Structure–activity studies of the role of aryl substituents were started only after the thorough pharmacological re-evaluation of TEA. Nador and Gyermek (*46*) suggested that in the case of monoquaternary ammonium compounds, in contrast to the requirements for curarelike action, the electronic charge density of the nitrogen atom of the blocking molecule should be below a certain limit. The ganglionic blocking characteristics of compounds with the formula **(1)**, where R_1 is alkyl, halogen, or phenyl, R_2 is methyl or ethyl, and X^- is halogen, were in contrast to those with unbranched chains, which were relatively inactive (*246*); see Tables 4.15 and 4.16. The alkyl and cycloalkyl types of compound, some with aralkyl quaternary groups and with α-branched aliphatic chains, were more potent also, according to studies of Winbury et al. (*251*). A long series of arylalkylamines of the structure **(9)**,

TABLE 4.16

Quaternary Derivatives of Piperidine[a]

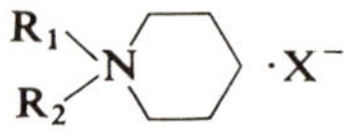

R_1	R_2	X	Ganglionic blocking potency[b]
CH_3	CH_3	I	<0.2
CH_3	C_2H_5	I	0.5
CH_3	$C_6H_5CH_2$	Br	0.3
CH_3	Br 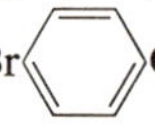 CH_2	Br	0.7
CH_3	$H_5C_2OCOCH_2$	Br	<0.2
C_2H_5	C_2H_5	Br	1.0
C_2H_5	$(CH_3)_2CH$	I	1.9
C_2H_5	$C_6H_5CH_2$	Br	0.3
C_2H_5	Br 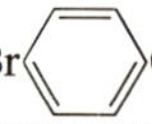 CH_2	Br	0.5
$(CH_3)_2CH$	$(CH_3)_2CH$	I	0.6
$(CH_3)_2CH$	Br 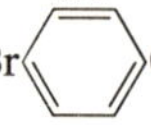 CH_2	Br	0.6
$(CH_3)_2CH$	CH_3	I	0.9
$(CH_3)_2CH$	CH_3 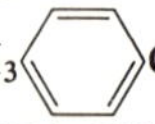 CH_2	I	0.8
CH_3	$(C_6H_5)_2CH$	I	<0.2
$C_6H_5CH_2$	$HOCH_2CH_2$	Br	<0.2
CH_3	$HOCH_2CH_2$	I	<0.1

[a] Data of Gyermek (*29*).
[b] Potency of TEA, 1.0.

where X represents different tertiary and quaternary amino groups, has been tested for ganglionic actions (Table 4.17). Most of these agents were tertiary amines. The results obtained with the few agents of the quaternary ammonium type indicate that the compounds that carried a triethyl- or diethylmethylammonium cationic group and were substituted at R with methyl or phenethyl groups, were as potent as, or somewhat more potent than, TEA on dog blood pressure and bladder and on cat nictitating membrane preparation. The tertiary amines of these series were considerably less potent (*255*).

3. ALICYCLIC MONOQUATERNARY AMMONIUM COMPOUNDS

Studies made about fifteen years ago, aiming at more potent ganglionic blocking agents than TEA (the prototype agent at that time), could utilize only limited amounts of information based on the structure–activity relationships of existing monoquaternary ganglionic blocking agents. Besides some new alkyl- and aralkyl-substituted aliphatic ammonium derivatives a series of alicyclic agents were synthesized by Robinson (*253*) at the same time that the ganglionic blocking properties of quaternary derivatives of the more complex alicyclic ring structure of tropane were also being recognized (*256*, *257*). A comprehensive study of monoquaternary derivatives of piperidine, pyrrolidine, and tetrahydroisoquinoline made by Winbury (*250*) and Winbury et al. (*251*) clarified to a great extent the structure–activity relationships of these classes of agents. The series all pointed to a common structural feature necessary for high ganglionic blocking potency: two short α-branched aliphatic chains that surround the central nitrogen atom. Classes of compounds in which this structural feature has been recognized are depicted in **(8)**.

Systematic studies with these and similar structures elucidated the role of different quaternary substituents and to some extent also the role of the substituent forming the branched chains alpha to the nitrogen atom (Table 4.18, A, B, C).

In the 2,5-dimethylpyrrolidinium and 2,6-dimethylpiperidinium series a sharp peak of ganglionic blocking potency appeared with the *N*,*N*-diethyl derivatives. In the isoquinolinium series the 1-benzyl-substituted compounds were the most active. In the latter, however, additional substituents (hydroxyl groups at 5 and 6) seem to be of a certain significance. Only one example is available regarding the position of the two methyl groups in the ring in addition to 2,6-dimethylpiperidinium derivatives; it concerns 2-methyl-5-ethylpiperidine and indicates that the positions of the methyl or alkyl groups in the ring are perhaps optimal for the α positions relative to nitrogen. Branching is essential for ganglionic blocking action in the cycloalkylammonium type of compound of small ring size, as simple piperidine derivatives are uniformly much less potent (*29*, *250*); see Table 4.16. Although it is possible that α

TABLE 4.17

Ganglionic Blocking Effects of Some Arylalkylamines[a]

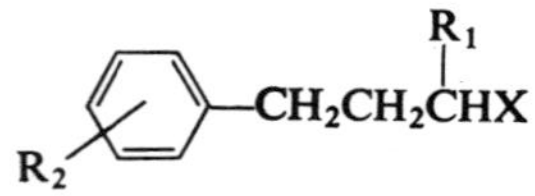

Code no.	R_1	R_2	X	Ganglionic blocking potencies (ED_{50}) mg/kg: Sympathetic: Against nicotine-induced blood pressure rise (dog)	Sympathetic: Against DMPP-induced blood pressure rise (dog)	Sympathetic: Against cat nictitating membrane contraction	Parasympathetic: Against DMPP-induced bladder contraction (dog)
1	H		$N(C_2H_5)_2$	20			
14	H		$N(C_4H_9)_2$	20	6.0		6.0
3	H		piperidine	20			
18	CH_3		NH_2	5[b]			
27	CH_3		$N(CH_3)_2$	10[b]			
44	CH_3		$N(C_2H_5)_2$	20	3.7	6.4	4.2
16	CH_3		piperidino	20			
19	CH_3		morpholino	20			
52	CH_3		$^{+}N(C_2H_5)_2CH_3$	5	1.4	1.0	1.7
45	CH_3		$^{+}N(C_2H_5)_3$	5	0.5	1.1	0.5
8	C_6H_5		NHC_2H_5	20			
41	C_6H_5		$N(CH_3)_2$	20			
43	C_6H_5		$N(C_2H_5)_2$	20	3.2		2.7
12	C_6H_5		piperidino	5			
4	C_6H_5		piperidino	20			
22	C_6H_5	*p*-OCH	$N(C_2H_5)_2$	20			
23	C_6H_5	*o*-Cl	$N(C_2H_5)_2$	20	5.7	7.0	3.3
20	C_6H_5	*o*-Cl	piperidino	20	2.5		6.9
50	C_6H_5	*p*-Cl	$N(C_2H_5)_2$	20			
39	$C_6H_5(CH_2)_2$		NHC_2H_5	20			
38	$C_6H_5(CH_2)_2$		$N(C_2H_5)_2$	20	13.9	15.0	6.7
53	$C_6H_5(CH_2)_2$		$^{+}N(C_2H_5)_2CH_3$	5	0.3	3.5	0.2
TEA					2.0	1.1	0.9
Hexamethonium					0.3	0.1	0.5

[a] Data of Pindell et al. (*255*).
[b] Ganglionic stimulation.

TABLE 4.18 A

Ganglionic Blocking Potencies of Monoquaternary Pyrrolidinium and Piperidinium Compounds[a]

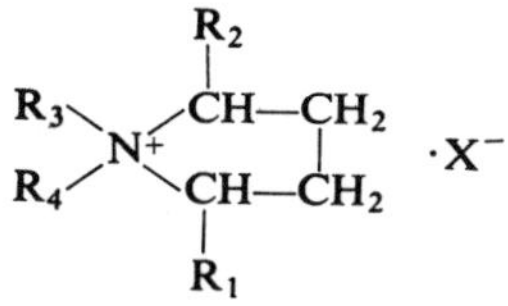

R_1	R_2	R_3	R_4	X	Ganglionic blocking potency[b]
CH_3	CH_3	C_2H_5	C_2H_5	Br	6.4
CH_3	CH_3	CH_3	C_2H_4OH	Br	0.36
CH_3	CH_3	C_2H_5	C_2H_4OH	Br	0.75
H	C_6H_5	C_2H_5	C_2H_5	Br	0.9
H	C_6H_5	CH_3	CH_3	I	1.1

[a] Data of Winbury (*250*).
[b] Potency of TEA on cat nictitating membrane, 1.0.

TABLE 4.18 B

Ganglionic Blocking Potencies of Monoquaternary Pyrrolidinium and Piperidinium Compounds[a]

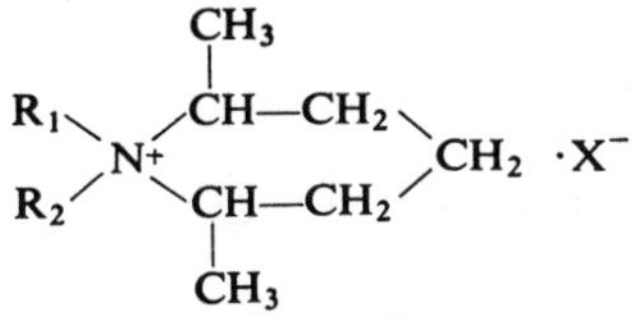

R_1	R_2	X	Ganglionic blocking potency[b]
CH_3	CH_3	Cl	2.0
CH_3	C_2H_5	Br	3.2
CH_3	$CH_3CH_2CH_2$	I	3.3
C_2H_5	C_2H_5	Br	9.5
C_2H_5	$C_6H_5CH_2$	Br	2.4
C_2H_5	$(CH_3)_2CH$ 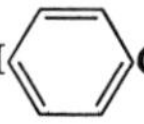 CH_2	Br	2.6
CH_3	C_2H_4OH	Br	2.4
C_2H_5	C_2H_4OH	Br	0.85
CH_3	$CH_2COOC_2H_5$	Br	1.9
CH_3	$C_2H_4COOCH_3$	Br	2.0

[a] Data of Winbury (*250*).
[b] Potency of TEA on cat nictitating membrane, 1.0.

TABLE 4.18 C

Ganglionic Blocking Potencies of Quaternary Isoquinoline Compounds[a]

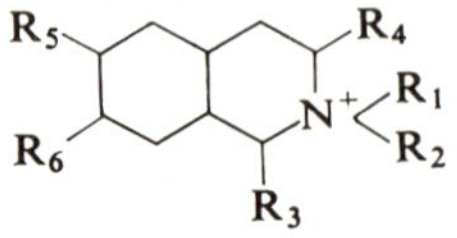

R_1	R_2	R_3	R_4	R_5	R_6	X	Ganglionic blocking potency[b] Symp.[c]	Para-symp.[d]
C_2H_5	C_2H_5	CH_3	H	H	H	Br	0.6	1.2
C_2H_5	C_2H_5	H	CH_3	H	H	Br	0.5	3.3
CH_3	C_2H_5	CH_3	CH_3	H	H	Cl	0.9	0.5
CH_3	CH_3	$CH(CH_3)_2$	H	H	H	I	1.9	4.4
CH_3	CH_3	$CH_2CH(CH_3)_2$	H	H	H	I	0.7	1.3
CH_3	CH_3	C_6H_5	H	H	H	I	1.6	1.6
CH_3	CH_3	$C_6H_5CH_2$	H	H	H	I	0.6	1.6
CH_3	CH_3	$CH_3(CH_2)_6$	H	OH	OH	Cl	3.8	4.1
CH_3	CH_3	$C_6H_5CH_2$	H	OH	OH	Cl	9.6	8.5
CH_3	C_2H_5	$C_6H_5CH_2$	H	OH	OH	Cl	7.8	4.3
C_2H_5	C_2H_5	$C_6H_5CH_2$	H	OH	OH	Cl	4.6	7.3
CH_3	CH_3	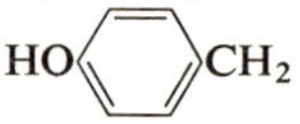	H	OH	OH	Cl	1.6	4.0
CH_3	CH_3	$CH_3(CH_2)_7$	H	CH_3O	CH_3O	I	0.9	7.9
CH_3	CH_3	$C_6H_5CH_2$	H	CH_3O	CH_3O	I	4.0	4.0
CH_3	CH_3	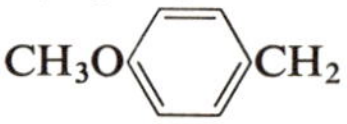	H	H	CH_3O	I	1.5	2.7
CH_3	CH_3	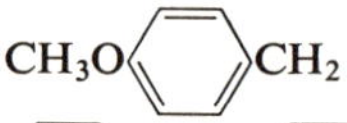	H	CH_3O	CH_3O	Cl	2.5	3.2
CH_3	CH_3	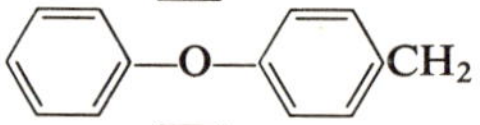	H	CH_3O	CH_3O	I	2.5	1.9
CH_3	CH_3	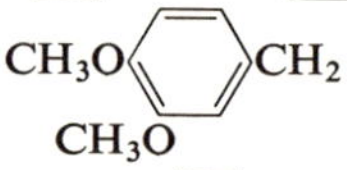	H	CH_3O	CH_3O	I	1.9	2.2
CH_3	CH_3	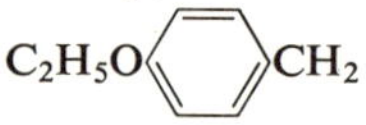	H	C_2H_5O	C_2H_5O	I	1.0	6.3

[a] Data of Winbury (*250*).
[b] Potency of TEA, 1.0.
[c] Cat nictitating membrane.
[d] Dog bladder.

branching is optimal for ganglionic blocking activity, there is some indication that the branching group also is longer. In addition, examples in the isoquinoline ring series show that the two α-methyl groups may not be optimal for ganglionic blocking activity. Several 1-benzyl-substituted isoquinolinium compounds show peak potency in that series. Thus, to explore compounds of the type **(10)**, where R_1 and R_2 are shorter alkyl groups and R_3 is a longer alkyl or aralkyl group, should be of interest.

The stereochemical considerations involving tropane compounds call attention to the fact that the steric conformation of the α,α′-methyl groups in the alicyclic rings is not uniform and that the stereochemical study of Winbury (*250*) is not conclusive. Stereospecific syntheses of 2,6-dimethylpiperidines led to the comparison of a few quaternary derivatives of *N*-methyl-2,6-(*cis*)- and *N*-methyl-2,6-(*trans*)-dimethylpiperidinium compounds carrying also different stereospecifically oriented quaternary groups. Not very marked, but measurable, differences between ganglionic blocking activities of the different isomers were found (Table 4.19). Owing to the possibility of restricted rotation the size of any substituent on the nitrogen atom may also influence the configuration of the α,α′-alkyl groups. Thus, the differences observed in pharmacological action reflect the difference in the stereochemistry only when the substituents on the nitrogen atom are small enough not to interfere with the steric orientation of the branching groups at the α positions.

TABLE 4.19

Comparison of the Ganglionic Blocking Activities of a Few *cis*- and *trans*-2,6-Dimethyl piperidinium Derivatives[a]

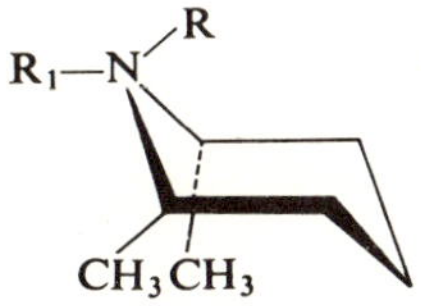

$CH_3, CH_3 = cis$

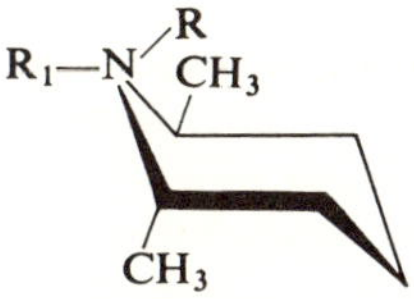

$CH_3, CH_3 = trans$

R	R_1	X	Ganglionic blocking potency[b]	R	R_1	X	Ganglionic blocking potency[b]
CH_3	$C_6H_5CH_2$	Br	3.4	CH_3	$C_6H_5CH_2$	Br	0.8
CH_3	CH_3	I	2.5	CH_3	CH_3	I	0.4
CH_3	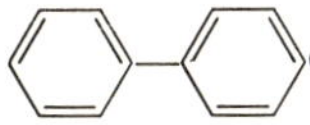 CH_2	Br	8.0	CH_3	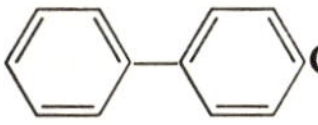 CH_2	Br	5.0

[a] Data of Gyermek (*29*).

[b] Potency of TEA on cat nictitating membrane preparation, 1.0.

4. ESTERS AND ETHERS OF ALKYLAMMONIUM COMPOUNDS

a. Choline, Homocholine, and Betaine Derivatives

The ganglionic blockade produced by ACh and its mechanism has been discussed by Takeshige et al. (*204*) and by Pappano and Volle (*180*), who compared its ganglionic blocking action with that of methacholine. A complex mode of action has been suggested, which is partly dependent on the preceding ganglionic stimulation these compounds produce. Ganglionic blockade against preganglionically induced potentials has been studied by Wurzel et al. (*127*) with acetylcholine, propionylcholine, butyrylcholine, benzoylcholine, and their thiocholine analogues. Holton and Ing (*120*) reported on the nicotinic blocking action of acetoxyethyltriethylammonium. The *N,N,N*-triethyl derivative of the reversed carboxyl analogue of acetylcholine produced a weak pressor effect and, in larger doses, a ganglionic blockade (*113*). Various agents of the choline ester and ether type are listed without detail in Table 4.20. A large number of esters of betaine (carboxymethyltrimethylammonium), choline, and homocholine have been investigated in the past in the autonomic nervous system. Data of these classes of agent derive from the studies of Hunt and Renshaw (*119*, *140*) in the early years of this century. Because of the simple investigational techniques used at that time, the only data are on a few animals injected intravenously, of which only blood pressure responses were measured. A quantitative evaluation of these agents is therefore difficult. Weak ganglionic blockade, as measured by the inhibitory action against the nicotinic rise in the

TABLE 4.20

Some Aliphatic Esters and Ethers of Ammonium Alkanols with Ganglionic Blocking Activity[a]

β-Acetoxyethyltriethylammonium
β-Butoxyethyltriethylammonium
Carbamoylmethyltrimethylammonium
N-Methylcarbamoylmethyltrimethylammonium
N-Ethylcarbamoylmethyltrimethylammonium
N-Propylcarbamoylmethyltrimethylammonium
N-Butylcarbamoylmethyltrimethylammonium
Acetylthioethyltrimethylammonium
Methylthiomethyltriethylcholine
Isopropylthiomethyltriethylcholine
Isobutylthiomethyltriethylcholine
Ethoxymethyltriethylammonium
Allyloxymethyltriethylammonium
γ-Homocholine methyl ether

[a] Data of Craig (*20*).

blood pressure of the cat, has been found with differently substituted carbamic acid esters in doses of 25 to 100 mg/kg (*119*). Methyl-, propyl-, *n*-butyl-, and phenyl-substituted ethyl esters of betaine showed, besides weak ganglionic stimulant properties, brief nicotinic blocking effects on the cat blood pressure (*119*). Some aliphatic ether derivatives of triethylammonium showed ganglionic blocking effects at about 10 mg/kg. A group of similar thioether derivatives was effective at the same dose range in the cat (*112*). A partial list of these different types of compound is given in Table 4.20.

b. Monoquaternary Ammonium Compounds of the Aromatic and Alicyclic Acid Ester Type

Many of the compounds that belong to the large class of aminoalkyl esters of the general type **(11)**, where R is H or OH, R_1 is one or two aryl or cycloalkyl groups, and R_2 and R_3 are alkyl or cycloalkyl groups, are pharmacologically known either as cholinolytic and spasmolytic agents or as local anesthetic drugs. Some quaternary salts of the aromatic acid esters of aminoalkanols were studied in recent years with the hope of finding agents which, besides blocking parasympathetic nerve endings, would inhibit ganglionic transmission. However, no such agents except propantheline bromide have been employed clinically. Since these agents possess atropinelike properties almost without exception, the evaluation of the degree of ganglionic blockade at parasympathetic ganglia presents a practical problem. Methodologic considerations for resolving such problems are outlined in Chapter 3. In this class of compounds the degree of ganglionic blockade obtained at a sympathetic ganglion is a more reliable indicator of activity. Unfortunately, several studies relied on preparations measuring parasympathetic functions, and thus a clear-cut picture of the potencies of these agents is usually not available. The studies of Cusic and Robinson (*258*), Gyermek et al. (*259*), Gyermek (*29*), and Winbury et al. (*251*) indicated that fairly potent ganglionic blocking compounds could be obtained in aromatic acid esters of type **(12)**, where R is H or OH, R_1 is one or two aryl or cycloalkyl groups, and R_2 is alkyl. These agents were usually inferior, however, in ganglionic blocking potency to those basic esters which carried tropane rings. An illustration of this relationship is given in Table 4.21 with the examples of benzoate and madelate esters of α-tropine and β-tropine and of 2,6-dimethyl-4-hydroxypiperidine. These piperidine and tropine derivatives differ by the presence of the 2,6-dimethyl substituent instead of the endoethylene bridge of the tropane ring, which may lead to a different configuration of the substituents on the nitrogen atom. Because of the presence of sterically less hindered 2,6-dimethyl groups there is a possible difference in conformational situation between the substituted piperidine ring and the tropane ring. In ganglionic blocking activity these

TABLE 4.21

Comparison of the Ganglionic Blocking Actions of Quaternary Ammonium Derivatives of Tropine Esters and of Corresponding 1,2,6-Trimethyl-4-acyloxypiperidinine Derivatives[a]

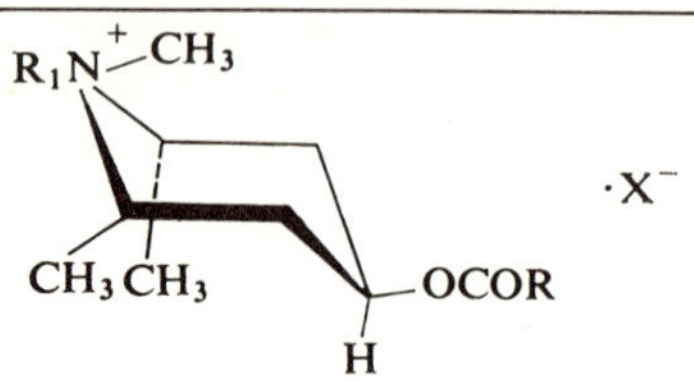

R	R_1	X	Gang. block. potency[b]
CH_3	C_6H_5	I	1.0
$C_6H_5CH_2$	C_6H_5	Br	0.5
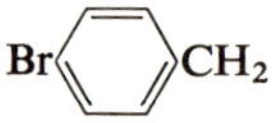	C_6H_5	Br	4.0
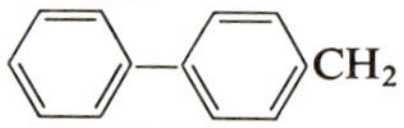	C_6H_5	Br	12.0
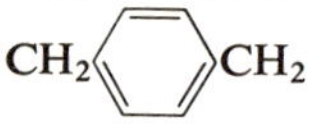	C_6H_5	2Br	0.3
CH_3	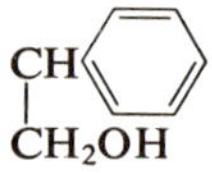	I	3.0
$C_6H_5CH_2$	”	Br	2.5

N—O = *cis* (β)

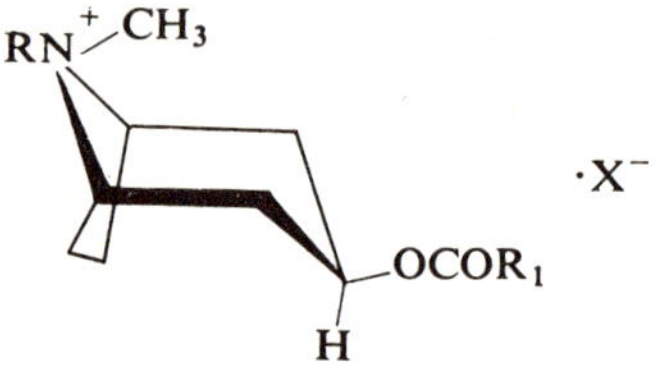

R	R_1	X	Gang. block. potency[b]
CH_3	C_6H_5	I	2.0
$C_6H_5CH_2$	C_6H_5	Br	3.0
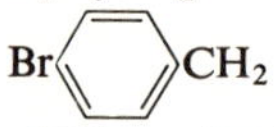	C_6H_5	Br	8.2
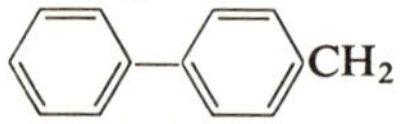	C_6H_5	Br	([c])
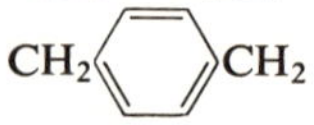	C_6H_5	2Br	0.4
CH_3	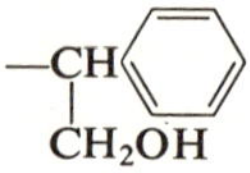	I	4.5
$C_6H_5CH_2$	”	Br	3.0

TABLE 4.21—*continued*

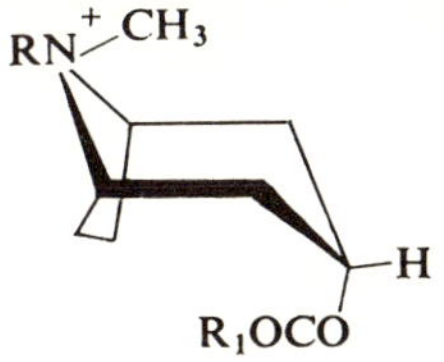

N—O = *trans* (α)

R	R_1	X	Gang. block. potency[b]
CH_3	C_6H_5	I	0.4
$C_6H_5CH_2$	C_6H_5	Br	0.5
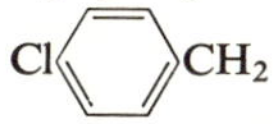	C_6H_5	Cl	3.0
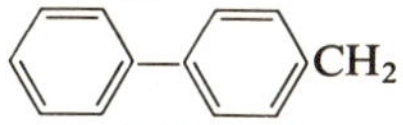	C_6H_5	Br	([c])
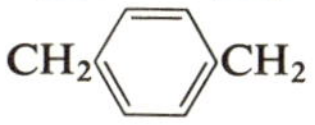	C_6H_5	Br	1.0

[a] Data of Gyermek (*29*).
[b] Potency of TEA, 1.0.
[c] Stimulant.

compounds do not markedly differ from either the benzoyl α-tropines or β-tropines. In their cholinolytic action, which seems to be more influenced by changes in the nitrogen-to-oxygen distances as a result of alterations in the conformation of the rings, these piperidine derivatives showed closer similarity to the benzoyl β-tropine esters than to the benzoyl α-tropine esters. Thus, from the pharmacological data it may be inferred that at least in these 1,2,6-trimethyl-4-acyloxypiperidines the conformation of the piperidine ring is represented by the boat form rather than the chair form (the latter being common with the tropane derivatives); on the other hand, the configuration of the 4-hydroxy group is *cis* and not *trans* (*29*).

Details of the study made by Winbury et al. (*251*) of several basic esters, evaluating the role of acidic groups, substituents on the terminal nitrogen atom, variations of the connecting chain, and the nature of this chain, are given in Tables 4.22 to 4.25. Of the similar compounds reported by Cusic and Robinson (*258*) the carbethoxymethyl bromide of *N*-piperidinoethyl 9-xanthenecarboxylate was 3.0 times more potent than TEA, the ethyl bromide of *N*,*N*-diethylaminoethyl 9-xanthenecarboxylate was 2.4 times more, the methyl bromide of *N*,*N*-diethyl-2,6-dimethylpiperidinium tropylate was 4.8 times more, and the methobromide of *N*-ethyl-2,6-dimethylpiperidinium diphenylacetate was 5.6 times more potent.

The highest ganglionic blocking potency was obtained with methyl quaternary salts of the *N*-(2-furfurylmethyl)-*N*-phenylcarbamate ester of diisopropylaminoethanol (*251*) and with N-420 (Table 4.21); both surpassed TEA by a factor of 12.

TABLE 4.22

Effect on Ganglionic Blocking Activity of Introducing Various Groups on Ethylmethyldiisopropylammonium[a]

$$RCH_2CH_2(CH_3)\overset{+}{N}(CH(CH_3)_2)_2$$

R	Molar potency[b]	R	Molar potency[b]
H	5.9	$C_6H_5-CH(CH_2OH)-COO$	3.5[c]
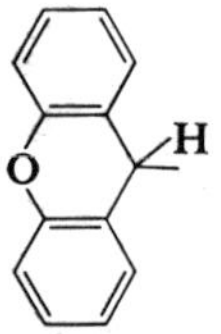	1.2	$(C_4H_9)_2NCOO$	6.7
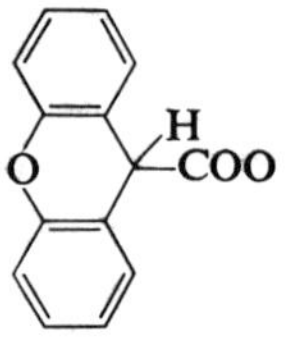	2.0+	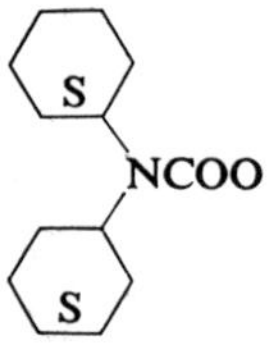	1.2
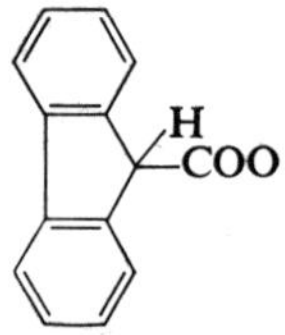	<0.1	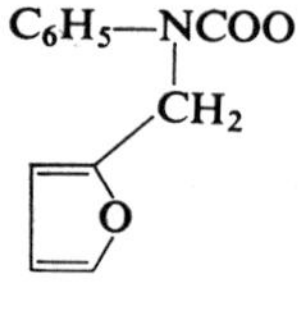	12.0[c]
$(C_6H_5)_2CHCOO$	1.8+	$C_6H_5-N(CH_2C_6H_5)COO$	7.3[c]
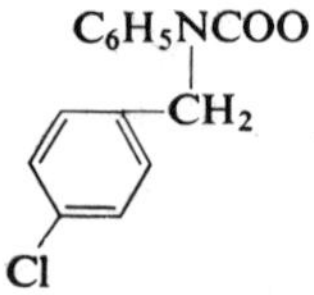	7.1+		

[a] Data of Winbury et al. (*251*).
[b] Potency of TEA, 1.0.
[c] Compound has parasympatholytic activity.

TABLE 4.23

Effect on Ganglionic Blocking Activity of Introducing Various Groups on the Ethylene Chain when the Quaternary Nitrogen Is in a Piperidinium or Pyrrolidinium Ring[a]

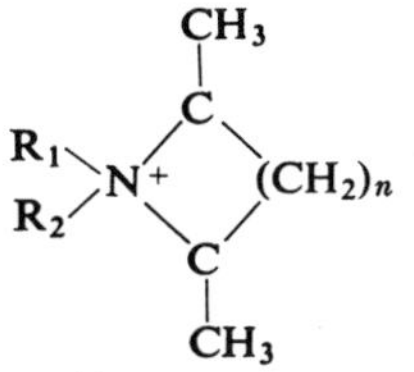

R_1	R_2	n	Molar potency[b]
$CH_3COOC_2H_4$	CH_3	3	2.0
	CH_3	2	1.0[c]
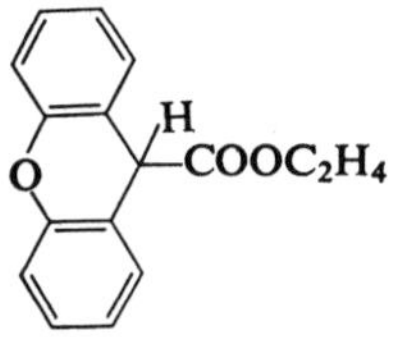	CH_3	3	2.3[c]
	C_2H_5	3	2.1[c]
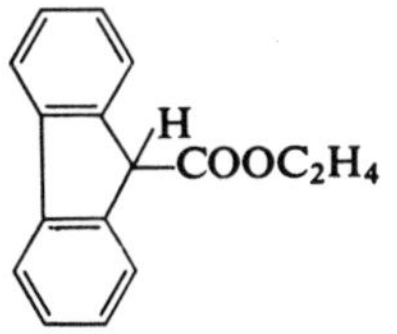	CH_3	3	0.2
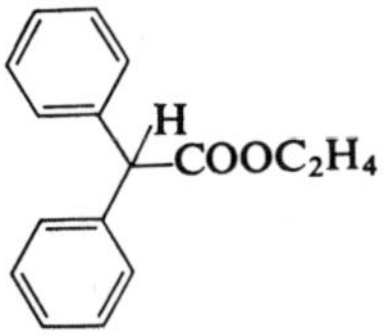	CH_3	3	4.5
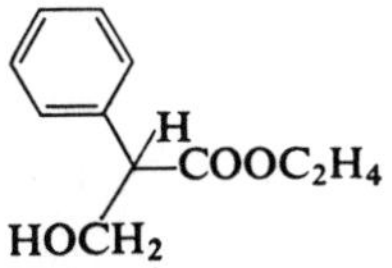	CH_3	2	1.6[c]
	CH_3	3	4.8[c]
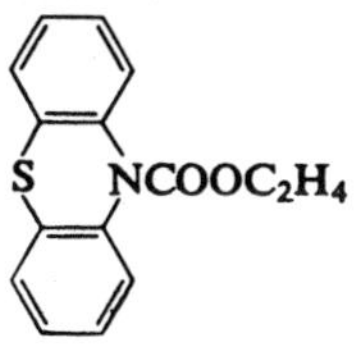	CH_3	2	3.5

[a] Data of Winbury et al. (*251*).
[b] Potency of TEA, 1.0.
[c] Compound has parasympatholytic activity.

TABLE 4.24

Effect on Ganglionic Blocking Activity of Various *N*-Alkyl Groups in the Presence of an *N*-Aralkyl Group[a]

R	Molar potency[b]	R	Molar potency[b]
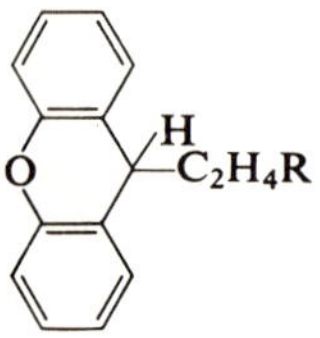		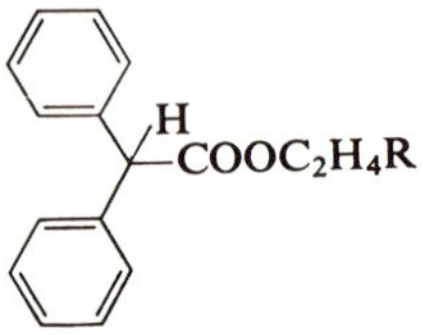	
$NCH_3, (C_2H_5)_2$	0.8	$N(CH_3)_3$	0.8
$NCH_3, [CH(CH_3)_2]_2$	1.2	$N(CH_3)_2, C_2H_5$	0.4
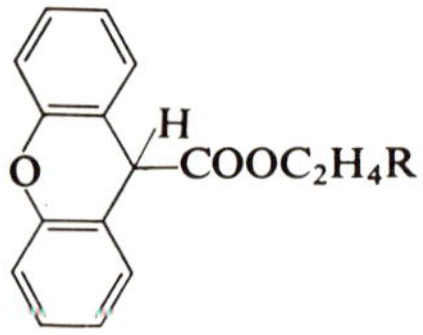		$NCH_3, [CH(CH_3)_2]_2$	1.8
		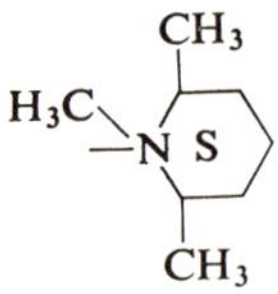	4.5
$N(CH_3)_3$	0.5		
$NCH_3, (C_2H_5)_2$	2.0	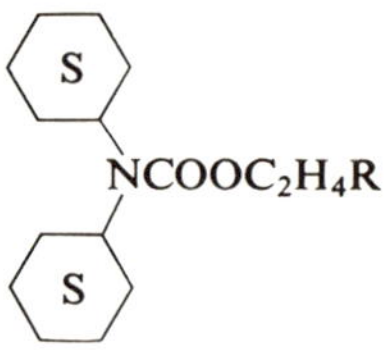	
$N(C_2H_5)_3$	1.7		
$N(CH_3)_2, CH(CH_3)_2$	1.9		
$NCH_3, C_2H_5, CH(CH_3)_2$	0.8		
$NCH_3[CH(CH_3)_2]_2$	2.0		
$NC_2H_5, [CH(CH_3)_2]_2$	3.4	$N(CH_3)_3$	0.8
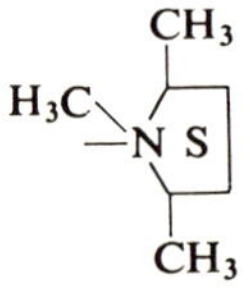	1.0	$NCH_3, [CH(CH_3)_2]_2$	1.2
		C_6H_5, $C_6H_5CH_2$ $NCOOC_2H_4R$	
		$N[(CH)_3]_3$	0.7
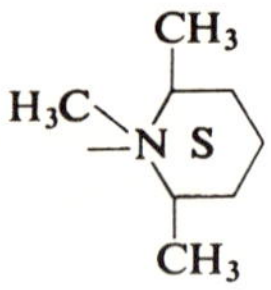	2.3	$NCH_3, (C_3H_5)_2$	1.7
		$N(C_2H_5)_3$	2.6
		$NCH_3, C_2H_5, CH(CH_3)_2$	2.9
		$NCH_3[CH(CH_3)_2]_2$	7.3
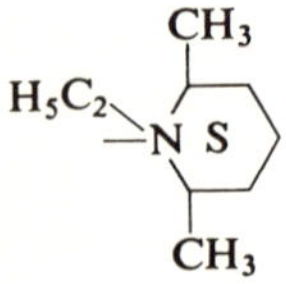	2.1	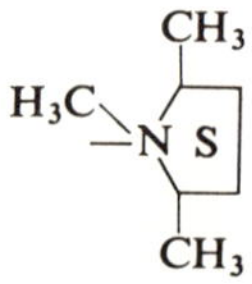	1.6

TABLE 4.24—*continued*

R	Molar potency[b]	R	Molar potency[b]
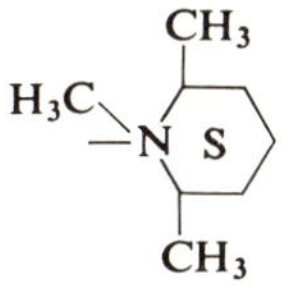	4.8	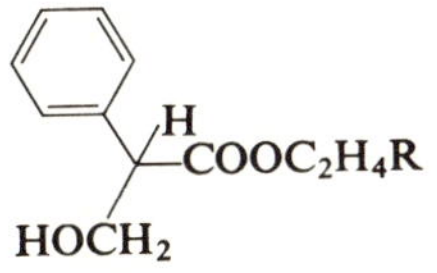	
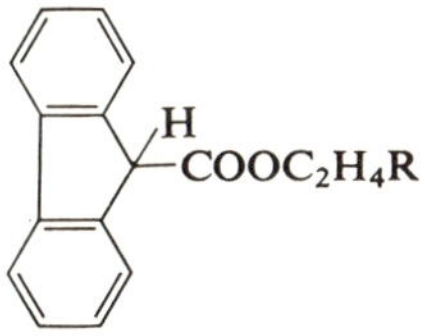		$N(CH_3)_2$, $CH(CH_3)_2$	0.4
		NCH_3, C_2H_5, $CH(CH_3)_2$	0.5
		$NCH_3[CH(CH_3)_2]_2$	3.5
$N(CH_3)_3$	0.7	C_6H_5(*p*-Cl$C_6H_4CH_2$)$NCOOC_2H_4$R	
NCH_3, $(C_2H_5)_2$	0.5		
NCH_3, $[CH(CH_3)_2]_2$	<0.1	NCH_3, $(n\text{-}C_3H_7)_2$	4.4
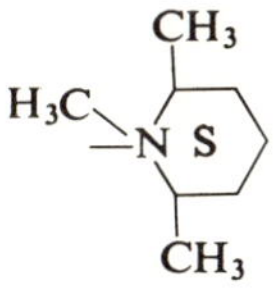	0.2	NCH_3, $[CH(CH_3)_2]_2$	7.1

[a] Data of Winbury (*251*).
[b] Potency of TEA, 1.0.

In a study designed to explore the degrees of ganglionic blockade of ester-type atropinelike cholinolytic compounds compared to typical ganglionic blocking agents with the cat superior cervical ganglion preparation the postganglionic action potential was recorded (*260*). Five synthetic atropinelike cholinolytic agents of the quaternary ammonium type that lacked the tropane ring system, were inferior to hexamethonium in potency. Methylatropinium bromide surpassed hexamethonium by a factor of 2, indicating the importance of the tropane ring for obtaining a high degree of potency. The ratio between ganglionic and peripheral parasympathetic blocking actions is approximately 1,000 with these agents. It therefore seems improbable that ganglionic block significantly contributes to their therapeutic action.

The relationship between chemical structure and spasmolytic and ganglioplegic actions was studied by Guyonneau (*32, 261*) with several compounds of

TABLE 4.25

Effect on Ganglionic Blocking Activity of Branched Alkylene Chains[a]

	$Ar—X—R_1, R_2, R_3$			
	X			
	$—CH_2CH_2N^+\equiv$	$—CH_2CH(CH_3)N^+\equiv$	$—CH(CH_3)CH_2N^+\equiv$	
Ar	Molar potency			R_1, R_2, R_3
$C_6H_5CH_2$	1.6	2.6		$(C_2H_5)_3$
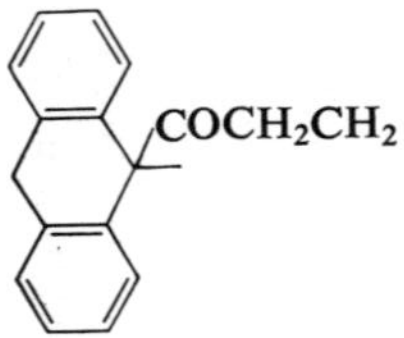	1.0	0.8		$(CH_3)_3$
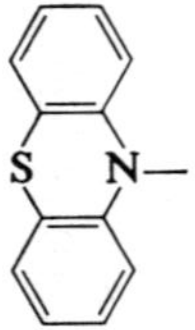	1.0	2.5		$(CH_3)_3$
	1.0	2.4		$(CH_3)_2, C_2H_5$
	1.2	1.8	1.2	$CH_3, (C_2H_5)_2$
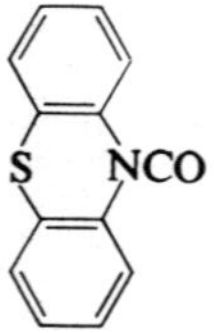	<0.1	1.2		$(CH_3)_3$
	0.2	1.5		$CH_3(C_2H_5)_2$
	0.6	2.2		CH_3, (N) S 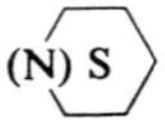

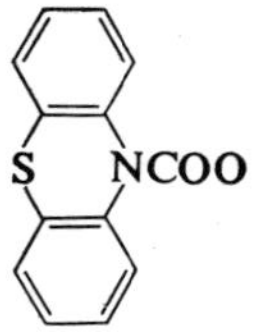	2.3	2.9		$CH_3, (C_2H_5)_2$
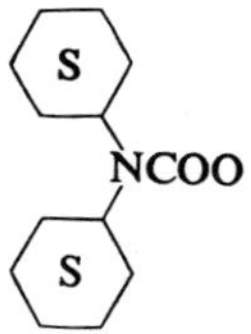	0.8	3.7	1.3	$(CH_3)_3$
C_6H_5NCOO / $C_6H_5CH_2$ (on N)	1.7	1.3		$CH_3, (C_2H_5)_2$
$(C_6H_5CH_2)_2NCOO$	2.7	1.1		$(CH_3)_3$
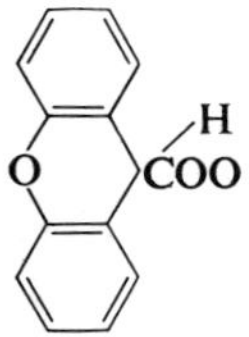	0.5	2.1		$(CH_3)_3$
	2.0	1.2		$CH_3, (C_2H_5)_2$
$(C_6H_5)_2CHCOO$	4.2	1.1		$(C_2H_5)_3$

[a] Data of Winbury et al. (*251*).
[b] Potency of TEA, 1.0.

the basic ester type. Only weak ganglionic blocking action was found with aminoalkyl esters of the formula **(13)**, where ring 1 is either saturated or unsaturated, *n* is 2 to 3, R_1 and R_2 are alkyl or cycloalkyl, and R_3 is H or alkyl. The tertiary amino compounds were 10 to 100 times less potent than the alkyl quaternary salts. The corresponding ketone and alkane derivatives were less potent than the ester compounds. Another series of spasmolytic agents of the tertiary and quaternary ammonium type, consisting of various aminoalkyl esters of isobutylphenylacetic acid, showed only moderate ganglionic blocking potency on the cat nictitating membrane preparation (*262*).

Aminoalkyl esters of piperidinecarboxylic acids and their "reversed" ester derivatives were studied only for hypotensive activity in dogs. The most potent member of the series was the bromide of *N*-methylmorpoliniumethyl 1-methyl-piperidine-3-carboxylate (*263*).

As an exception, a very high degree of ganglionic blocking potency was reported for the diethylmethylammoniumethyl ester of 1,1,6-trimethyl-piperidinium-2-carboxylic acid and its corresponding α-quinuclidinecarboxylic acid analogue. Both agents markedly surpassed hexamethonium in potency (*264*).

Aminoalkyl esters of *p*-diphenylacetic acid with the general structure **(14)**, where R_1, R_2, and R_3 are lower alkyl groups, have been reported by Cavallini et al. (*217*) to have ganglionic blocking properties.

Three series of basic esters with alkylamino and piperidino groups were studied by Gyermek (*29*). In the first two series with the structures **(15)**, where R_1 is alkyl or aralkyl and R_2 is acetyl, benzoyl, or diphenylglycolyl groups, a weak ganglionic blocking action was observed in several compounds. Of these only one, the *p*-phenylbenzyl quaternary salt of piperidinoethyl diphenyl-glycolate, was slightly more potent than TEA. In another series of a few quaternary ammonium derivatives of type **(16)**, where R is methyl or aralkyl, the benzyl and *p*-bromobenzyl derivatives showed significant ganglionic blocking potency, surpassing that of TEA by a factor of 4 to 5.

In the following paragraphs are given some miscellaneous ester types of spasmolytics, which were studied for ganglionic blocking action.

Diethylaminopropyl diphenylethoxyacetate (Ethpenal), which shows peripheral cholinolytic action and local anesthetic properties, also exhibits ganglionic blockade and blocks chemoreceptors at moderate doses (*265*).

N-Diphenylacetyl-*N'*-piperidinoethyl hydrazide shows ganglionic blockade at 5 to 20 mg/kg in the cat nictitating membrane and on dog blood pressure (*266*). 2-Benzyloxyethyldimethyl-*N*-octylammonium bromide, primarily a spasmolytic agent, showed moderate ganglionic blocking action in the dog bladder preparation (*267*). 2-Benzoyloxy-1-phenyl-3-(1,4-dimethylpiperazi-nium)propane iodide blocks the nicotinic pressor effect in the dog (*268*).

Procaine blocks the effect of ACh and KCl on the cat nictitating membrane

Guyonneau (*32*) studied the activity of quaternary ammonium derivatives of the type **(19)** in dog blood pressure experiments against phenoxycholine-induced pressor responses. Only moderate activity (effective doses ranged from 7 to 12 mg/kg intravenously administered) was observed with those compounds carrying various proportions of methyl and ethyl substituents on the nitrogen atom.

A mixed ganglionic blocking and adrenolytic action has been demonstrated with 6-oxythymoxyethyltrimethylammonium bromide (*226*).

Fakstorp and Pedersen (*283a*) studied a series of choline phenyl ethers substituted in the benzene nucleus by an amino group carrying alkyl substituents. The structure and pharmacological potencies on parasympathetic and sympathetic ganglia of these agents are presented in Table 4.26. These compounds showed structural similarity to the bisammonium phenylalkanes described by Wien and Mason. In ganglionic blocking potency, however, they were inferior to them.

5. TROPANE COMPOUNDS

The intensive pharmacological actions of atropine, of related tropine esters, and of their quaternary ammonium derivatives at the postganglionic parasympathetic receptor sites have been known for a long time. Demonstrations of an action of the quaternary salts of atropine and homatropine at the myoneural junctions of striated muscles, made by Crum, Brown, and Fraser in 1869, by Hildebrandt in 1906, by Issekutz in 1917, and by Kimura, Unna, and Pfeiffer in 1948 (*30*), and, finally, the discovery of the ganglionic blocking action of quaternary salts of atropine and tropine by Gyermek et al. (*256*, *257*) added new aspects to the spectrum of action of those compounds whose basic structure is the tropane ring system. With a wide spectrum of activity against different cholinergic receptor sites these compounds seemed to offer unique possibilities for structure–activity studies; the studies were reviewed in 1957 by Gyermek and Nador (*30*). The actions of the peripheral sites could be assessed with relative ease and, in addition, the rigid structure of the tropane ring system offered further advantage regarding structure–activity studies with respective receptor sites. The difficulty with regard to the limited knowledge of the stereochemistry of tropane alkaloids and tropane itself was largely overcome by the studies of Fodor in the last decade (cited in *30*). According to these fundamental studies the absolute configuration of the 3-OH group in *trans*-α-tropane and in *cis*-β-tropine (pseudotropine) has been clarified, and consequently the exact steric positions of the acid ester groups of different tropane alkaloids and synthetic derivatives have been established. Conformational studies indicated that the tropane ring should be assigned the chair rather than the boat form. The steric conformation of the epoxy group of scopolamine has also been determined, and the configuration 6,7β-epoxy-3α-tropyloxytropane was assigned to scopolamine, while 3α-*dl*-tropyloxy-tropane was assigned to atropine. In addition to these findings an important aspect of stereoisomerism about the nitrogen atom of the tropane ring has been clarified; it indicates that the first substituent on the nortropane nitrogen assumes an angular position facing toward the piperidine component of the tropane ring system and that the second (quaternary) substituent orients itself into an equatorial position. Thus, the absolute position of every substituent of the tropane ring and the conformation of the rigid-ring system became well characterized and adaptable to structure–activity studies. The relation between the ganglionic and related anticholinergic activities of this class of agents and the chemical structure will be discussed within the framework of these stereochemical considerations.

a. Ganglionic Blocking Tropane Compounds

Early pharmacological studies showed a vasodepressor effect of tropine. In view of the potent ganglionic blocking action of some tropine esters, a

TABLE 4.27

Ganglionic Blocking Action of Derivatives of Tropane[a]

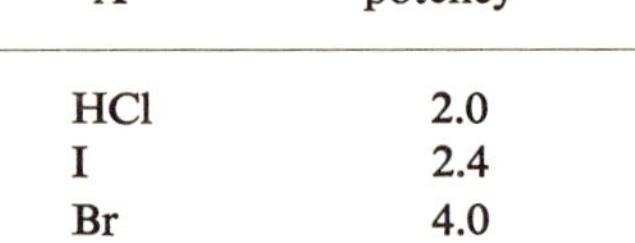

R	X	Ganglionic blocking potency[b]	Antinicotinic potency on isolated rabbit ileum (ED_{50}), μg/ml
	HCl	2.0	
CH_3	I	2.4	5.0
$C_6H_5CH_2$	Br	4.0	1.0
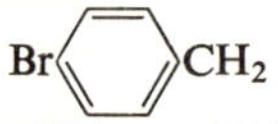	Br	17.0	0.2
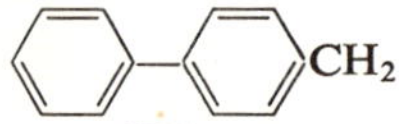	Br	28.0	0.1
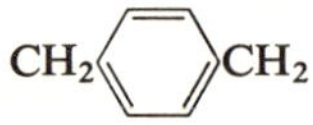	2 Br	2.0	1.0
$H_5C_2OOCCH_2$	Br	1.0	1.0

[a] Data of Gyermek (*29*).
[b] Potency of TEA, 1.0.

TABLE 4.28

Comparison of Ganglionic Blocking Potencies of Derivatives of α-Tropine, Tropane, and Mandelyl-α-Tropine

N substituent	X	α-Tropine	Tropane	Mandelyl-α-tropine
H	HCl	0.5	2.0	0.2
CH_3	Br	1.0	2.4	4.5
$C_6H_5CH_2$	Br	0.8	4.0	3.0
p-$BrC_6H_4CH_2$	Br	2.5	17.0	19.0
p-$C_6H_5C_6H_4CH_2$	Br	6.0	28.0	40.0

pertinent study with tropine was carried out. In the cat nictitating membrane preparation tropine was found to be approximately two times weaker than TEA and showed a slightly longer duration of action. Methyl and ethyl quaternization only slightly increased the ganglionic blocking action.

Structural relationships of tropine to some highly potent tropine esters and 2,6-dimethylpiperidinium compounds suggested that the weak potency of tropine derivatives was due to the presence of the hydroxyl group. In fact, tropane showed a higher degree of ganglionic blocking potency (*257*). A ganglionic blocking effect of tropine and pseudotropine and of methyl- and ethyltropinium halides has also been reported recently by Freiss et al. (*283b*).

Tropane derivatives having various substituents on carbons such as aryl, alkylaryl, carboxy, hydroxy, and carbalkoxy groups were claimed to have analgetic, anticholinergic, and ganglionic blocking activity (*284*). Data on the ganglionic blocking efficiency of quaternary derivatives of tropine and tropane are listed in Tables 4.27 and 4.28, where it is indicated that the highest potency was obtained with the *p*-phenylbenzyl quaternary derivative of tropane.

b. Atropine and Monoquaternary Derivatives of Tropines

After earlier indications that atropine had a ganglionic site of action Konzett and Rothlin (*54*) provided evidence with the perfused denervated superior cervical ganglion that the ganglionic response to ACh is depressed by as little as 0.3 μg of atropine. This observation was in contrast to that of Feldberg and Vartiainen (*53*), who found that only large (100 μg) doses of atropine could inhibit the synaptic response to injected ACh. Kewitz (*55*) also found that on this preparation atropine and scopolamine block the ganglionic effects of ACh. It is also effective against the action of muscarine (*7*, *174*, *175*), McN-A-343 (*285*), Tremorine (*198*), and nicotine monomethiodide (*152*) in the ganglia. The pressor response of neostigmine, elicited under ganglionic blockade in dogs, is sensitive to small doses of atropine (*166*, *171*). It was also found that atropine interferes with ACh at a ganglionic receptor site by producing restoration of ganglionic conduction that has previously been depressed by ACh (*180*, *204*). Like ganglionic blocking agents, atropine enhances the cardiovascular responses to norepinephrine, to angiotensin, and to 5-HT (*286*).

Comparison of the ganglionic blocking potencies of the tertiary and the methyl quaternary derivatives of atropine, homatropine, and benzoyl tropine (*287*) indicated that the actions on the postganglionic parasympathetic nerve endings and motor end plates are largely independent. The ganglionic blocking effects of *N*-allylnoratropine (dog bladder, superior cervical ganglion, DMPP stimulation on the isolated guinea pig ileum) are similar to that of atropine (*288*).

By recording postganglionic nerve activity on the superior cervical ganglion of the cat atropine was found to be equipotent with TEA, but methylatropine surpassed the potency of TEA by a factor of 10, which corresponds fairly well with the earlier findings of Gyermek (*287*) and Fink and Cervoni (*289*) with the cat nictitating membrane. In spite of the relatively high ganglionic blocking potency of methylatropine and a few other atropinelike agents, Bainbridge et al. (*260*) are of the opinion that the ratio between the ganglionic and peripheral parasympathetic blocking actions is still too high with these agents and that it is improbable that ganglionic block contributes to the therapeutic action.

The fairly potent ganglionic blocking action of methyl quaternary salts of atropine, homatropine, and benzoyltropine led to a systematic study of quaternizing groups and esterifying acidic groups and of correlations between cholinergic blocking actions and stereochemical factors of the tropane group. The structure–activity relations are outlined in Tables 4.29 to 4.37 and cover most of the reported monoquaternary tropane derivatives.

Several of the monoquaternary tropine esters were studied beyond the scope of the usual structure–activity studies. Of the aliphatic quaternary ammonium compounds of atropine *n*-octylatropinium bromide showed the most significant potency. On the cat superior cervical ganglion and on the dog pelvic ganglia it was many times more potent than TEA (*290*, *291*). This agent is very similar in its over-all anticholinergic spectrum of action to *p*-phenylbenzyl-*dl*-tropyl-α-tropinium bromide (N-399).

The study of Hermann et al. (*292*) merits attention, because besides determining the ganglionic blocking action on the cat superior cervical ganglion it compares the capacities of different atropinelike agents for producing blockade of gastric secretion in the Shay rat preparation. It was concluded that ganglionic blocking efficacy is more important than the cholinolytic activity in preventing gastric hypersecretion. Atropine methylbromide, propionyltropine methonitrate, and valeryltropine methylbromide were only slightly less potent than

TABLE 4.29

Ganglionic Blocking Activity of Acetyl- and Dimethylcarbamoyl Tropine Derivatives

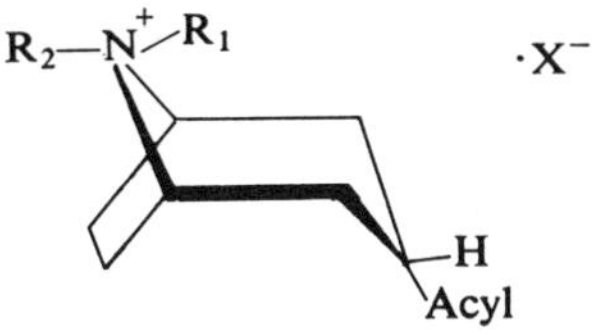

Code no.	R_1	R_2	X	Potency ([a])	Potency ([b])	Ref.
		Acyl = —OCO—CH_3				
N-180	CH_3	CH_3	I	<0.30	stimul.	*297, 298*
N-604	C_2H_5	CH_3	I	0.34	0	*297, 298*
N-242	CH_3	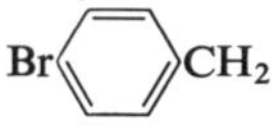	Br	1.5		*297, 298*
N-605	C_2H_5	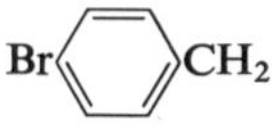	Br	3.9	0	*297, 298*
N-228	CH_3	$C_6H_5CH_2$	Br	2.0	stimul.	*29*
N-418	CH_3	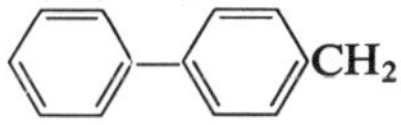	Br	12.0	stimul.	*141*
		Acyl = $OCON(CH_3)_2$				
N-258	CH_3	H	HCl	<0.1	0	*741*
N-277	CH_3	CH_3	I	<0.2		*297*
N-268	CH_3	$C_6H_5CH_2$	Br	3.0		*297*

[a] Ganglionic blocking potency of TEA on cat nictitating membrane, 1.0.
[b] Cholinolytic potency of atropine against ACh on cat blood pressure, 1.0.

pentamethonium, which was the most potent agent studied. Hyoscine methylbromide proved to be somewhat less potent than the atropine derivatives mentioned.

A study on the cat superior cervical and ciliary ganglia was carried out with methylscopolamine; no difference between their sensitivities was observed (*85*). Another quaternary ammonium derivative of scopolamine, *N*-butylscopolaminium bromide, has been suggested as blocking ganglia, because it inhibits the pilocarpine-induced blood pressure rise in the atropinized cat. In addition to its relatively moderate ganglionic blocking action (*141*) it exhibits a fairly marked spasmolytic and atropinelike activity (*293*).

N-Benzylatropinium chloride, besides having a hypotensive action, prevents the effect of preganglionic stimulation of the superior cervical ganglion. A more marked hypotensive action has been found with phenacylatropinium bromide (*294*).

TABLE 4.30

Ganglionic Blocking Activity of Benzoyl Tropine Derivatives

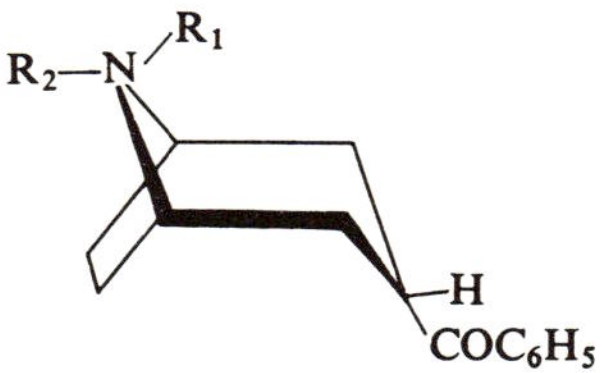

Name or code no.	R_1	R_2	Acyl[a]		Ganglionic block. potency[b]	Cholinolytic potency[c]	Ref.
Benzoyl tropine	CH_3	H		HCl	0.1		*464, 465*
Benzoyl pseudotropine	CH_3	H	β	HCl	0.1		*464, 465*
N-160	CH_3	CH_3		I	(3.2)	< 0.0003	*297, 298, 464*
N-293	CH_3	CH_3	β	I	< 0.4		*464, 465*
	CH_3	C_2H_5		Br	3.0 (4.8)	0.01	*290, 291, 464, 465*
	CH_3	C_2H_5	β	Br	6.7		*464, 465*
	CH_3	n-C_3H_7		Br	2.8 (4.0)	0.002	*290, 291, 464, 465*
	CH_3	n-C_3H_7	β	Br	6.0		*464, 465*
	CH_3	n-C_4H_9		Br	6.0 (3.6)	0.0005	*290, 291, 464, 465*
	CH_3	n-C_4H_9	β	Br	4.6		*464, 465*
	CH_3	n-C_5H_{11}		Br	(3.4)	0.00025	*290, 291, 464, 465*
	CH_3	i-C_5H_{11}	β	I	0.2		*464, 465*
	CH_3	n-C_6H_{13}		Br	(9.2)	0.004	*290, 291*
	CH_3	n-C_7H_{15}		Br	(6.0)	0.007	*290, 291*
	CH_3	n-C_8H_{17}		Br	(4.8)	0.015	*290, 291*
	CH_3	n-C_9H_{19}		Br	(3.2)	0.02	*290, 291*

	CH_3	n-$C_{10}H_{21}$		Br	(<1.6)	0.03	*290, 291*
	CH_3	n-$C_{11}H_{23}$		Br	(<1.6)	0.05	*290, 291*
	CH_3	n-$C_{12}H_{25}$		Br	(<1.6)	0.01	*290, 291*
N-601	C_2H_5	CH_3		I	2.1	0.0007	*298*
N-220	CH_3	$C_6H_5CH_2$		Br	3.0	<0.01	*297, 298, 464*
N-294	CH_3	$C_6H_5CH_2$	β	Br	0.5		*464*
N-501	$C_6H_5CH_2$	CH_3		Br	0.7		*29*
N-594	C_2H_5	$C_6H_5CH_2$		Br	5.7	0	*298*
N-262	CH_3	Br 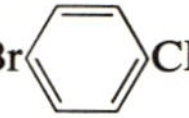 CH_2		Br	8.2		*29, 297, 298*
N-602	C_2H_5	Br 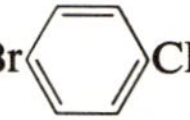 CH_2		Br	9.2	0	*298*
N-863	CH_3	H_3C 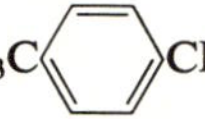 CH_2		Br	10.0	0.016	*29, 463*
N-867	CH_3	H_3C 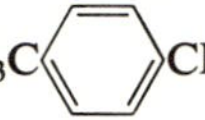 CH_2	β	Br	<1.0	0.014	*463*
N-706	CH_3	H_5C_2 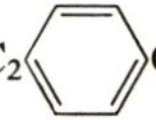 CH_2		Br	13.3	0.004	*463*
N-848	CH_3	H_5C_2 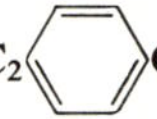 CH_2	β	Br	<1.0	0.001	*463*
N-705	CH_3	i-C_3H_7 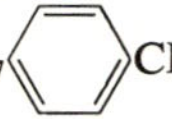 CH_2		Br	8.28	<0.01	*463*
N-703	CH_3	n-C_4H_9 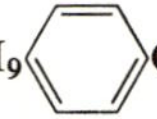 CH_2		Br	2.67	0.009	*463*
N-707	CH_3	t-C_4H_9 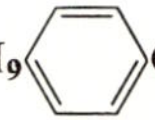 CH_2		Br	2.28	<0.1001	*463*
N-712	CH_3	C_5H_{11} 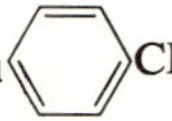 CH_2		Br	<0.5	0.04	*463*

TABLE 4.30—*continued*

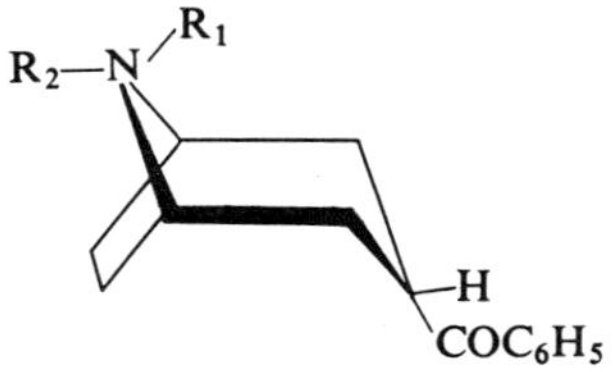

Name or code no.	R_1	R_2	Acyl[a]		Ganglionic block. potency[b]	Cholinolytic potency[c]	Ref.
N-710	CH_3	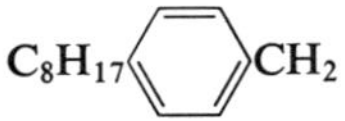		Br	< 0.25	0.018	*463*
N-361	CH_3	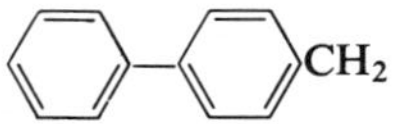		Br	gang. stimul.		*29, 95, 298*
N-406	CH_3	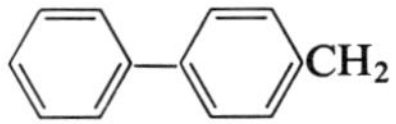	β	Br	2.0		*29*
N-949	C_2H_5	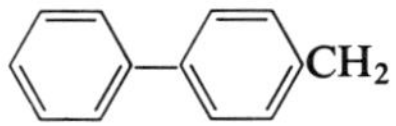		Br	gang. stimul.	0	*298*
N-718	CH_3	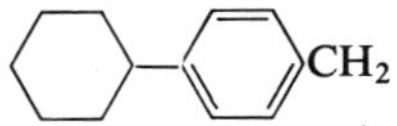		Br	1.3	0	*107*
N-833	CH_3	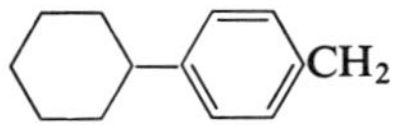	β	Br	2.0	< 0.001	*462*
N-830	C_2H_5	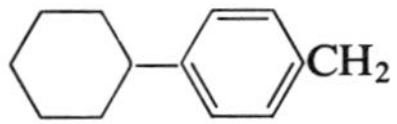		Br	1.2	0	*107, 462*
N-917	i-C_3H_7	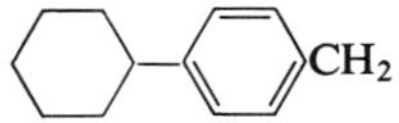		Br	0		*462*

N-858	CH_3	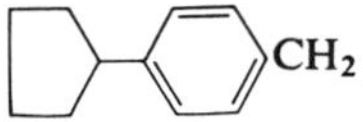		Br	3.2	0	*462*
N-871	CH_3	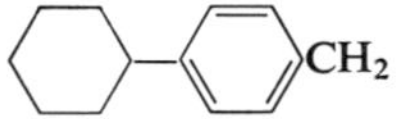		Br	0.5	0	*462*
N-925	CH_3	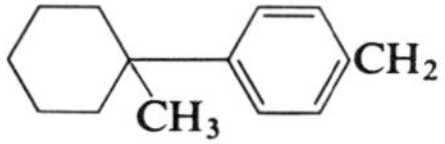		Br	0.5		*462*
N-856	CH_3	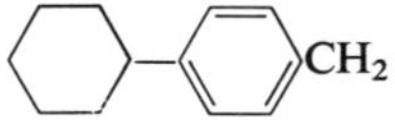	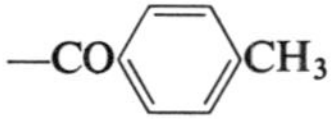	Br	2.0	0	*107, 462*
N-901	CH_3	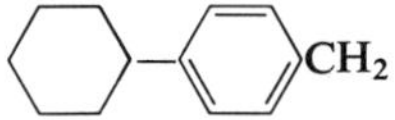	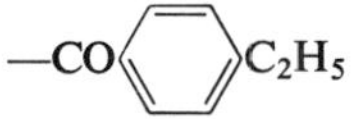	Br	4.8		*462*
N-447	CH_3	CH_3	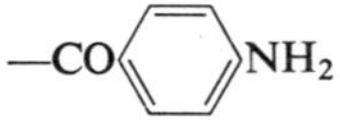	Br	4.0		*29*
N-234	CH_3	$C_6H_5CH_2$	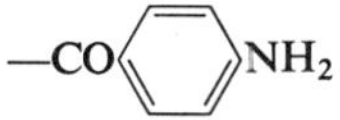	Br	8.0		*29, 297*
N-266	CH_3	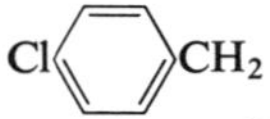	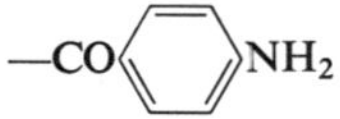	Br	22.0		*297*
N-267	CH_3	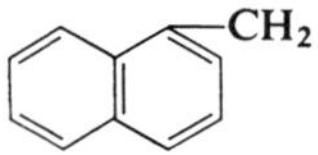	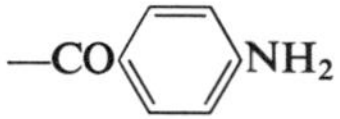	Cl	10.0		*29, 297*
N-261	CH_3	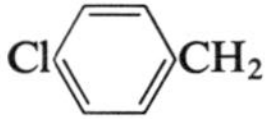	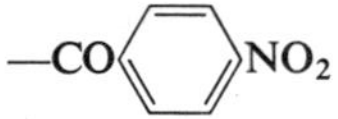	Br	8.0		*297*
N-451	CH_3	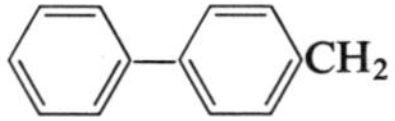	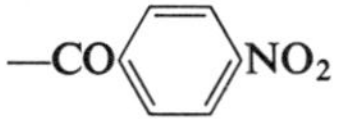	Br	1.5		*29, 95*
N-284	CH_3	$C_6H_5CH_2$	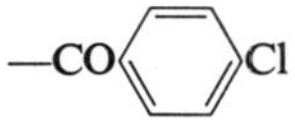	Br	2.6		*29, 297*
N-857	CH_3	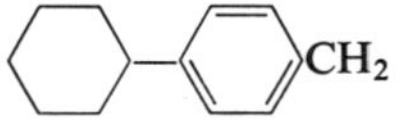	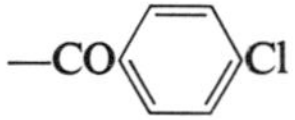	Br	0.63	0	*462*

TABLE 4.30—*continued*

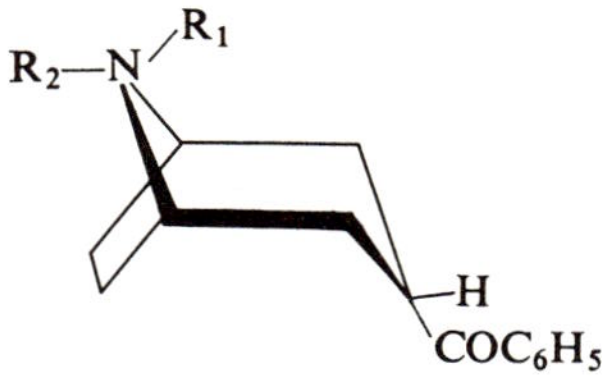

Name or code no.	R_1	R_2	Acyl[a]		Ganglionic block. potency[b]	Cholinolytic potency[b]	Ref.
N-903	CH_3	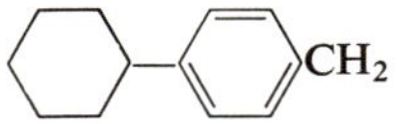	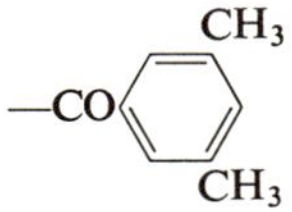	Br	0		*462*
N-842	CH_3	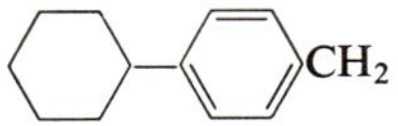	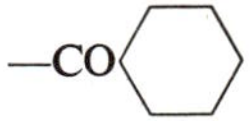	Br	0.5	< 0.001	*462*
N-931	CH_3	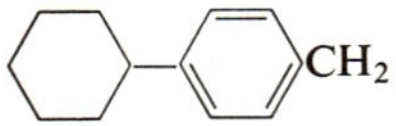	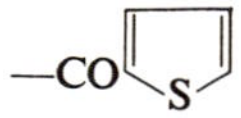	Br	1.6		*462*

[a] Steric position of the acyl group on the C-3 atom of the tropane ring is α relative to the ring except in those cases marked with β.
[b] Cat nictitating membrane; potency of TEA, 1.0; values in parentheses, dog bladder preparation, TEA, 1.0.
[c] Cat blood pressure against ACh; potency of atropine, 1.0; values in parentheses, dog bladder preparation, TEA, 1.0.

TABLE 4.31

Ganglionic Blocking Activity of Phenylacetyl Tropine Derivatives

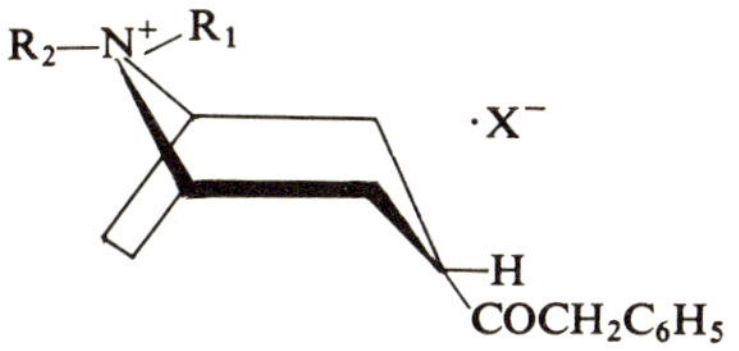

Code no.	R_1	R_2	X	Gang. block. potency[a]	Cholinolyt. potency[b]	Ref.
	CH_3				<0.10	
N-308	CH_3	CH_3	I	3.0		*29, 297*
N-309	CH_3	$C_6H_5CH_2$	Br	4.8		*29, 297*
N-340	CH_3	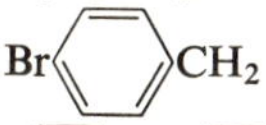	Br	9.0		*29, 297*
N-351	CH_3	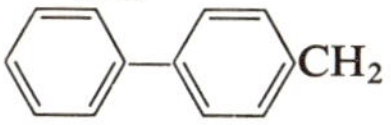	Br	10.0		*29, 297*

[a] Cat nictitating membrane; potency of TEA, 1.0.
[b] Cat blood pressure against ACh; potency of atropine, 1.0.

A pharmacological description of *p*-phenylbenzyl-*dl*-tropyl-α-tropinium bromide (N-399, gastropin), a ganglionic blocking and cholinolytic compound that in animal experiments seems to unite these pharmacological properties in a nearly optimal ratio, was given by Gyermek and Nador (*295*). The ganglionic blocking components in this compound markedly surpass that of other cholinolytic agents with mixed cholinolytic and ganglionic blocking properties (methantheline, propantheline, oxyphenonium, methatropine). *p*-Bromobenzyl-*dl*-mandelyltropinium bromide (N-239) was an active ganglionic blocking agent on the cat nictitating membrane and against carotid occlusion at 0.5 mg/kg, but considerably higher doses were necessary to depress the nicotine-induced blood pressure rise in the cat. N-239 is about as potent as pentamethonium and is antagonized by neostigmine (*296*).

The *p*-phenylbenzyl group forming the quaternary group on the tropane nitrogen atom has been found to be optimal for obtaining high ganglionic blocking potency. *p*-Phenylbenzyl-*dl*-mandelyl-α-tropinium bromide, N-310 (*297*) and $N_{(a)}$ ethyl-$N_{(b)}$-(*p*-phenylbenzyl)-*dl*-mandelyl-α-nortropinium bromide, N-760 (*298*) were 40 and 104 times more potent, respectively, than TEA on a weight basis. As measured by moles of active cation, these compounds are more than 100 to 200 times as potent as TEA, and are thus the most active ganglionic blocking agents of the monoquaternary ammonium type.

TABLE 4.32

Ganglionic Blocking Activity of *dl*-Mandelyl Tropine Derivatives

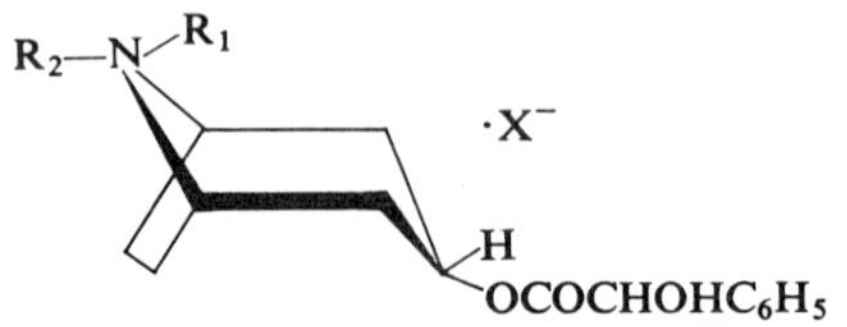

Name or code no.	R_1	R_2	X	Gang. block. potency[a]	Cholinolyt. potency[b]	Ref.
Homatropin	CH_3		HBr	0.3	0.02	*287, 298*
N-608	C_2H_5		HBr		0.0015	*298*
Novatropin	CH_3	CH_3	Br	4.5	0.038	*29, 287, 298, 358, 468*
N-763	C_2H_5	CH_3	Br	4.0	0.12	*298, 468*
N-146	CH_3	C_2H_5	Br	2.2	0.05	*29, 298, 468*
N-188	CH_3	i-C_3H_7	Br	0.8		*29, 279*
N-762	C_2H_5	C_2H_5	I	0.77	0.003	*298*
N-190	CH_3	$C_6H_5CH_2$	Br	3.0	0.005	*298*
N-955	C_2H_5	$C_6H_5CH_2$	Br	6.8	0.02	*298*
N-295	CH_3	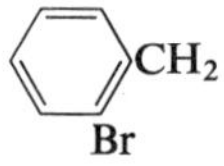	Br	4.1		*29, 297*
N-300	CH_3	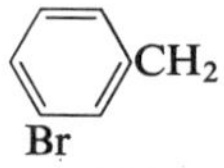	Br	6.8		*29, 297*
N-239	CH_3	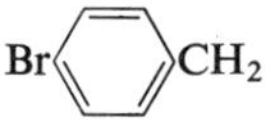	Br	19	0.015	*29, 296, 297, 468*
N-781	C_2H_5	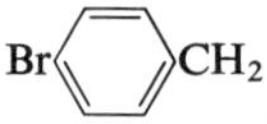	Br	23.8	0.003	*298*
N-252	CH_3	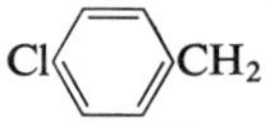	Br	16.0		*29, 297*
N-272	CH_3	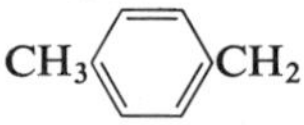	Br	14.0	<0.05	*29, 297*
N-253	CH_3	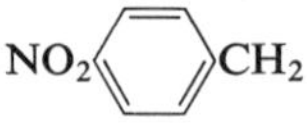	Br	16.0		*29, 297*
N-296	CH_3	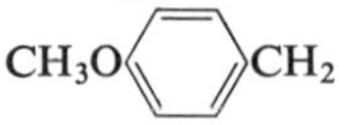	Br	8.0		*29, 297*
N-915	CH_3	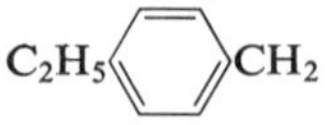	Br	7.3	0.008	*463*

TABLE 4.32—*continued*

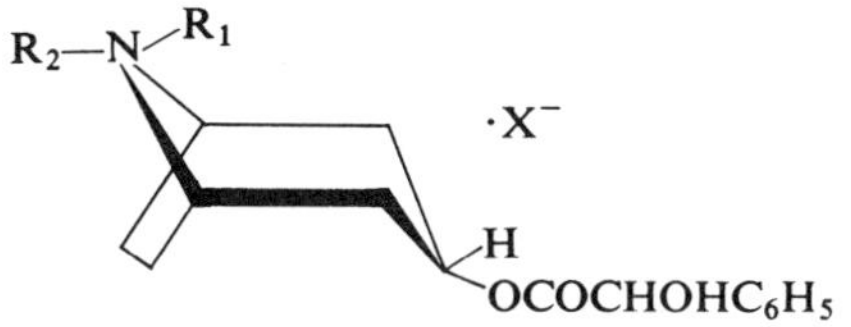

Name or code no.	R_1	R_2	X	Gang. block. potency[a]	Cholinolyt. potency[b]	Ref.
N-922	CH_3	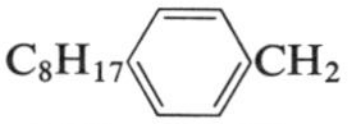	Br	0.13	0.02	*463*
N-310	CH_3	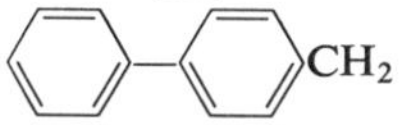	Br	40.0	0.015	*466, 468*
N-760	C_2H_5	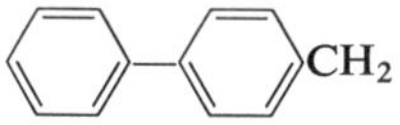	Br	104.0	0	*298*
N-720	CH_3	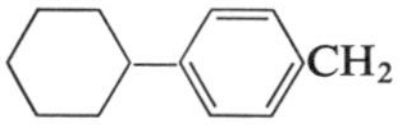	Br	4.1		*462*
N-248	CH_3	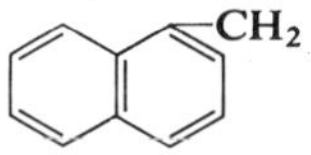	Cl	7.0	0.05	*29, 297*
N-263	CH_3	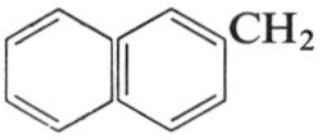	Br	4.0	<0.05	*29, 297*
N-241	CH_3	$(C_6H_5)_2CH$	Br	0.7	0.02	*29, 297*
N-271	CH_3	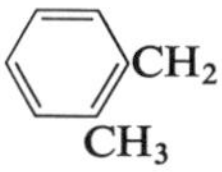	Br	1.6	0.05	*29, 297*
N-213	CH_3	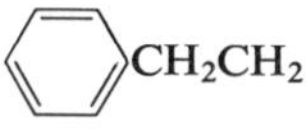	Br	1.0	0.02	*297*
		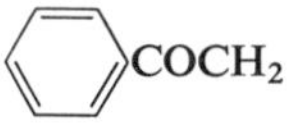	Br			*63, 297, 300*
N-237	CH_3	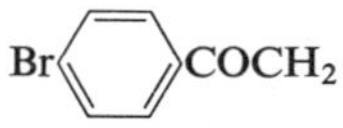	Br	4.0	<9.10	*297*

[a] Cat nictitating membrane; potency of TEA, 1.0.
[b] Cat blood pressure against ACh; potency of atropine, 1.0.

A more recent tropine derivative, *N-p*-ethylbenzyl-*dl*-α-tropyltropinium bromide, N-685, was about ten times more potent than TEA. A special characteristic of this compound and some of the spasmolytic and parasympatholytic compounds of this series was a satisfactory degree of oral adsorption. It seems that the *p*-alkylbenzyltropinium moiety is important for

TABLE 4.33

Ganglionic Blocking Activity of *dl*-Tropyl Tropine Derivatives

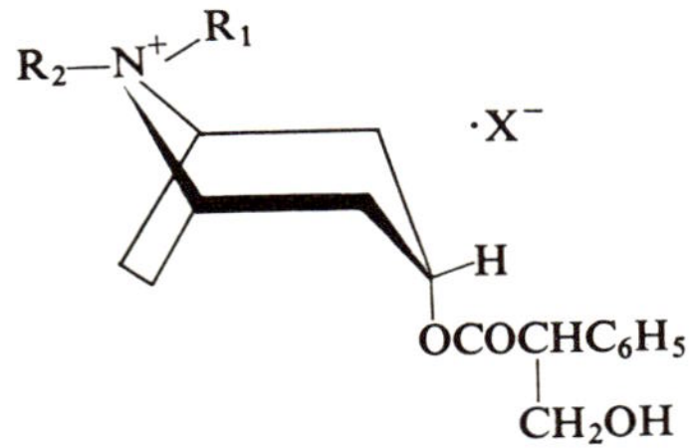

Name or code no.	R_1	R_2	X	Gang. block. potency[a]	Cholinolytic potency[b]	Ref.
Atropin	CH_3		HBr	0.3	1.0	*29, 287, 298*
N-678	C_2H_5		HBr		0.038	*298*
N-allyl-noratropine	$CH_2CH{=}CH_2$		Base	0.3		*467*
Atropine methobromide	CH_3	CH_3	Br	(4.0)	9.3	*29, 291, 292, 298, 466*
	CH_3	C_2H_5	Br	(4.0)	0.3	*29, 291*
	CH_3	n-C_3H_7	Br	(7.2)	0.05	*290, 291*
	CH_3	n-C_4H_9	Br	(8.0)	0.02	*290, 291*
	CH_3	n-C_5H_{11}	Br	(13.2)	0.03	*290, 291*
	CH_3	n-C_6H_{13}	Br	(27.0)	0.1	*290, 291*
	CH_3	n-C_7H_{15}	Br	(27.0)	0.2	*290, 291*
	CH_3	n-C_8H_{17}	Br	(40.0)	1.0	*290, 291*
	CH_3	n-C_9H_{19}	Br	(9.6)	0.2	*290, 291*
	CH_3	n-$C_{10}H_{21}$	Br	(5.2)	0.1	*290, 291*
	CH_3	n-$C_{11}H_{23}$	Br	(<4.0)	0.2	*290, 291*
	CH_3	n-$C_{12}H_{25}$	Br	(<0.8)	0.25	*290, 291*

N-960	C_2H_5	CH_3	Br	0.46	1.07	
A-60	CH_3	$C_6H_5CH_2$	Br	2.1, 7.4	0.25	*29, 297, 463*
N-243	CH_3	Br–C_6H_4–CH_2 *dl-*	Br	8.5	0.15	*29, 297, 466*
N-825	C_2H_5	Br–C_6H_4–CH_2 *dl-*	Br	13.8	0.055	*298*
N-259	CH_3	Br–C_6H_4–CH_2 *l-*	Br	8.5	0.15	*297*
N-866	CH_3	CH_3–C_6H_4–CH_2	Br	7.8	0.16	*29, 463*
N-685	CH_3	C_2H_5–C_6H_4–CH_2 α	Br	9.92	0.14	*463*
N-784	CH_3	C_2H_5–C_6H_4–CH_2 β	Br	1.9	0.035	*463*
N-683	CH_3	i-C_3H_7–C_6H_4–CH_2	Br	5.71	0.41	*463*
N-682	CH_3	*n*-C_4H_9–C_6H_4–CH_2	Br	3.04	0.51	*463*
N-680	CH_3	*t*-C_4H_9–C_6H_4–CH_2	Br	2.52	0.18	*463*
N-730	CH_3	C_5H_{11}–C_6H_4–CH_2	Br	0.20	0.39	*463*
N-815	CH_3	$(C_2H_5)_2CHCH_2$–C_6H_4–CH_2	Br	0.16	0.31	*463*
N-724	CH_3	C_8H_{17}–C_6H_4–CH_2	Br	0	0.07	*463*
Gastripon (N-399)	CH_3	C_6H_5–C_6H_4–CH_2	Br	26.0	0.009	*298, 466*

TABLE 4.33—*continued*

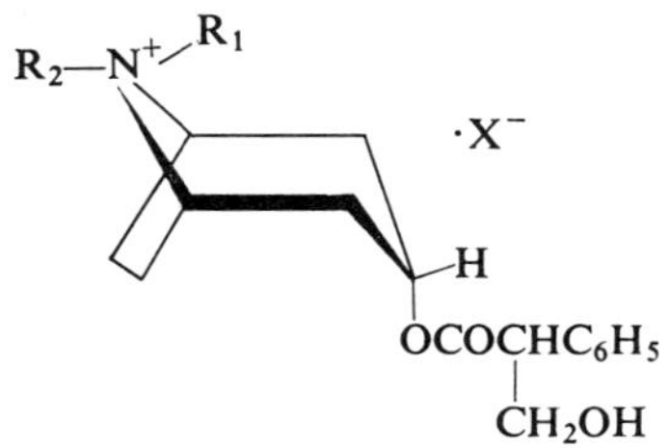

Name or code no.	R_1	R_2	X	Gang. block. potency[a]	Cholinolytic potency[b]	Ref.
N-814	C_2H_5	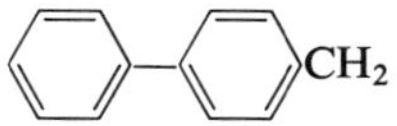	Br	110.5	0.045	*298*
N-238	CH_3	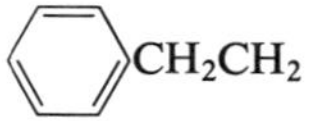	Br	0.7	>0.5	*297*
IN-618	CH_3	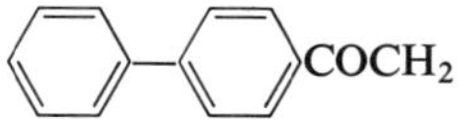	Br	10 (5)		*141*
IN-620	CH_3	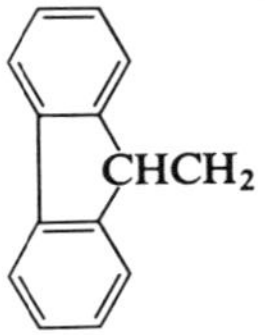	Br	(2)		*141*

[a] Cat nictitating membrane; potency of TEA, 1.0; values in parentheses, dog bladder preparation.
[b] Cat blood pressure against ACh; potency of atropine, 1.0; values in parentheses, dog bladder preparation, TEA, 1.0.

TABLE 4.34

Ganglionic Blocking Activity of Diphenylacetyl Tropine Derivatives

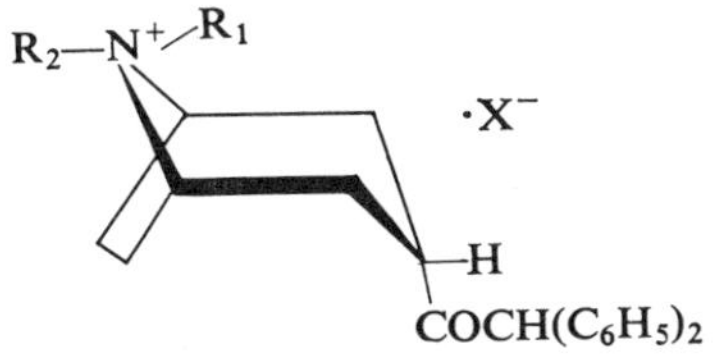

Code no.	R_1	R_2	X	Gang. block. potency[a]	Cholinolyt. potency[b]	Ref.
N-148	CH_3		HBr		0.045	*298*
N-676	C_2H_5		HCl		0.0006	*298*
N-278	CH_3	CH_3	I	5.3	0.08	*29, 297*
N-299	CH_3	CH_2	Br	2.0		*29, 297*
N-350	CH_3	CH_2	Br	10.0		*29, 297*

[a] Cat nictitating membrane; potency of TEA, 1.0.
[b] Cat blood pressure against ACh; potency of atropine, 1.0.

this action (*299*). N-Phenacylhomatropinium was found to be a potent ganglionic blocking agent, producing hypotension at 0.1 mg/kg in the cat. Its action is of short duration. It has been successfully used as a hypotensive agent during surgery with minimal atropinelike side effects (*300*). It was found to have effect, although of a much shorter duration than found with hexamethonium, on the rabbit ear preparation (*63*). Quaternary tropines that are potent ganglionic blocking agents, such as N-239 and N-310, are capable of inhibiting the TEA-produced adrenal medullary stimulation; the effect cannot be blocked by hexamethonium. This observation leads to the conclusion that different ganglionic blocking agents differ widely in their potency of blocking the autonomic (i.e., vagus) ganglia and the adrenal medulla (*99*). A study of the mode of action of tropane types of ganglionic blocking agent, in which methylhomatropinium bromide and N-310 were used, indicated that the effect of these tropane derivatives is directed toward the activated ganglionic receptors, whereas the ganglionic stimulation produced by ACh is unaffected (*205*). A nonganglionic hypotensive action of newer atropine derivatives through inhibition of adrenergic neurons must be mentioned: three tropane derivatives showed predominantly adrenergic and neuron-blocking effects in addition to a slight ganglionic blockade and parasympatholytic action. All three compounds belong to the *p*-cyclohexylbenzyltropinium group (*107*).

TABLE 4.35

Ganglionic Blocking Activity of Xanthene-9-Carboxylic Acid Derivatives

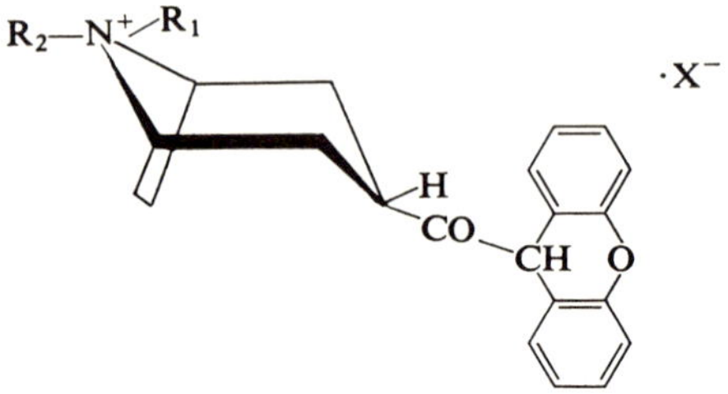

Code no.	R_1	R_2	X	Gang. block. potency[a]	Cholinolyt. potency[b]	Ref.
NA-145	CH_3		HCl		0.25	*298*
N-947	C_2H_5		HBr		0.029	*298*
N-640	CH_3	CH_3	Br	4.5	0.55	*298, 466*
N-968	C_2H_5	CH_3	Br	2.2	10.5	*298*
N-738	CH_3	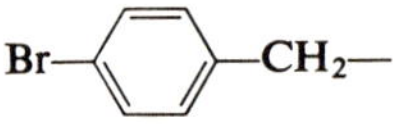	Br	1.2	0.029	*298, 466*
N-981	C_2H_5	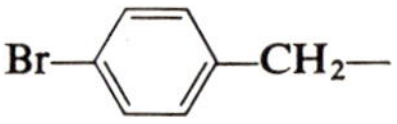	Br	3.4	0.15	*298*
N-864	CH_3	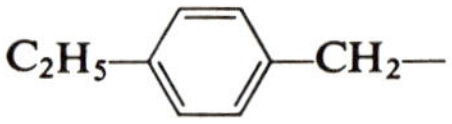	Br	<1.0	0.02	*463*
N-865	CH_3	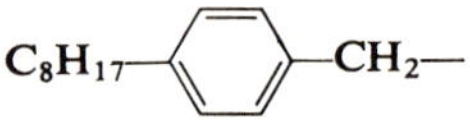	Br	<1.0	0.002	*463*
N-665	CH_3	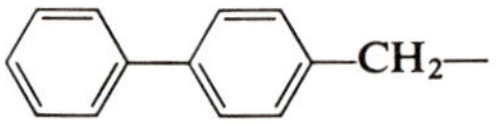	Br	1.0	0.016	*298, 466*
N-967	C_2H_5	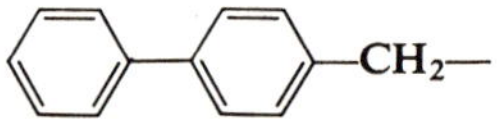	Br	2.1	0.0036	*298*

[a] Cat nictitating membrane; potency of TEA, 1.0.
[b] Cat blood pressure against ACh; potency of atropine, 1.0.

In a comparative study with atropine sulfate it was shown that tropine benzhydryl ether methanesulfonate was slightly more effective than atropine on the superior cervical ganglion. *N*-Ethylnortropine benzhydryl ether hydrobromide, up to the low toxic level of 4 mg/kg ,did not show ganglionic blockade (*301*).

TABLE 4.36

Ganglionic Blocking Activity of Diphenylglycolic Acid Derivatives

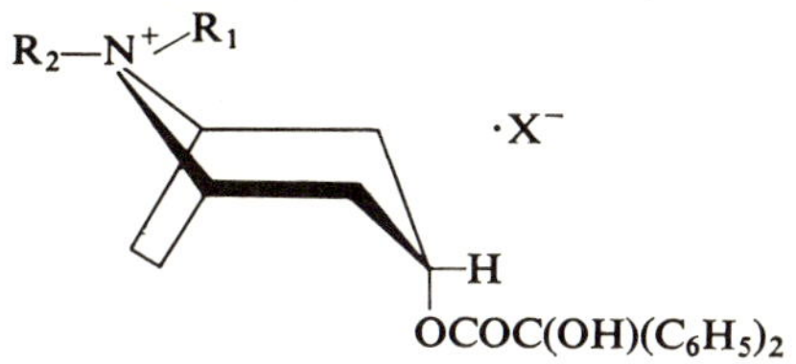

Code no.	R_1	R_2	X	Gang. block. potency[a]	Cholinolyt. potency[b]	Ref.
Na-154	CH_3		HBr		3.06	*298*
N-679	C_2H_5		HBr		0.045	*298*
Na-158	CH_3	CH_3	Br	1.6	28.8	*298*
N-990	C_2H_5	CH_5	Br	1.0	1.0	*298*
N-956	CH_3	C_2H_5	Br	1.4	0.14	*298*
N-808	C_2H_5	C_2H_5	Br	0.99	0.11	*298*
N-747	CH_3	$C_6H_5CH_2$	Br	1.3	0.007	*298*
N-789	C_2H_5	$C_6H_5CH_2$	Br	3.2	0.0004	*298*
N-611	CH_3	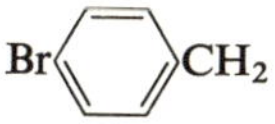	Br	1.5	0.0057	*298*
N-790	C_2H_5	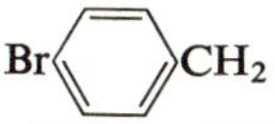	Br	4.4	0.012	*298*
N-610	CH_3	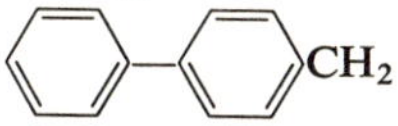	Br	5.2	0.0023	*298*
N-824	C_2H_5	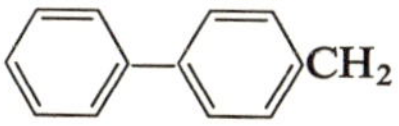	Br	4.4	0.001	*298*

[a] Cat nictitating membrane; potency of TEA, 1.0.
[b] Cat blood pressure against ACh; potency of atropine, 1.0.

A study with the cat nictitating membrane and dog bladder preparations indicated that tropyl chromone-2-carboxylate methobromide and tropyl chromone-2-carboxylate methiodide at 1 to 5 mg/kg produced ganglionic blockade without producing atropinelike or adrenolytic actions (*302*). Relatively few studies were made with compounds substituted on atoms of the tropane ring other than nitrogen. Compounds with substituents at C-6 (6-methoxytropine benzoate, benzylate, and their methyl quaternary salts) showed no greater activity against vagus stimulation on the dog than against pilocarpine, indicating very little ganglionic blocking effect with these compounds. Larger doses of 6-methoxytropinebenzylate methobromide showed a

TABLE 4.37

Effect of Different Quaternary Ammonium Groups on Ganglionic and Other Peripheral Blocking Actions of Tropine Esters[a]

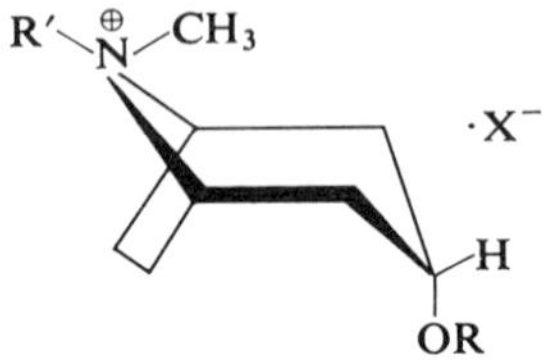

R	R′	X	Gang. block. potency[b]	Parasymp. block. potency[c]	Curarelike potency[d]
C_6H_5CO	H	HCl	0.1	0.006	
C_6H_5CO	CH_3	Br	2.0	0.04	0.01
C_6H_5CO	$C_6H_5CH_2$	Br	3.0	0.004	0.1
C_6H_5CO	*p*-$BrC_6H_4CH_2$	Br	8.2	0.003	0.07
C_6H_5CO	*p*-$C_6H_5C_6H_4CH_2$	Br	stimul.		
$C_6H_5CHOHCO$	H	HCl	0.35	0.08	
$C_6H_5CHOHCO$	CH_3	Br	4.5	0.3	0.07
$C_6H_5CHOHCO$	$C_6H_5CH_2$	Br	3.0	0.005	0.1
$C_6H_5CHOHCO$	*p*-$BrC_6H_4CH_2$	Br	19.0	0.015	0.12
$C_6H_5CHOHCO$	*p*-$C_6H_5C_6H_4CH_2$	Br	40.0	0.015	0.12
$C_6H_5CH(CH_2OH)$	H	H_2SO_4	0.35	1.0	
	CH_3	Br	4.0	1.0	0.15
	$C_6H_5CH_2$	Br	2.1	0.1	0.18
	p-$BrC_6H_4CH_2$	Br	8.5	0.07	0.17
	p-$C_6H_5C_6H_4CH_2$	Br	28.0	0.15	0.10

[a] Data of Gyermek and Nador (*30*).
[b] Cat nictitating membrane preparation; potency of TEA, 1.0.
[c] Isolated rabbit intestine; potency of atropine, 1.0.
[d] Frogs: potency of tubocurarine, 1.0.

ganglionic blocking effect (*303*). Modifying the tropane ring by extending the endoethylene bridge to an endopropylene bridge, such as in granatanium derivatives, did not yield potent compounds. For example, methyl and ethyl quaternary salts of acetyl and benzoylgranatanol showed only moderate ganglionic blocking action. Similar compounds containing quaternizing groups (longer alkyl or *para*-substituted benzyl), suitable for obtaining high ganglionic potency, were not available. It seems that the granatane ring structure offers no advantage over the tropane ring structure (*141*).

The extensive structure–activity studies with tropane compounds indicate that the different cholinergic receptor sites can be blocked to a rather selective extent mainly by variations in the quaternizing materials and in the ester

TABLE 4.38

Selectivity of Ganglionic Blocking Actions of Some Quaternary Tropine Esters Compared with Standard Blocking Agents of Cholinergic Pathways[a]

Compound	Ratio gang. block. potency[b] to: Atropinelike potency[c]	Curarelike potency[d]
Methylatropinium bromide	4.0	20
p-Phenylbenzylatropinium bromide	280.0	168
p-Brombenzyl (±)-mandelyl-α-tropinium bromide	1,250.0	160
p-Chlorbenzyl-(*p*-aminobenzoyl)-α-tropinium bromide	8,800.0	55
N_a-ethyl, N_b-(*p*-phenylbenzyl)-*O*-*dl* (±)mandelyl-α-nor-tropinium bromide	100,000.0[e]	
TEA		15
Atropine sulfate	0.3	
Tubocuarine		3

[a] Data of Gyermek and Nador (*30*).
[b] Cat nictitating membrane; potency of TEA, 1.0.
[c] Isolated rabbit gut; potency of atropine, 1.0.
[d] Frog; potency of tubocurarine, 1.0.
[e] Cat blood pressure; antiacetylcholine potency of atropine, 1.0; data of Doda et al. (*298*).

groups. Examples illustrating selectivity to these receptor sites are given in Tables 4.29 to 4.38. A summary of the structural requirements for blockade of different cholinergic sites is included in Table 4.39.

6. MONOQUATERNARY AMMONIUM COMPOUNDS WITH COMPLEX RING SYSTEMS OTHER THAN TROPANE

Fewer compounds of this class are known than are those of the asymmetric bisquaternary type, of which many possess fairly large complex rings.

Endo-exo-cyclohexane amino alcohol methiodides of the general formula $RCH_2N^+(R_1)R_2Me \cdot I^-$, where R is 2-hydroxymethyl-*endo*-*exo*-cyclohexane and R_1 and R_2 are methyl, ethyl, piperidyl, or morpholinyl, were weaker blocking agents than TEA (*304*). Bicyclic spiroquaternary salts of formula **(20)** and tricyclic spiroquaternary salts of type **(21)** were tested as possible ganglionic blocking agents for their hypotensive effects on dogs (*305*).

Methyl ammikhelline, 2-methyl-5-hydroxy-2-(β-diethylaminoethyl) furanochromone methobromide and ethobromide showed ganglionic blocking potency on the cat nictitating membrane preparation in the same range of magnitude as TEA. The tertiary amine analogues of these agents were considerably less potent (*306*). Q-160, a compound with a complex structure **(22)** was claimed to possess ganglionic blocking potency in addition to its atropine-like and local anesthetic actions; if so, the potency may influence its spectrum of action so that a selectivity to parasympathetic ganglia is apparent (*307*). However, the selectivity was not proved, according to the results of a detailed study made by Holtz and Schümann (*226*).

TABLE 4.39

Structural Requirements for Blockade of Different Types of Cholinergic Receptor Site by Tropane Compounds

Structural factor	Autonomic ganglia	Postganglionic parasympathetic receptors, atropinelike action	Myoneural junctions, curarelike action
Acid ester group attached to tropane ring	Not necessary	Essential	Essential
Type of esterifying acidic group	If present, important; not identical with acids found optimal for blocking postganglionic parasympathetic receptors	Important, including requirements for specific optical rotation (i.e., *l* vs. *d*, tropic, mandelic acid)	Important; not identical with those found essential for blocking postganglionic parasympathetic receptors
Site of substitution of ester group to tropane ring	?	C_3 is favorable to C_2, but ester groups attached to N are also highly potent	?
Alteration of the ring by addition substituents	Second quaternary ammonium alkyl group attached to C_3 favorable; 3-hydroxy group unfavorable; 6,7-epoxy group unfavorable: expansion of the ring (granatane) unfavorable	6,7-epoxy group (scopolamine) favorable	?

TABLE 4.39—*continued*

Structural factor	Autonomic ganglia	Postganglionic parasympathetic receptors, atropinelike action	Myoneural junctions, curarelike action
Steric position of ester group at C_3	Not important	Important; α-tropine esters are superior to β-tropine esters	Not important
Number of substituents of N atom	Quaternary ≫ tertiary	Quaternary ≧ tertiary > secondary	Quaternary ≫ tertiary
Steric constellation[a] around the N atom	Important	Important	Important
Nature of onium salt forming substituent	Important; aralkyl > alkyl > asymmetric bisquaternary > symmetric bisquaternary	Important; small alkyl and symmetric bisquaternaries of certain chain length are optimal; > larger alkyl > arakyl	Important; symmetric bisquaternaries of certain aliphatic chain length and aralkyl groups are optimal; > asymmetric bisquaternaries > aralkyl and alkyl monoquaternaries
Nature of tertiary substituent on the N atom	?	Important; optimal = methyl	?
Presence of tropane ring	Important (α-branching alicyclic ring system); tropane; 2,6-dimethyl piperidine; aliphatic α-branched quaternary compounds > simple piperidinium and straight-chain quaternary compounds	Not important	Important for tubocurarine type of action; bisquaternary tropane derivatives > bisquaternary piperidine derivatives

[a] Of tertiary and quaternary substituents.

7. SYMMETRIC POLYMETHYLENE BISAMMONIUM COMPOUNDS

a. Hexamethonium and Pentamethonium

Studies made by Barlow and Ing (*308*) and Paton and Zaimis (*79*) in 1948 led to the discovery of hexamethonium, which since has become the most frequently used ganglionic drug, at least in pharmacologic studies. For several reasons hexamethonium may be considered an ideal reference drug; it is fairly potent and also very selective in its action on autonomic ganglia. Its pharmacology, including its structure–activity relationships with a large number of related bisquaternary ammonium compounds, has been widely explored.

The first studies indicated that among polymethylene α,ω-bistrimethylammonium compounds with chain lengths of C_2 to C_{12} a sharp peak of ganglionic blocking potency appears with chain lengths of C_5 to C_6. A similar peak for neuromuscular blocking activity is manifested at lengths between C_8 and C_{12}. Hexamethonium, the most potent ganglionic blocking agent in the series, was substantially more effective than TEA on several preparations (*79*) and also showed a considerably longer duration of action. Correlations between chain length and ganglionic blocking efficacy in the polymethylene bistrimethylammonium series are illustrated in Table 4.40.

The criteria of an ideal ganglionic blocking agent as laid out by Paton and Zaimis (*201*) were met by hexamethonium. According to these criteria such a

TABLE 4.40

Polymethylene Bistrimethylammonium Salts[a]

	Ganglionic blocking potency[b]	
	Cat nictitating membrane	Peristaltic reflex preparation (rabbit ileum)
Ethylene bistrimethylammonium diodide		0.21[c]
Trimethylene bistrimethylammonium diodide	0.2[c]	0.31[c]
Tetramethylene bistrimethylammonium diodide	0.4	0.42
Pentamethylene bistrimethylammonium diodide	16.0	2.4
Hexamethylene bistrimethylammonium diodide	20.0	7.1
Heptamethylene bistrimethylammonium diodide	2.0	1.2
Octamethylene bistrimethylammonium diodide	0.4	
TEA	1.0	1.0

[a] Data of Paton and Zaimis (*79*).
[b] Potency of TEA, 1.0.
[c] Data of Paton and Zaimis (*201*).

compound should interfere only with ganglionic transmission, and block should ensue without previous excitation and without interference with the release of the synaptic neurotransmittor substance. Lack of effect of hexamethonium on release of ACh was later reconfirmed and contrasted with the effect of nicotine, which in its postdepolarizing blocking phase suppresses release of ACh (*207*). However, an interference with this release from mammalian neuromuscular junctions has been noted (*309*).

Hexamethonium blocks sympathetic and parasympathetic ganglia to the same extent when tested on the two divisions of autonomic ganglia of cat heart (*85*, *94*). Blockade with hexamethonium occurs exclusively at the ganglionic level, as demonstrated on the isolated superior cervical ganglion of the rabbit (*60*).

The degree of blockade is dependent on the frequency of preganglionic electrical stimulation in the cat superior ganglion preparation. This property is shared with several other types of ganglionic blocking agents (*210*). However, differences in the slopes of the dose–response-frequency curves of different compounds indicate that characteristic and individual receptor affinities or intrinsic activities exist among the different types of agents.

Hexamethonium on the guinea pig ileum is a surmountable, nondepolarizing type of ganglionic blocking agent against DMPP, as are chlorisondamine and mecamylamine (*208*). The early phase of stimulation of ACh in the ganglia, but not the late stage, is sensitive to hexamethonium blockade. The last stage is sensitive to atropine (*40*). Its blocking action at the superior cervical ganglion of the cat is inhibited by potassium, rhodium, and cesium salts. The blockade produced by other ganglionic blocking agents is influenced in a similar fashion. On the other hand, the stimulant action of K^+ is not influenced by hexamethonium on this preparation (*310*). When other types of preparation are employed, the K^+ effect is either slightly (guinea pig ileum) or markedly (rabbit intestine) depressed by hexamethonium (*311*).

Various additional ganglionic and nonganglionic actions of hexamethonium may be summarized as follows: depression of ganglionic after-discharges (*67*), effect on innervated, as compared to denervated, rabbit ear (*63*), decreasing ganglionic blocking efficacy with repeated doses in rats (*312*), inhibition of oxygen consumption in the superior cervical ganglia (*299*), increase of gastrointestinal motility and excitation of parasympathetic spinal centers (*313*), action on the urinary bladder against atropine-resistant contractions (*72*), and effects on local application to the superior cervical ganglion (*243*).

The following ganglionic effects should be noted as hexamethonium-resistant: eserine stimulation of the superior cervical ganglion (*40*) and pressor response to neostigmine (*166*).

Its actions other than ganglionic are action against nicotinic convulsions (*314*, *315*, *246*), action against ACh in postganglionic sympathetic fibers, preventing its entry into the nerve fibers (*316*), potentiation of pressor amines in the cat (*234*) and on isolated arterial strips (*317*, *318*) and, finally, an anti-arrhythmic action (*249*).

The studies in which hexamethonium was used as a reference standard are too numerous to be discussed in detail. The following outlines the types of compounds and the nature of the techniques used.

Different bisquaternary ammonium compounds: Hypotensive activity in rabbits, mouse mydriasis (*319*); mydriatic activity in mice (*320*); vagal ganglia, salivary glands of the cat (*321*); seven different animal tests for ganglion blocking activity (*322*); human studies (*323*); hypertensive patients (*324–326*).

Hexamethylene bistrialkylammonium compounds: Cat nictitating membrane, isolated guinea pig ileum (*221*).

Polymethylene and azapentylene bisammonium compounds: Cat nictitating membrane, bladder, mouse mydriasis, isolated rabbit ileum (*327*).

N-Methoxy-, ethoxy-, and carbethoxy-substituted hexamethylene bis-ammonium compounds: Hypotensive and ganglionic blocking activity in the dog and rabbit (*328*).

Pentolinium: Superior cervical ganglion and peristaltic reflex preparations (*80*).

Phenylalkane bisammonium compounds: Cat nictitating membrane, isolated guinea pig ileum (*329*).

Bisammonium alkyl ethers and thioethers: Cat nictitating membrane, isolated guinea pig ileum (*48*, *49*, *330*, *331*).

Thiapolymethylene bisammonium salts: Sympathetic and parasympathetic ganglia of the cat (*219*).

Various types of ganglionic blocking agents: Cat nictitating membrane, nicotine convulsions in mice (*315*); stellate and superior cervical ganglion of the cat (*241*); celiac ganglion (splenic volume changes) (*240*); isolated vagus-stomach preparation of the rat (*322*); hypertensive patients (*26*).

The second most explored ganglionic blocking agent of the methonium series is *pentamethonium*. It is fairly close in type and potency of action to hexamethonium (*79*, *110*, *201*, *320*), although there is some evidence that this compound may, in certain preparations, block predominantly the parasympathetic ganglia. On the cat's heart preparation, pentamethonium blocked 10 times more readily the parasympathetic ganglia, whereas other ganglionic agents, including hexamethonium, did not show any major difference in blocking the two different divisions of ganglia (*94*). In a manner similar to hexa- and heptamethonium, pentamethonium blocks nicotine convulsion in mice and rats; shorter C_{3-4} chain members of the series, together with TEA, are inactive in this respect (*314*).

Pentamethonium, like hexamethonium, depresses the tissue respiration of the superior cervical ganglion (*229*), produces sensitization to adrenergic vascular mechanisms (*234*), and elicits increased motility in the gastrointestinal tract of the dog (*245*).

Decamethonium, a potent neuromuscular blocking agent which belongs to the depolarizing type of paralyzants of the motor end plates was not tested first for ganglionic-blocking activity probably because of the predominance of curarelike actions. However, it was found recently that it has considerable ganglionic blocking activity, approaching that of hexamethonium (*333*). This action, unlike the blockade at the motor end plates, is of a competitive nature, at least on the superior cervical ganglion. Decamethonium also shows blockade at postganglionic sites (*202*).

b. Replacement of the Terminal Methyl Group with Other Alkyl or Alkoxy Groups in the Polymethylene Bisammonium Series

Several studies have dealt with the relationships between biological activity and changes at the terminal methyl group of methonium compounds. Replacement of the terminal methyl groups with ethyl groups in tetra-, penta-, hexa-, and heptamethylene bisammonium compounds was analyzed by Wien (*110*). The changes in ganglionic blocking potency of these compounds, brought about by introducing ethyl groups, greatly depends on the chain length of the compounds (Table 4.41). In the tetramethylene series a very marked increase in potency occurs by exchanging one or two methyl groups for ethyl. A smaller increase occurs in the pentamethylene series. In the hexamethylene series the introduction of only one ethyl group is optimal. The *N,N'*-diethyl analogue of hexamethonium, when compared in seven different ganglionic preparations, showed a potency one to three times that of hexamethonium (*322*), whereas in the heptamethylene series ethyl substitution is no longer effective. Replacement of all methyl groups by ethyl results in compounds of very low potency (*110*) in all cases.

Relatively low activities in a fairly small series of polymethylene bistriethylammonium compounds have been observed by Chou and De Elio (*334*). Ethylene, trimethylene, and pentamethylene bistriethylammonium salts were all considerably weaker than TEA. However, the corresponding decamethylene analogue was twice as potent as TEA on the superior cervical ganglion of the cat.

A systematic study with a larger series of *long-chain bistriethylammonium salts* in comparison with the similar bistrimethylammonium series has been carried out recently by Barlow and Zoller (*333*). Both series of compounds showed a peak activity at a chain length of C_{15} to C_{18}, and no major difference in ganglionic blocking potency between the trimethyl and triethyl series was noticed with these long-chain compounds. Members of the series extending from pentadecamethylene to octadecamethylene exhibited remarkable degrees

TABLE 4.41

Effect of Successive Replacement of Methyl with Ethyl Groups on Nitrogen Atoms in Polymethylene Bisammonium Compounds on Ganglionic Blocking Activity[a]

$$(R_1)(R_2)(R_3)N^+(CH_2)_nN^+(R_1)(R_2)(R_3) \cdot 2Br^-$$

				Relative potency[b]	
n	R_1	R_2	R_3	Sympath. (cat superior cervical)	Parasymp. (guinea pig ileum)
4	Me	Me	Me	0.01	0.05
	Et	Me	Me	0.10	0.25
	Et	Et	Me	1.00	0.25
	Et	Et	Et	0.05	0.05
5	Me	Me	Me	0.65	0.75
	Et	Me	Me	1.50	1.50
	Et	Et	Me	1.25	1.00
	Et	Et	Et	0.07	0.10
6	Me	Me	Me	1.00	1.00
	Et	Me	Me	1.50	2.00
	Et	Et	Me	0.75	1.00
	Et	Et	Et	<0.05	<0.02
7	Me	Me	Me	0.12	0.30
	Et	Me	Me	0.10	0.30
	Et	Et	Me	0.15	0.02
	Et	Et	Et	0.02	<0.02

[a] Data of Wien (*110*).
[b] Potency of hexamethonium, 1.0.

of ganglionic blocking potency on the superior cervical ganglion, surpassing hexamethonium by a factor of 2 to 6. The degree of neuromuscular blockade ran parallel with the ganglionic blocking potency in the bistrimethylammonium series, but not in the bistrimethyl compounds (Table 4.42).

The role of substitution of methyl groups by alkyls other than ethyl has been studied in detail only in the hexamethonium series. Longer chains than ethyl uniformly caused marked loss of potency (*221*, *328*); see Tables 4.43 and 4.44. Substituents at each end of the terminal methyls (oxyalkyl, alkyl ether, alkyl ester, carbamoyl methyl, carbamoyl ethyl, phenyl, benzyl, phenethyl, and amyl ether groups) usually gave less potent agents than hexamethonium.

TABLE 4.42

Ganglionic Blocking Activity of Polymethylene Bis-*N*,*N*′-Trimethyl- and Bis-*N*,*N*′-Triethylammonium Compounds on the Cat Superior Cervical Ganglion Preparation[a]

BTM series		BTE series		Hexadecamethylene compounds	
n	Molar potency[b]	*n*	Molar potency[b]	*n*	Molar potency[b]
10	0.45	10	0.25		
11	0.24	11	0.25	BEDM 16	3.1
12	0.27	12	0.5	BMDE 16	3.3
13	0.46	13	1.1		
14	0.85	14	2.2		
15	2.8	15	3.3		
16	3.8	16	5.0		
17	3.8	17	6.2		
18	4.2	18	2.0		
19	1.9	19	0.5		
20	0.85	20	0.28		
21	0.35	21	0.06		

[a] BTM = polymethylene bis-*N*,*N*′-trimethylammonium series, BTE = polymethylene bis-*N*,*N*′-triethylammonium series, BEDM 16 = hexamethylene bis-*N*,*N*′-ethyldimethylammonium, BMDE 16 = hexamethylene bis-*N*,*N*′-methyldiethylammonium, *n* = carbon units in polymethylene chain. Data of Barlow and Zoller (*333*).

[b] Potency of hexamethonium, 1.0.

One compound, hexamethylene-bis(dimethyl-β-hydroxyethylammonium) dibromide, was reported to be as potent as hexamethonium but to have a lower degree of acute toxicity. The *N*,*N*′-phenoxymethyl and phenoxypropyl analogues of hexamethonium were about as potent as the parent compound at the ganglionic sites but also showed curarelike and anticholinesterase properties; see Table 4.44.

The effect of the change in size of the substituents of the terminal nitrogen atoms on the chain length of flexible polymethylene bisammonium compounds has been studied by Elworthy (*335*, *336*). Measurements of the conductances in water of polymethylene bistrimethyl- and triethylammonium compounds were made for estimations of the structural changes in the shape of the polymethylene chain as influenced by the energy of the hydrocarbon–water interphase. The measurements indicated that the internitrogen distances are markedly shorter than had been estimated from extended molecular

TABLE 4.43

Ganglionic Blocking Activity of Hexamethylene Bisammonium Compounds with Various Substituents on the Terminal N Atoms[a]

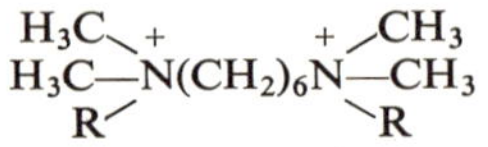

$\cdot 2X^-$

Code no.	R	X	Ganglionic blocking potency[b]: Vagus blockade in dogs	Antinicotine potency in rabbits
1248	C_2H_5	I	1.0	0.2
1249	n-C_3H_7	I		0.1
1200	n-C_3H_7	Br	1.0	0.2
1277	$CH_2CHOHCH_3$	Br		0.4
1247	$CH_2CH_2OC_2H_5$	I	0.05	0.04
1138	$CH_2COOC_2H_5$	Br		0.1
1246	CH_2OCH_3	I	0.10	0.2
1142	CH_2CONH_2	Br	0.10	0.04
1141	$CH_2CH_2CONH_2$	Br		0.10
1140	$CH_2CON(CH_3)_2$	I	0.10	0.04
1229	$CH_2CON(C_2H_5)_2$	I	0.25	0.10
1279	C_6H_5	I		0.20
1250	$CH_2C_6H_5$	I	0.10	0.4
1278	$CH_2CH_2C_6H_5$	Br	0.25	0.10
1294	$CH_2CH_2OC_6H_5$	Br		0.20
1253	$C_3H_5OC_6H_5$	Br	0.25	1.0
1208	$CH_2OC_6H_5$	Br	2.5	0.4
Hexamethonium bromide			1.0	1.0

[a] Data of Palazzo and Virno (*328*).
[b] Potency of hexamethonium, 1.0.

models. For example, in hexamethonium the calculated distance is 6.3 A, which is about 3 A less than the model indicated; the difference in the case of decamethonium amounts to 4 A. The steric arrangements of the terminal alkyl substituents influences the fit of the cationic group to the receptor and the flexibility of the polymethylene chain. Thus, for example, complete exchange of the terminal methyls for ethyl groups in the tetramethyl bisammonium compounds presumably decreases the degree of fit to the receptor site, as judged from the biological activities. This may be a suitable explanation because, in spite of the favorable change in the internitrogen distance produced by the introduction of the larger ethyl group (resulting in a calculated increase of this distance by 2.2 A, which yielded an over-all length of 6.4 A, the optimal internitrogen distance for ganglionic blocking activity) the tetramethylene bistriethylammonium compound is quite inactive.

These studies also suggested that bulkiness of the cationic head should have

TABLE 4.44

Hexamethylene Bisammonium Compounds with Various Alkyl Substituents on the Terminal N Atoms[a]

$RN^+(CH_2)_6N^+R \cdot 2Br$

R	Relative potency: Cat nict. membrane	Relative potency: Guinea pig ileum
MeMeMe	1.00	1.00
EtMeMe	1.50	2.00
n-Propyl MeMe	<0.05	<0.05
Isopropyl MeMe	0.15	0.10
n-Butyl MeMe	<0.04	<0.02
Isobutyl MeMe	<0.04	0.04
Allyl MeMe	0.04	0.04
MeEtEt	0.75	1.00
EtEtEt	<0.05	<0.50

[a] Data of Wien (*221*).

a more significant effect on the fit of short-chain molecules than on that of long-chain ones. Not only the size of the terminal substituents, but configurational changes in the steric position of the terminal (ethyl groups) may notably influence ganglionic blocking action. Canepa (*51*) questioned the general validity of two-point attachment in respect to the bisquaternary ammonium type of ganglionic blocking agent because of crystallographic measurements of pentamethonium. Although the blocking activity of compounds with methyl quaternary groups seems to be a function of chain length, bulkier groups on the nitrogen atoms seem to act independently of chain length by shielding one receptor area rather than by allowing a complete fit to two receptors separated by a distinct interreceptor distance.

Recently an attempt was made to decrease the flexibility of the polymethylene chain by replacing it with a cyclopropane polymethylene bridge, where the cyclopropane moiety is located in the middle of the chain. In this series of compounds ganglionic blocking action was observed with the isomers of 1,2-di(β-trimethylammoniumethyl) cyclopropane diiodide. The other members of the group were predominantly curarelike in their action (*337*).

c. Polymethylene Bisalicyclicammonium Compounds

Wien and Mason (*322*) observed that the terminal alkylammonium groups can be replaced successfully with alicyclic groups, resulting in some agents that significantly surpass hexamethonium in potency and duration of action.

Systematic structure–activity studies were therefore conducted with polymethylene biscycloalkylammonium compounds.

(1) *Polymethylene Bispyrrolidinium, Bispiperidinium, and Bismorpholinium Compounds.* The pharmacology of these series was explored by Mason and Wien (*222*). While the peak activity of the piperidinium series appeared with the C_4 to C_6 chain length and, in the *N*-morpholinium series, with the C_5 to C_7 chain length and did not surpass that of hexamethonium (Table 4.45), the penta- and hexamethylene members of the *N*-methylpyrrolidinium series were significantly more potent than hexamethonium in a variety of test organs (*322*) and in man (*323*). Similarly, ganglionically active hexamethylenebispyrrolidinium, bispiperidinium, -morpholinium, and -isoquinolinium derivatives were reported by Phillips (*200*).

Pentamethylenebis-*N*-methylpyrrolidinium (pentapyrrolidinium, pentolinium) was 1.5 to 5 times as potent as hexamethonium in different animal preparations (*322*, *327*) and exhibited a duration of action 2 to 4 times longer, whereas hexamethylenebis-*N*-ethylpyrrolidinium was about twice as potent. Pentolinium, like hexamethonium and mecamylamine, antagonizes nicotine convulsions in mice (*246*). Comparisons of several other different types of ganglionic blocking agent were done with pentolinium on the celiac ganglion (*240*) and on the superior cervical ganglion and stellate ganglia (*241*). Its action on the gastrointestinal motility was studied by Shuster and Polyakov (*338*). Like hexamethonium, it makes certain effector cells sensitive to epinephrine

TABLE 4.45

Comparison of Ganglionic Blocking Potencies of Polymethylene Bis-*N*-pyrrolidinium, Bis-*N*-piperidinium, and Bis-*N*-morpholinium Compounds[a]

		Ganglionic blocking potency[b]					
		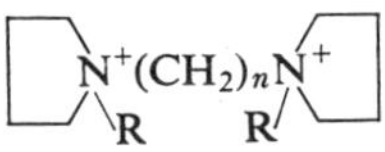 $\cdot 2X^-$		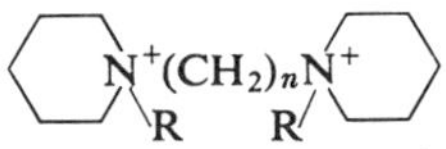 $\cdot 2X^-$		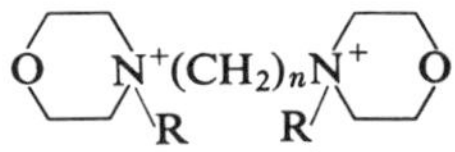 $\cdot 2X^-$	
R	*n*	Pot.[b]	2X	Pot.[b]	2X	Pot.[b]	2X
CH_3	3	0.05	I	0.07	I		
CH_3	4	0.5	I	0.8	I	0.2	Br
CH_3	5	5.0	I	0.9	Br	1.0	Br
CH_3	6	3.0	Br	0.8	I	1.0	I
C_2H_5	6	0.6	Br	<0.1	I	0.06	I
CH_3	7			0.3	I	0.8	I
CH_3	10	0.75	I	0.05	I	0.6	I
C_2H_5	10			<0.01	Br		
CH_3	12	0.1	I			1.0	I

[a] Data of Mason and Wien (*222*).

[b] Cat nictitating membrane preparation; potency of hexamethonium, 1.0.

and norepinephrine on blood vessels and on the nictitating membrane of the cat (*318*), but is inactive as a sensitizing agent on isolated rabbit arterial strips (*317*). Because pentolinium and hexamethonium block the action of bretylium on the postganglionic sympathetic fibers, probably by inhibiting its entry into the fiber, a postganglionic effect of these agents might also be suggested (*316*). In the rat the hypotensive effect of pentolinium is attributable about equally to a decrease of peripheral resistance and a decrease of cardiac output (*339*). In isolated guinea pig ileum pentolinium behaves like hexamethonium in blocking the effect of different types of ganglionic stimulants (*164*). In comparison with other ganglionic blocking agents mecamylamine and pempidine surpassed pentolinium in potency on the vagal ganglia of the heart and parasympathetic ganglia of the salivary glands (*321*). Major differences were found between the mydriatic potency of pentolinium-type ganglionic blocking agents and that of other types of ganglionic blocking drugs. In conventional ganglionic preparations pentolinium is three to five times as potent as hexamethonium, but its dilating action on the mouse pupil is much more pronounced. Some pentolinium-type agents surpassed hexamethonium by a factor of 50 (*327*). Pentapyrrolidinium is a highly potent and less abruptly acting hypotensive agent than TEA or hexamethonium and has a fairly long-lasting effect. It has been the subject of several animal and human studies, which cannot be discussed here in detail. A few comparative data on clinical vagolytic and hypotensive potencies obtained with pentolinium-type and several bisammonium-type ganglionic blocking agents were obtained in the study of Maxwell and Campbell (*323*). Besides a high absolute potency, the dose ratios between side effects and vasodilation were most favorable with pentolinium. In this study the potency was 10 times higher and the duration of action 2 times longer than with hexamethonium. Pentolinium was employed with favorable effects as compared with hexamethonium in clinical studies (*324*, *326*). The treatment of hypertension by means of a combination of Rauwolfia preparations, pentolinium, or mecamylamine was superior to treatment by means of combinations with hexamethonium and chlorisondamine as ganglionic blocking agents (*340*). Like the polymethylenebistrimethylammonium series, decamethylenebis-*N*-methylpyrrolidinium was primarily curarelike. Introducing an α-branched alkyl moiety into the alicyclic terminal groups, which makes for a structural factor found favorable in the monoquaternary ammonium type (2,6-dimethylpiperidinium and 2,5-dimethylpyrrolidinium), reduces activity in the bisquaternary series (*341*). A series of cyclizable haloalkyl-substituted bisamines were studied with special emphasis on their intestinal adsorptive capacity. A considerably more favorable ratio of adsorption has been noted, for example, with the pentamethylene bis-ω-bromopentylmethylamine than with the preformed pentamethylene-bis-*N*-methylpiperidinium analogue. This study also covered the cyclizable haloalkylamine congener of pentolinium, which was equipotent with it but showed a less favorable ratio of oral to parenteral dose, probably because its transformation into the cyclic quaternary analogue (pentolinium) took place too rapidly. It was concluded that for best oral adsorption a slow degree of cyclization of suitable tertiary amines into quaternary ammonium ions is necessary (*342*).

(2) *Symmetric Polymethylene Bis-N-isoquinolinium and Quinuclidinium Compounds.* The first class reported by Smith et al. (*343*) showed predominantly curarelike actions, and only as a side effect was ganglionic blockade detected. This was usually manifested at doses producing a significant degree of neuromuscular paralysis. Polymethylenebis-*N*-quinuclidine derivatives with a connecting chain of three to ten carbon atoms and with or without substituents at the C-3 atom of the quinuclidine ring were also studied for the same actions (*344*). Of a series of twenty-five compounds the most active ganglionic blocking agent was *N,N'*-heptamethylenebisquinuclidinium, and the corresponding C_9 derivative showed the peak curarelike effect within the group.

8. BISAMMONIUM COMPOUNDS WITH CONNECTING ALKYL ETHER OR ESTER CHAINS

In addition to the variations on the terminal nitrogen atoms an important structural element to be studied in connection with the structure–activity relationships of hexamethonium-type agents is the connecting chain between the ammonium groups. The majority of compounds in this group belong to the ether type, $R_1R_2R_3N^+(CH_2)_x—O—(CH_2)_y—N^+R_1R_2R_3 \cdot 2X^-$. A relatively smaller group represents diammonio esters of the type $R_1R_2R_3N(CH_2)_2COO$-$(CH_2)_2NR_4R_5R_6 \cdot 2X^-$ and bischoline derivatives of dicarboxylic acids of the general structure $(CH_3)_3N^+C_2H_4OOCRCOOC_2H_4N^+(CH_3)_3 \cdot 2X^-$. The first symmetric bisammonium aliphatic ether type of compound reported as a ganglionic blocking agent was bis-γ,γ'-1-trimethylammonium propyl ether (Mc-2444), which was found to be about as potent as hexamethonium. In dogs Mc-2444 was eleven times as potent as TEA in inhibiting the nicotine-induced blood pressure rise (*345*).

Comparison of the abilities of polymethylene alkyl ether and alkyl thioether chains to produce ganglionic blockade in the bistrialkylammonium series resulted in the following order of potency: $—(CH_2)_5— > —(CH_2)_2—S—(CH_2)— > —(CH_2)_3—O—(CH_2)_3— > C_4 = C_6 > —(CH_2)_2—O—(CH_2)_2—$ (*346*). Systematic studies with a large number of bisammoniumalkyl ethers and thioethers were conducted by Fakstorp et al. (*48*, *49*, *347*, *348*). In these studies they made quantitative assessments of ganglionic blocking potencies on sympathetic ganglia (cat nictitating membrane) and parasympathetic ganglia (isolated guinea pig ileum) and of the role of alkyl and thioalkyl ether chain length and terminal alkyl substituents. Among the symmetric ethyl ether and ethyl thioether types of agent optimal potency was obtained with dimethylethyl or diethylmethyl terminal groups. These agents approached hexamethonium in potency. The thioether class, particularly the bistrimethylammonium compounds, showed a higher degree of activity. The structure–activity relations of these agents are shown in Table 4.46. Optimal potency

TABLE 4.46

Ganglionic Blocking Activity of Symmetric Bisquaternary Ammonium Compounds with Heteroatoms in the Polymethylene Connecting Chain[a]

$R_3(R_1)_2N^+(CH_2)_2—Y—(CH_2)_2—N^+(R_2)_2R_3 \cdot 2X^-$

			Ganglionic blocking potency[c]							
			Y=O		Y=S		Y=SS		Y=SO	
R_1	R_2[b]	R_3[b]	Symp.	Paras.	Symp.	Paras.	Symp.	Paras.	Symp.	Paras.
Et	Et	Et	0.056	0.056	0.059	0.39	0.17	ϕ	0.17	ϕ
Me	Et	Et	1.18	1.40	1.39	2.09			<0.05	0.42
Et	Me	Et	0.41	0.36						
Et	Et	Me			0.96	0.68	0.97	0.41	<0.05	0.009
Me	Et	Me	0.53	0.28						
Me	Me	Et	0.32	0.23	0.84	1.24	0.46	0.62	1.15	0.84
Me	Me	Me	0.10	0.019	0.67	0.75	0.69	0.37	<0.05	0.019
Et	Pyr	Et	1.03	1.45						
Me	Pyr	Me	<0.05	0.15						
Me	Pip	Et	1.31	1.49						
Et	Pip	Et	0.22	0.10						
Et	Mo	Me	1.12	0.33						
Me	Mo	Me	<0.05	0.026						
Me	Me	Pr	0.05	0.008						
Me	Me	Bu	0.098	0.009						
Me	Me	Allyl	0.05	0.022						
Me	Me	Oc	0.16	0.025						
Me	Me	Bu		0.020						
Me	Me	Carb	0.05	0.05						
Me	Et	Bu	0.10	0.01						
Me	Et	Hy	1.00	1.13						
Me	Et	Pr	0.82	0.89						
Me	Et	BuEt	1.07	1.87						
Me	Et	Hept	0.14	46						

[a] Data of Fakstorp and Pedersen (*48*).

[b] Pyr=pyrrolidine, Pip=piperidine, Mo=morpholine, Carb=carbethoxyethyl, Hy=hydroxyethyl.

[c] Parasympathetic ganglion blockade, guinea pig ileum, sympathetic ganglion blockade, cat nictitating membrane; potency of hexamethonium, 1.0.

occurs with derivatives that carry different alkyl substituents at the ends of the chain; thus, they usually belong to the asymmetric bisquaternary class. A symmetric propyl ether series of the general formula $R_1R_2R_3N(CH_2)_3—O—(CH_2)_3—NR_1R_2R_3 \cdot 2X^-$ yielded fairly weak ganglionic blocking compounds (Table 4.47). Here again, different alkyl substitutions on the two nitrogen atoms improved ganglionic blocking efficacy. Introducing an asymmetric link of ethyl-propyl ether resulted in optimal potency within the series (*49*). Branched-chain derivatives (diisopropylammonio ethers) were less potent than any of the straight-chain ether analogues (*49*); see Table 4.48.

Two other structural variations of the connecting chain of ether-type bisammonium agents were studied: the introductions of a sulfur atom into ether-type agents and into thioether-type compounds. In the first group with $—(CH_2)_2—S—S—(CH_2)_2—$ connecting chains the ganglionic blocking potency was approximately equal to that of the thioether group. The $—(CH_2)_2—SO—(CH_2)_2—$ chain, except in the bisdimethylethyl and bisdiethyl-methylammonium derivatives, resulted in compounds of quite low potency (*25, 48, 331*).

Bisquinuclidine derivatives with connecting methyl and ethyl ether chains were reported recently by Sadritdinov (*349*). Of these the *N*-bisquinuclidine methyl ether showed the highest ganglionic blocking activity. The high potency with the relatively short connecting chain in this series indicates that

TABLE 4.47

Ganglionic Blocking Activity of Bisquaternary Ammonium Compounds with Symmetric and Asymmetric Alkyl Ether Connecting Chains

$R_3(R_1)_2N^+(CH_2)_mO(CH_2)_nN^+(R_2)_2R_3 \quad \cdot 2X^-$

					Gang. block. potency[b]							Gang. block. potency[b]	
R_1	R_2	R_3	*m*	*n*	Symp.	Paras.	R_1	R_2	R_3	*m*	*n*	Symp.	Paras.
Me	Me	Me	3	2	1.84	1.02	Me	Me	Me	3	3	0.13	0.019
Me	Me	Et	3	2	1.46	1.45	Me	Me	Et	3	3	<0.05	0.12
Me	Et	Me	2	3	1.50	2.45	Et	Et	Me	3	3	<0.05	0.96
Et	Me	Et	2	3	1.98	1.40	Et	Et	Et	3	3	<0.05	0.14
Et	Me	Et	2	3	0.61	0.59	Me	Et	Me	3	3	0.33	0.10
Et	Me	Et	3	2	0.63	0.52	Me	Et	Et	3	3	0.73	0.35
Et	Et	Et	3	2	<0.045	0.01							
Et	Me	Me	3	2	0.46	0.46							

[a] Data of Fakstorp and Pedersen (*347*).
[b] Potency of hexamethonium, 1.0.

TABLE 4.48

Ganglionic Blocking Activity of Bisquaternary Ammonium Compounds with Branched Asymmetric Alkyl Ether Connecting Chains[a]

$R_3(R_1)_2N^+CH_2CH(R_4)OCH(R_5)CH_2N^+(R_2)_2R_3 \cdot 2X^-$

				Gang. block. potency[b]	
R_1	R_2	R_3	$\cdot 2X^-$	Symp.	Paras.
			R_4=Me, R_5=H		
Me	Me	Me	I	0.18	0.21
Me	Me	Et	Br	0.85	0.45
Me	Et	Me	I	<0.086	0.20
Et	Me	Et	Br	0.05	0.023
			R_4, R_5=Me		
Me	Me	Me	I	0.05	0.05
Me	Me	Et	Br	0.05	0.05

[a] Data of Fakstorp et al. (*49*).
[b] Potency of hexamethonium, 1.0.

the bulkiness of the terminal groups is probably an important contributing factor in the attachment to the receptor sites and in influencing the flexibility of the connecting chain.

In a series of over forty diammonio esters of the general formula $R_1R_2R_3N(CH_2)_nCOO(CH_2)_mNR_1R_2R_3$ the presence of one ester group created a certain degree of asymmetry, which is increased further by branching on one side of the alkylene chain. This series of compounds was tested for hypotensive activity and screened for ganglionic blocking action against DMPP-produced spasms in the isolated guinea pig ileum. The peak potency with the latter test object was obtained with an asymmetric ester analogue resembling pentolinium **(23)**, which was one and a half times as potent as pentolinium (*330*). In vivo, however, hexamethonium was superior to all members of the series in inhibition of the intestinal motility of rat.

A bisquaternary bisammonio ester, β-triethylammonium(β′-triethylammoniumethyl)propionate, with a chain length comparable to that of hexamethonium, was found to be a relatively weak ganglionic blocking agent, approximately as potent as TEA. The corresponding bistrimethyl analogue was a ganglionic stimulant (*133*, *263*).

Symmetric dicarboxylate esters of choline have been described primarily as curarelike agents; in these compounds the length of the connecting chain between the terminal trimethylammonium group varied with the carbon chain length of the acidic moiety. None of these esters showed ganglionic blockade except carbonyldicholine, which exhibited a low degree of activity. The acid esters ranging from succinyl- to sebacyldicholine were ganglionic stimulants (*135*). Practically no ganglionic blocking activity was found in another study with suxamethonium and succinyl disulfocholine (*332*).

3-Thiopentylene-bis-*N*-methylpyrrolidinium, 3-thiopentylene-bis-*N*-piperidinium, and diethylmethylammonium were compared with pentolinium. A favorable therapeutic index has been found for the third of these compounds (*350*).

The 3,4-dithio analogue of hexamethonium and the 4,5-dithio analogue of decamethonium were about three times less potent than hexamethonium in cat experiments. Both of these exhibited pronounced curarelike activity (*219*).

In addition to the majority of symmetric bisquaternary ammonium derivatives with polymethylene, alkyl ether, phenylalkane, and azaalkane chains a few bisammonium compounds with different connecting chains were reported to possess ganglionic blocking activity. Dimethylaminoalkyl derivatives of malonic acid, urea, and malonyl urea were described by Gerazzani et al. (*351*). Optimal ganglionic blocking activity was obtained with dimethylaminoethyl or dimethylaminopropyl chains attached to the nitrogen atoms of these derivatives.

N,N'-Dimethylbipyridylium, diethyl-α,α'-bipyridylium, and bipiperidylium derivatives with the general structure **(24)** were reported by Beyerman and Bontekoe (*352*, *353*) to have ganglionic blocking actions.

An attempt was made to prepare active bisquaternary ammonium compounds with a rigid connecting chain structure of the general formula **(25)**, but ganglionic blocking activity was not found with this type of agent (*50*).

9. BISQUATERNARY AMMONIUM COMPOUNDS WITH OTHER TYPES OF CONNECTING CHAIN

Besides bisammonium ethers and thioethers there are two major groups of bisquaternary compounds in which the connecting chain is composed of elements other than polymethylene; these are discussed below.

a. Azapentylene Derivatives

Compounds of the structure shown in Figure 4.26, where *n* was usually 2 and R_1, R_2, and R_3 were methyl or ethyl groups, were reported shortly after the introduction of hexamethonium as a hypotensive agent. Of these compounds azamethonium, *N,N,N',N'*-3-pentamethyl-*N,N*-diethyl-3-azapentylene dibromide (Pendiomid, C-92295), was the most active, approaching the potency of hexamethonium in several ganglionic preparations (*354*). A detailed pharmacologic description of this agent was given by Bein and Meier (*355*). Besides the fairly high degree of potency and specificity a wide therapeutic index was reported. Quantitative evaluations with azamethonium were made with the superior cervical and stellate ganglion of the cat (*241*), vagal ganglia, and ganglia of the salivary glands (*321*). No difference in sensitivity between the sympathetic and parasympathetic heart ganglia was found (*94*). A clinical comparison in hypertensive patients also showed close similarity to hexamethonium (*325*). A paradoxical effect on vagus stimulation in the isolated guinea pig stomach preparation was equally inhibited by azamethonium and hexamethonium (*356*). Potassium salts antagonize its ganglionic blocking effect (*310*).

A review of hypotensive agents has dealt in detail with the structure–activity relationships of azamethonium and numerous similar azapentanediammonium salts. The following relationships have been established: (a) for terminal alkyl substituents, optimal activity was obtained with dimethylethyl and with pyrrolidine groups; (b) for substitution on the central nitrogen, hydrogen instead of methyl slightly reduced activity; (c) for the connecting chain, the nature of the connecting chain between the two quaternary centers had a definite influence on the activity. Replacement of the 3-azapentylene chain with 3,6-diazaoctylene, 4-azaheptylene, or 4-aza-α,ω-isoheptylene chains resulted in curarelike agents. Introducing other heteroatoms into the chain instead of nitrogen caused the thiapentylene diammonium derivative to display a somewhat weaker potency than azamethonium. Replacement of the *N*-methyl group with oxygen led to a marked decrease of activity. A hydrazine group in the middle of the connecting chain also resulted in an inactive compound. Introduction of phenyl rings in compounds of the polyamine type leads in every case to a significant loss of potency. Acylation of the central nitrogen atom of the chain resulted in an elimination of ganglionic blocking activity (*25*). Correlations between chain length and terminal groups, made with 3-azapentylene bisammonium compounds and polymethylene bisammonium derivatives of similar chain length, were studied by Gyermek (*320*). Considering that the internitrogen distances of the 3-azapentylene chain are somewhat smaller than in pentamethylene, and assuming that the degree of bending of the chain is not markedly affected by the NCH_3 group, the ganglionic potencies agree well with the estimate that the interprosthetic distances of 3-azapentylene derivatives correspond to that of a C_4 or C_5 polymethylene chain. There was a reciprocal correlation between chain length and the size of the bisammonium groups. In general, azapentylene and pentamethylene bis(*N*-methylpyrrolidinium) salts were about three to five and a half times as active as hexamethonium. The activity of the various compounds differed for various ganglia. For example, in paralyzing the ciliary ganglion of mice (mydriasis) 1,5-(3-azapentylene)bis(*N*-methylpiperidinium) diiodide was fifty times more potent than hexamethonium, but its effect on the superior cervical ganglion was only about equal to that of hexamethonium. The structure–activity relationships of these compounds are represented in Table 4.49

TABLE 4.49

Ganglionic Blocking Action of Polymethylene and Azapentylene Bisammonium Compounds and Related Tertiary Amines[a]

	Ganglionic blocking potency[b]			
	Sup. cerv. gang.[c]	Pelv. nerve bladd.[d]	Anti-nicotine activ.[e]	Mydriatic effect[f]
Ethylene bis-*N*-methylpiperidinium dibromide	0.2			
Ethylene bis-*N*-ethylpiperidinium dibromide	0.2			
Trimethylene bis-*N*-methylpiperidinium diiodide	0.3	0.4		
Trimethylene bis-*N*-ethylpiperidinium dibromide	0.2		0.2	
Tetramethylene bis-*N*-methylpiperidinium diiodide	0.5	0.5	2.0	28
Tetramethylene bis-*N*-ethylpiperidinium dibromide	0.3			
Pentamethylene bis-*N*-methylpyrrolidinium dibromide	5.5		5.0	17
Hexamethylene bistrimethylammonium dibromide	1.0	1.0	1.0	1.0
Hexamethylene bisdimethylethylammonium dibromide	2–3		2.0	
Hexamethylene bisdimethylbenzylammonium dibromide	<0.1		<0.15	
Hexamethylene bis-*N*-methylpiperidinium dibromide	0.7	1.0	1.2	28
Hexamethylene bis-*N*-ethylpiperidinium dibromide	0.2			
N,N,N,N',N',N'-Hexamethyl-3-aza-pentylene-1,5-diammonium dichloride 3-hydrochloride	<0.1		0.07	
1,5-(3-Azapentylene) bis-*N*-dimethylethylammonium dibromide	0.6		0.6	
1,5-(3-Azapentylene) bis-*N*-methylpyrrolidinium dichloride	5.0		3.5	14
1,5-(3-Azapentylene) bis-*N*-methylpyrrolidinium diodide	3.2		4.0	
1,5-(3-Azapentylene) bis-*N*-methylpiperidinium diodide	1.1	1.5	2.5	50
Bis-(*N,N'*-β-Dimethylaminoethyl)amine trihydrochloride	<0.15		<0.05	
Tris-(β-dimethylaminoethyl)amine trihydrochloride	1.0		0.58	

[a] Data of Gyermek (*320, 327*).
[b] Potency of hexamethonium, 1.0.
[c] Cat nictitating membrane.
[d] Dog bladder.
[e] Rabbit ileum.
[f] Mouse.

(*327*). Bis(piperidinoethyl)methylamine dimethiodide and the corresponding trimethiodide, the latter being identical with some piperidine derivatives investigated by Gyermek (*327*) and Schlittler et al. (*25*), were studied by Voigtlaender et al. (*357*). Ganglionic blocking and hypotensive activity was claimed for only the first compound.

b. 1,4-Xylylene Bisammonium Compounds

The observation that a C_8, C_9, or C_{10} polymethylene chain can be successfully replaced with a diphenylmethane group separating the terminal alkyl-substituted quaternary nitrogen atoms and can retain high curarelike potency was the basis of an attempt to replace the shorter aliphatic chain of hexamethonium with a *p*-xylylene group. A series of compounds with different substituents at the terminal quaternary nitrogen have been studied, but none of the compounds showed a significant ganglionic blocking potency in the cat (*16, 47, 358*); see Table 4.50.

Similar *p*-xylylene bisammonium compounds with alkyl, cycloalkyl, and oxyalkyl substituents were reported more recently to be without significant ganglionic blocking activity (*200, 319, 350*). Other 1,4-xylylene bisquaternary ammonium compounds, in which the onium groups are formed by more complex rings or by amines having appendages of substantial size, have also been studied (*29, 141*) without their showing significant ganglionic blocking

TABLE 4.50

Ganglionic Blocking Potency of Some 1,4-Xylylene Bisammonium Salts[a]

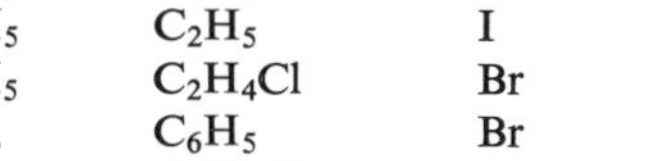

R_1	R_2	R_3	X	Gang. block. potency[b]
CH_3	CH_3	CH_3	Br	<0.3
C_2H_5	C_2H_5	C_2H_5	I	0.5
CH_3	C_2H_5	C_2H_5	I	0.8
C_2H_5	C_2H_5	C_2H_4Cl	Br	0.3
CH_3	CH_3	C_6H_5	Br	<0.1
CH_3	CH_3	$C_6H_5CH_2$	Br	0.2
C_2H_5	C_2H_5	$C_6H_5CH_2$	Br	<0.1
CH_3	CH_3	$C_6H_5CH_2CH_2$	Br	0.5

[a] Data of Gyermek and Nador (*358*) and Nador (*16*).
[b] Cat nictitating membrane preparation; potency of TEA, 1.0.

potency. These agents included bisquaternary ammonium derivatives of tropane, tropine, different tropine esters, *N,N*-diethylaminoethyl-2-phenylvalerate, piperidinoethyl acetate and benzoate, *N*-methyl-*N*-ethylaminoethanol acetate, and *N,N*-diethylaminoethylphenylpropylacetate.

In conclusion, it seems that the symmetric 1,4-xylylene bisquaternary ammonium derivatives as a class are much inferior in ganglionic blocking potency to those isosteric phenethyl-*p*-ω-bisammonium compounds, which are discussed with the asymmetric class of ganglionic blocking agents.

10. BISQUATERNARY TROPANE COMPOUNDS

A series of unsymmetric bisammonium salts, which on one end of the molecule carry a small cationic group (trimethyl, methylpyrrolidino, or methylpiperidino) and on the other a bulky tropane ring system (tropane, tropine, tropinone, atropine), has shown moderate hypotensive action in dogs. The short duration of action of some of the tropinone derivatives was suggested to be due to the instability of this structure (*359*). A larger group of unsymmetric bisquaternary tropane derivatives (Table 4.51) has been described

TABLE 4.51

Ganglionic Blocking Activity of Some Asymmetric Bisquaternary Tropane Derivatives[a]

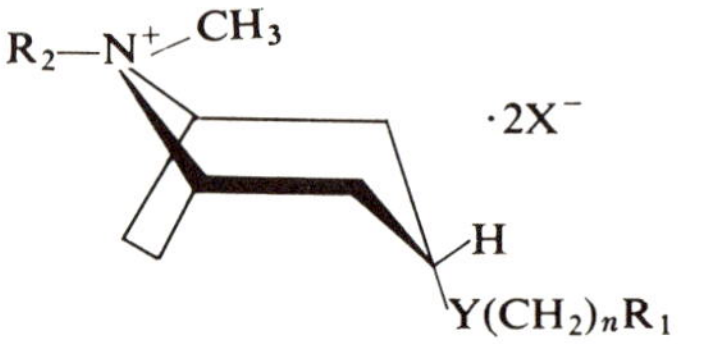

R_1	n	Y	R_2	Gang. block. potency[b]: Dog blood press. carotid occl.	Cat nict. membrane
$N^+CH_3(C_2H_5)_2$	2	O	CH_3	0.8	0.09
$N^+(CH_3)_2C_2H_5$	2	O	C_2H_5	0.11	0.06
$N^+(CH_3)_3$	2	O	CH_3	0.10	0.10
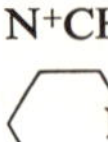 N^+CH_3	2	O	CH_3	0.06	0.12
$N^+CH_3(C_2H_5)_2$	3	O	CH_3	0.23	0.16
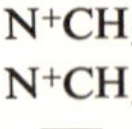 N^+CH_3	3	O	CH_3	1.0	0.40
$N^+CH_3(C_2H_5)_2$	2	NH	CH_3	0.02	0.04
$N^+CH_3(C_2H_5)_2$	2	NCH_3	CH_3	0.48	1.03
O^- NCH_3	2	NCH_3	CH_3	>2.0	0.4

TABLE 4.51—*continued*

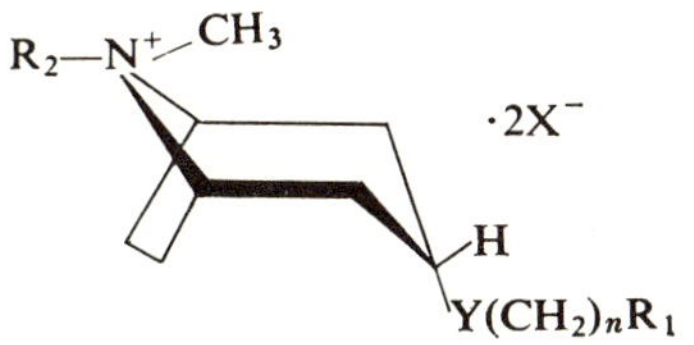

R_1	n	Y	R_2	Gang. block. potency[b] Dog blood press. carotid occl.	Gang. block. potency[b] Cat nict. membrane
$N^+(C_2H_5)_3$	2	NCH_3	C_2H_5	> 1.0	> 3.2
$N^+(CH_3)_3$	2	NCH_3	CH_3	0.65	0.3
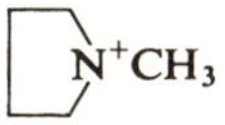	2	NCH_3	CH_3	0.24	0.14
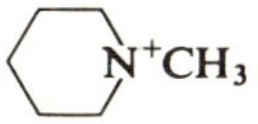	2	NCH_3	CH_3	0.17	0.30
$N^+CH_3(C_2H_5)_2$	3	NCH_3	CH_3	0.45	0.30
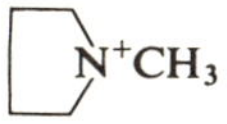	3	NCH_3	CH_3	0.20	0.25
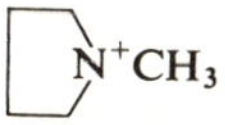	3	NH	CH_3	0.20	0.04
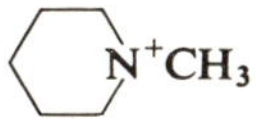	2	NH	CH_3	0.59	0.38
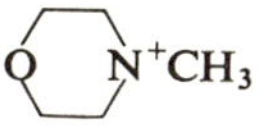	2	NH	CH_3	0.21	0.22
$N^+CH_3(C_2H_5)_2$	2	NH	CH_3	0.18	0.09
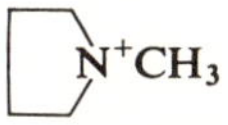	2	NH	CH_3	0.11	0.06
$N^+CH_3(C_2H_5)_2$	2	NC_2H_5	CH_3	> 1.0	> 2.0
$N^+CH_3(C_2H_5)_2$	2	NC_3H_7	CH_3	> 1.0	> 1.0
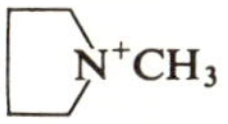	2	O	CH_3	>0.5	0.5

[a] Data of Lape et al. (*360*).
[b] ED_{50} in milligrams per kilogram.

by Lape et al. (*360*); diethylamino-8-(2-chlorobenzyl) nortropane bismethobromide proved to be the most potent, significantly surpassing the ganglionic potency of hexamethonium in cat and dog experiments (*361*). The discrepancy between the blocking potencies of the carotid sinus reflex depressor action and the ganglionic depression on the nictitating membrane and cross-circulation experiments indicated that some of these agents may show, in addition to a peripheral ganglionic blockade, a damping effect on central vasomotor regulating mechanisms (*360*).

Symmetric bisquaternary ammonium derivatives of different tropine esters (succinyl and phthaloyl tropines) exhibited marked neuromuscular blocking and a less pronounced ganglionic blocking action. These two actions seem to vary somewhat parallel with each other. In this series aralkyl quaternary groups were favorable for both synaptic actions (*362*); see Tables 4.52. 1,4-Xylylene bisquaternary salts of different tropine esters were also predominantly curarelike agents. Another group of symmetric polymethylene bisquaternary derivatives of homatropine showed neuromuscular and ganglionic blocking properties that did not vary parallel with each other. Peak activity for the curarelike action was found with the heptamethylene derivative, whereas the highest ganglionic blocking potency was obtained with the pentamethylene member of the series (*363*). In the groups of different bisquaternary ammonium compounds the mutual interactions between the

TABLE 4.52 A

Comparison of Ganglionic Blocking, Neuromuscular Blocking, and Cholinolytic Potencies of Some Symmetrical Bisquaternary Tropane Compounds[a]

Compound	Gang. block. potency[b]	Neuromusc. block. potency[c]	Cholinolyt. potency[d]
1,2-Ethylene-bis(*dl*-mandelyl tropinium)	0.3	<0.04	0.2
1,3-Trimethylene-bis(*dl*-mandelyl tropinium)			0.1
1,4-Tetramethylene-bis(*dl*-mandelyl tropinium)	<0.1		0.2
1,5-Pentamethylene-bis(*dl*-mandelyl tropinium)	2.2	0.1	<0.01
1,6-Hexamethylene-bis(*dl*-mandelyl tropinium)	<0.1	1.1	0.01
1,7-Heptamethylene-bis(*dl*-mandelyl tropinium)		2.0	0.02
1,8-Octamethylene-bis(*dl*-mandelyl tropinium)	0.1	1.7	0.1
1,9-Nonamethylene-bis(*dl*-mandelyl tropinium)			0.1
1,10-Decamethylene-bis(*dl*-mandelyl tropinium)	0.5	3.7	0.2
1,12-Dodecamethylene-bis(*dl*-mandelyl tropinium)		1.7	0.25
1,6-Hexamethylene bis(benzoyl β-tropinium) bromide[e]	<0.5	3.0[f]	0.002[g]

[a] Data of Haining and Johnston (*363*).
[b] Cat nictitating membrane; potency of TEA, 1.0.
[c] In the cat; potency of tubocurarine, 1.0.
[d] In guinea pig ileum; potency of atropine, 1.0.
[e] Data of Gyermek and Nador (*30*).
[f] In the rabbit.
[g] In rabbit ileum.

TABLE 4.52 B

Code no.	Compound	Gang. block. pot.[b]	Neuromusc. block. pot.[c]	Cholinol. pot.[d]	Curarelike pot.[e]
N-138	1,4-Xylylene-bisatropinium bromide	0.3	1.3	0.15	
N-141	1,4-Xylylene-bis-*dl*-mandelyl-tropinium bromide	0.5	0.8	0.03	
N-147	1,4-Xylylene-bis-benzoyltropinium bromide	0.4	1.3	0.01	
N-181	1,4-Xylylene-bisacetyltropinium bromide	2.5	0.2		
N-276	1,4-Xylylene-bis(dimethyl-carbamoyl)tropinium bromide	0.2	0.3		
N-297	Methylsuccinyltropinium diiodide	0.5			0.5
N-298	*p*-Methylbenzylsuccinyltropinium dibromide	2.0			1.0
N-307	*m*-Bromobenzylsuccinyltropinium dibromide	3.6			2.5
N-305	Methyl-phthaloyltropinium diiodide	0.5			0.3
N-306	Benzyl-phthaloyltropinium dibromide	1.8			5.0

[a] Data of Gyermek and Nador (*30, 358, 362*).
[b] In cat nictitating membrane; potency of TEA, 1.0.
[c] In the frog; potency of tubocurarine, 1.0.
[d] In rabbit ileum; potency of atropine, 1.0.
[e] Potency of *d*-tubocurarine, 1.0.

terminal quaternary ammonium groups, the length of the connecting chain between these onium groups, and the bulk and steric constellation around the terminal groups do not influence uniformly ganglionic blocking activity. For example, in the polymethylene bistrialkylammonium series the size of the alkyl substituents is of marked significance. In the asymmetric aryl or cyclo-alkyl polymethylenetrialkylammonium series the size and electronic structure of both terminal groups is important, whereas in the bistropine ester type of compound other steric factors seem also to be of significance, such as chain length and onium cation.

The structure–activity relationships of most of the available mono- and bisquaternary tropane derivatives are presented in Table 4.52, which includes data on potency relative to TEA or hexamethonium, variations of optimal structures for different cholinergic receptor sites, and degrees of selectivity toward ganglionic receptors in series of selected compounds. A summary of structural requirements for cholinergic receptor sites is outlined in Table 4.39. Besides several established points a few "blank spaces" still need additional exploration.

In summing up the structure–activity relationships of tropane compounds the advantages deriving from the elucidation of stereochemical aspects of a relatively rigid ring system in evaluating correlations between structure and activity must be stressed again.

11. ASYMMETRIC BISQUATERNARY AMMONIUM DERIVATIVES WITH CONNECTING POLYMETHYLENE CHAINS

Where the *y* and *z* substituents can be hydrogen, chlorine, alkyl, phenyl, methoxy, or a second ring (naphthyl), compounds of the structure **(27)** are the simplest representatives of the derivatives of substituted *N*-benzylalkylenediamines. They have shown ganglionic blocking potencies up to twenty times that of hexamethonium (*364*); however, no mention was made of the method used for determining ganglionic blocking activity. A broad class of asymmetric bisammonium compounds was reported by Adamson et al. (*365*); it consisted of different subclasses: bisquaternary amino carbinols, alkenes, alkanes, nitriles, ethers, and esters. The general structure of these compounds is $R_1R_2X(CH_2)_m—N^+—(CH_2)_nN^+$, where X is $C(OH)CH_2$, C═CH, $CHCH_2$, $C(CN)CH_2$, CHO, or CHCOO, and where R_1 and R_2 are phenyl or cyclohexyl groups. Ganglionic blockade was also present when R_1 and R_2 consisted of a pyridyl or thienyl ring. The ganglionic blocking activity reaches a maximum at a chain length of $m=3$ or $m=4$. One compound, pentacynium, went through clinical trial. Its structure is depicted in formula **(28)**. Oral absorption was generally poor throughout the series. A more detailed pharmacological evaluation of pentyacynium and an analogue with a chain length of four carbons (Presidal) was reported by Locket (*366*). Both compounds were active clinically in severe hypertension (*366*, *367*).

Unsymmetric bisquaternary derivatives of substituted pyridine bases were reported as potent and selective hypotensive agents by Gray et al. (*368*). In this group the large cationic head is derived from substituted pyridine or piperidine bases. The ganglionic blocking efficacy as compared to that of hexamethonium is presented in Table 4.53. The most active members of the series (2-(1-naphthylethyl)pyridinium and indolylethyl pyridinium) had large cationic groups, which were connected through a propyl chain to a small cationic head with three methyl groups. The pharmacology of these asymmetric pyridine and piperidine derivatives was reported in more detail by O'Dell and Napoli (*369*).

In another series some unsymmetric bisquaternary salts that derive from decahydroquinoline and decahydroisoquinoline were prepared by the same investigators (*370a*). Some of these compounds possessed marked hypotensive activity but only weak peripheral ganglionic blocking action. Structure–activity relationships in regard to the ability of this type of molecule to approach the surface of receptors have been discussed. The structural characteristics and ganglionic blocking capacities of this group of agents are presented in Tables 4.54 and 4.55 (*370a*, *370b*). Ethiquinium (IN-292), formula **(29)**, an asymmetric bisquaternary ammonium salt, has been studied clinically.

TABLE 4.53

Ganglionic Blocking and Hypotensive Activity of Asymmetric Bisquaternary Ammonium Compounds with Pyridine and Piperidine Rings[a]

Substituted pyridinium salts,

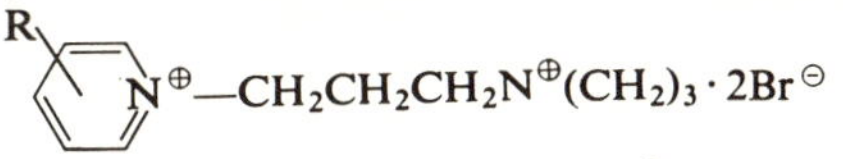

R				Relative gang. block. potency[b]	Hypotensive activity in dogs
Hydrogen					0
4-Methyl					0
4-Benzyl					0
4-Phenylethenyl					0
4-Diphenylmethyl				0.5	+
2-(1-Naphthylethyl)				2.0	+++
4-(1-Naphthylethenyl)					+
2-(3-Indenylethyl)				1.0	++
4-(3-Indenylethyl)				1.0	++
2-(3-Indolylethyl)				3.0	++
4-(3-Indolylethyl)				3.0	++
4-(1-Indolylethyl)				2.0	+++
4-(3-Indolylethenyl)				1.0	+
2-(1-Methyl-3-indolylethyl)				1.0	++
4-(1-Methyl-3-indolylethyl)				1.0	++
4-(1-Benzyl-3-indolylethyl)					+
2-(1-Methyl-3-indolylethyl)-5-ethyl				0.5	+++
3-(2-Indolyl)					0
4-(2-Indolyl)					+
4-(3,3′-Diindolylmethyl)					+
4-(Phthalimidoethyl)					+

Substituted piperidine salts,

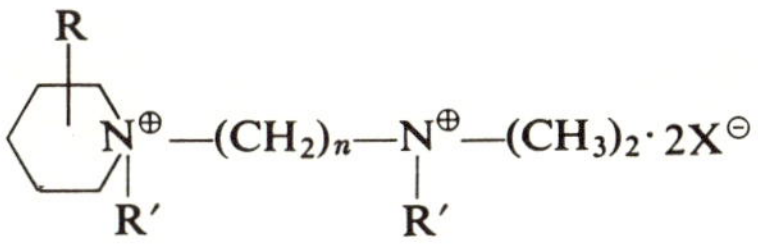

R	R′	n	X	Relative gang. block. potency[b]	Hypotensive activity in dogs
Hydrogen	CH_2	3	Br		ϕ
4-Benzyl	CH_2	3	Br		+
4-Benzyl	CH_3	2	I		+
4-Benzyl	H	2	Cl	0.5	ϕ

[a] Data of Gray et al. (*368*).

[b] Cat nictitating membrane; potency of hexamethonium, 1.0.

The compound appeared to be an effective and safe hypotensive agent having only moderate side effects (*371a*).

Unsymmetric bisammonium salts in which one ammonium group was incorporated into tropane, tropine, and tropinone rings have been described.

TABLE 4.54

Ganglionic Blocking Activity of Some Unsymmetrical Bisquaternary Compounds[a]

Code no.	$R^{\oplus}(CH_2)_3N^+Me_3 \cdot 2Br^{\ominus}$ $R^{\oplus}$	Symp. gang. block,[b] dose/degree/duration
IN 278	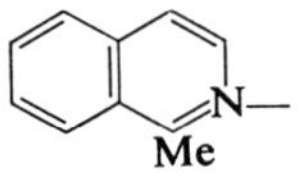 ([c])	0.1/0/0 0.25/+/0.1 0.5/++/0.5 1.0/++/0.75
IN 270	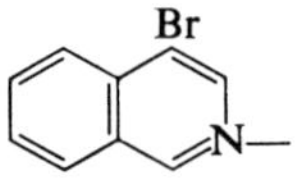	0.5/++/0.5 1.0/+++/0.5
IN 260	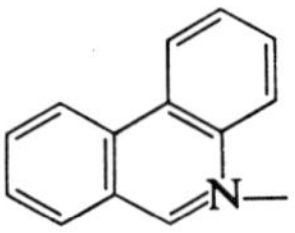 ([c])	0.5/+/0.2
IN 261	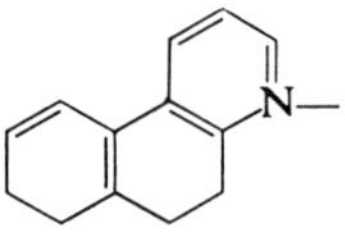 ([c])	0.25/0/0 0.5/+/0.2
IN 243	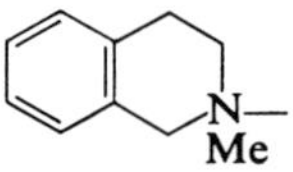	0.25/+/0.1 0.5/+++/0.5 1.0/+++/>0.5
IN 298	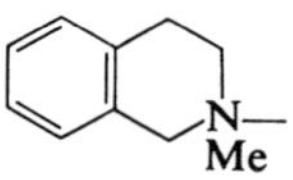 ([c])	0.25/0/0 0.5/+/0.1 1.0/++/?
IN 321	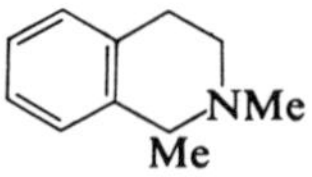	0.25/0/0 0.5/++/0.3 1.0/+++/1.0
IN 292	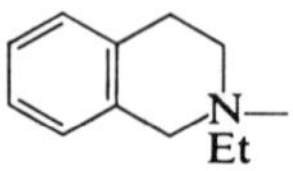	0.25/0/0 0.5/+/0.2 1.0/++/0.25 2.0/++++/0.5

TABLE 4.54—*continued*

Code no.	$R^{\oplus}(CH_2)_3N^+Me_3 \cdot 2Br^{\ominus}$ $R^{\oplus}$	Symp. gang. block,[b] dose/degree/duration
IN 253	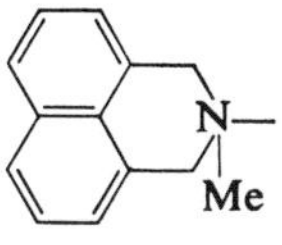	0.15/0/0 0.5/0/0 2.0/+ +/0.75
IN 317	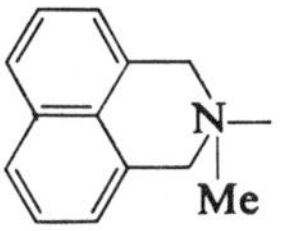 (c)	0.25/0/0 0.5/+ +/0.25
IN 316	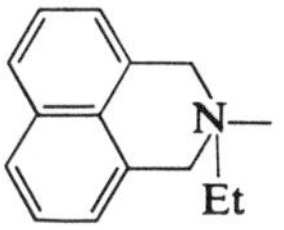 (d)	0.25/0/0 0.5/+/0.25

[a] Data of Gray et al. (*370*).
[b] Cat superior cervical ganglion; dose in milligrams per kilogram, intravenous; degree of block, 0 to + + + + (zero to complete blockade); duration, recovery in hours.
[c] The small cationic head is 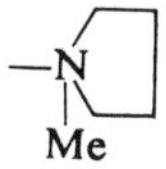
[d] The small cationic head is NMe_2Et.

These agents were moderately inactive hypotensive agents, some of them with a short duration of action. Characteristics of these compounds are presented in Table 4.56 (*371b*).

Unsymmetrical derivatives of β-carbolines, including derivatives of norharmane, harmane, and α-carboline, have been detailed with respect to their preparation and pharmacology by Gray et al. (*372*) and O'Dell et al. (*373*). All had an alkyl chain at either the pyridine nitrogen or indole nitrogen of the β-carboline system. The pyridine N-substituted carbolinium salts, particularly those in which the cations are separated by a three-carbon chain, produced intensive hypotensive activity but, again, this potency was not associated directly with the ganglionic blocking properties. Data on these agents are presented in Table 4.57.

The whole class of unsymmetric trimethylene-1,3-bisquaternary ammonium derivatives was reviewed by Cavallito et al. (*374*). The general structure of

TABLE 4.55

Ganglionic Blocking Activity of Some Unsymmetric Bisquaternary Isoquinolinium Compounds[a]

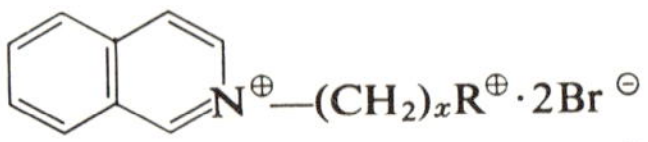

Code no.	R⊕	X	Symp. gang. block,[b] dose/degree/duration
IN-206	NMe_3	3	2.0/+/0.25
IN-181	NMe_3	6	2.0/0/0
IN-239	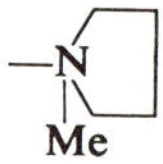	3	1.0/+/0.3 2.0/+++/0.6
IN-306	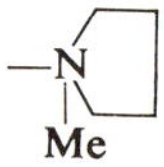	4	0.25/0/0 0.5/+/0.2 1.0/++/0.75
IN-265	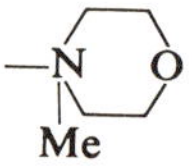	3	0.5/++/0.1 1.0/+++/0.75 2.0/+++/?
IN-257	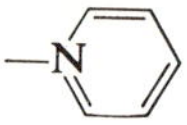	3	2.0/0/0
Hexamethonium bromide			2.0/++++/2

[a] Data of O'Dell et al. (*370b*).

[b] Cat superior cervical ganglion; dose in milligrams per kilogram, intravenous; degrees of block, 0 to ++++ (zero to complete blockade); duration, recovery in hours.

these compounds is A—$CH_2CH_2CH_2$—B, where A is a large bulky nucleus connected through the nitrogen to B, which is a small cationic group. At group B the alkyl substituents had to be smaller than ethyl to cause a high degree of hypotensive activity. Some of these compounds show a predominantly central hypotensive action with varying degrees of peripheral ganglionic blockade. A few of them also block the parasympathetic nerve endings. A detailed discussion of their structure–activity relationships with reference to the accessibility to different cholinergic receptor sites has been given, and the conclusion was reached that the structural requirements for obtaining the hypotensive, ganglionic blocking, curarelike, and parasympathetic nerve-ending blocking actions are strictly different. Phillips (*375*) described 3-substituted or 4-substituted 3′-aminopropylpiperidine derivatives of structure **(30)**, where R_1 is dimethyl or diethyl, pyrrolidino, piperidino, or morpholino

TABLE 4.56

Hypotensive Activity of Some Asymmetric Bisquaternary Tropane Derivatives[a]

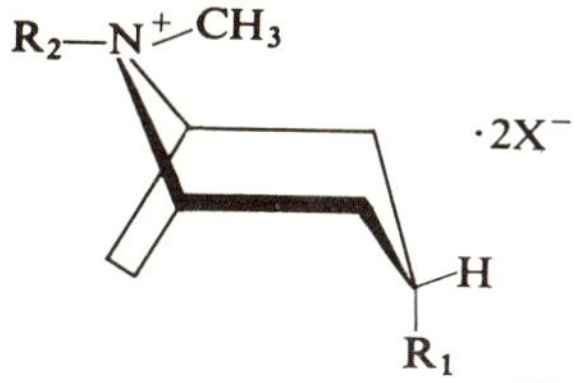

R_1	R_2	Blood pressure lowering dose in dogs, mg/kg
$OCOCH(CH_2OH)C_6H_5$	$(CH_2)_2N^+Me_3$	1
OH	$(CH_2)_2N^+Me_3$	2
OH	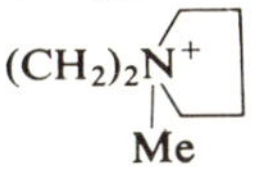	0.5
OH	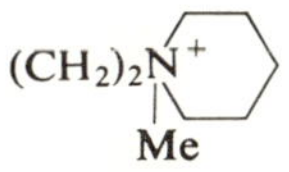	1
$HR_2{=}O$ (tropinone)	$(CH_2)_2N^+Me_3$	2
H	$(CH_2)_2N^+Me_3$	1[b]

[a] Data of Archer et al. (*371b*).
[b] Long-acting.

and R_2 is hydrochloric acid or metho and etho salts. Several of these compounds in the cat showed equal or higher ganglionic blocking action than hexamethonium. The most active compounds were the bismetho and etho salts of 3-(3-aminopropyl) and 3-(3-pyrrolidinopropyl) piperidines; they were about four times more potent than hexamethonium. Phillips (*376*) reported on another series containing some powerful ganglionic blocking agents that had the structure shown **(31)**, where R is H, CH_3, C_2H_5, n-C_3H_7, n-C_4H_9, and benzyl. The methyl quaternary salts were effective and long-lasting ganglionic blocking agents in the cat, but some of the corresponding tertiary amines were also potent. Colville and Fanelli (*377*) described 4-aminoethylpiperidine derivatives with the structure **(32)**, where R_2 is pyrrolidine, piperidine, or morpholine, R_1 is methyl or hydrogen, and R_x is methiodide, ethiodide, n-propyl iodide, or hydrochloric acid. The most active member of the group was approximately equipotent with hexamethonium in its hypotensive ganglionic blocking potency. Unsymmetrically substituted acetylenic

TABLE 4.57

Ganglionic Blocking Activity of Some Unsymmetric Bisquaternary Compounds[a]

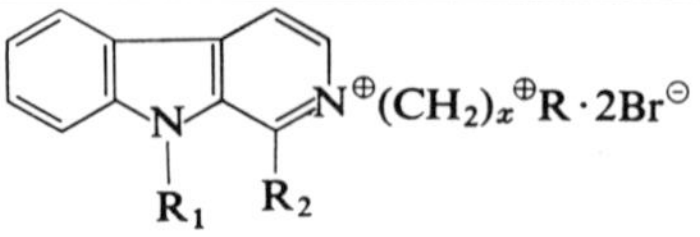

Code no.	R⊕	x	R_1	R_2	Symp. gang. block,[b] dose/deg./duration
205	NMe_3	3	H	Me	0.5/+/0.5 1.0/++++/2–3
216	NMe_3	5	H	Me	([c])
178	NMe_3	6	H	Me	0.5/++/0.5 1.0/++++/?
208	NMe_3	10	H	Me	([c])
116	$NMeEt_2$	3	H	Me	0.5/+/0.5 1.0/+++/0.75 2.0/++++/2–3
182	NEt_3	3	H	Me	2.0/+/0.5
215	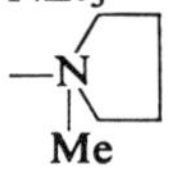	3	H	Me	0.5/+/0.75 1.0/++/0.75
221	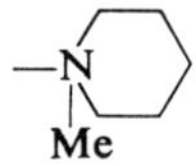	3	H	Me	0.5/+/0.5 1.0/++/1.5
217	$NMe_2(CH_2C_6H_5)$	3	H	Me	([c])
279	NMe	3	Me	Me	0.1/±/0.1 0.25/+++/0.75 0.5/++++/>1
203	NMe_3	3	Me	Me	0.5/0/0 1.0/+/0.75
226	NMe_3	3	H	H	1.0/±/0.1 2.0/+/0.25
274	NMe_3	3	([d])	([d])	0.1/+/0.1 0.25/+++/? 0.5/++++/2.5
264	NMe_3	3	([e])	([e])	([c])
Hexamethonium bromide					2.0/++++/2

[a] Data of O'Dell et al. (*373*).

[b] Cat superior cervical ganglion; dose in milligrams per kilogram, intravenous; degree of block, 0 to ++++ (zero to complete blockade; duration in hours).

[c] Slight hypotensive action in dogs.

[d] The large cationic head is 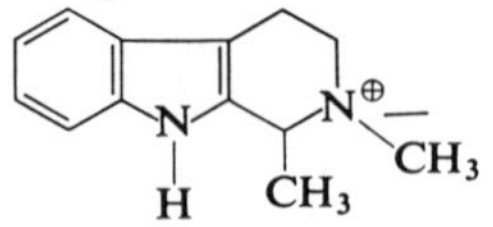

[e] The large cationic head is 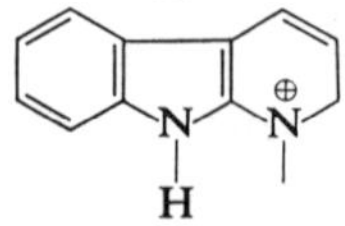

bisquaternary ammonium compounds were studied with the aim of producing compounds having a limited degree of free rotation of the biquaternary ammonium groups; compared with simple aliphatic compounds they should force the quaternary groups into a more rigid orientation. An evaluation of this series is hindered by the fact that only hypotensive potencies and not ganglionic blocking activities were reported. The compounds belonged to the two different types **(33)**, where R_1 is $—CH{=}CH(CH_2)_nN(CH_3)_3$ or $—C{\equiv}C—(CH_2)_n—N(CH_3)_3$, R_2 is H or CH_3O, and *n* is 2 to 3. According to measurements of hypotensive activity none of the compounds reached the potency of chlorisondamine. Activity generally increased with the introduction of a double bond and, even more, of a triple bond. In certain cases there was an indication that the compounds even surpassed in duration of action the long-acting asymmetric bisquaternary ammonium compounds (*378*).

a. Chlorisondamine

This agent (Table 4.58) was one of the first of the asymmetric bisquaternary ammonium types of compounds that achieved therapeutic recognition.

TABLE 4.58

Ganglionic Blocking Activity of Asymmetric Bisquaternary Agents of the Chlorisondamine Class[a]

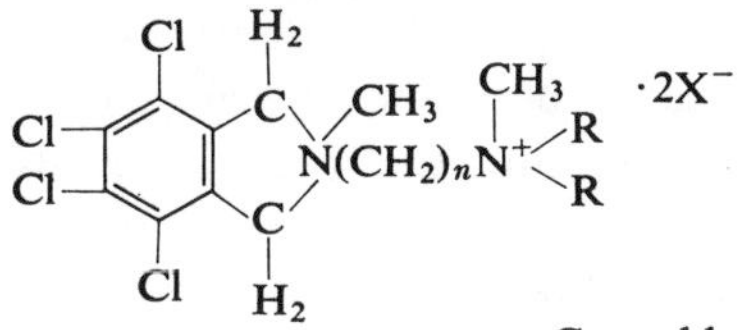

R	*n*	X	Gang. block. potency[b]	Duration of action
C_2H_5	2	I[c]	0.06	++
C_2H_5	2	I[d]	0.32	+
CH_3	2	I[c]	1.07	+
C_2H_5	2	I	1.14	++++
CH_3	2	Cl	6.40	++++
C_2H_5	4	I	1.07	+
C_2H_5	5	I	3.76	+
Hexamethonium			1.00	++
Pentolinium			3.20	+++

[a] Data of Plummer et al. (*379*).
[b] Cat superior cervical ganglion.
[c] No substituents on the aromatic nucleus.
[d] Bromine substituents instead of chlorine.

Structurally it is characterized by the bulky chlorinated isoindole group, which provides one of the onium groups, a short connecting ethylene chain, and a small cationic trimethylammonium group. Methyl substituents on the small cationic group and a methyl quaternary group on the isoindole nitrogen were required for maximal activity in a series of seven compounds, in which limited variations in the substituents of the quaternary groups (methyl versus ethyl) and in the length of connecting chain were made (*379*); see Table 4.58. Not only the selectivity and potency of this agent, but also the duration of action, which was maximal with chlorisondamine, changed markedly with the structural variations mentioned and with chlorination of the isoindoline ring. A general pharmacologic description of chlorisondamine (*379*) and a neuropharmacologic study of its actions, comparing the functions on the superior cervical with those on the ciliary ganglion, has been reported and includes differences in duration of action and in capacity of blockade as influenced by electric stimulus frequencies (*84*). Chronic oral administration of chlorisondamine and mecamylamine leads to an abnormally elevated blood pressure in dogs, probably by upsetting the adjustment of the blood pressure regulatory mechanisms through mechanoreceptors. This type of hypertension is amenable to treatment with other types of hypotensive agents, such as reserpine or phenoxybenzamine (*380*).

In its actions against nicotine convulsions chlorisondamine does not seem to be identical with mecamylamine, pentolinium, or hexamethonium, because it offers protection only against a tonic phase of convulsion (*246*). Chlorisondamine did not potentiate peripheral vasocostrictor mechanisms on isolated arterial strips. A discrepancy between different ganglionic blocking agents is noted in this test: hexamethonium and pentolinium behaved like chlorisondamine, whereas TEA and mecamylamine potentiated the actions of many vasoactive agents (*317*). Clinical studies with hypertensive patients and Rauwolfia alkaloids included observations on chlorisondamine. The results obtained with pentolinium and mecamylamine, however, were more favorable than with chlorisondamine (*340*).

b. Trimethidinium (Camphidonium)

N-(γ-Trimethylammoniumpropyl)*N*-methylcamphidinium dimethyl sulfate (*34*) is one of the newest and therapeutically most used ganglionic blocking agents. The structure of this compound fits well into the general formula of many asymmetric ganglionic blocking agents, in that it carries a small cationic group with three methyl groups, a connecting propyl chain between the ammonium groups, and a bulky cationic group with a complex ring system. The pharmacologic properties are also typical of this class of agents. Its potency, depending on the test object, is equal to, or higher than, that of hexamethonium; however, owing to its much more prolonged action it is difficult to make a correct comparison with hexamethonium. The oral-to-parenteral dose ratio is relatively low, indicating a considerable degree of intestinal absorption. Its ganglionic blocking actions and general pharmacology were evaluated by Klupp (*381*). Long-lasting hypotensive action was observed in normotensive rats (*382*), and a favorable ratio between its ganglionic blocking and acute toxic doses in cats (LD_{50}, 250 mg/kg) was reported (*383*).

Results of clinical studies with trimethidinium parallel the animal data, in that a favorable oral absorption rate and long-lasting hypotensive action were obtained with hypertensive patients (*382*). The compound was reported to be effective and to be devoid of a common side effect of ganglionic blocking agents, that of constipation. Ambulatory treatment of hypertensive patients with daily varying oral doses was effective (*384*).

12. ASYMMETRIC BISQUATERNARY AMMONIUM COMPOUNDS WITH CONNECTING CHAINS OTHER THAN ALKANE OR ALKENE

Of the asymmetric bisquaternary ammonium compounds with connecting chains other than alkane or alkene, one group contains connecting aliphatic ether chains that are unsymmetric in the sense that one side of the chain is longer than the other with reference to the position of the ether oxygen, or the chains are branched on one side only. Furthermore, there may be a lack of symmetry in this class of compounds in respect to the placement of alkyl substituents on the terminal nitrogen atoms. Compounds belonging to these groups (Table 4.59) were described by Fakstorp et al. (*49*) and Lenke (*331*); they have been given with the corresponding symmetric derivatives in Table 4.48. Some of them were highly potent.

2-Methyl-3-thiapentane 1,5-bis(trimethylammonium iodide) is twice as potent a ganglionic blocking agent as hexamethonium. The β-branching methyl group seems to be responsible for this increase of activity (*385a*).

Of a series of about 150 agents β-*N*-diethylamino-β′-*N*′-pyrrolidino diethyl ether diodomethylate (Plegarol, SY-108) was selected for a detailed pharmacology study. This compound showed typical ganglionic blocking properties (*385b*). Its potency was comparable to hexamethonium and azamethonium in certain tests; for example, it suppressed epinephrine-induced bradycardia and it blocked the nicotinic blood pressure rise in atropinized dogs. Duchene-Marullaz et al. (*386*) studied the pharmacodynamics of the hypotensive and ganglionic blocking action of this agent, and Vogrin (*387*) reported on its long-lasting hypotensive effect in patients. The compound was claimed to be superior to trimethaphane and azamethonium and to be stronger than hexamethonium. The ganglionic blocking potency of asymmetric bisquaternary

TABLE 4.59

Ganglionic Blocking Activity of Bisquaternary Ammonium Compounds with Branched Asymmetric Alkyl Ether Chains[a]

$(R_1)_2N^+CH_2CHOCH_2CH_2N^+(R_2)_2 \cdot 2X^-$ (with R_3 on the first N, R_4 on the CH, R_3 on the second N)

R_1	R_2	R_3	R_4	ED_{50} against nicotinic blood pressure rise in cats, mg/kg
Me	Me	Me	Me	12.5
Me	Me	Et	Et	0.3
Et	Et	Me	Me	0.95
Et	Et	Et	Me	> 10.0
Me	Et	Me	Me	4.0
Me	Et	Et	Me	> 10.0
Et	Me	Me	Me	0.16
Et	Me	Et	Me	0.12
Et	Me	Et	H	0.11

[a] Data of Lenke (*331*).

ammonium derivatives of tetrahydrofuran of structure **(35)** was reported by Mndzhoyan and Ordzhanyan (*388*).

Few of the symmetric ester type of compound with piperidine and quinuclidine rings on one side and a small cationic group on the other are known. Of the first group, Phillips (*389*) described esters of *N*-methylnipecotic acid. The compound having structure **(36)** was almost as potent as hexamethonium. Horowitz et al. (*390*) reported on the similar *ortho* ester derivative, which was considerably weaker than chlorisondamine. Dimecoline, a more recently developed pipecolinic acid ester of structure **(37)** was reported to be highly potent in animals (*391*). The only quinuclidine type of compound, dioquine, also was described by Sharapov (*392*). This agent was structurally closely related to the former series depicted in formula **(38)**. It was claimed to have therapeutically useful ganglionic blocking actions.

One of the first of the asymmetric bisquaternary ammonium ganglionic blocking compounds was a series of phenylalkane *p*-ω-bis(trialkylammonium) derivatives. In contrast to the ganglionically weak, symmetric *p*-xylylene bistrialkylammonium compounds, several of those having the structure **(39)**, where n is 0 to 6 and R_1, R_2, and R_3 are methyl or ethyl, were potent blocking agents. The peak potency was reached with trimethyl or dimethylethyl terminal groups and with $n=2$ (Table 4.60). These compounds were 2.5 to 3 times more potent than hexamethonium, and a more detailed pharmacologic analysis with several ganglionic preparations was performed with them (*322*). The bistrimethylammonium derivative was found to be a competitive-type antagonist and was also tested clinically (*323*). Significant is the tremendous

TABLE 4.60

Ganglionic Blocking Activity of Phenylalkane Bistrialkylammonium Compounds[a]

					Gang. block. potency[b]	
Code no.	R_1	R_2	R_3	*n*	SCG[c]	PRP[d]
		Phenyl alkane *p*-ω-bistrimethylammonium compounds				
1878	CH_3	CH_3	CH_3	0	<0.02	<0.05
1899	CH_3	CH_3	CH_3	1	0.005	0.05
1950	CH_3	CH_3	CH_3	2	3.00	2.50
2072	CH_3	CH_3	C_2H_5	2	3.30	2.50
2175	CH_3	C_2H_5	C_2H_5	2	1.80	1.00
2132	C_2H_5	C_2H_5	C_2H_5	2	<0.02	0.10
2034	CH_3	CH_3	CH_3	3	0.25	0.50
2056	CH_3	CH_3	C_2H_5	3	0.50	1.00
2278	CH_3	C_2H_5	C_2H_5	3	0.15	0.50
2184	C_2H_5	C_2H_5	C_2H_5	3	<0.04	0.15
2071	CH_3	CH_3	CH_3	4	<0.05	0.33
2082	CH_3	CH_3	C_2H_5	4	0.10	0.25
2297	CH_3	C_2H_5	C_2H_5	4	0.05	0.25
2272	C_2H_5	C_2H_5	C_2H_5	4	<0.03	<0.05
2268	CH_3	CH_3	CH_3	5	<0.05	0.02
2363	C_2H_5	C_2H_5	C_2H_5	5	<0.05	<0.02
2357	CH_3	CH_3	CH_3	6	0.20	1.00
2362	C_2H_5	C_2H_5	C_2H_5	6	<0.12	1.25
Hexamethonium bromide					1.00	
		Phenyl alkane-*m*-ω-bistrimethylammonium compounds				
2030				1	<0.05	<0.05
2064				2	1.5	1.25
2090				3	1.0	0.50
2139				4	1.0	1.0

Structure, *p*-ω compounds:

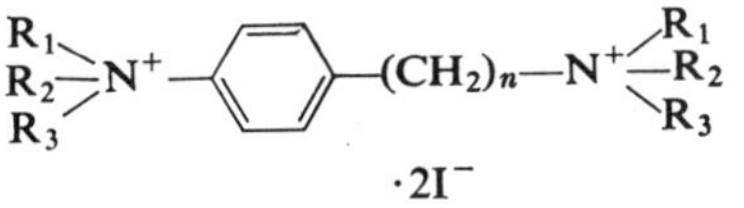

Structure, *m*-ω compounds:

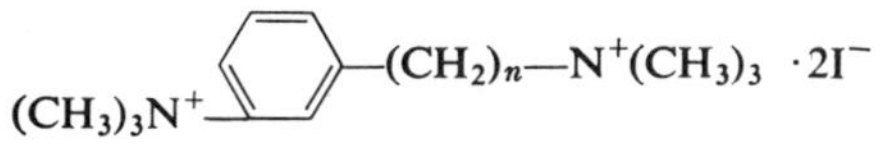

[a] Data of Wien and Mason (*322*, *329*).
[b] Potency of hexamethonium, 1.0.
[c] Superior cervical ganglion, cat.
[d] Peristaltic reflex preparation, guinea pig ileum.

drop in activity effected by shortening the chain length by one methylene unit. The similar *m*-ω-bistrialkylammonium series with alkyl chains of two to four methylene units and with trimethylammonium end groups also yielded fairly potent compounds, the range of potency being equal to that of hexamethonium (*392*); see Table 4.60.

13. ONIUM COMPOUNDS OTHER THAN AMMONIUM

a. Sulfonium Compounds

Two very weak ganglionic blocking sulfonium compounds, carbethoxymethyl-di-*n*-propylsulfonium bromide and methyl-dibenzylsulfonium nitrate, were described by Hunt and Renshaw (*393*). The only potent ganglionic blocking sulfonium derivative with a single sulfur atom is *d*-3,4-(1,3-dibenzyl-2-ketoimidazolino)-1,2-trimethylenethiophanium-*d*-camphorsulfonate (trimethaphan camphorsulfonate, Arfonad), which is structurally related to biotine. This agent is very potent, producing in different animal species short-lasting hypotension which, in the case of the dog, is largely independent of its ganglionic blocking action (*394*). Ganglionic blocking potency as measured in the cat, dog, and monkey amounts to 30 times that of TEA. The *l* isomer of these agents was half as potent as TEA, the monobenzyl analogue only twice as potent, and another derivative, 3,4-(2-ketoimidazolino)-1,2-trimethylenethiophanium bromide, even weaker (*78*).

Bissulfonium derivatives were subjects of several studies. Della Bella (*395*) and D'Amico and Busaccio (*396*) reported on the pharmacology of the sulfonium analogue of hexamethonium and the hexamethylene-1,6-bis(dimethylsulfonium) halides, which were found to be five to ten times less potent than hexamethonium on different preparations. A better absorption from the gastrointestinal tract than with hexamethonium has been observed. A comparison of three hexamethylene bissulfonium compounds indicated that the optimal potency in this series is found in the bisdiethyl derivative, which was only about one-half as potent as hexamethonium. The bisethylmethyl analogue was slightly less potent, and the bisdimethyl derivative was markedly less potent (*397*). Penta- and hexamethylene bisdimethylsulfonium were found to be inactive in the cat against the reflex blood pressure rise produced by carotid occlusion (*341*). Hexamethylene bisthiuronium compounds were described by Williams et al. (*341*). Only short-lasting hypotensive action has been reported. Weak vagolytic and sympathetic ganglion blocking action in the cat has been reported with hexamethylene 1,6-bisthiuronium (*398*).

b. Phosphonium Compounds

Hunt and Renshaw (*118*) reported on the nicotinic blocking action in cat blood pressure experiments with the three triethylphosphonium compounds

TABLE 4.61

Ganglionic Blocking Action of Polymethylene Bisphosphonium Compounds[a]

$(R)_3P^+(CH_2)_nP^+(R)_3 \cdot 2Br^-$

Code no.	R	*n*	ED,[b] mg/kg
Q-3	C_2H_5	4	4
Q-6	C_2H_5	5	4
Q-7	C_2H_5	6	4
Q-8	C_2H_5	10	1
Q-11	C_6H_5	5	1
Q-12	C_6H_5	6	>1

[a] Data of Ginzel et al. (*399*).
[b] Effective ganglionic blocking doses in cat nictitating membrane.

hydroxyethyltriethylphosphonium bromide, acetoxyethyltriethylphosphonium bromide, and carbethoxymethyltriethylphosphonium bromide, which were effective in 50 mg/kg doses. A series of polymethylene bisphosphonium derivatives with a chain length of C_4 to C_{10} were studied by Ginzel et al. (*399*). Data on their ganglionic blocking potency are shown in Table 4.61. The most potent member of this series, the pentamethylene derivative, produced blockade of vagal ganglia in 0.1 to 0.2 mg doses, whereas the minimal effective dose for suppressing sympathetic vasomotor ganglia (splanchnic stimulation) was established at 0.5 mg/kg. This compound was calculated to be 25 to 50 times as potent as TEA. Data obtained on isolated guinea pig ileum suggest the existence of additional cholinolytic action. In contrast to ammonium-type ganglionic blocking agents, it does not inhibit the reflex respiratory arrest produced by nicotinic stimulants and does not produce intestinal stimulation in the cat.

In most instances sulfonium and phosphonium compounds yielded only weak ganglionic blocking agents. However, ten thiophanium and bisphosphonium compounds point to a possibility of developing highly active and valuable agents in the nonnitrogenic onium class.

14. TERTIARY AND SECONDARY AMINES

Tertiary and secondary amines are in general much weaker ganglionic blocking agents than the corresponding quaternary derivatives. A few exceptions, however, exist when quaternary salts of certain tertiary amines are the less potent species. Ganglionically active tertiary and secondary amines belong mainly to three chemical classes: trialkylaminoalkylamines, piperidine derivatives, and azabicycloalkanes. Besides these, several miscellaneous tertiary and secondary amines were reported to have ganglionic blocking action, but the lack of a marked degree of activity and of structure–activity studies make them of minor importance.

The first group was studied by Mizzoni et al. (*400*), who dealt with the structure–activity relationships of thirty compounds of the general type $A{-}N{<}^{B}_{C}$, where A, B, and C are alkylamino or cycloalkylamino groups. Nine (see Table 4.62) were analyzed pharmacologically by Plummer et al. (*401*), who found that bis(diethylaminoethyl)(diethylaminopropyl)amine is highly effective in the dog in blocking autonomic ganglia upon oral administration. Surprisingly, the ganglionic blocking efficacy of this compound is eliminated by quaternization. Trisammonium compounds of the general structure $A{-}C{<}^{B}_{C}$, where A, B, and C are alkylammonium groups, were also very weak as ganglionic blocking agents (*402*). The analogous tris(dimethylaminoethyl)-amine was found to possess similar blocking properties (*320*, *403*). This compound was four times more potent than the TEA on the cat nictitating membrane and showed longer duration of action. It was orally active and showed a favorable ratio between the mydriatic response in mice as compared with

TABLE 4.62

Ganglionic Blocking Action of Tris(dialkylamine alkyl)amines[a]

$$(R_1)_2N(CH_2)_{n_3}N[(CH_2)_{n_1}NEt_2](CH_2)_{n_2}NEt_2 \cdot 3HCl$$

R_1	n_1	n_2	n_3	Potency[b]
Et	2	2	2	+++
Et	3	2	2	++++[c]
Et	4	2	2	+++
Et	5	2	2	0
Me	3	2	2	+++
n-Pr	3	2	2	+
n-Bu	3	2	2	0
Et	3	3	2	+
Et	3	3	3	+

[a] Data of Plummer et al. (*401*).
[b] Cat nictitating membrane.
[c] Effective dose 1 mg/kg.

other therapeutically useful (sympathetic) ganglionic blocking effects. However, such a favorable ratio may merely indicate a difference in species rather than in ganglionic sensitivity. In contrast to tris(dimethylaminoethyl) amine, bis(dimethylaminoethyl) amine was ganglionically inactive. Similar patterns in hypotensive action and in increasing intestinal motility were reported for tris(dimethylaminoethyl) amine, TEA, and hexamethonium (*313*).

Simple substituted piperidine derivatives (the 2,3- and 2,4-dimethylpiperidines) were first reported to show ganglionic blocking activity, but a more detailed pharmacologic analysis was not made (*404*). Recently 2,6-dimethylpiperidine was found to have similar action (*405*). Of the similar tertiary piperidines, 1,2,6-*cis*-trimethylpiperidine showed an activity twice that of TEA, whereas its 1-benzyl analogue was considerably weaker (*29*).

The first study with tertiary bisamines containing one piperidine group was made by Norton and Phillips (*406*). Of the compounds tested, 1-methyl-3-(dimethylaminobutyl)piperidine dihydrochloride was reported to be equipotent with hexamethonium and also acted longer orally. The possibility that ganglionic blocking agents exist in the tertiary amine class was emphasized relatively early in this study. Similar piperidine compounds with aminoalkyl side chains were reported more recently to be quite potent ganglionic blocking agents. Dialkylaminoalkoxyalkylpiperidines belong to this group. In this class also several compounds were more potent, or only potent in the tertiary and not in the quaternary form (*407*). The most significant tertiary amine type of ganglionic blocking agent, pempidine, and the best-known secondary amine derivatives, mecamylamine and its analogues, will be discussed separately in the next section.

Several series of compounds, which were tertiary amines and had complex ring systems consisting of seven-, eight-, or nine-membered rings, were reported to have hypotensive activity, but specific tests for determining ganglionic blockade were not conducted with these agents. In the azabicyclo[3.2.0]-heptane series the bisquaternary salts showed hypotensive activity (*408*). Azabicyclo[3.2.1]octanes, which were tested for hypotensive activity on dogs, were described by Grogan and Rice (*409*). A series of bicyclo[2.2.2]octane derivatives and their bisquaternary salts were listed in the patent literature (*410*), and antihypertensive properties were claimed. 3-Azabicyclo[3.3.1]-nonane derivatives were also tested but found to be inactive in dogs as hypotensive agents (*411*). Similar azabicyclo[3.3.1]nonanes were described as ganglionic blocking agents. In the first series the nitrogen atom occupied the 3 position, forming a ring system isomeric with that of granatane (**40**), where R is methyl, ethyl, propyl, allyl, *tert*-butyl, isobutyl, and isoamyl (*412*). Ganglionic blocking properties, but no atropinelike actions, were observed with these compounds. In 9-methyl-3,9-diazabicyclo[3.3.1]nonanes substituted at C-3 with alkyl groups the ganglionic blocking actions were more pronounced with the 3-alkyl than with the 3-aminoacyl substituents. Bisquaternary ammonium derivatives of this ring system showed marked curare-like actions (*413*).

Structurally different tertiary amines are shown in the last class. Of the aliphatic amine types, Pardo et al. (*218*) described the pharmacologic characteristics of ethylmethylisooctenylamine. Besides ganglionic blockade, which was more manifest at vagal than at sympathetic ganglia, a spasmolytic effect was noted. Secondary and tertiary aliphatic and alicyclic amines of the general structure $CR_1R_2R_3N(CH_3)R$ were described by Kharkevich (*414*); the secondary and tertiary amines $(C_2H_5)_3CNCH_2H_5$ and $(CH_3)_3CC(CH_3)_2N(CH_3)_2$ surpassed hexamethonium in potency and also showed favorable toxicity ratios.

About forty compounds of the tertiary phenylalkylamine class were of the types **(41)** and **(42)**, where X is *N*-alkyl, *N*-piperidino, *N*-morpholino, or *N*-pyrrolidino, R is H, OH, or O, R_1 is H, alkyl, aryl, or aralkyl, and R_2 is H, alkoxy, or halogen. None of the tertiary amines of these types showed ganglionic blocking potency reaching that of TEA. Some quaternary derivatives of this series were somewhat more potent (*255*). Usually the *N*-diethyl-substituted amines and ethyl quaternary salts were superior to the others. Clear-cut structure–activity studies, however, could not be made because of the over-all weak activity observed in both series of compounds.

Twelve different types of hexamethylene-1,6-bis(*t*-amine), in which part of the six-carbon chain is also a part of a six-membered ring, were studied by McMillan et al. (*415*). Three orally active compounds showed ganglionic blocking potency equal to that of hexamethonium [**(43)**, **(44)**, **(45)**].

It is interesting that, although the *p*-xylylenebisdimethylamine proved to be effective, its quaternary derivatives showed hardly any ganglionic blocking potency (*29*); see Table 4.50. 1-[(2-(2-Diethylaminoethoxy)phenyl)]-2-methylphenylpyrrole was reported to have ganglionic blocking, spasmolytic, and local anesthetic properties and also to exhibit low toxicity (*416*). Guyonneau (*32*) reported that in a series of basic amino esters, ethers, and alkanes **(46)**, where ring 1 is saturated or unsaturated, R is an alkyl ester, alkyl ether, or alkane moiety of chain length 0 through 2, and R_1 and R_2 are alkyl or cycloalkyl groups, there was hypotensive action on the rat blood pressure and ganglionic blockade on the isolated rat duodenum. Some of the compounds also showed stimulant action, and the ganglionic blocking potency in general was not impressively high. Structure–activity studies here were hindered by the relatively low efficacy of the compounds. Basically substituted azepine compounds derived from 5*H*-dibenz(b,f)azepine were claimed to possess ganglionic blocking activity in addition to other (antihistamine, spasmolytic) actions (*417*). Some benzodioxanes belonging to a group of adrenolytic agents —that is, diethylaminomethyl-3-benzodioxane (F-883), and piperidinomethyl-

3-benzodioxane (F-933)—were shown to have blocking properties on the superior cervical ganglion when applied locally to the ganglion (*196*).

a. Mecamylamine

Mecamylamine, described in 1956, was the first long-lasting, secondary amine type of ganglionic blocking agent of considerable potency that became fairly widely used clinically. In the first study on mecamylamine, Stone et al. (*418*, *419*) reported on its long-lasting action, which markedly surpassed that of hexamethonium and pentolinium. A comparison of its relative potency on the cat nictitating membrane and against nicotine pressor response indicated a relatively large difference between them. In the former test it was much less potent than in the latter, whereas the two reference agents showed only small differences in their respective effective doses. Although some curarelike action was noted, no other major pharmacologic actions were ascribed to the agent at that time. The low ratio of oral-to-intravenous mouse LD_{50} values indicated a good oral absorption. A comparison of mecamylamine with several ganglionic blocking agents showed that it has a longer-lasting effect on parasympathetic ganglia (vagal ganglia and parasympathetic ganglia of the salivary gland of the cat) than the other ganglionic blocking agents, except pempidine (*321*). Mecamylamine does not act by competition with ACh for ganglionic receptor sites. It has a distinctly different type of action from hexamethonium or pentolinium. The compound readily enters into cells, and so its action is not restricted to the ganglia. It extends also to the neuromuscular junctions, CNS, intestine, and heart. In the mechanism of hypotensive action of mecamylamine in man several factors other than ganglionic blockade (e.g., local anesthetic action) are involved. This is indicated by the minimal hypotensive dose, which is considerably lower than the minimal ganglionic blocking dose. Mecamylamine was also shown to be a noncompetitive ganglionic blocking and antinicotinic agent at ganglia of the isolated guinea pig ileum (*208*, *212*). A considerable difference was demonstrated between mecamylamine and some other well-known ganglionic blocking agents in their actions against nicotine convulsions. Mecamylamine, pentolinium, and hexamethonium were effective against all phases of nicotine convulsions, whereas chlorisondamine, nicotine, and TEA were either incompletely active or inactive. The potencies of these ganglionic blocking agents against nicotine convulsions and in blocking autonomic ganglia were not alike (*246*).

Mecamylamine produces mydriasis in the mouse through a ganglionic blocking action that is considerably more intensive than that of hexamethonium (*69*). In a study comparing the potency of different classes of ganglionic blocking agents on the superior cervical and stellate ganglia of the cat mecamylamine was surpassed by only one agent, chlorisondamine (*241*), an unsymmetric quaternary ammonium type of agent (see above).

A detailed pharmacologic study of mecamylamine in different species (*420*) indicated wide differences in the effective dose levels, depending on the test object.

(1) *Effects Other Than Ganglionic.* Mecamylamine depresses the vasomotor center independently of its ganglionic blocking action (*421*). On chronic oral administration it produces a sustained increase of systolic and diastolic blood pressure in dogs. The possible mechanism of this rise in blood pressure is an offsetting of the regulatory mechanisms, which operate through mechanoreceptors; similar hypertensive reactions were reported with mecamylamine in patients (*380*). Mecamylamine and pempidine can abolish the response to stimulation of postganglionic sympathetic fibers (*316*). Mecamylamine, but

TABLE 4.63

Influence of Variation of Substituents on the 3-Amino Group of Mecamylamine-Type Compounds[a]

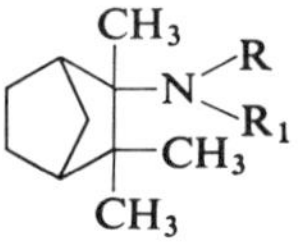

Code no.	R	R_1	Activity against:[b] Nicot. convuls. (ED_{50}), mg/kg	Pupil dilat. (ED), mg/kg	CNM effect. dose range[c] (intraven.), mg/kg
IX-1	H	H	2.8	5.2	
III-2	H	CH_3 (mecamylamine)	0.78	1.3	0.25–1.0
III-3	H	C_2H_5	1.3	1.6	
III-4	H	$(CH_2)_2CH_3$	6.4	7.5	
III-5	H	$(CH_2)_3CH_3$	toxic	toxic	
III-6	H	$(CH_2)_4CH_3$	11.0	>13.5	
III-7	H	$CH(CH_3)_2$	4.9	5.2	
III-8	H	$CH_2CH{=}CH_2$	5.8	8.5	
III-9	H	$(CH_2)_2C(CH_3)_3$	26.5	43.0	
III-10	H	C_6H_{13}	24.0	40.0	
III-11	H	$C_6H_5CH_2$	48.0	83.0	
III-12	H	$C_6H_5CH_2CH_2$	15.0	36.0	
III-13	H	$C_6H_5(CH_2)_3$	45.0	37.0	
III-14	CH_3	CH_3	0.71	1.5	0.25–1.0
III-15	C_2H_5	C_2H_5	3.2	3.8	

[a] Data of Stone et al. (*424*).

[b] ED, effective dose producing dilatation of 10 units; intraperitoneal administration.

[c] CNM, cat nictitating membrane; to produce 20 to 80% blockade of contractions.

not pempidine, potentiates morphine analgesia in rats (*422*). Like other ganglionic blocking agents, it sensitizes the effector cells to catecholamines (*225*), and this sensitization may mask the manifestation of the ganglionic blocking effect. Mecamylamine and a few other ganglionic blocking agents do not influence the activity of different enzymes that are important in nervous functions, such as specific and nonspecific cholinesterase, acid and alkaline phosphatase, and succinic dehydrogenase (*423*).

There is a potentiation, caused by mecamylamine and TEA, of the effects of several spasmogenic agents (catecholamines, angiotensin, 5-HT, histamine, and $BaCl_2$) on isolated arterial strips. The potentiating action was found to be independent of the degree of ganglionic blockade (*317*). Mecamylamine potentiated the action of epinephrine in decreasing the spleen volume (*240*) and the peripheral effects of catecholamines on isolated aortic strips of rabbits (*235*). However, other ganglionic blocking agents, such as hexamethonium, pentolinium, and pempidine, did not share this property.

TABLE 4.64

Influence of Ring Methyl and Bridge Methylene Groups on Activity of Compounds Related to Mecamylamine[a]

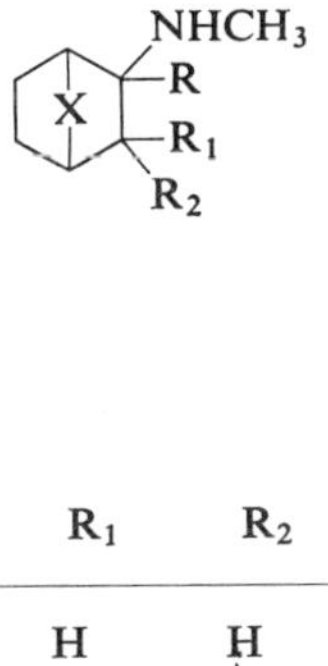

Code no.	X	R	R1	R2	Activity against:[b] Nicot. convuls. (ED_{50}), mg/kg	Activity against:[b] Pupil dilat. (ED), mg/kg	CNM effect. dose range[c] (intraven.), mg/kg
III-16		H	H	H	70.0	48.0	
III-17		CH_3	H	H	6.6	21.0	
III-18		CH_3	CH_3	H	1.1	3.1	
III-19		CH_3	CH_3	CH_3	0.96	2.7	1.0–2.0
III-2	CH_2	CH_3	CH_3	CH_3	0.78	1.3	0.25–1.0
XIII-20	CH_2	CH_2CH_3	CH_3	CH_3	4.2	7.0	
XIII-21	CH_2	$CH_2CH_2CH_2$	CH_3	CH_3	39.0	50.0	
XIII-22		H	CH_3	H	17.0	22.0	
XIII-23		H	CH_3	CH_3	9.2	12.0	
XIII-24	CH_2	H	CH_3	CH_3	1.3	2.9	1.0–2.0

[a] Data of Stone et al. (*424*).
[b] ED, effective dose producing dilatation of 10 units; intraperitoneal administration.
[c] CNM, cat nictitating membrane; to produce 20 to 80% blockade of contractions.

(2) *Derivatives of Mecamylamine.* The first pharmacologic studies of mecamylamine were followed only considerably later by a rather detailed structure–activity study made by Stone et al. (*424*), of analogues and derivatives of mecamylamine. Results of these studies with the mouse nicotine

TABLE 4.65

Comparison of Activity of Geometric and Other Stereoisomers of Mecamylamine[a]

Compound	Configuration	Activity against:[b] Nicotine convuls. (ED_{50}), mg/kg	Activity against:[b] Pupil dilat. (ED), mg/kg	CNM effect. dose range[c] (intraven.), mg/kg
d,l-mecamylamine	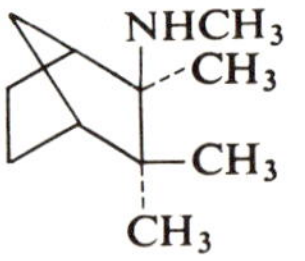	0.78	1.3	0.25–1.0
d-mecamylamine		0.92	1.0	
d,l-exo form	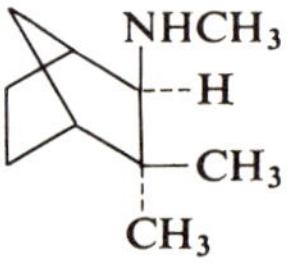	1.3	2.9	
d,l-endo form	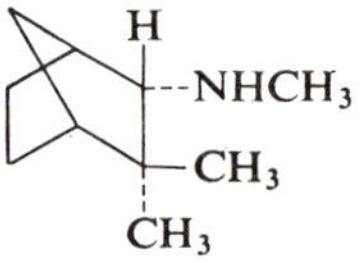	2.0	4.6	
d,l-exo form	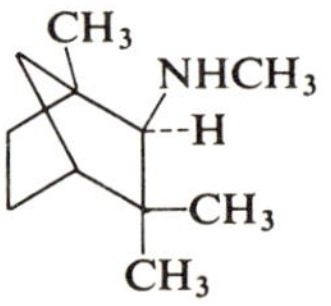	1.0	2.2	0.5–1.0
d,l-endo form	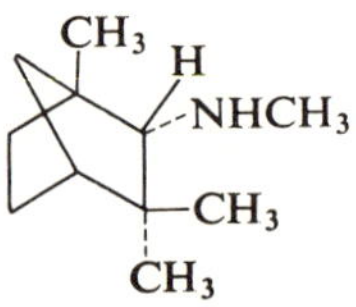	3.0	5.2	

[a] Data of Stone et al. (*424*).
[b] ED, effective dose producing dilatation of 10 units; intraperitoneal administration.
[c] CNM, cat nictitating membrane; to produce 20 to 80% blockade of contractions.

convulsion test as a screening procedure and with the mouse pupil dilatation and the cat nictitating membrane as additional supportive methods are presented in Tables 4.63 to 4.65. The conclusions of these studies (*424*) are as follows.

Mecamylamine and its dimethylamino analogue were the most active members of the groups of secondary and tertiary amines studied for the following structure–activity aspects: influence of various alkyl and arylalkyl substituents on the 3-amino group of mecamylamine, influence of ring methyl and bridge methylene groups, role of geometric and optical isomerism, and potency of partial structures related to mecamylamine.

These studies indicated that an angular methyl at position 3, methyl groups substituted at position 2, and a bridge methylene group enhance potency in this class of agents. Of the *exo-endo* isomeric pairs the *exo* isomer was the more potent. Methyl or dimethyl substitution on the amino group was optimal for activity. One of the partial structures without the ring system of mecamylamine was only slightly less potent than the parent compound (Tables 4.65 and 4.66).

A steric hindrance developing around an amino group corresponding to that of mecamylamine is important for maximal activity. A similar situation exists both with piperidines and pyrrolidines having α-branched chains and with tropanes.

Several of the structure–activity aspects of the mecamylamine group correspond to those ascribed to the pentamethylpiperidine (pempidine) series of compounds.

Within a series of derivatives of mecamylamine the relative potency of

TABLE 4.66

Relative Activity of Partial Structures of Mecamylamine[a]

		Activity against:[b]		
Compound	Structure	Nicot. convuls. (ED_{50}), mg/kg	Pupil dilat. (ED), mg/kg	CNM effect. dose range[c] (intraven.), mg/kg
30	$CH_3CH(CH(CH_3)_2)NHCH_3$	4.9	13.0	5.0–10.0
31	$(CH_3)_2C(C(CH_3)_3)NHCH_3$	0.96	4.9	10.0–2.0
III-2	Mecamylamine	0.78	1.3	5.0–10.0

[a] Data of Stone et al. (*424*).

[b] ED, effective dose producing dilatation of 10 units; intraperitoneal administration.

[c] CNM, cat nictitating membrane; to produce 20 to 80% blockade of contractions.

antagonizing nicotine convulsions parallels ganglionic blockade, as measured with the cat nictitating membrane. However, the authors well recognized that this within-a-series correlation may not hold true for between-series comparisons (*424*).

A group of analogues of mecamylamine has been studied by Rubinstein et al. (*425*) and by Edge et al. (*426*), who characterized the structural requirements for optimal mecamylaminelike ganglionic blocking action. In a series of 3-aminoisocamphanes illustrated below it was found that R_2 must carry a methyl group for maximal potency but that the presence of the methyl groups at R_3 and R_4 are not essential. Relative potencies of this series are indicated in Table 4.67. The 2,3-dimethyl derivative of this series was tested clinically and was described as a ganglionic blocking agent of long-lasting action that was potent orally and subcutaneously in the same dose range and also showed less parasympathetic blocking side effects than mecamylamine. However, both compounds produced CNS side effects (tremors, ataxia, and hallucinations).

The structural requirements for strong ganglionic blocking activity and long duration of action among some lower homologues of mecamylamine and

TABLE 4.67

Ganglionic Blocking Activity of Methyl-Substituted 3-Aminonorcamphanes[a]

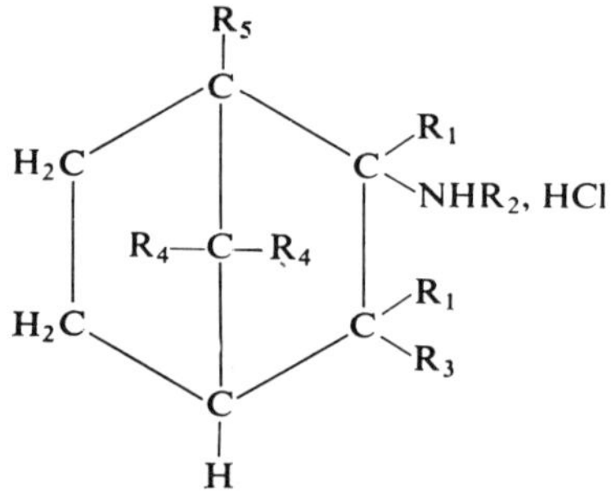

R_1	R_2	R_3	R_4	R_5	Ganglionic blocking action: Parasymp.[b]	Ganglionic blocking action: Symp.[c]
H	Me	H	H	H	0.10	(+)
H	Me	Me	H	H	3.00	+++
Me	Me	Me	H	H	4.50	+++
H	H	Me	H	H	0.40	+
H	Me	H	Me	Me	1.30	+
H	Me	Me	H	Me	1.35	++

[a] Data of Rubinstein et al. (*425*).
[b] Potency of hexamethonium, 1.0.
[c] Degree of blockade.

similar activities among isomers with enlarged ring structures were recorded by Edge et al. (*426*). In both series of compounds the successive introduction of C-methyl groups surrounding the nitrogen atom resulted in an increase of ganglionic blocking activity and duration of action. When tested on the nictitating membrane of the cat, the activity of these compounds was only 4 to 7% that of hexamethonium. Changing the structure of aminobicycloheptanes, in which the nitrogen atom is exocyclic, to that of bicycloazaoctanes, in which the nitrogen atom is endocyclic, resulted in no loss of ganglionic blocking potency. These findings are outlined in Table 4.68.

TABLE 4.68

Blocking Activity of Isomers of Mecamylamine on Preganglionically Stimulated Cat Nictitating Membrane[a]

Name or code no.	Structure	Potency[b]
N-Methyl-(−)-isobornylamine	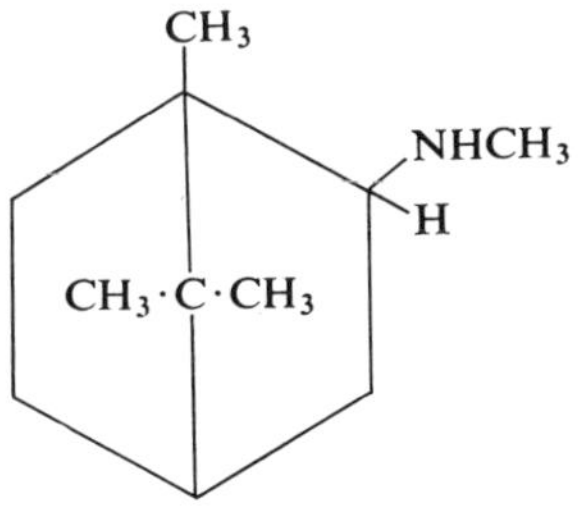	0.05
N-Methyl-(+)-bornylamine	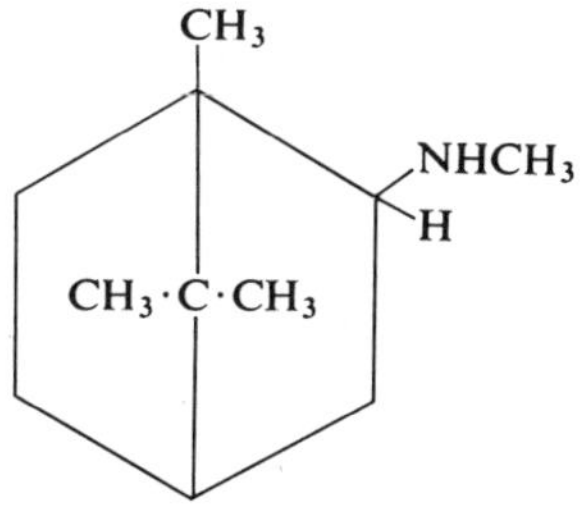	0.04
N-Methylfenchyl-amine	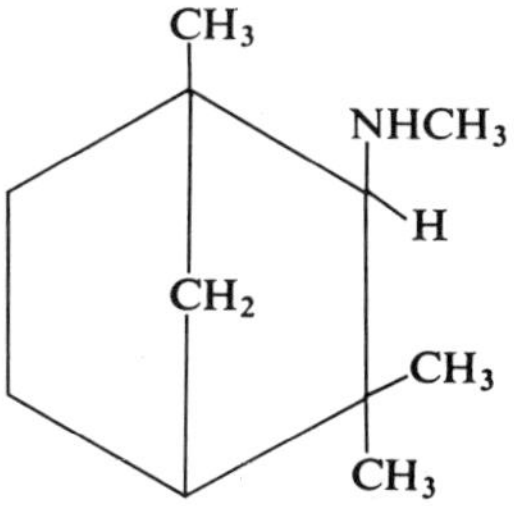	0.07

TABLE 4.68—*continued*

Name or code no.		Structure	Potency[b]
N-Methylcamphidine		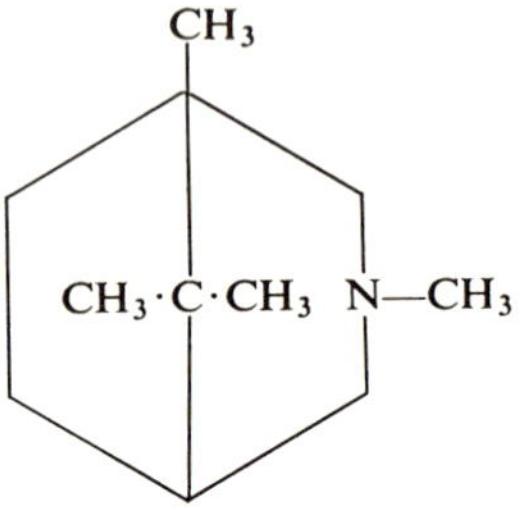	0.06
Mecamylamine,		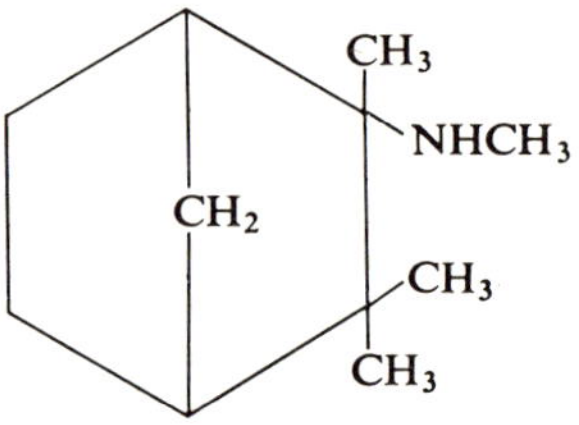	1.2
556	R=H	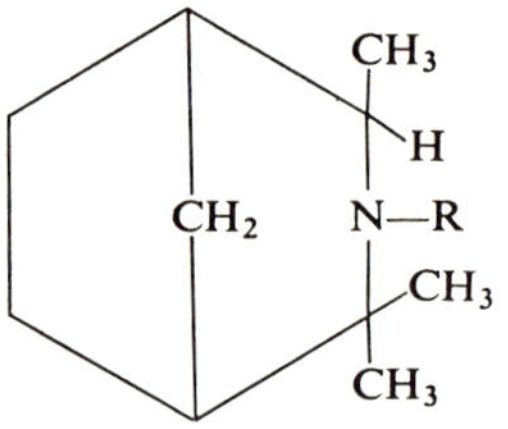	1.34
5199	$R=CH_3$		1.00
5562	R=H	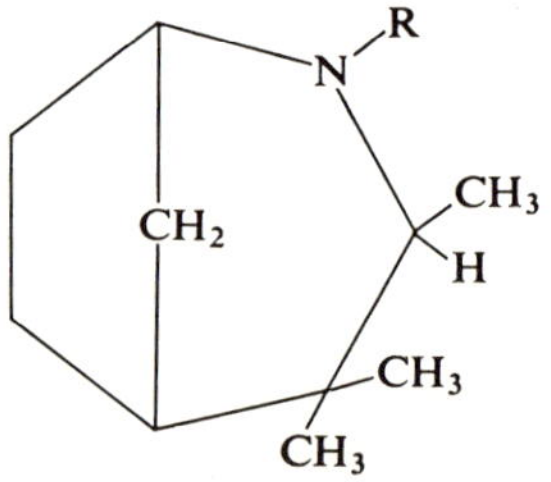	0.75
5200	$R=CH_3$		0.40
4315		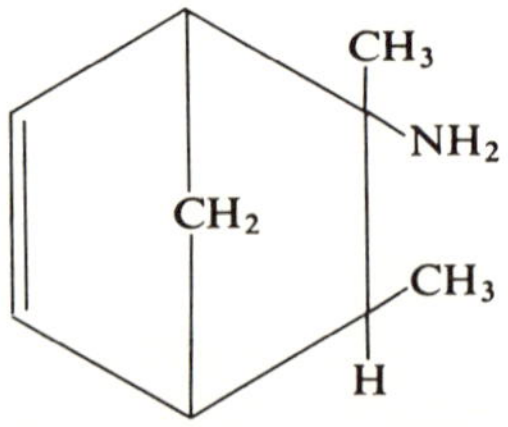	0.15

TABLE 4.68—*continued*

Name or code no.		Structure	Potency[b]
4058	$R_1=R_2=H$	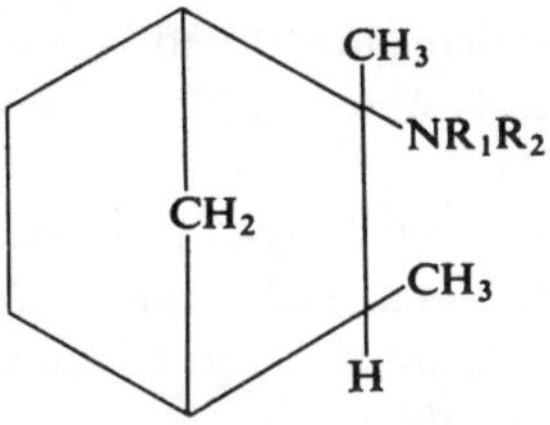	0.15
4086	$R_1=CH_3$, $R_2=H$		0.35
4620	$R_1=R_2=CH$		0.50
4126	$R_1=CH_2C_6H_5$, $R_2=H$		<0.01
4387		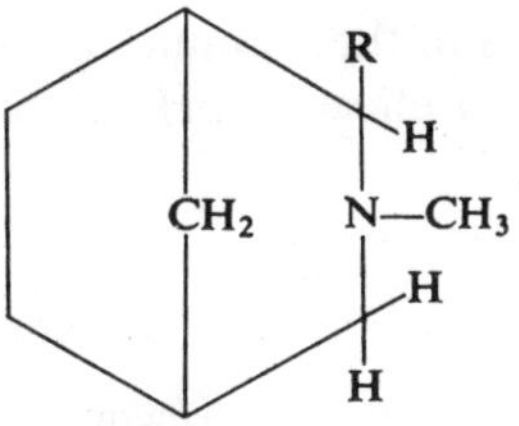	0.50
4188	$R=CH_3$	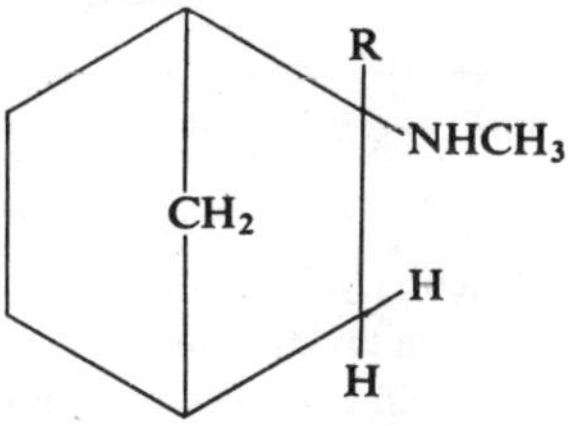	0.25
4269	$R=C_2H_5$		0.25
4443	$R=CH_3$	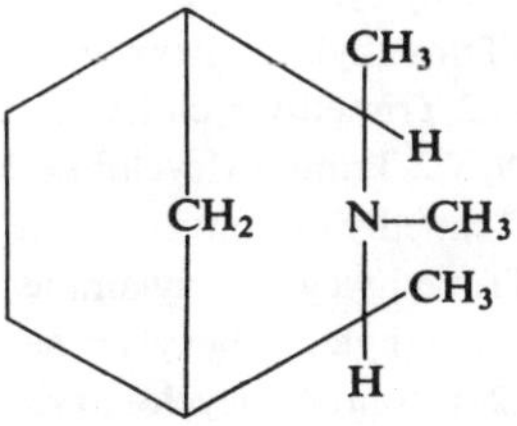	0.25
4442	$R=C_2H_5$		0.20–0.25
4280		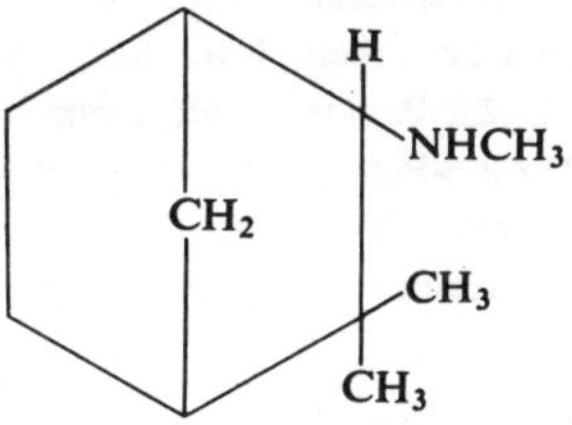	0.15

[a] Data of Edge et al. (*426*).
[b] Potency of hexamethonium, 1.0.

Other structure–activity studies of the mecamylamine type of compound resulted in simplified structural analogues. Aliphatic amines modeling the branched-chain structure in mecamylamine were studied by Stone et al. (*424*). Some of the similar substituted *t*-hexylamine derivatives, such as *N*,*N*,2,2,3-pentamethylbutylamine-3 and penbutamine, were equipotent with mecamylamine (*427*, *428*).

In a series of polymethylcyclohexylamines a few of the fifteen derivatives studied by Protiva et al. (*429*), the 1,2,2-trimethyl- and *N*,*N*,1,2,2-pentamethylcyclohexylamines, were found to show degrees of potency similar to that of mecamylamine (Table 4.69).

In studies with the quaternary metho salts of mecamylamine, dimecamine, and pempidine in neuromuscular junction preparations it was suggested that the active species of these amines is a cationic form which acts extracellularly (*430*). The lack of effect of pH on the blockade by mecamylamine supports this hypothesis.

TABLE 4.69

Polymethylcyclohexylamines[a]

Compound	Gang. block. action[b]
N,1-Dimethylcyclohexylamine	+++[c]
cis-*N*,2-Dimethylcyclohexylamine	0
trans-*N*,2-Dimethylcyclohexylamine	+
2,2-Dimethylcyclohexylamine	++
N,*N*,1-Trimethylcyclohexylamine	++++
cis-*N*,*N*,2-Trimethylcyclohexylamine	++
trans-*N*,*N*,2-Trimethylcyclohexylamine	0
N,2,2-Trimethylcyclohexylamine	+
1,2,2-Trimethylcyclohexylamine	++++
2,2,6-Trimethylcyclohexylamine	0
N,*N*,2,2-Tetramethylcyclohexylamine	++
N,1,2,2-Tetramethylcyclohexylamine	++++
2,2,6,6-Tetramethylcyclohexylamine	+++[c]
N,*N*,1,2,2-Pentamethylcyclohexylamine	++++
N,*N*,2,2,6-Pentamethylcyclohexylamine	+++
Mecamylamine·HCl	++++
Dimecamine·HBr	++++

[a] Data of Protiva et al. (*429*).
[b] Cat nictitating membrane; 5 mg/kg intravenous.
[c] Action of short duration.

b. Pempidine and Related Compounds

Pempidine (1,2,2,6,6-pentamethylpiperidine) is a tertiary amine more recently developed as a ganglionic blocking agent (*431, 432*). It shows a certain structural similarity to mecamylamine, to the branched-chain substituted aliphatic ammonium compounds, and to 2,6-dimethylpiperidine derivatives. According to a detailed comparative pharmacologic study (*220, 315*), pempidine ranks close to mecamylamine in its type of action. A long-lasting blockade of autonomic ganglia is characteristic of pempidine. This effect was demonstrated on the cat superior cervical ganglion and nictitating membrane preparation and by recording the ganglionic action potentials of the cervical sympathetic. Furthermore, in the cardiovascular system of the cat it depresses the pressor responses to nicotine, DMPP, ACh, carotid occlusion, and electric stimulation of the splanchnic nerves. The inhibition of parasympathetic ganglia was shown on the sympathetically denervated iris and against vagus stimulation and ganglionic stimulation of the urinary bladder. Efficacy on the guinea pig ileum against ganglionic and other stimulants was also explored. Comparisons with mecamylamine and *N*-ethylpempidine showed a potency of approximately the same magnitude without marked differences in blockade at different ganglia (nictitating membrane as compared with urinary bladder). Several nonganglionic actions also were reported for pempidine (*220, 315*). More favorable ratios between hypotensive and toxic doses than with hexamethonium were reported in rabbits (*433*). The p*K* values for both pempidine and mecamylamine are similar; the two compounds seem to be about equally lipid-soluble, which may account for the similar distributions and excretion patterns of these agents. However, pempidine shows a lesser degree of protein-binding than mecamylamine and is therefore of shorter duration of action. While the conventional ganglionic blocking actions of pempidine are about equal to those of hexamethonium, pempidine is considerably more potent against nicotine convulsions in the mouse (Table 4.70). Lawrence and Stacey (*315*) believe that the action of the quaternary ammonium type of ganglionic blocking agents against nicotine convulsions may be attributed to a peripheral sympatholytic action, that is, inhibition of epinephrine release by nicotine. The antinicotine action of pempidine and mecamylamine-like agents is predominantly a central antinicotinic effect. Indication of a central vasomotor effect is offered in the study of Dhawan and Bhargava (*434*).

Pempidine was a significant product of a broad search in England for new ganglionic blocking agents, the search covering about 2400 compounds, mostly of the nonquaternary type. Some characteristic compounds of this series, represented by branched-chain aliphatic amines and substituted piperidines, are shown in formulas **(47)** to **(50)** and in Table 4.71. While piperidine was without any ganglionic blocking potency, aliphatic ammonium compounds,

TABLE 4.70

Comparison of Potencies of Some Therapeutically Used Ganglionic Blocking Drugs

	Relative potency[a]			Parasymp. gang.	Cat nicot. pressor response[d]	Mouse nicot. convuls.[b]
	([b])	([c])	([d])			
TEA			0.52	0.4		
Hexamethonium	1.0	1.0		1.0	1.0	1.0
Pentolinium	4.0		4.2		3.9	6.0
Mecamylamine	1.2	1.3	1.1	0.8[c]	3.0	13.9
Pempidine	1.3	3.3		1.9		16.7

[a] Cat nictitating membrane; potency of hexamethonium, 1.0.
[b] Data of Corne and Edge (*315*).
[c] Data of Nador (*16*).
[d] Pentolinium and mecamylamine; data of Stone et al. (*418*).

such as 25645 **(47)** and 25635 **(48)** and piperidine derivatives with similar α-branched aliphatic side chains, showed considerable ganglionic blocking potency in the cat nictitating membrane preparation, which served as a screening test procedure. The results obtained in the same study, concerning the role of substitution of the nitrogen atom of the potent derivative 25636 **(50)** are shown in Table 4.71. Another detailed study (*435*) of pempidine analogues of the general structure **(51)** covered 150 compounds, 34 of which were pharmacologically explored. The role of changes in the molecular structure at the nitrogen atom (introducing 3,4 and 5,6 double bonds, changing the piperidine ring to a pyrrolidine ring and opening the ring structure to produce *t*-butylamines) was investigated. Several compounds derived from these molecular modifications showed a somewhat higher potency than pempidine itself on the cat nictitating membrane. The *N*-ethyl analogue and the quarternary *N*,*N*-dimethyl analogue of pempidine were highly potent, although the latter showed a characteristically short, quaternary ammonium type of blocking effect. The structural alterations listed above were generally favorable for retention or increase of ganglionic blocking action.

Several derivatives of pempidine were studied by Philippot et al. (*436*) and were found to be less potent than pempidine. Substitution of the piperidine ring for a pyrrolidine ring resulted in a series of tetramethyl-, pentamethyl-, and hexamethylpyrrolidine derivatives with different alkyl substituents at the nitrogen atom. These compounds were claimed to be useful as ganglionic blocking agents (*437*).

Bis-tertiary amines of type **(52)**, where *n* is 2 to 4 and R_1, R_2, and R_3 are H or lower alkyl, were derived from pempidine (*438*). These also showed hypotensive and ganglionic blocking properties.

TABLE 4.71

Ganglionic Blocking Activity of Piperidine Derivatives Related to Pempidine[a]

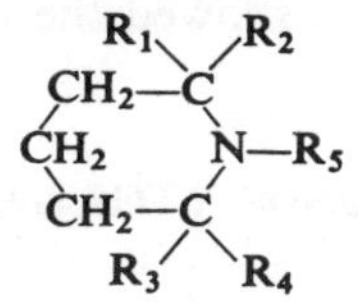

R_1	R_2	R_3	R_4	R_5	Gang. block. potency[b]	Hypotensive ED in man[c]
H	H	H	H	H	0	
CH_3	H	H	H	H	0	
CH_3	H	CH_3	H	H	0	
CH_3	CH_3	CH_3	H	H	0.50	23.2
CH_3	CH_3	CH_3	CH_3	H	2.40	3.4
CH_3	CH_3	CH_3	CH_3	CH_3	3.0	4.2
CH_3	CH_3	CH_3	CH_3	C_2H_5	3.6	
CH_3	CH_3	CH_3	CH_3	$n\text{-}C_3H_7$	2.4	
CH_3	CH_3	CH_3	CH_3	$n\text{-}C_4H_{9n}$	1.8	
CH_3	CH_3	CH_3	CH_3	$CH_2{=}CH{-}CH_2$	1.5	
CH_3	CH_3	CH_3	CH_3	$C_6H_5CH_2$	0.18	
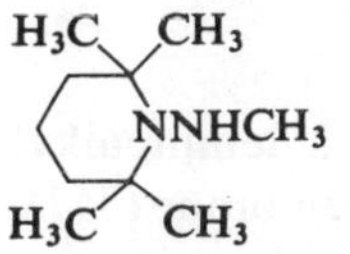			M & B 5409A			4.2
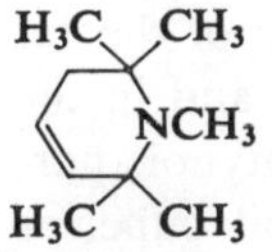			M & B 4577A			6.3
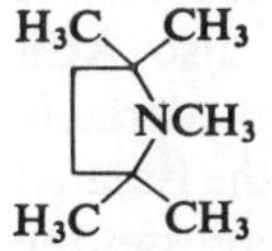			M & B 4859A			11.1

[a] Data of Spinks et al. (*220*).
[b] Cat nictitating membrane; potency of hexamethonium, 1.0.
[c] ED, effective dose in milligrams per subject; data of Smirk (*439*).

A comparative clinical study with pempidine and six analogues with variations on the nitrogen atom (introducing a 3,4 double bond, reducing the size of the piperidine ring, expanding it, and eliminating one methyl substituent at C-2) indicated that the first two variations were favorable whereas the second two resulted in compounds considerably weaker than pempidine. Norpempidine, being slightly more effective than pempidine itself, was reported to be the most potent ganglionic blocking drug available in 1960 (*439*, *440*). All these compounds showed the usual side effects characteristic of ganglionic blocking agents.

15. MISCELLANEOUS COMPOUNDS WITH GANGLIONIC BLOCKING ACTION

a. Sympathomimetic Amines

Epinephrine, norepinephrine, phenethylamine, tyramine, 5-HT, ephedrine, and mescaline (*38*) block the cat superior cervical ganglion. In the perfused cat superior cervical ganglion several sympathomimetic amines block the transmission at doses about ten times higher than those of epinephrine (*215*, *441*). Epinephrine is four times more potent than norepinephrine in inhibiting single, evoked ganglionic potentials in the superior cervical ganglion. DHE antagonizes the inhibitory effect of epinephrine (*422*). Epinephrine and other catecholamines produce blockade of transmission also in the ciliary ganglion. The order of decreasing efficacy is: epinephrine, norepinephrine, isoproterenol, amphetamine, ephedrine, phenylephrine, and isometheptene (*227*).

b. Hypnotic and Sedative Drugs

Malonic acid, urea, and malonylurea derivatives with dimethylaminoalkyl side chains produce ganglionic blockade on the cat nictitating membrane (*351*). Pentobarbital, chloral hydrate, hexobarbital, and urethane, in that order, were increasingly depressant on the perfused superior cervical ganglion of the cat (*443*). Pentobarbital on the perfused stellate ganglion of the cat and in the excised superior cervical ganglion of the rabbit (*59*), methylpentynol, paraldehyde, amylbarbital, and procaine amide on cat and rabbit superior cervical ganglia (*60*, *230*, *231*) were reported to show blocking action. Different centrally depressant drugs inhibit ganglionic transmission and also ACh output in the perfused superior cervical ganglion (*236*, *444*). A moderately selective action of amylbarbital and paraldehyde was observed on the isolated rat superior cervical ganglion (*61*). Hydroxydione in large doses depresses the superior cervical ganglion and blocks the effect of nicotine on the blood pressure of the cat (*445*).

c. Guanidine Derivatives

Guanethidine is a ganglionic depressant on the cat superior cervical ganglion and vagal cardiac ganglia of the dog (*446*). Guanethidine (*447*) and *N*,*N*-diethylguanidine (*448*) were also shown to have blocking properties at the ganglia.

d. Phenothazines

Chlorpromazine and *N*-methylpiperidyl-3-phenothiazine (Mepazine) were found to have ganglionic blocking properties on the cat superior cervical ganglion (*238*, *449*, *450*).

e. Antihistamines

Mild ganglionic blocking action was found with diphenhydramine and antazoline on the superior cervical ganglion of the cat (*451*).

f. Monoamine Oxidase Inhibitors

Harmine, 2-phenylcyclopropylamine, pheniprazine, phenelzine, iproniazide, nialamide (*452*), and *N*-diphenylacetyl-N′-piperidylethyl hydrazide (*453*, *454*) were reported to have ganglionic blocking properties.

16. ANTAGONISTS OF THE GANGLIONIC ACTIONS OF HISTAMINE AND 5-HT

Histamine and 5-HT are known to stimulate receptor sites of autonomic ganglia other than those sensitive to ACh. The ganglionic stimulation of these amines is resistant to typical ganglionic blocking agents that inhibit the effects of ACh or of electric stimulation. This indicates that, at least under normal circumstances and on the mammalian ganglion preparations used for this purpose, they are probably not involved in the phenomena of neurotransmission across autonomic synapses. Specific blocking agents against these amines may, however, be of significance as pharmacologic tools in analyzing the receptor sites of ganglia, and they may also yield practical applications in pathologic phenomena, in which abnormal oversecretion or interference with metabolic inactivation may bring about effects attributable to these ganglionically active amines.

a. Antagonists of Histamine

The ganglionic stimulant action of histamine is abolished on the cat superior cervical ganglion by cocaine, morphine, and methadone (*13*). That the same blocking agents are also effective against 5-HT and pilocarpine suggests that these ganglionic stimulants act at similar receptor sites. The antihistaminic agent pyrilamine is potent only against the ganglionic action of histamine (*13*); this seems to accord with the earlier findings of Gyermek and Sztanyik (*94*), which indicated selective blocking of histamine stimulation in the adrenal medulla of the cat by tripelennamine.

b. Antagonists of 5-HT

The majority of conventional antagonists of 5-HT that are effective almost exclusively against the smooth-muscle effects of 5-HT are either weak or inactive against the ganglionic stimulation produced by 5-HT. The description of M-receptors (morphine-sensitive, neural) and D-receptors (Dibenzyline-sensitive, muscular) given by Gaddum (*455*) for the guinea pig ileum clearly indicates that significantly different receptor sites must be considered. The first blocking agents of the M-receptors of the guinea pig ileum, morphine and cocaine, although potent in inhibiting the 5-HT-induced ganglionic stimulation, also exhibit other significant pharmacologic actions. Therefore, a search for more potent and more selective neurotropic antagonists of 5-HT has been

TABLE 4.72

Ganglionic Action of Quaternary Indolealkylammonium Compounds Against 5-HT[a]

Compound	Minim. effect. dose against 5-HT, μg/kg ([b])	Minim. effect. dose against 5-HT, μg/kg ([c])
N-(Benzyl)-*N*,*N*-dimethyl-β-(3-indolylethyl)ammonium bromide	30.0	11.0
N-(*o*-Xylyl)-*N*,*N*-dimethyl-β-(3-indolylethyl)ammonium bromide	80.0	20.0
N-(*o*-Chlorbenzyl)-*N*,*N*-dimethyl-β-(3-indolylethyl)ammonium bromide	50.0	20.0
N-(*m*-Xylyl)-*N*,*N*-dimethyl-β-(3-indolylethyl)ammonium bromide	20.0	8.0
N-(*m*-Chlorbenzyl)-*N*,*N*-dimethyl-β-(3-indolylethyl)ammonium bromide	7.0	1.0
N-(*m*-Nitrobenzyl)-*N*,*N*-dimethyl-β-(3-indolylethyl)ammonium bromide	20.0	2.5
N-(*p*-Xylyl)-*N*,*N*-dimethyl-β-(3-indolylethyl)ammonium bromide	80.0	20.0
N-(*p*-Bromobenzyl)-*N*,*N*-dimethyl-β-(3-indolylethyl)ammonium bromide	20.0	20.0
N-(*m*-Chlorbenzyl)-*N*,*N*-diethyl-β-(3-indolylethyl)ammonium bromide	80.0	20.0
N-(Benzyl)-*N*,*N*-dimethyl-β-(5-hydroxy-3-indolylethyl)ammonium bromide	4.2	2.0
N-(*m*-Xylyl)-*N*,*N*-dimethyl-β-(5-hydroxy-3-indolylethyl)ammonium bromide	8.3	0.3
N-(*m*-Chlorbenzyl)-*N*,*N*-dimethyl-β-(5-hydroxy-3-indolylethyl)-ammonium bromide	0.66	0.04

[a] Data of Gyermek (*33*).
[b] Inferior mesenteric ganglion of the cat.
[c] Pelvic ganglia of the dog.

indicated. The first such agent fulfilling the criteria was 5-hydroxyindole-3-acetamidine. Its prominent action is inhibition of the ganglionic and chemoreceptor stimulating effects of 5-HT. Indole-3-acetamidine was less potent (*184*). The result of a more detailed analysis of several types of agent effective against the ganglionic stimulation of 5-HT was a new classification of its antagonists, advanced by Gyermek (*33*, *456*). The "A" receptor type in the smooth muscle can be characterized by conventional 5-HT blocking agents which inhibit the smooth muscle actions. The "B" receptors situated in autonomic ganglia and at chemoreceptors are sensitive to the "neurotropic" classes of 5-HT antagonists (morphine, cocaine, indoleacetamidines), and to two new classes of agents (quaternary indolylalkylammonium compounds and arylguanidines).

A few characteristics of these two newer types of agents are outlined in Tables 4.10 and 4.71, indicating values of potency and/or selectivity as obtained on two ganglionic preparations. Some of the quaternary indolylalkylammonium types of compounds, i.e., *N*-*m*-bromobenzyl-*N*,*N*-dimethyl-5-hydroxy-3-indolylethylammonium bromide, proved to be extremely potent against the ganglionic stimulant action of 5-HT; the compound, however, also showed cholinergic type of ganglionic stimulant properties (*76*).

Some arylguanidine compounds, particularly 2-anthrylguanidine, selectively block the effects of 5-HT and of stimulant-type guanidines such as phenyldiguanide which seems to act at the same ganglionic receptors as 5-HT. Relationships between these neurotropic classes of blocking agents to 5-HT and other anti-5-HT agents have been discussed in detail by Gyermek (*33*).

4.5. CLINICAL ASPECTS OF GANGLIONIC AGENTS

The possible therapeutic uses of ganglionic stimulant agents are not well recognized. The usually mild and also variable effects of different amounts of nicotine on the autonomic nervous system produced through inhaling cigarette smoke should be considered significant enough to contribute to the almost habit-forming effect of smoking. Nevertheless, these actions are not thought to be of any therapeutic value.

The only agent used for its chemoreceptor-stimulant action that is closely related to ganglionic stimulation is lobeline, but the extent of its use is very limited, particularly in North America.

It seems that not enough attention has been paid to the possibility of using ganglionic stimulant agents in combating symptoms of certain types of cardiovascular shock, in which an increase of endogenous sympathomimetic amine output may be of value.

Three major clinical groups of pathologic conditions are amenable to therapy with drugs that block autonomic ganglionic functions: the cardiovascular, the gastrointestinal, and the genitourinary. Of these, hypertension, peptic ulcer, spasms, and colic pains have been explored to a great extent.

Promising results as far as hypotensive action is concerned were obtained with the first clinically applied ganglionic blocking agents. However, problems related to duration of action, lack of efficacy or inconsistent efficacy with the quaternary ammonium type of compound, autonomic and other side effects, and development of tolerance on chronic administration, have limited the clinical applications of this class of agents until recently. With the emerging of new types of drugs, such as bretylium and guanethidine, which act at the postganglionic sympathetic fibers by interfering with the release of the sympathetic transmitter substances, and α-methyldopa, which interferes with the formation of norepinephrine, only a few of the newer, long-lasting, and orally fairly active compounds have survived as therapeutic agents in the treatment of hypertension. Even these few (pentolinium, mecamylamine, and pempidine) are recommended now exclusively for combination with a background drug therapy of Rauwolfia alkaloids and diuretic agents (*457*).

A few compounds, including some whose action is of shorter duration, are used in producing hypotension during surgery. For this purpose hexamethonium, trimethaphan camphorsulfonate (Arfonad), and an asymmetric bisquaternary ammonium compound (Plegarol, SY-108) have been used (*387*). Promising results superior to those obtained with Arfonad have been reported with a monoquaternary homatropinium derivative, tropenium (*214*, *300*). This class of agents can also be employed in symptomatic therapy in acute hypertensive crisis (toxemia of pregnancy). The intravenous use of TEA as a diagnostic agent in pheochromocytoma is generally known.

Theoretically it is possible to use pure ganglionic blocking agents for suppressing smooth-muscle spasms and hypersecretion of the gastrointestinal tract and alleviating spasms of the genitourinary tract. Several human studies indicate that ganglionic blocking agents are effective in this regard (*232*, *459*, *460*). The hypotensive effect of these agents limits their application for this purpose. As outlined before, attempts to develop agents with selective action at one division of the autonomic ganglia have been without much success, and thus the application of these agents does not seem to be feasible.

Although the use of generalized ganglionic blockade alone is not ideal for combatting gastrointestinal spasm and hypersecretion, the desirability of agents that combine ganglionic blocking action with peripheral cholinolytic properties has been advanced, and a few pharmacologic and clinical studies were made in this direction. As discussed before, a great number of quaternary salts of atropinelike aminoalkanol esters exhibit both these types of property; however, usually a preponderance of the atropinelike effect exists. Therapeutically used agents that exhibit moderate ganglionic blockade in addition to marked atropinelike actions are methantheline bromide, propantheline bromide, and methylhomatropinium bromide. *p*-Phenylbenzyl-(*dl*-tropyl tropinium)bromide, or gastropin, seems to be the only agent in which both the ganglionic blocking and cholinolytic components are represented in favorable ratio. Satisfactory clinical results were obtained with it (*16*, *461*).

4.6. CONCLUSIONS

Agents that affect the functions of autonomic ganglia are very numerous and fall into the fairly broad category of onium (mostly ammonium) and ionizable amine-type compounds that mimic, potentiate, or inhibit the ganglionic actions of ACh, the neurotransmitter substance. The same general chemical and structural features, however, are also related to actions that influence other, peripheral neural elements sensitive to ACh (postganglionic parasympathetic receptor sites, motor end plates). Further structural requirements, which frequently but not exclusively distinguish ganglionic agents from other cholinergic drugs may be outlined as follows.

Ganglionic stimulants

A. A cationic group containing at least two methyl groups (TMA, DMPP).

B. An alkyl appendage of approximately five carbon atoms (amyltrimethylammonium).

C. An aromatic ether group with suitable electronegative substituents in the nucleus (choline phenylethers).

D. A trimethylammonium, pyrrolidinium, or ionizable amine group attached in a specific structural relation to a pyridine ring moiety (nicotine and analogues, cytisine).

E. A *p*-phenylbenzyl group as the quaternizing moiety, attached to certain stereospecifically characterized cycloalkyl compounds [*p*-phenylbenzyl(*p*-aminobenzoyl-α-tropinium) bromide, N-417].

Ganglionic blocking agents

A. Monoquaternary ammonium compounds: (1) a cationic group with at least two ethyl groups (TEA); (2) α-branched short aliphatic chains in aliphatic or cycloalkyl compounds of certain stereochemical configuration (diethyl- and diisopropylammonium, *N*,*N*-diethyl- and 2,6-dimethylpiperidinium, and tropane compounds); (3) an alkyl quaternizing group of the size of a C_7 to C_9 chain length or *p*-substituted aralkyl quaternizing groups attached to the nitrogen atom of suitably built alicyclic ring systems (tropane, 2,6-dimethylpiperidine compounds).

B. Symmetric bisquaternary compounds: (1) trimethyl, dimethylethyl, or small alicyclic groups forming the terminal cationic groups (hexamethonium, pentolinium); (2) polymethylene or similar flexible connecting chains of five or six carbon atoms (hexamethonium, pentolinium).

C. Asymmetric bisquaternary compounds: (1) a bulky cationic group, i.e., two- or three-ring heterocyclic systems (chlorisondamine); (2) a relatively short connecting chain, i.e., C_2 or C_3 (chlorisondamine).

D. Tertiary and secondary amines, various structures: (1) branched aminoalkane chains [tris-(dialkylaminoalkyl)amines]; (2) α-branched methyl groups in aliphatic or alicyclic amines (pempidine, mecamylamine).

E. Onium compounds other than ammonium, specific steric arrangements and substituents surrounding a sulfonium group (trimetaphan camphorsulfonate).

These cover the most important chemical structural features that are typical of highly potent ganglionic stimulant and blocking agents. The nature of structure–activity studies, however, does not permit the use of such an outline as a set of rules or even of definite guidelines. Each individual class of agents has to be looked upon as an entity of structural complexities. Tropane compounds, whose structure–activity relationships were treated in a more comprehensive fashion, would be a proper example (Table. 4.39). Structural aspects of the drug molecules comprise only the first part of the problems in such studies. The extremely complex series of events that represent functional changes in the living tissue are still very much beyond our comprehension. The few biological parameters that can be analyzed with the existing methods give only superficial information, often really inadequate for relating even the structural changes to the "effect," since the effect is often far from being equivalent to the product of the kinetic interactions between the drug and receptor. This inherent difficulty cannot be resolved at present, and structure–activity studies based on the information so far available have proceeded toward the solving of basic relationships between drug and receptor molecules by small and often indirect steps.

The oversimplified, practical approach to exploring the biological activity of ganglionic stimulant and blocking agents is similar to that used in the study of other classes of drugs and consists of determining potency in a few limited test preparations and selectivity, again with the use of only a few organs or receptor types. Biological exploration of this scope merely allows classification of the pharmacologic agents.

Most of the structure–activity studies conducted with ganglionic stimulant and blocking agents have hardly allowed our present knowledge to exceed this classifying stage. Nevertheless, proper classification itself is significant for further exploration. Pharmacologic studies so far indicate that many ganglionic stimulant and blocking agents primarily affect autonomic ganglia as distinguished from other nonnervous and nervous tissue elements. A further degree of separation of the possible sites of action is available through the numerous studies that have proved that these agents substitute, release, or inhibit ACh at autonomic ganglionic sites. However, these agents do not influence the activity of ACh at other nerve elements, or they do so to a much smaller degree.

Thus, a relatively high selectivity of most of these agents toward cholinergic ganglionic receptor sites, as distinguished from cholinergic nonganglionic and noncholinergic ganglionic sites, is now known. This feature is of obvious theoretical and practical interest and can be utilized in future studies aiming at the exploration of ganglionic functions and of new therapeutic agents. Structural changes in ganglionic drugs, no matter how delicate, have nevertheless not been able to yield selective stimulant or blocking agents at sympathetic ganglia rather than at parasympathetic ganglia or at a particular set of ganglia of one division. It seems that the drug–receptor interactions at the surface of all autonomic ganglion cells are extremely similar. The expected therapeutically important selectivity toward one group of ganglia can thus be approached through utilizing extraganglional biological factors, that is, transport and penetration to active sites. The reason why not much success has been achieved in producing selectively acting agents according to these criteria seems to be that structural requirements influencing these factors have practically not been explored. To find structures that will provide for optimal access to one site and not to another while retaining high activity at the ganglionic receptors is a rather demanding proposition. Nevertheless, it seems to be the most reasonable avenue to developing selective agents for certain groups of autonomic ganglia.

It is also recognized that there is more than one type of ganglionic receptor site. ACh, the neurotransmitter substance, seems to act at two different kinds of ganglionic receptor, of which one resembles the postganglionic parasympathetic receptor sites. These latter ones may have only limited significance.

Besides the ACh-sensitive receptor sites, however, there are other ganglionic sites that are highly sensitive to biogenic amines other than ACh. These amines, although not liberated at the presynaptic nerve endings, are available to the ganglionic cells at various concentrations, depending on other factors. Their modulatory, secondary role in ganglionic transmission should therefore not be dismissed. Pathologic changes in these modifying influences may lead to alterations of ganglionic transmissions that could be influenced, for example, by new classes of ganglionic blocking agents of the noncholinergic type.

LIST OF CHEMICAL FORMULAS

1.
$$\begin{array}{l} \qquad\quad\;\; \text{—CH—} \\ \qquad\qquad\;\; | \\ \text{Aryl-CH}_2\overset{}{\text{N}}^{+}\text{CH}_3 \text{ (or } C_2H_5) \cdot X^- \\ \qquad\qquad\;\; | \\ \qquad\quad\;\; \text{—CH—} \end{array}$$

2. 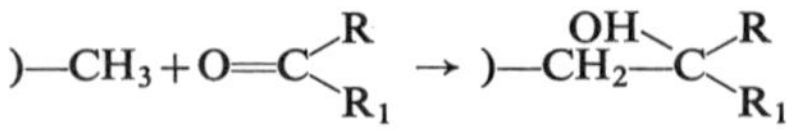

3. 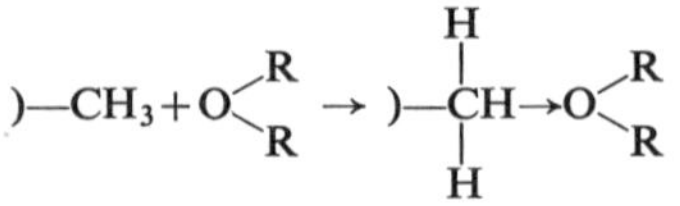

4. 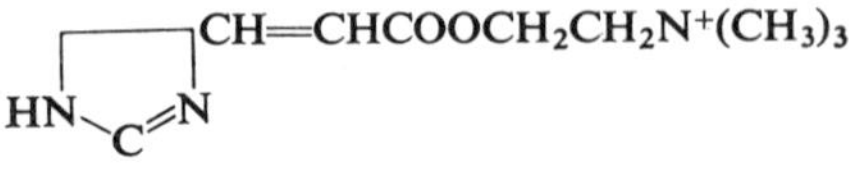

5. 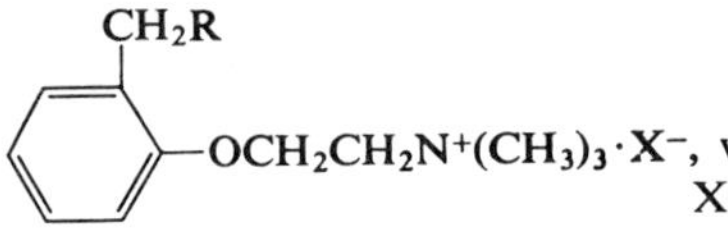 where $R = C_6H_5$, $p\text{-}FC_6H_4$ and 2-thienyl, X = halogen

6. 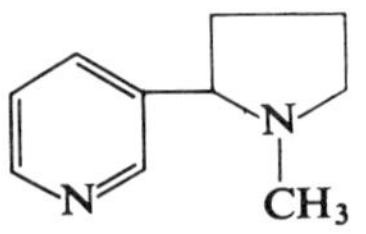

Nicotine

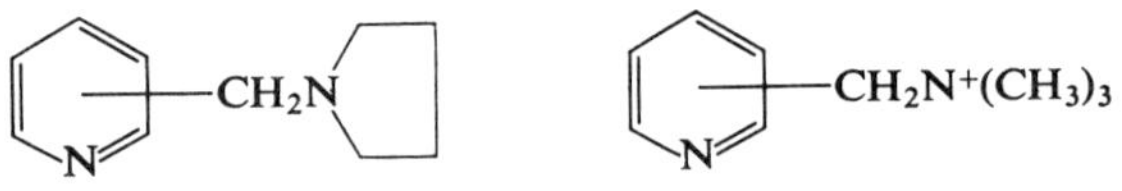

Potent synthetic derivatives

7. 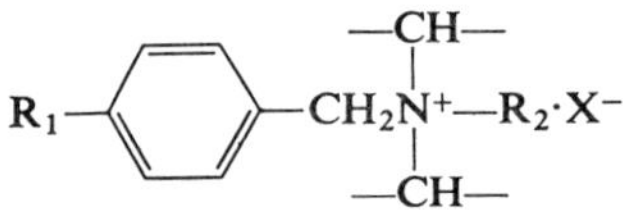

8. 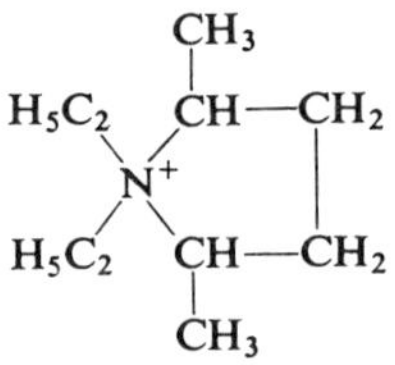

1,1-Diethyl-2,5-dimethylpyrrolidinium ion

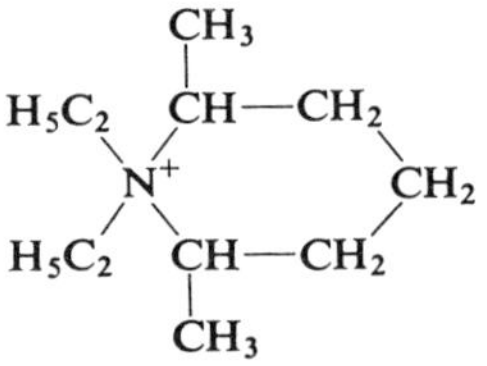

1,1-Diethyl-2,6-dimethylpiperidinium ion

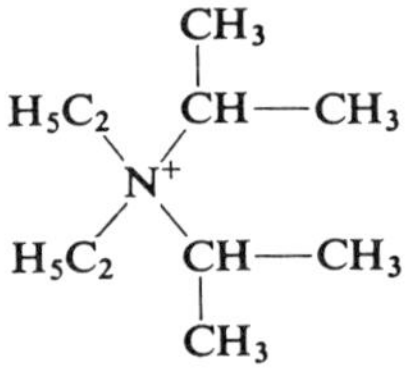

Diethyl, diisopropyl ammonium ion

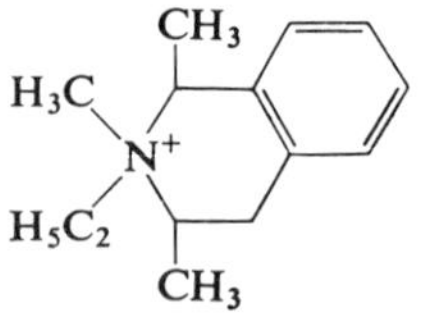

N-Ethyl-*N*-methyl-1,3-dimethyltetrahydroisoquinolinium ion

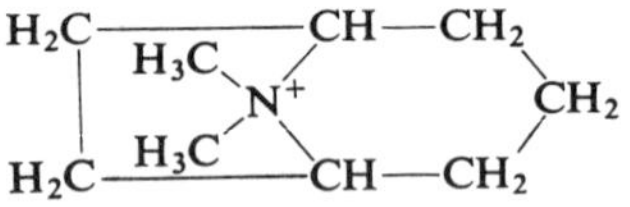

N-Methyltropanium ion

9. 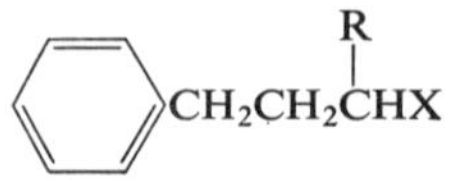

10. 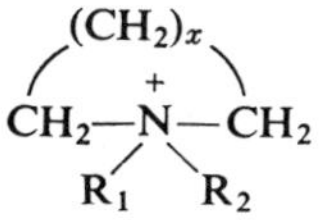

11. RR_1COO-Alkyl-NR_2R_3

12. $RR_1COOC_2H_4R_2$ $\quad$ $R_2 = N^+R_3$

$N^+(i\text{-}C_3H_7)_2R_3$

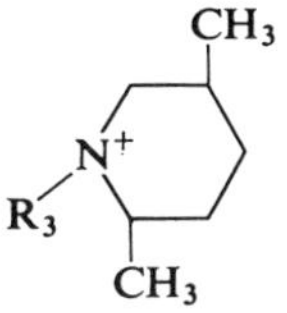

13. 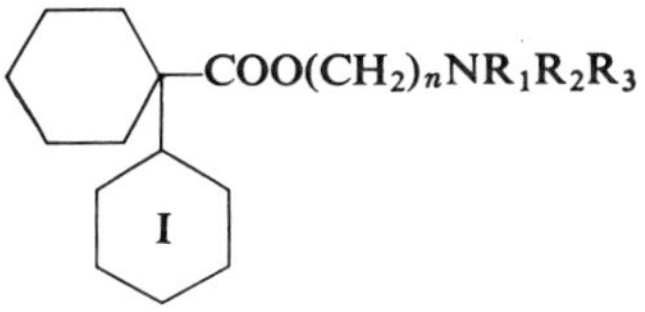

14. 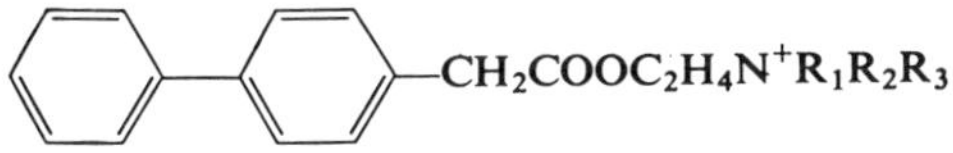

15. 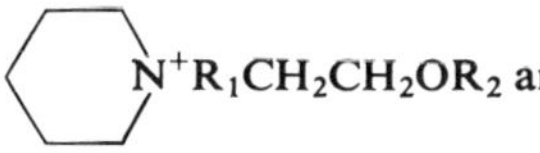 and $(R_1)_3NCH_2CH_2OR_2$

16. 

17. $ArNHCO(CH_2)_nNR_1R_2R_3$ where Ar=

R_1R_2=alkyl or cycloalkyl

R_3=H or alkyl

n=1–3

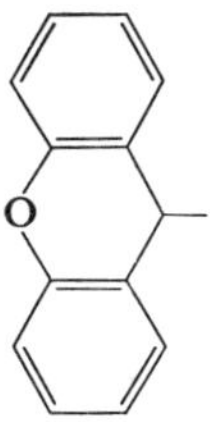

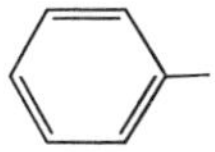

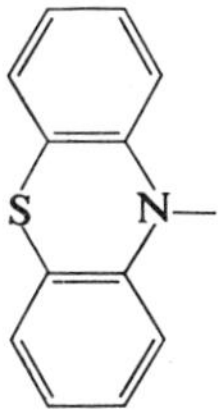

18. 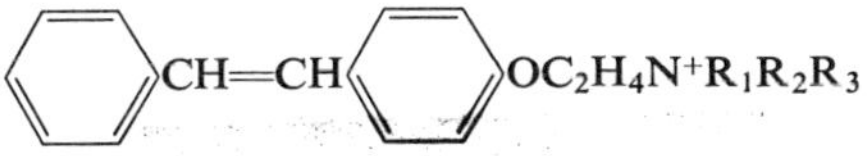

19. 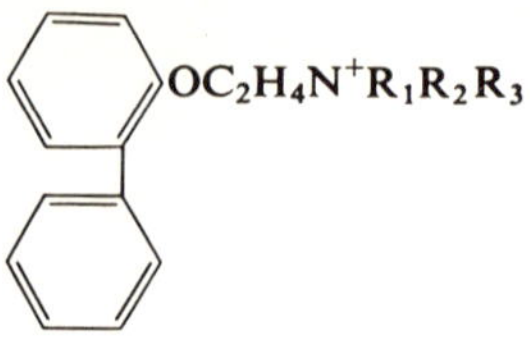

20. 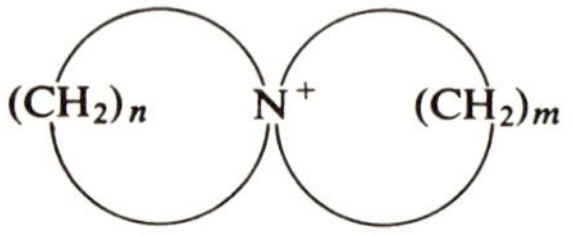 where $n = 4–6$, $m = 4–8$

21. 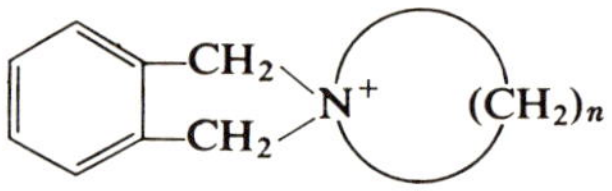 where $n = 6–8$

22. 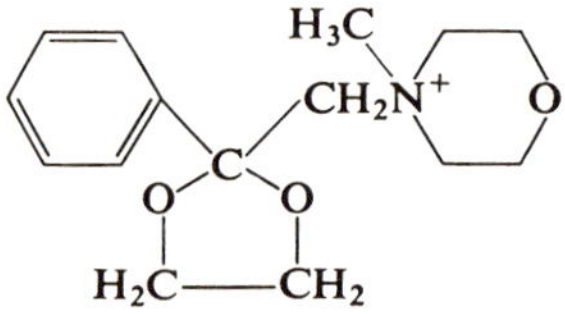

23. 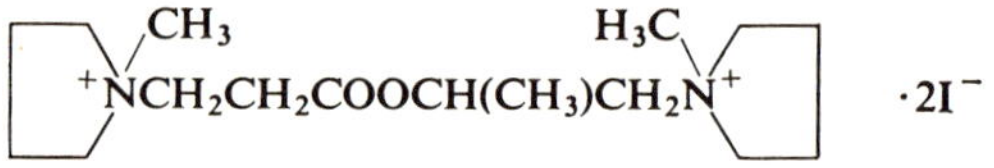

24. 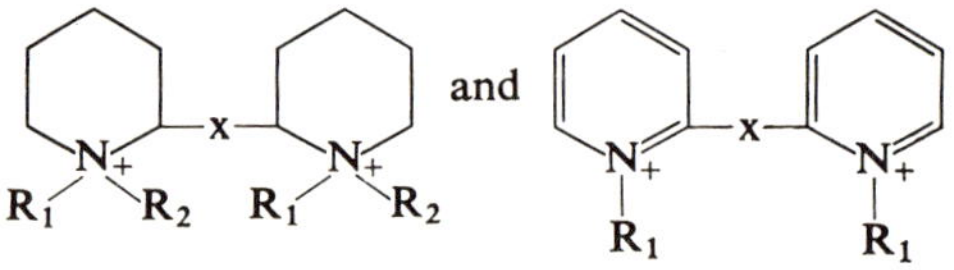 where R_1 and R_2 are methyl or ethyl x = O or $(CH_2)_n$

25. 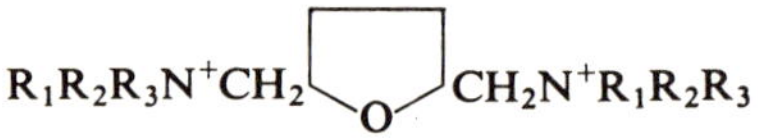 where R_1 = methyl; R_2, R_3 = methyl or ethyl groups

26. $R_1R_2R_3N(CH_2)_nN(CH_3)(CH_2)_nNR_1R_2R_3 \cdot 2Br$

27. $R(CH_2)_nN^+(CH_3)_2(CH_2)_{2-3}N^+(CH_3)_3$ R = 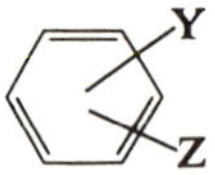

28. 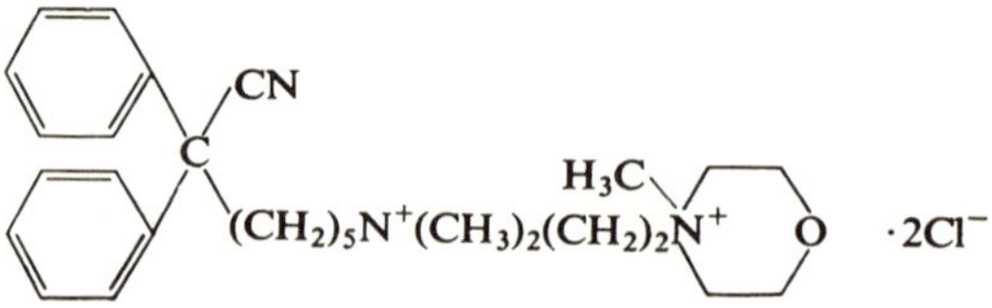

29.

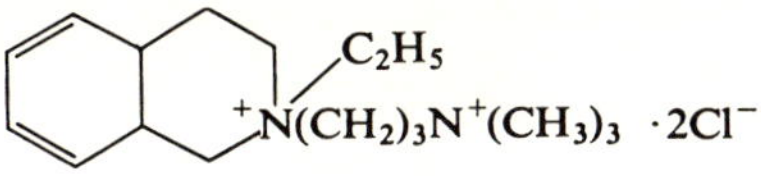

30.

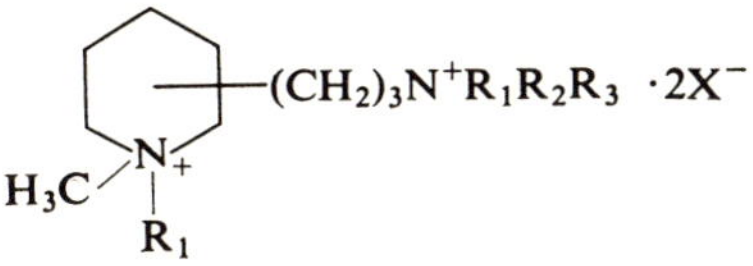

31.

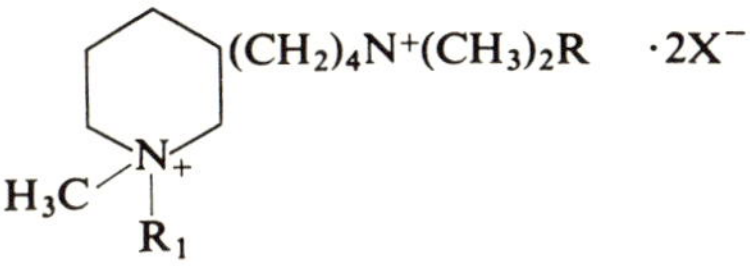

32.

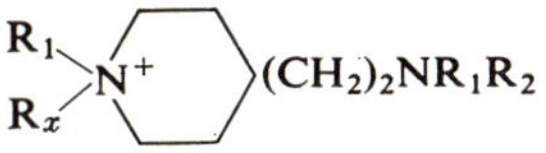

33.

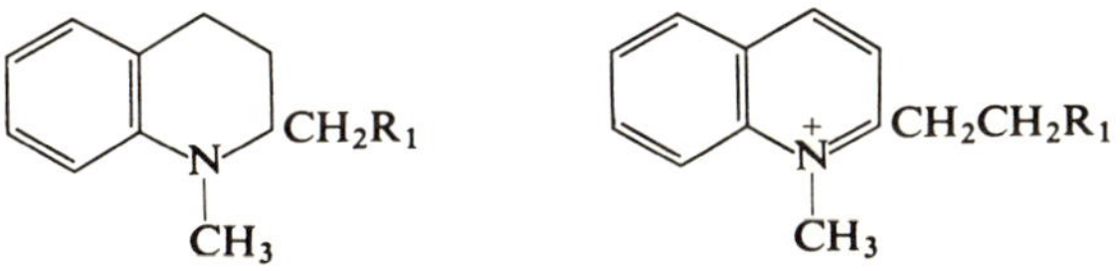

34.

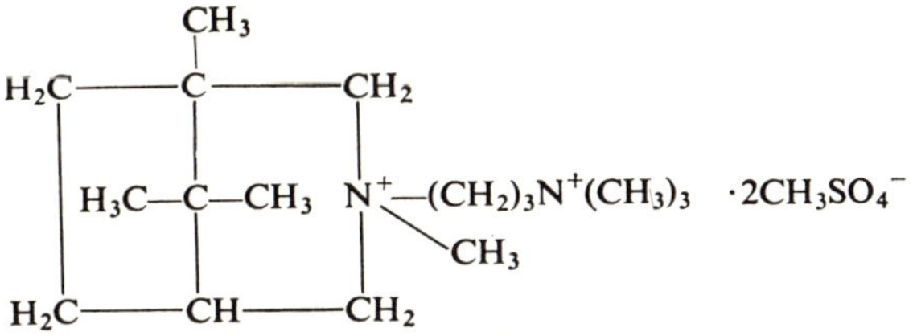

35.

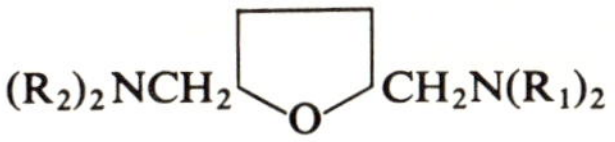

where $R_1 = CH_3$, C_2H_5, C_3H_7; $R_2 = CH_3$–C_4H_9

36.

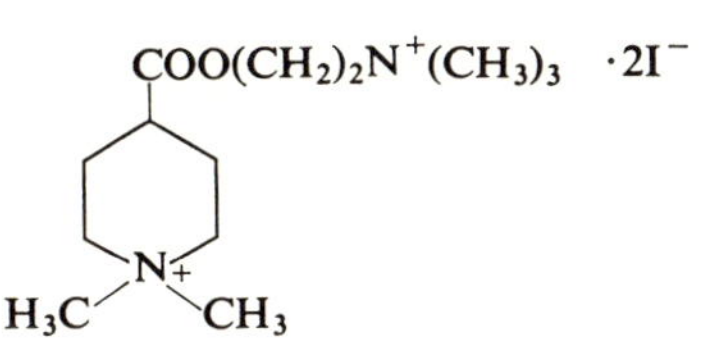

37.

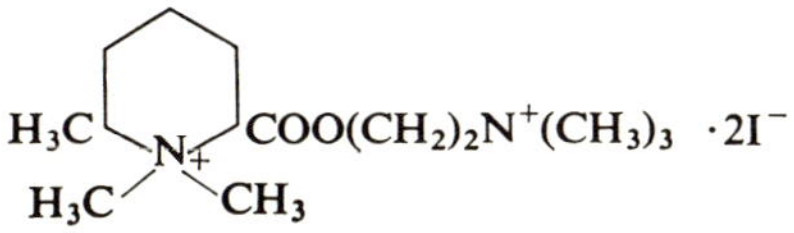

38. 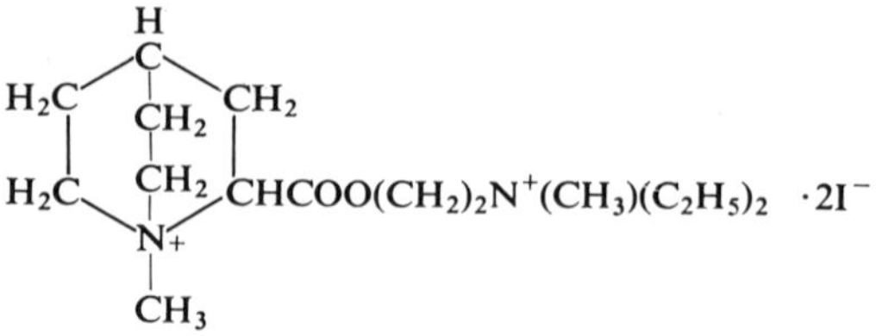

39. 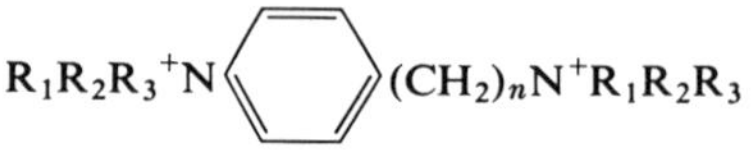

40. 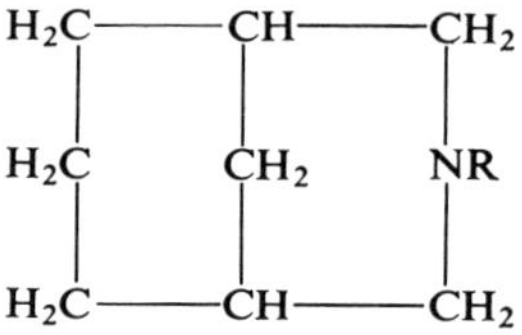

41. 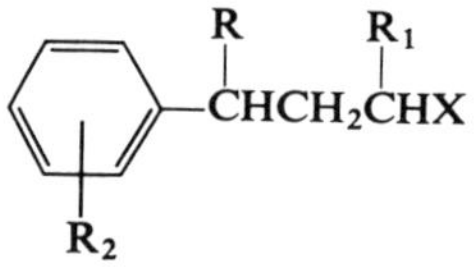

42. 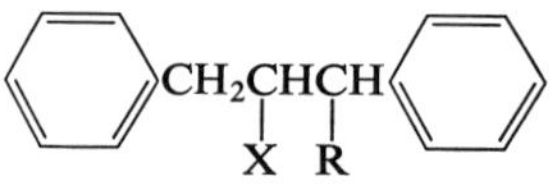

43. 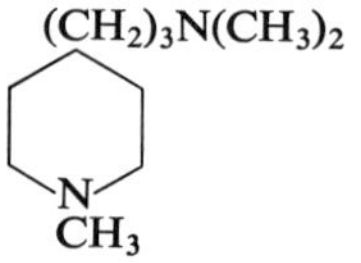

44. 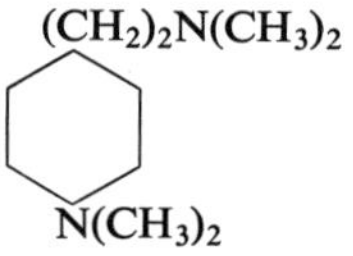

45. 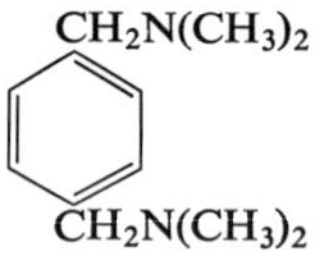

46. 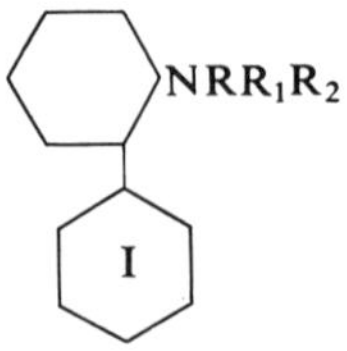

47. 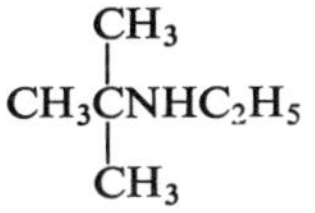 No. 25645

48. 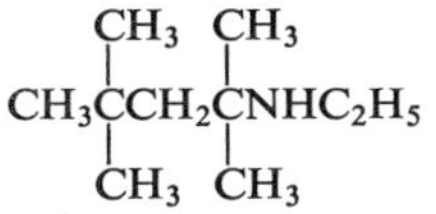 No. 25635

49. 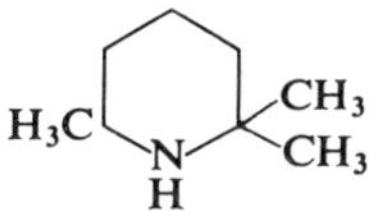 No. 26725

50. 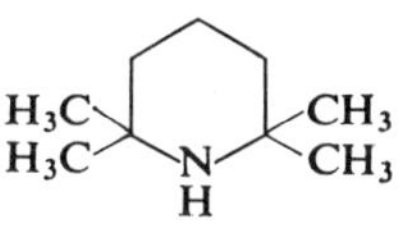 No. 25636

51. 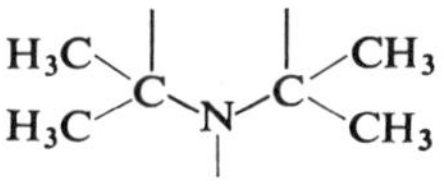

52. 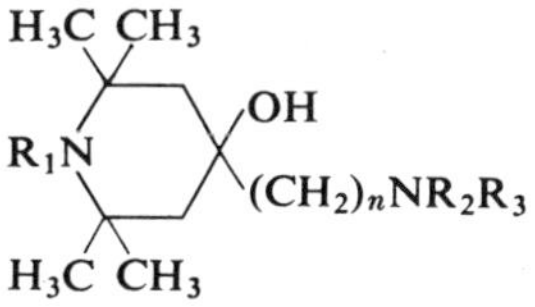

REFERENCES

1. J. C. Eccles, *The Physiology of Synapses*, Academic Press, New York, 1964.
2. G. H. Acheson and G. K. Moe, *J. Pharmacol. Exptl. Therap.*, **87**, 220 (1946).
3. A. Rosenblueth, *The Transmission of Nerve Impulses at Neuroeffector Junctions and Peripheral Synapses*, Wiley, New York, 1950.
4. R. M. Eccles and B. Libet, *J. Physiol.* (*London*), **157**, 484 (1961).
5. G. B. Koelle, *Nature*, **190**, 208 (1961).
6. R. L. Volle, *J. Pharmacol. Exptl. Therap.*, **135**, 54 (1962).
7. N. Ambache, W. L. M. Perry, and P. A. Robertson, *Brit. J. Pharmacol.*, **11**, 442 (1956).
8. A. P. Roszkowski, *J. Pharmacol. Exptl. Therap.*, **132**, 156 (1961).
9. W. D. M. Paton, *Ann. Rev. Physiol.*, **20**, 431 (1958).
10. W. L. M. Perry, *Ann. Rev. Physiol.*, **18**, 279 (1956).
11. H. Konzett and E. Rothlin, *Experientia*, **9**, 405 (1953).
12. U. Trendelenburg, *Ann. Rev. Pharmacol.*, **1**, 219 (1961).
13. U. Trendelenburg, *Federation Proc.*, **18**, 1001 (1959).
14. E. J. Ariëns and A. M. Simonis, *J. Pharm. Pharmacol.*, **16**, 137 (1964).
15. R. B. Barlow, *Biochem. Soc. Symp.*, **19**, 46 (1960).

16. K. Nádor, *Progr. Drug Res.*, **2**, 303 (1960).
17. C. J. Cavallito and A. P. Gray, *Progr. Drug Res.*, **2**, 135 (1960).
18. M. Guggenheim, *Die biogenen Amine*, Karger, Basel, 1940, p. 138.
19. D. Bovet and F. Bovet-Nitti, *Structure et activité pharmacodinamique des médicaments du systéme nerveux végétatif*, Karger, Basel, 1948, p. 366.
20. L. E. Craig, *Chem. Rev.*, **42**, 285 (1948).
21. C. Heymans, *Arch. Intern. Physiol.*, **59**, 561 (1951).
22. L. Gyermek, *Mod. Hosp.*, **92**, 122 (1959).
23. R. Wien, *Progr. Med. Chem.*, **1**, 53 (1961).
24. P. F. D'Arcy and E. P. Taylor, *J. Pharm. Pharmacol.*, **14**, 129 (1962).
25. E. Schlittler, J. Druey, and A. Marxer, *Progr. Drug Res.*, **4**, 306 (1962).
26. A. N. Brest and J. H. Moyer, *Angiology*, **14**, 64 (1963).
27. G. K. Moe and W. A. Freyburger, *Pharmacol. Rev.*, **2**, 61 (1950).
28. N. Ambache, *Pharmacol. Rev.*, **7**, 467 (1955).
29. L. Gyermek, Habilitation dissertation, Budapest, 1954 (in Hungarian).
30. L. Gyermek and K. Nador, *J. Pharm. Pharmacol.*, **9**, 209 (1957).
31. A. S. Spinks, E. H. P. Young, J. A. Farrington, and D. Dunlop, *Brit. J. Pharmacol.*, **13**, 501 (1958).
32. M. Guyonneau, *J. Physiol (Paris)*, **54** (Suppl. IV), 1 (1962).
33. L. Gyermek, in *Heffters Handbuch der exp. Pharmakologie Ergänswk.*, Vol. XIX (Erspamer, ed.), Springer, Heidelberg, 1964, p. 471.
34. W. L. M. Perry, *Brit. Med. Bull.*, **13**, 220 (1957).
35. A. Lundberg, *Acta Physiol. Scand.*, **26**, 254 (1952).
36. E. Costa, A. M. Revzin, R. Kuntzman, S. Spector, and B. B. Brodie, *Science*, **133**, 1822 (1961).
37. E. Muscholl and M. Vogt, *J. Physiol (London)*, **141**, 132 (1958).
38. H. Reinert, *J. Physiol. (London)*, **167**, 18 (1963).
39. J. C. Eccles, *J. Physiol. (London)*, **85**, 179 (1935).
40. C. Takeshige and R. L. Volle, *J. Pharmacol. Exptl. Therap.*, **141**, 206 (1963).
41. C. Takeshige and R. L. Volle, *Brit. J. Pharmacol.*, **23**, 80 (1964).
42. R. L. Volle, *J. Pharmacol. Exptl. Therap.*, **136**, 68 (1962).
43. R. L. Volle, *J. Pharmacol. Exptl. Therap.*, **135**, 45 (1962).
44. S. Ehrenpreis, *Georgetown Med. Bull.*, **16**, 148 (1963).
45. F. Bergel, *J. Pharm. Pharmacol.*, **3**, 385 (1951).
46. K. Nádor and L. Gyermek, *Acta Chim. Acad. Sci. Hung.*, **2**, 95 (1952).
47. P. E. B. Holmes, D. J. Jenden, and D. B. Taylor, *Nature*, **159**, 86 (1947).
48. J. Fakstorp and J. G. A. Pedersen, *Acta Pharmacol. Toxicol.*, **14**, 148 (1957).
49. J. Fakstorp, J. G. A. Pedersen, E. Poulsen, and M. Schilling, *Acta Pharmacol. Toxicol.*, **13**, 52 (1957).
50. E. W. Gill and H. R. Ing, *J. Chem. Soc.*, **(1958)**, 4728.
51. F. G. Canepa, *Nature*, **195**, 573 (1962).
52. A. W. Kibjakow, *Pflinger Arch.*, **232**, 432 (1933).
53. W. Feldberg and A. Vartiainen, *J. Physiol. (London)*, **83**, 103 (1935).
54. H. Konzett and E. Rothlin, *Helv. Physiol. Pharmacol. Acta*, **7**, 46 (1949).
55. H. Kewitz, *Arch. Exptl. Pathol. Pharmakol.*, **222**, 323 (1954).
56. H. Kewitz and H. Reinert, *Arch. Exptl. Phatol. Pharmakol.*, **215**, 547 (1952).
57. S. B. Gertner, *Nature*, **183**, 750 (1959).
58. R. L. Volle, *J. Pharmacol. Exptl. Therap.*, **135**, 45 (1962).
59. M. G. Larrabee and D. A. Holaday, *J. Pharmacol. Exptl. Therap.*, **105**, 400 (1952).
60. R. C. Elliott and J. P. Quilliam, *Brit. J. Pharmacol.*, **23**, 222 (1964).

61. J. P. Quilliam and D. G. Shand, *Brit. J. Pharmacol.*, **23**, 273 (1964).
62. E. Hertzler, *Brit. J. Pharmacol.*, **17**, 406 (1961).
63. H. Giono and L. Chevillard, *Compt. Rend. Soc. Biol.*, **156**, 1048 (1962).
64. J. A. Bevan, *J. Pharmacol. Exptl. Therap.*, **140**, 193 (1963).
65. G. A. Bentley and J. R. Sabine, *Brit. J. Pharmacol.*, **21**, 190 (1963).
66. E. Kreppel, *Med. Exp.*, **7**, 223 (1962).
67. D. A. Kharkevich, *Byul. Eksperim. Biol. Med.*, **49**, 62 (1960); through *CA*, **55**, 14710 (1961).
68. G. P. Shafer, *J. Pharmacol. Exptl. Therap.*, **67**, 341 (1939).
69. L. Gyermek, *Am. J. Physiol.*, **204**, 68 (1963).
70. R. C. Ursillo and B. B. Clark, *J. Pharmacol. Exptl. Therap.*, **114**, 54 (1955).
71. L. Gyermek, *Am. J. Physiol.*, **201**, 325 (1961).
72. G. Stille and H. Hilfiker, *Arch. Intern. Pharmacodyn.*, **130**, 211 (1961) (in German).
73. G. R. Chandrasekhar, L. F. Soyka, and L. Gyermek, *Physiologist*, **2**, 23 (1959).
74. L. Gyermek, *Arch. Intern. Pharmacodyn.*, **137**, 137 (1962).
75. L. Gyermek, *Arch. Intern. Pharmacodyn.*, **150**, 570 (1964).
76. L. Gyermek, *J. Med. Pharm. Chem.*, **7**, 280 (1964).
77. D. Della Bella, F. Rognoni, and U. N. Teotino, *J. Pharm. Pharmacol.*, **14**, 701 (1962).
78. G. A. Thomas and J. R. Trounce, *Guy's Hosp. Rept.*, **109**, 21 (1960).
79. W. D. M. Paton and E. J. Zaimis, *Brit. J. Pharmacol.*, **4**, 381 (1949).
80. R. Wien and D. F. J. Mason, *Lancet* **1953–I**, 454.
81. M. Day and J. R. Vane, *Brit. J. Pharmacol.*, **20**, 150 (1963).
82. J. Harry, *Brit. J. Pharmacol.*, **20**, 399 (1963).
83. J. Levy, N. Mathieu, and E. Michel-Ber, *J. Physiol.* (*Paris*), **50**, 1043 (1958).
84. J. A. Schneider and R. F. Moore, Jr., *Proc. Soc. Exptl. Biol. Med.*, **89**, 450 (1955).
85. F. A. De Florida, J. Cato, L. Ramirez, and E. G. Pardo, *J. Pharmacol. Exptl. Therap.*, **129**, 433 (1960).
86. L. Gyermek and K. Nádor, unpublished, 1953.
87. K. C. Wong and J. P. Long, *Pharmacol. Exptl. Therap.*, **137**, 70 (1962).
88. P. Hey, *Brit. J. Pharmacol.*, **7**, 117 (1952).
89. J. H. Welsh and R. Taub, *J. Pharmacol. Exptl. Therap.*, **99**, 334 (1950).
89a. W. E. Ormerod, *Brit. J. Pharmacol.*, **11**, 267 (1956).
90. H. R. Ing, *Science*, **109**, 264 (1949).
91. H. H. Dale, *J. Pharmacol. Exptl. Therap.*, **6**, 147 (1914).
92. J. H. Burn and H. H. Dale, *J. Pharmacol. Exptl. Therap.*, **6**, 417 (1914).
93. J. A. B. Gray and J. Diamond, *Brit. Med. Bull.*, **13**, 185 (1957).
94. L. Gyermek and L. Sztanyik, *Kiserl. Orvostud.*, **4**, 241 (1952).
95. L. Gyermek and K. Nádor, *Pharmazie*, **10**, 238 (1955).
96. M. Penna and D. M. Aviado, *Arch. Intern. Pharmacodyn.*, **140**, 269 (1962).
97. E. Göres, *Arch. Exptl. Pathol. Pharmakol.*, **236**, 1 (1959).
98. R. Schneider and A. R. Timms, *Brit. J. Pharmacol.*, **12**, 30 (1957).
99. L. György, J. Porszász, and E. Zsigmond, *Acta Phys. Acad. Sci. Hung.*, **10**, 113 (1956).
100. S. Loewe and S. L. Puttuck, *Arch. Exptl. Pathol. Pharmakol.*, **215**, 525 (1952).
101. J. H. Burn, E. H. Leach, M. J. Rand, and J. W. Thompson, *J. Physiol.* (*London*), **148**, 332 (1959).
102. A. Bucknell and B. Whitney, *J. Physiol.* (*London*), **172**, 50–51 (1964).
103. J. Weis, *Acta Pharmacol. Toxicol.*, **19**, 121 (1962).
104. A. B. Wilson, *J. Pharm. Pharmacol.*, **14**, 700 (1962).
105. J. A. Bevan, T. Hughes, and T. M. Murphy, *Arch. Intern. Pharmacodyn.*, **146**, 285 (1963).
106. S. Schapiro, *Acta Physiol. Scand.*, **52**, 146 (1961).
107. M. Dóda, O. Fehér, L. György, and K. Nádor, *Brit. J. Pharmacol.*, **21**, 10 (1963).

108. R. Hunt, *J. Pharmacol. Exptl. Therap.*, **28**, 367 (1926).
109. R. Hunt and R. R. Renshaw, *J. Pharmacol. Exptl. Therap.*, **25**, 315 (1925).
110. R. Wien, *Brit. J. Pharmacol.*, **7**, 534 (1952).
111. M. J. Dallemagne and E. Philippot, *Arch. Intern. Pharmacodyn.*, **84**, 189 (1950).
112. J. Jacob, I. Marszak, R. Epsztein, M. Olomucki, and J. P. Guermont, *Compt. Rend.*, **237**, 1289 (1953).
113. J. Jacob, I. Marszak, M. Olomucki, and R. Epsztein, *Compt. Rend.*, **238**, 290 (1954).
114. J. Jacob, I. Marszak, R. Epsztein, and J. P. Guermont, *Compt. Rend.*, **234**, 1230 (1952).
115. I. Marszak, J. P. Guermont, R. Epsztein, and J. Jacob, *Compt. Rend.*, **233**, 530 (1951).
116. J. Jacob, I. Marszak, L. Bardisa, A. Marszak-Fleury, and R. Epsztein, *Arch. Intern. Pharmacodyn.*, **91**, 303 (1952).
117. I. Marszak, R. Epsztein, and J. Jacob, *Compt. Rend.*, **231**, 1578 (1950).
118. R. Hunt and R. R. Renshaw, *J. Pharmacol. Exptl. Therap.*, **29**, 17 (1926).
119. R. Hunt and R. R. Renshaw, *J. Pharmacol. Exptl. Therap.*, **35**, 99 (1929).
120. P. Holton and R. H. Ing, *Brit. J. Pharmacol.*, **4**, 190 (1949).
121. G. L. Willey, *Brit. J. Pharmacol.*, **10**, 466 (1955).
122. A. M. Lands and C. J. Cavallito, *J. Pharmacol. Exptl. Therap.*, **110**, 369 (1954).
123. I. Marszak, A. Marszak-Fleury, J. Jacob, and G. Montezin, *Compt. Rend.*, **231**, 186 (1950).
124. H. Kreitmair, *Arch. Exptl. Pathol. Pharmakol.*, **164**, 346 (1932).
125. K. B. Augustinsson, T. Fredriksson, A. Sundwall, and G. Jonsson, *Biochem. Pharmacol.*, **3**, 68 (1959).
126. D. B. Sprinson, *J. Am. Chem. Soc.*, **63**, 2249 (1941).
127. M. Wurzel, A. G. Efird, and L. I. Goldberg, *Arch. Intern. Pharmacodyn.*, **148**, 53 (1964).
128. F. F. Cowan, *Federation Proc.*, **19**, 285 (1960).
129. A. Heusner and H. Wick, *Z. Physiol. Chem.*, **320**, 246 (1960).
130. E. T. Eckhardt and F. W. Schueler, *J. Pharmacol. Exptl. Therap.*, **141**, 345 (1963).
131. U. G. Bijlsma, *Arch. Exptl. Pathol. Pharmakol.*, **241**, 369 (1961).
132. A. A. Sekul and W. C. Holland, *J. Pharmacol. Exptl. Therap.*, **132**, 171 (1961).
133. F. W. Schueler, H. H. Keasling, and R. M. Featherstone, *Science*, **113**, 512 (1951); F. W. Schueler and H. H. Keasling, *J. Pharmacol. Exptl. Therap.*, **103**, 222 (1951).
134. W. B. Bass, F. W. Schueler, R. M. Featherstone, and E. G. Gross, *J. Pharmacol. Exptl. Therap.*, **100**, 465 (1950).
135. F. Brucke, *Pharmacol. Rev.*, **8**, 265 (1956).
136. A. Simonart, *Arch. Intern. Pharmacodyn.*, **48**, 328 (1934).
137. R. Hunt and R. R. Renshaw, *J. Pharmacol. Exptl. Therap.*, **44**, 151 (1932).
139. R. Hunt and R. R. Renshaw, *J. Pharmacol. Exptl. Therap.*, **37**, 193 (1929).
139. J. Jacob, I. Marszak, S. Cruck, and J.-P. Guermont, *Compt. Rend.*, **239**, 1151 (1954).
140. R. Hunt and R. R. Renshaw, *J. Pharmacol. Exptl. Therap.*, **58**, 140 (1936).
141. L. Gyermek, unpublished, 1954.
142. R. Hunt and M. de Taveau, *Publ. Hlth. Hyg. Lab. Bull., Wash.*, **73**, 1 (1911).
143. A. Akcasu, Y. K. Sinha, and G. B. West, *Brit. J. Pharmacol.*, **7**, 331 (1952).
144. R. Hazard, J. R. Boissier, Ch. Malen, and A. Renier-Cornec, *Compt. Rend.*, **249**, 792 (1959).
145. J. Porszász, K. Porszász-Gibiszer, S. Földeák, S. Matkovics, and J. Czombos, *Kiserl. Orvostud.*, **16**, 348 (1964).
146. V. Erspamer and A. Glasser, *Brit. J. Pharmacol.*, **13**, 378 (1958).
147. I. I. A. Tabachnick, F. E. Roth, J. Mershon, A. A. Rubin, E. T. Eckhardt, and W. M. Govier, *J. Pharmacol. Exptl. Therap.*, **123**, 98 (1958).

148. M. M. Winbury, J. K. Wolf, and I. I. A. Tabachnick, *J. Pharmacol. Exptl. Therap.*, **123**, 104 (1958).
149. D. B. Taylor, *Pharmacol. Rev.*, **3**, 412 (1951).
150. R. B. Barlow and J. T. Hamilton, *Brit. J. Pharmacol.*, **18**, 510 (1962).
151. R. B. Barlow and N. A. Dobson, *J. Pharm. Pharmacol.*, **7**, 27 (1955).
152. C. N. Gillis and J. J. Lewis, *J. Pharm. Pharmacol.*, **8**, 46 (1956).
153. G. Chen and R. F. Parcell, *Arch. Intern. Pharmacodyn.*, **97**, 186 (1954).
154. G. Chen, R. Portman, and A. Wickel, *J. Pharmacol. Exptl., Therap.*, **103**, 330 (1951).
155. F. Herr and L. Gyermek, *J. Pharmacol. Exptl. Therap.*, **129**, 338 (1960).
156. J. Sanghvi, S. Murayama, C. M. Smith, and K. R. Unna, *J. Pharmacol. Exptl. Therap.*, **142**, 192 (1963).
157. G. M. Maxwell, G. M. Kneebone, and R. B. Elliott, *Arch. Intern. Pharmacodyn.*, **143**, 431 (1963).
158. J. M. Van Rossum, *J. Pharm. Pharmacol.*, **15**, 285 (1963).
159. H. W. Ling, *Brit. J. Pharmacol.*, **14**, 505 (1959).
160. G. Chen and R. F. Parcell, *Arch. Intern. Pharmacodyn.*, **97**, 186 (1954).
161. A. M. Lands, and S. Archer, *J. Med. Pharm. Chem.*, **2**, 449 (1960).
162. B. Levy and R. P. Ahlquist, *J. Pharmacol. Exptl. Therap.*, **137**, 219 (1962).
163. B. Jones, A. B. Gomez, and U. Trendelenburg, *J. Pharmacol. Exptl. Therap.*, **139**, 312 (1963).
164. G. Brownlee and E. S. Johnson, *Brit. J. Pharmacol.*, **21**, 677 (1962).
165. J. P. Kalbermatten, *Helv. Phys. Acta*, **20**, 294 (1962).
166. J. G. Hilton, *J. Pharmacol. Exptl. Therap.*, **132**, 28 (1961).
167. J. P. Long and J. W. Eckstein, *J. Pharmacol. Exptl. Therap.*, **133**, 216 (1961).
168. D. F. J. Mason, *Brit. J. Pharmacol.*, **18**, 76 (1962).
169. C. Takeshige and R. L. Volle, *Brit. J. Pharmacol.*, **20**, 214 (1963).
170. D. F. J. Mason, *Brit. J. Pharmacol.*, **18**, 572 (1962).
171. P. A. Fenner and J. G. Hilton, *Brit. J. Pharmacol.*, **21**, 323 (1963).
172. K. Minker and M. Koltai, *Acta Phys. Acad. Sci. Hung.*, **20**, 411 (1961).
173. K. Kamijo and G. B. Koelle, *J. Pharmacol. Exptl. Therap.*, **105**, 349 (1952).
174. H. Konzett and P. G. Waser, *Helv. Physiol. Pharmacol. Acta*, **14**, 202 (1956).
175. L. Gyermek, E. B. Sigg, and E. Bindler, *Am. J. Physiol.*, **204**, 68 (1963).
176. L. Gyermek and K. R. Unna, *Proc. Soc. Exptl. Biol. Med.*, **98**, 882 (1958).
177. F. Herr and L. Gyermek, *J. Pharmacol. Exptl. Therap.*, **129**, 338 (1960).
178. U. Trendelenberg, *J. Pharmacol. Exptl. Therap.*, **131**, 65 (1961).
179. I. M. Van Rossum, *Experientia*, **16**, 373 (1960).
180. A. J. Pappano and R. L. Volle, *Life Sciences*, **1**, 677 (1962).
181. S. Murayama and R. K. Unna, *J. Pharmacol. Exptl. Therap.*, **140**, 183 (1963).
182. B. V. Franko, J. W. Ward, and R. S. Alphin, *J. Pharmacol. Exptl. Therap.*, **139**, 25 (1963).
183. A. Jones, *J. Pharmacol. Exptl. Therap.*, **141**, 195 (1963).
184. L. Gyermek, *Nature*, **192**, 465 (1961).
185. L. Gyermek and E. Bindler, *J. Pharm. Exptl. Therap.*, **135**, 344 (1962).
186. L. Gyermek and E. Bindler, *J. Pharm. Exptl. Therap.*, **138**, 150 (1962).
187. L. Gyermek, E. Bindler, and L. Soffer, *Federation Proc.*, **21**, 335 (1962).
188. L. Gyermek and K. R. Unna, *J. Pharmacol. Exptl. Therap.*, **128**, 30 (1960).
189. L. Gyermek and K. R. Unna, *J. Pharmacol. Exptl. Therap.*, **128**, 37 (1960).
190. H. R. Ing, P. Kordick, and D. P. H. T. Williams, *Brit. J. Pharmacol.*, **7**, 103 (1952).
191. U. Schmidt and A. Enders, *Naturwiss.*, **40**, 292 (1953).
192. A. Vartiainen, *J. Pharmacol. Exptl. Therap.*, **54**, 265 (1935).

193. G. Bertaccini and T. Vitali, *J. Pharm. Pharmacol.*, **16**, 441 (1964).
194. V. Erspamer and A. Glasser, *Brit. J. Pharmacol.*, **15**, 14 (1960).
195. M. F. Cuthbert, *Brit. J. Pharmacol.*, **23**, 55 (1964).
196. Z. M. Bacq, *Arch. Intern. Pharmacodyn.*, **52**, 471 (1936).
197. W. C. Bowman and I. S. Sanghvi, *J. Pharm. Pharmacol.*, **15**, 1 (1963).
198. A. H. Friedman and C. M. Smith, *J. Pharmacol. Exptl. Therap.*, **135**, 62 (1962).
199. A. K. Cho, W. L. Haslett, and D. J. Jenden, *J. Pharmacol. Exptl. Therap.*, **138**, 249 (1962).
200. W. C. DeGroot and R. L. Volle, *Life Sciences*, **4**, 618 (1963).
201. W. D. M. Paton and E. J. Zaimis, *Brit. J. Pharmacol.*, **6**, 155 (1951).
202. W. D. M. Paton and W. L. M. Perry, *J. Physiol.* (*London*), **119**, 43 (1953).
203. T. Koppanyi, J. M. Dille, and C. R. Linegar, *J. Pharmacol. Exptl. Therap.*, **58**, 105 (1936).
204. C. Takeshige, A. J. Pappano, W. C. DeGroot, and R. L. Volle, *J. Pharmacol. Exptl. Therap.*, **141**, 333 (1963).
205. O. Fehér, E. Labos, G. Mozsik, and T. Szabo, *Acta Phys. Acad. Sci. Hung.*, **20**, 177 (1961).
206. J. C. Eccles, *J. Physiol.* (*London*), **85**, 207 (1935).
207. E. W. Pelikan, *Ann. N.Y. Acad. Sci.*, **90**, 52 (1960).
208. U. Trendelenburg, *Arch. Exptl. Pathol. Pharmakol.*, **241**, 452 (1961).
209. J. H. van Rossum and E. J. Ariëns, *Arch. Intern. Pharmacodyn.*, **118**, 447 (1959).
210. W. K. Riker and A. Komalahiranya, *J. Pharmacol. Exptl. Therap.*, **137**, 267 (1962).
211. R. J. McIsaac and N. R. Millerschoen, *J. Pharmacol. Exptl. Therap.*, **139**, 18 (1963).
212. G. Bennett, C. Tyler, and E. Zaimis, unpublished results, 1957.
213. C. Bennett, C. Tyler, and E. Zaimis, *Lancet*, **1957–II**, 218.
214. B. L. Ginsborg and S. Guerrero, *J. Physiol.* (*London*), **172**, 189 (1964).
215. D. Gold and H. Reinert, *J. Physiol.* (*London*), **151**, 3 (1960).
216. A. Komalahiranya and R. L. Volle, *J. Pharmacol. Exptl. Therap.*, **139**, 304 (1963).
217. G. Cavallini, P. Montegazza, E. Massarani, and R. Tommasini, *Farmaco.* (*Pavia*) *Ed. Sci.*, **8**, 317 (1953).
218. E. G. Pardo, J. Mendez, R. Vargas, J. Cato, and J. Laguna, *J. Pharmacol. Exptl. Therap.*, **116**, 377 (1956).
219. M. D. Mashkovsky and B. A. Medvedev, *Byul. Eksperim. Biol. Med.*, **49**, 66 (1960); through *CA*, **55**, 8630*f* (1961).
220. A. Spinks, E. H. P. Young, J. A. Farrington, and D. Dunlop, *Brit. J. Pharmacol.*, **13**, 501 (1958).
221. R. Wien and D. F. J. Mason, *Brit. J. Pharmacol.*, **6**, 611 (1951).
222. D. F. J. Mason and R. Wien, *Brit. J. Pharmacol.*, **10**, 124 (1955).
223. J. Garrett, *Arch. Intern. Pharmacodyn.*, **144**, 381 (1963).
224. F. W. Schueler and H. H. Keasling, *J. Am. Pharm. Assoc.*, **43**, 98 (1954).
225. E. Zaimis, *Hypotensive Drugs*, Pergamon, London, 1956.
226. P. Holtz and H. J. Schumann, *Arch. Exptl. Pathol. Pharmakol.*, **229**, 101 (1956).
227. E. G. Pardo, J. Cato, E. Gijon, A. de Florida, *J. Pharmacol. Exptl. Therap.*, **139**, 296 (1963).
228. L. Gyermek, *Acta Phys. Acad. Sci. Hung.*, **8**, 43 (1954).
229. N. B. Vysotskaya, *Farmakol. i Toksikol.*, **25**, 160 (1962).
230. D. A. Brown and J. P. Quilliam, *Brit. J. Pharmacol.*, **23**, 257 (1964).
231. D. A. Brown and J. P. Quilliam, *Brit. J. Pharmacol.*, **23**, 241 (1964).
232. S. J. Corne and H. D. Edge, *Brit. J. Pharmacol.*, **13**, 339 (1958).
233. J. E. Gardiner, *Nature*, **184**, 71 (1959).

234. S. Mawji and M. F. Lockett, *J. Pharm. Pharmacol.*, **15**, 45 (1963).

235. V. V. Kelkar, O. D. Gulati, and S. D. Gakhale, *Arch. Intern. Pharmacodyn.*, **149**, 209 (1964).

236. P. Mantegazza, C. Tyler, and E. Zaimis, *Brit. J. Pharmacol.*, **13**, 480 (1958).

237. A. G. H. Blakeley, G. L. Brown, and C. B. Ferry, *J. Physiol.* (*London*), **167**, 505 (1963).

238. H. Budde and E. Witzleb, *Arch. Intern. Pharmacodyn.*, **102**, 126 (1955).

239. G. K. Moe, L. R. Capo, and R. Braulio Peralta, *Am. J. Physiol.*, **153**, 601 (1948).

240. H. Saito, *Nippon Yakurigaku Zasshi*, **57**, 32 (1961); through *CA*, **56**, 7957*b* (1962).

241. K. Yanagiya, *Nippon Yakurigaku Zasshi*, **56**, 69 (1960); through *CA*, **55**, 21371 (1961).

242. J. V. Luco and J. Marconi, *J. Pharmacol. Exptl. Therap.*, **95**, 171 (1949).

243. R. Marlier, *Arch. Intern. Pharmacodyn.*, **129**, 371 (1960).

244. J. A. Bevan, *J. Pharmacol. Exptl. Therap.*, **140**, 193 (1963).

245. M. R. Gavend, M. Gavend, and J. Mercier, *J. Physiol.* (*Paris*), **52**, 643 (1960).

246. C. A. Stone, K. L. Meckelnburg, and M. L. Torchiana, *Arch. Intern. Pharmacodyn.*, **117**, 419 (1958).

247. H. E. Lape and J. O. Hoppe, *J. Pharmacol. Exptl. Therap.*, **116**, 453 (1956).

248. G. Dastague, M. Lavedrine, G. Costerizant, P. Hospital, and J. C. Moinet, *Trav. Soc. Pharm. Montpellier*, **19**, 30 (1959).

249. G. F. Kareva and Z. P. Senova, *Farmakol. i Toksikol.*, **25**, 434 (1962); through *CA*, **56**, 12246*i* (1962).

250. M. M. Winbury, *J. Pharmacol. Exptl. Therap.*, **105**, 326 (1952).

251. M. M. Winbury, D. L. Cook, and W. E. Hambourger, *Arch. Intern. Pharmacodyn.*, **97**, 125 (1954).

252. D. L. Cook, W. E. Hambourger, and R. G. Bianchi, *J. Pharmacol. Exptl. Therap.*, **99**, 435 (1950).

253. R. A. Robinson, *J. Org. Chem.*, **16**, 1911 (1951).

254. J. Levy and E. M. Ber, *Compt. Rend. Soc. Biol.*, **149**, 1356 (1955).

255. M. H. Pindell, J. K. Finnegan, and J. D. Smith, *J. Med. Pharm. Chem.*, **3**, 167 (1961).

256. L. Gyermek and L. Sztanyik, *Acta Phys. Acad. Sci. Hung.*, **2**, 41 (1951).

257. L. Gyermek, *Acta Phys. Acad. Sci. Hung.*, **2**, 175 (1951).

258. J. W. Cusic and R. A. Robinson, *J. Org. Chem.*, **16**, 1921 (1951).

259. L. Gyermek, E. Kasztreiner, and K. Nádor, *Acta Phys. Acad. Sci. Hung.*, **5**, (Suppl.), 41 (1954).

260. J. G. Bainbridge and D. M. Brown, *Brit. J. Pharmacol.*, **15**, 147 (1960).

261. M. Guyonneau, *Med. Exp.*, **6**, 245 (1962).

262. K. Formanek and W. Weis, *Arzneimittel-Forsch.*, **13**, 66 (1963).

263. F. W. Schueler and H. H. Keasling, *J. Am. Pharm. Assoc.*, **43**, 98 (1954).

264. I. M. Sharapov, *Pharmacol. Toxicol.* (*USSR*) (*English Transl.*), **20**, 501 (1957); through Ref. *17*.

265. U. V. Samvelyan, *Izv. Akad. Nauk. Arm. SSR, Biol. Nauk.*, **16**, 41 (1963).

266. A. I. Popa, *Acad. Rep. Populare Romine, Studii Cercetari Fiziol.*, **8**, 125 (1963).

267. E. B. Sigg, *Toxicol. Appl. Pharmacol.*, **5**, 225 (1963).

268. A. Lespagnol, R. Hazard, A. Renier-Cornec, C. Lespagnol, and J.-C. Cazin, *Compt. Rend.*, **252**, 808 (1961).

269. R. Hazard and A. Renier-Cornec, *Compt. Rend. Soc. Biol.*, **154**, 533 (1960).

270. V. M. Vinogradov, *Tr. Leningr. Khim.-Farmatsevt. Inst.*, **13**, 193 (1961).

271. J. W. Cusic, U.S. Pat. 2,627,517 (1953).

272. R. O. Clinton and S. Laskowski, U.S. Pat. 2,642,434 (1953).

273. J. W. Cusic, U.S. Pat. 2,714,594.

274. U. Schaeppi and P. Waser, *Arzneimittel-Forsch.*, **8**, 107 (1958).

275. W. W. Jenkins, U.S. Pat. 2,673,873 (1954).
276. W. D. M. Paton and J. W. Thompson, *Brit. J. Pharmacol.*, **22**, 143 (1964).
277. R. C. Ursillo and B. B. Clark, *J. Pharmacol. Exptl. Therap.*, **114**, 54 (1955).
278. J. W. Cusic, U.S. Pat. 2,715,645 (1955).
279. J. H. Burn and H. Froede, *Brit. J. Pharmacol.*, **20**, 378 (1963).
280. K. A. Exley, *Brit. J. Pharmacol.*, **12**, 297 (1957).
281. E. Bülbring and F. Depierre, *Brit. J. Pharmacol.*, **4**, 22 (1949).
282. J. Jacob and F. Depierre, *Arch. Intern. Pharmacodyn.*, **83**, 1 (1950).
283a. J. Fakstorp and J. G. A. Pedersen, *Acta Pharmacol. Toxicol.*, **13**, 359 (1957).
283b. S. L. Friess, L. J. Reber, W. C. Thommesen, L. J. Greenbaum, F. G. Standaert, and W. V. Hudak, *Toxicol. Appl. Pharmacol.*, **2**, 574 (1960).
284. S. Archer and M. R. Bell, U.S. Pat. 3,058,984 (1962).
285. S. Murayama and K. R. Unna, *Federation Proc.*, **21**, 322 (1962).
286. I. H. Page and F. Olmsted, *Am. J. Physiol.*, **204**, 582 (1963).
287. L. Gyermek, *Acta Phys. Acad. Sci. Hung.*, **2**, 511 (1951).
288. L. F. Soyka and K. R. Unna, *Federation Proc.*, **20**, 307 (1961).
289. L. D. Fink and P. Cervoni, *J. Pharmacol. Exptl. Therap.*, **109**, 372 (1953).
290. H. Wick and A. Engelhardt, *Arzneimittel-Forsch.*, **7**, 217 (1957).
291. L. F. Soyka and L. Gyermek, *J. Med. Pharm. Chem.*, **2**, 361 (1960).
292. L. Hermann, F. H. Shaw, and E. J. Rosenblum, *J. Pharm. Pharmacol.* **10**, 348 (1958).
293. H. Wick, *Arch. Exptl. Pathol. Pharmakol.*, **213**, 485 (1951).
294. A. M. Kunkel, J. H. Wills, and A. H. Dikemus, *Proc. Soc. Exptl. Biol. Med.*, **96**, 791 (1957).
295. L. Gyermek and K. Nador, *Arch. Intern. Pharmacodyn.*, **113**, 1 (1957).
296. B. Issekutz, *Arch. Exptl. Pathol. Pharmakol.*, **215**, 283 (1952).
297. L. Gyermek and K. Nador, *Acta Phys. Acad. Sci. Hung.*, **4**, 341 (1953).
298. M. Doda, L. Gyorgy, and K. Nador, *Arch. Intern. Pharmacodyn.*, **145**, 264 (1963).
299. L. Decsi, M. K. Varszegi, and K. Nador, *Arzneimittel-Forsch.*, **13**, 776 (1963).
300. J. D. Robertson, J. Gillis, and K. E. V. Spencer, *Brit. J. Anaesthesia*, **29**, 342 (1957).
301. T. J. Haley, A. M. Flesher, N. Komesu, and E. Lee, *Arch. Intern. Pharmacodyn.*, **144**, 555 (1963).
302. K. Vidal-Beretervide and M. Monti, *Arzneimittel-Forsch.*, **13**, 452 (1963).
303. E. Rothlin, M. Taeschler, H. Konzett, and A. Cerletti, *Experientia*, **10**, 142 (1954).
304. Y. Shuster, *Sb. Nauchn. Rabot, Rizhskii Med. Inst.*, **11**, 155 (1961); through *CA*, **58**, 10626*f* (1963).
305. F. F. Blicke and E. B. Hotelling, *J. Am. Chem. Soc.*, **76**, 5099 (1954).
306. K. Vidal-Beretervide and M. Monti, *Med. Exp.*, **11**, 1 (1964).
307. R. Kadatz and H. Klupp, *Arch. Exptl. Pathol. Pharmakol.*, **227**, 382 (1956).
308. R. B. Barlow and H. R. Ing, *Nature*, **161**, 718 (1948).
309. L. Beani, C. Bianchi, G. Bieber, and F. Ledda, *J. Pharm. Pharmacol.*, **16**, 557 (1964).
310. E. Minker and M. Koltai, *Acta Phys. Acad. Sci. Hung.*, **20**, 187 (1961).
311. W. Feldberg, *J. Physiol.* (*London*), **113**, 483 (1951).
312. J. G. Blackman and R. Laverty, *Brit. J. Pharmacol.*, **17**, 124 (1961).
313. B. Juhász, B. Szegedi, and M. Gertner, *Acta Phys. Acad. Sci. Hung.*, **21**, 225 (1962).
314. D. R. Laurence and R. S. Stacey, *Brit. J. Pharmacol.*, **7**, 80 (1952).
315. S. J. Corne and N. D. Edge, *Brit. J. Pharmacol.*, **13**, 339 (1958).
316. J. H. Burn and W. R. Gibbons, *Brit. J. Pharmacol.*, **22**, 549 (1964).
317. K. B. Lum and L. Rashleigh, *J. Pharmacol. Exptl. Therap.*, **132**, 13 (1961).
318. P. Mantegazza, C. Tyler, and E. Zaimis, *Brit. J. Pharmacol.*, **13**, 480 (1958).

319. J. G. Blackman, F. M. Fastier, C. M. Patel, and L. C. K. Wong, *Brit. J. Pharmacol.*, **11**, 282 (1956).
320. L. Gyermek, *Acta Phys. Acad. Sci. Hung.*, **5**, 163 (1954).
321. K. Horiuchi, *Nippon Yakurigaku Zasshi*, **56**, 784 (1960); through *CA*, **55**, 22605*e* (1961).
322. R. Wien, D. F. J. Mason, N. D. Edge, and G. T. Langston, *Brit. J. Pharmacol.*, **7**, 534 (1952).
323. R. D. H. Maxwell and A. J. M. Campbell, *Lancet*, **264**, 455 (1953).
324. F. H. Smirk, *Lancet*, **264**, 457 (1953).
325. F. H. Smirk, *Lancet*, **263** (II), 1002 (1952).
326. O. S. Hetherington, *Lancet*, **265** (II), 391 (1953).
327. L. Gyermek, *Acta Phys. Acad. Sci. Hung.*, **8**, 49 (1954).
328. G. Palazzo and M. Virno, *Farmaco. Ed. Sci.*, **9**, 3 (1954).
329. R. Wien and D. F. J. Mason, *Brit. J. Pharmacol.*, **8**, 306 (1953).
330. J. Hidalgo, W. Wilken, and V. P. Seeberg, *Arch. Intern. Pharmacodyn.*, **118**, 210 (1959).
331. D. Lenke, *Arzneimittel-Forsch.*, **7**, 616 (1957).
332. D. Della Bella, F. Rognoni, and U. M. Teotino, *J. Pharm. Pharmacol.*, **14**, 701 (1962).
333. R. B. Barlow and A. Zoller, *Brit. J. Pharmacol.*, **23**, 131 (1964).
334. T. C. Chou and F. J. De Elio, *Brit. J. Pharmacol.*, **2**, 268 (1947).
335. P. H. Elworthy, *J. Pharm. Pharmacol.*, **16**, 375 (1964).
336. P. H. Elworthy, *J. Pharm. Pharmacol.*, **15**, 137 (1963).
337. A. Burger and G. R. Bedford, *J. Med. Pharm. Chem.*, **6**, 402 (1963).
338. Y. Shuster and A. L. Polyakov, *Sb. Nauchn. Rabot, Rizhskii Med. Inst.*, **11**, 159 (1961); through *CA*, **58**, 6094*d* (1963).
339. R. Van den Brink, R. Rosas, P. Blaquier, and D. B. Bohr, *Proc. Soc. Exptl. Biol. Med.*, **113**, 652 (1963).
340. J. H. Moyer and A. N. Brest, *Arch. Internal Med.*, **108**, 231 (1961).
341. A. R. Williams, J. Hidalgo, and I. F. Halverstadt, *J. Am. Pharm. Assoc.*, **45**, 423 (1956).
342. R. R. Levine, J. Weinstock, C. S. Zirkle, and R. McLean, *J. Pharmacol. Exptl. Therap.*, **131**, 334 (1961).
343. C. M. Smith, E. W. Pelikan, L. R. Maramba, and K. R. Unna, *J. Pharmacol. Exptl. Therap.*, **108**, 317 (1953).
344. F. Sadritdinov, *Farmakol. i Toksikol.*, **25**, 327 (1962).
345. J. L. Morrison, C. Heymans, and A. D. Richardson, *Arch. Intern. Pharmacodyn.*, **86**, 203 (1951).
346. A. M. Kunkel, A. H. Oikemus, and J. H. Wills, *Federation Proc.*, **11**, 365 (1952).
347. J. Fakstorp and J. G. A. Pedersen, *Acta Pharmacol. Toxicol.*, **10**, 7 (1954).
348. J. Fakstorp, E. Poulsen, W. Richter, and M. Schilling, *Acta Pharmacol. Toxicol.*, **11**, 319 (1955).
349. F. Sadritdinov, *Farmakol. i Toksikol.*, **25**, 428 (1962).
350. B. Bobranski, T. Jakobiec, and D. Prelicz, *Arch. Immunol. Terapii Doswiadczalnej*, 383 (1956); through *CA*, **52**, 3156 (1958).
351. E. Gerazzani, A. Bianchi, and M. de Maio, *Giorn. Ital. Chir.*, **13**, 204 (1957).
352. H. C. Beyerman and J. S. Bontekoe, *Rec. Trav. Chim.*, **74**, 1395 (1955).
353. H. C. Beyerman and J. S. Bontekoe, *Rec. Trav. Chim.*, **74**, 1395 (1955); through *CA*, **50**, 10718 (1955).
354. H. J. Bein and R. Meier, *Experientia*, **6**, 351 (1950).
355. H. J. Bein and R. Meier, *Schweiz. Med. Wochschr.*, **81**, 446 (1951).
356. K. Greef, H. Kasperat, and W. Osswald, *Arch. Exptl. Pathol. Pharmakol.*, **243**, 528 (1962).

357. W. Voigtlaender, H. Wunderlich, E. Carstens, and F. Hausschild, German (East) Pat. 21,823 (1961).

358. L. Gyermek and K. Nador, *Acta Phys. Acad. Sci. Hung.*, **3**, 183 (1952).

359. W. L. Archer, C. J. Cavallito, and A. P. Gray, *J. Am. Chem. Soc.*, **78**, 1227 (1956).

360. H. E. Lape, D. J. Fort, and J. O. Hoppe, *J. Pharmacol. Exptl. Therap.*, **116**, 462 (1956).

361. J. O. Hoppe, H. E. Lape, and D. J. Fort, *J. Pharmacol. Exptl. Therap.*, **116**, 30 (1956).

362. L. Gyermek and K. Nádor, *Acta Phys. Acad. Sci. Hung.*, **4**, 159 (1954).

363. C. G. Haining and R. G. Johnston, *Brit. J. Pharmacol.*, **18**, 275 (1962).

364. R. Pinson, D. E. Hutcheon, and S. Y. P'an, Abstracts, 132nd Meeting, American Chemical Society, Sept., 1957, p. 190.

365. D. W. Adamson, J. W. Billinghurst, A. F. Green, and S. Locket, *Nature*, **177**, 523 (1956).

366. S. Locket, *Brit. Med. J.*, **1956** (II), 116.

367. C. S. McKendrick and P. O. Jones, *Lancet*, **1958** (I), 340.

368. A. P. Gray, W. L. Archer, E. E. Spinner, and C. J. Cavallito, *J. Am. Chem. Soc.*, **79**, 3805 (1957).

369. T. B. O'Dell and M. D. Napoli, *J. Pharmacol. Exptl. Therap.*, **120**, 438 (1957).

370a. A. P. Gray, D. E. Heitmeier, and C. J. Cavallito, *J. Am. Chem. Soc.*, **81**, 728 (1959).

370b. T. B. O'Dell, C. Luna, and M. D. Napoli, *J. Pharmacol. Exptl. Therap.*, **114**, 317 (1955).

371a. B. M. Cohen, *New Engl. J. Med.*, **257**, 971 (1957).

371b. W. L. Archer, C. J. Cavallito, and A. P. Gray, *J. Am. Chem. Soc.*, **78**, 1227 (1956).

372. A. P. Gray, E. E. Spinner, D. C. Schlieper, and C. J. Cavallito, *J. Am. Chem. Soc.*, **77**, 3533 (1955).

373. T. B. O'Dell, C. Luna, and M. D. Napoli, *J. Pharmacol. Exptl. Therap.*, **114**, 306 (1955).

374. C. J. Cavallito, A. P. Gray, and T. B. O'Dell, *Arch. Intern. Pharmacodyn.*, **101**, 38 (1955).

375. A. P. Phillips, *J. Am. Chem. Soc.*, **79**, 5754 (1957).

376. A. P. Phillips, *J. Am. Chem. Soc.*, **76**, 2211 (1954).

377. K. I. Colville and R. V. Fanelli, *J. Am. Pharm. Assoc.*, **45**, 727 (1956).

378. J. L. Neumeyer, J. G. Cannon, and J. P. Buckley, *J. Med. Pharm. Chem.*, **5**, 784 (1960).

379. A. J. Plummer, J. H. Trapold, J. A. Schneider, R. A. Maxwell, and A. E. Earl, *J. Pharmacol. Exptl. Therap.*, **115**, 172 (1955).

380. E. G. Pardo and H. Vidrio, *J. Pharmacol. Exptl. Therap.*, **144**, 127 (1964).

381. H. Klupp, *Arzneimittel-Forsch.*, **7**, 123 (1957).

382. G. Bilecki, *Med. Klin.*, **51**, 1516 (1956).

383. A. M. Rusanov and G. A. Bol'shakova, *Farmakol. i Toksikol.*, **25**, 163 (1962); through *CA*, **57**, 15756*b* (1962).

384. R. A. Dunsmore, L. D. Dunsmore, A. Goldman, M. Elias, and R. S. Warner, *Am. J. Med. Sci.*, **236**, 483 (1958).

385a. K. J. M. Andrews, F. Bergel, and A. L. Morrison, *J. Chem. Soc.*, **1961**, 3483.

*385*b. E. Frommel, D. Vincent, D. Melkonian, C. Raduco-Thomas, M. Meyer, M. B. DeQuay, and F. Vallette, *Helv. Physiol. Phramacol. Acta*, **13**, 217 (1955).

386. P. Duchene-Marullaz, S. Blaise, and J. Berthelay, *Path.-Biol.*, **7**, 2101 (1959).

387. G. Vogrin, *Muench. Med. Wochschr.*, **105**, 531 (1963).

388. A. L. Mndzhoyan and N. M. Ordzhanyan, *Izv. Akad. Nauk Arm. SSR.*, *Khim. Nauki*, **15**, 173 (1962) (in Russian); through *CA*, **52**, 4493*d* (1958).

389. A. P. Phillips, *J. Am. Chem. Soc.*, **78**, 1930 (1956).

390. Z. P. Horovitz, E. C. Reif, and J. P. Buckley, *J. Am. Pharm. Assoc.*, **47**, 718 (1958).

391. I. M. Sharapov, *Farmakol. i Toksikol.*, **25**, 533 (1962).

392. I. M. Sharapov, *Khim. i Med.*, **15**, 39 (1960).

393. R. Hunt and R. R. Renshaw, *J. Pharmacol. Exptl. Therap.*, **44**, 63 (1932).

394. J. W. McCubbin and I. H. Page, *J. Pharmacol. Exptl. Therap.*, **105**, 437 (1952).

395. D. Della Bella, *Arch. Exptl. Pathol. Pharmakol.*, **226**, 335 (1955).
396. A. D'Amico and C. G. Busacca, *Farmaco*, **10**, 192 (1955).
397. R. B. Barlow and R. J. Vane, *Brit. J. Pharmacol. Chem.*, **11**, 198 (1956).
398. D. Della Bella and R. Villani, *Bull. Soc. Ital. Biol. Sper.*, **31**, 703 (1955).
399. K. H. Ginzel, H. Klupp, O. Kraupp, and G. Werner, *Arch. Exptl. Pathol. Pharmakol.*, **221**, 336 (1954).
400. R. H. Mizzoni, M. A. Hennessey, and C. R. Scholz, *J. Am. Chem. Soc.*, **76**, 2414 (1954).
401. A. J. Plummer, J. A. Schneider, and W. E. Barrett, *Arch. Intern. Pharmacodyn.*, **97**, 1 (1954).
402. C. J. Kensler, C. L. Zirkle, A. Matallana, and G. Condouris, *J. Pharmacol. Exptl. Therap.*, **112**, 210 (1954).
403. L. Gyermek, *Orv. Hetilap.*, **94**, 381 (1953).
404. T. Koppanyi and A. E. Vivino, *Federation Proc.*, **5**, 185 (1946).
405. V. V. Solovev and E. F. Saikina, *Sov. Med.*, **22**, 66 (1958).
406. S. Norton and A. P. Phillips, *Nature*, **172**, 867 (1953).
407. S. L. Shapiro, H. Soloway, and L. Freedman, *J. Am. Chem. Soc.*, **80**, 2743 (1958).
408. L. M. Rice and C. H. Grogan, *J. Org. Chem.*, **22**, 1100 (1957).
409. C. H. Grogan and L. M. Rice, *J. Org. Chem.*, **22**, 1223 (1957).
410. Shionogi & Co., Ltd., Brit. Pat. 876,686.
411. L. M. Rice and C. H. Grogan, *J. Org. Chem.*, **23**, 844 (1958).
412. S. Rossi and C. Valvo, *Farmaco. Ed. Sci.*, **12**, 1008 (1957).
413. M. V. Rubtsov, M. D. Mashkovskii, E. S. Nikitskaya, B. A. Medvedev, and V. S. Usovskaya, *J. Med. Pharm. Chem.*, **3**, 441 (1961).
414. D. A. Kharkevich, *Farmakol. i Toksikol.*, **25**, 151 (1962).
415. F. H. McMillan, K. A. Kun, C. B. McMillan, and J. A. King, *J. Am. Chem. Soc.*, **78**, 4077 (1956).
416. P. Magnin, R. Rips, B. Nicod, and J. P. Ergetaeu, *Ann. Sci. Univ. Besancon, Med.*, **6**, 105 (1962).
417. W. Schindler and F. Häfliger, U.S. Pat. 2,965,639 (1960); *CA*, **55**, 12437*g* (1961).
418. C. A. Stone, M. L. Torchiana, G. Q. O'Neill, and K. H. Beyer, *J. Pharmacol. Exptl. Therap.*, **116**, 54 (1956).
419. C. A. Stone, M. L. Torchiana, A. Navarro, and K. H. Beyer, *J. Pharmacol. Exptl. Therap.*, **117**, 169 (1956).
420. P. Lechat, M. Lamarche, and C. A. Renier, *Therapie*, **16**, 252 (1961).
421. K. P. Bhargava and K. N. Dhawan, *Brit. J. Pharmacol.*, **21**, 39 (1963).
422. G. P. Gupta and B. N. Dhawan, *Arch. Intern. Pharmacodyn.*, **134**, 54 (1961).
423. N. B. Vysotskaia, E. I. Iliina, and D. A. Kharkevich, *Fiziol. Zh. SSSR*, **46**, 1076 (1960).
424. C. A. Stone, M. L. Torchiana, K. L. Mecklenberg, J. Stavorski, M. Sletzinger, G. A. Stein, W. V. Ruyle, D. F. Reinhold, W. A. Gaines, H. Arnold, and K. Pfister, III. *J. Med. Pharm. Chem.*, **5**, 665 (1962).
425. K. Rubinstein, J. G. A. Pedersen, and J. Fakstorp, *Experientia*, **14**, 222 (1958).
426. N. D. Edge, S. J. Corne, G. E. Lee, and W. R. Wragg, *Brit. J. Pharmacol.*, **15**, 207 (1960).
427. Z. J. Vejdelek and V. Trcka, *Experientia*, **15**, 215 (1959).
428. Z. J. Vejdelek, Czech. Pat. 96,100 (1960).
429. M. Protiva, J. Rajsner, V. Trcka, M. Vanecek, and Z. J. Vejdelek, *Experientia*, **15**, 54 (1959).
430. J. G. Blackman and C. Ray, *Brit. J. Pharmacol.*, **22**, 56 (1964).
431. G. E. Lee, W. R. Wragg, S. J. Corne, N. D. Edge, and H. W. Reading, *Nature*, **181**, 1717 (1958).
432. A. Spinks and E. H. P. Young, *Nature*, **181**, 1397 (1958).

433. A. M. Dombrovskaya, V. A. Krementulo, and A. I. Cherkes, *Vrachebnoe Delo*, **12**, 102 (1960); *CA*, **55**, 27653*i* (1961).
434. K. N. Dhawan and K. P. Bhargava, *Brit. J. Pharmacol.*, **15**, 215 (1960).
435. L. Bretherick, G. E. Lee, E. Lunt, W. R. Wragg, and N. D. Edge, *Nature*, **184**, 1707 (1959).
436. E. Philippot, W. Denys, and M. J. Dallemagne, *Arch. Intern. Pharmacodyn.*, **135**, 273 (1962).
437. W. R. Wragg and L. Bretherick, Brit. Pat. 857,426 (1960).
438. G. E. Lee and W. R. Wragg, U.S. Pat. 3,060,143 (1962).
439. A. Simonart, *Arch. Intern. Pharmacodyn.*, **48**, 328 (1934).
440. F. H. Smirk and J. V. Hodge, *New Zealand Med. J.*, **59**, 253 (1960).
441. H. Kewitz and H. Reinert, *Arch. Exptl. Pathol. Pharmakol.*, **222**, 311 (1954).
442. A. Lundberg, *Acta Physiol. Scand.*, **26**, 254 (1952).
443. F. Brücke, W. Macho, and G. Werner, *Klin. Wochschr.*, **59**, 537 (1947).
444. E. Marley and W. D. M. Paton, *Brit. J. Pharmacol.*, **14**, 303 (1959).
445. L. H. Lerman and W. D. M. Paton, *Brit. J. Pharmacol.*, **15**, 458 (1960).
446. R. A. Maxwell, A. J. Plummer, F. Schneider, H. Poralski, and A. I. Daniel, *J. Pharmacol. Exptl. Therap.*, **128**, 22 (1960).
447. F. B. Giller and W. W. Baker, *Am. J. Pharm.*, **135**, 334 (1963).
448. F. Barzaghi, P. Mantegazza, and M. Riva, *Brit. J. Pharmacol.*, **19**, 414 (1962).
449. O. Neischulz, K. Popendiker, and I. Hoffmann, *Arzneimittel-Forsch.*, **5**, 680 (1955).
450. M. A. F. Sherif, M. K. Chata, and M. K. Madkour, *Arch. Intern. Pharmacodyn.*, **115**, 269 (1958).
451. N. K. Dutta, *Brit. J. Pharmacol.*, **4**, 281 (1949).
452. S. B. Gertner, *J. Pharmacol. Exptl. Therap.*, **131**, 223 (1961).
453. A. I. Popa, *Acad. Rep. Populare Romine, Stud. Cercetari Fiziol.*, **8**, 137 (1963).
454. X. Urquiaga, J. Villarreal, F. Alonso-deFlorida, and E. G. Pardo, *Arch. Intern. Pharmacodyn.*, **146**, 126 (1963).
455. J. H. Gaddum and Z. P. Picarelli, *Brit. J. Pharmacol.*, **12**, 323 (1957).
456. L. Gyermek and L. Sztanyik, *Acta Phys. Acad. Sci. Hung.*, **2**, 41 (1951).
457. H. Smirk, *Current Therapy* (H. F. Conn, ed.), Saunders, Philadelphia, 1964, p. 150.
458. A. Bourmanne, *Acta Anesthesiol. Belg.*, **12**, 1348 (1961–62).
459. T. G. Masevich, *Tr. Leningr. Sanit-Gigien. Med. Inst.*, **59**, 285 (1960).
460. F. Claudio and R. Cerra, *Gazz. Med. Ital.*, **117**, 18 (1958).
461. J. Toth and F. Fürst, *Orvosi Hetilap*, **101**, 1280 (1960).
462. K. Nádor, L. György, M. Dóda, II, *Conf. Hung. Therap. Invest. Pharmacol.*, **1963**, 232.
463. L. Decsi and K. Nádor, *Arch. Intern. Pharmacodyn.*, **144**, 404 (1963).
464. L. Gyermek, *Nature*, **171**, 788 (1953).
465. L. Gyermek, *Acta Phys. Acad. Sci. Hung.*, **4**, 333 (1953).
466. L. György, M. Dóda, and K. Nádor, *Arzneimittel-Forsch.*, **11**, 444 (1961).
467. L. F. Soyka and K. R. Unna, *Federation Proc.*, **20**, 307 (1961).
468. K. Nádor and L. Gyermek, *Arzneimittel-Forsch.*, **8**, 336 (1958).
469. J. K. Mohanty, *Brit. J. Pharmacol.*, **10**, 279 (1955).
470. K. Shimamoto, K. Inoue, and K. Ogiu, *J. Pharmacol. Exptl. Therap.*, **7**, 135 (1958).
471. F. H. Longino, J. R. Chittum, and K. S. Grimson, *Proc. Soc. Exptl. Biol.*, **70**, 467 (1949).
472. R. C. Ursillo, *J. Pharmacol. Exptl. Therap.*, **131**, 231 (1961).
473. E. G. Pardo, J. Cato, E. Gijon, and F. Alonso-deFlorida, *J. Pharmacol. Exptl. Therap.*, **139**, 296 (1963).
474. J. R. Cummings, J. L. Grace, and C. N. Latimer, *J. Pharmacol. Exptl. Therap.*, **141**, 349 (1963).

CHAPTER 5

DRUGS ACTING AT NERVE–SKELETAL–MUSCLE JUNCTIONS*

J. J. LEWIS† *and T. C. MUIR*

DIVISION OF EXPERIMENTAL PHARMACOLOGY
INSTITUTE OF PHYSIOLOGY
UNIVERSITY OF GLASGOW, SCOTLAND

5.1. INTRODUCTION

Neuromuscular blocking agents have been extensively investigated, and numerous comprehensive reviews cover the field (*1–5*). No purpose would be served by repeating what has already been accomplished adequately, nor is

* Literature survey completed in June 1965.

† Deceased.

there need for a detailed catalogue of all the compounds that have been synthesized, isolated, and tested for neuromuscular blocking activity. The principle adopted in this article, therefore, has been to outline what is known of the events that take place during neuromuscular transmission and then to describe how they may be modified by means of drugs. Chemical structure will thus be related to the ability to influence physiological events.

5.2. HISTORY

The history of the discovery of curare, its early scientific investigation, and its acceptance as an essential adjunct to surgical anesthesia have been well documented (*1*, *6*, *7*).

The first mention of curare was probably that in *De Orbe Novo* written by the Italian, Peter Martyr d'Anghera, in 1516 (*6*); the earliest scientific experiments were those made by de la Condamine in the 18th century (*8*, *9*). The mode of action of curare was first demonstrated in the classic experiments of Claude Bernard in 1856 (*10*). Curare was first used in modern medicine in 1940–1941 as a biologically standardized extract of *Chondrodendron tomentosum* for reducing the incidence of sprains and fractures in electroshock therapy (*11–13*). The determination of the chemical structure of tubocurarine, which had been shown already to be contained in *Chondrodendron tomentosum* (*14*) by King in 1935 (*15*, *16*), made available the pure alkaloid and led eventually to the syntheses of other compounds. The use of neuromuscular blocking agents in anesthetic practice, initially the work of Griffith and Johnson (*17*), has now gained almost universal acceptance.

5.3. THE NEUROMUSCULAR JUNCTION

A. Microanatomy

A wealth of literature pertains to microanatomical studies of the neuromuscular junction; for reviews of the earlier work see Hinsey (*18*) and Tiegs (*19*). The classic light-microscopic and histochemical studies of Couteaux (*20–22*), confirmed and extended by electron microscopy (*23–25*) with the use of a variety of species including man (*26–28*), have established the basic anatomical features of this synapse; a recent monograph by Zacks (*29*) also concerns this subject. The morphological individuality of presynaptic and postsynaptic components persists at the neuromuscular junction, and there is no direct cytoplasmic continuity between nerve and muscle fiber.

Where contact between a portion of the axon terminal and the sarcolemma surface does not take place, the upper portions of the axon termination are protected by a Schwann cell. In close proximity to the synapse the nerve fiber is unmyelinated, the terminal branchlets, each containing "synaptic vesicles" (*30*, *31*) and mitochondria embedded in axonal cytoplasm, arborizing in grooves in the thickened sarcolemma surface. The intervening gap between the motor nerve termination and the muscle fiber end plate is known as the synaptic cleft. Structures similar to synaptic vesicles may exist postsynaptically (*32–35*) and at nonsynaptic sites (*36*), although their functions may be different (*24*, *37*). The term "synaptic vesicles" has been justified, however, by their profusion at presynaptic nerve terminals in close proximity to postsynaptic thickenings of the sarcolemma (*24*). The sarcoplasmic structure immediately underlying the interface, the subneural apparatus (*22*), is formed by infoldings of the surface membrane, called junctional folds (*23*). A reconstructed motor end plate, prepared from a series of electron micrographs by Andersson-Cedergren (*24*), is shown in Figure 5.1.

Attempts at correlating morphological features with the results of physiological and histochemical experimentation have been a significant consequence of electron microscope studies (*38–40*). The function of synaptic vesicles in the storage, synthesis, and transfer of acetylcholine (*23*, *25*, *30*), based upon their origin from (*41*) and close association with the presynaptic membranes (*42*), their identification within the synaptic space (*31*), and the effects upon them of nerve fiber (*37*) and "synaptic" stimulation (*44*) and degeneration (*45*, *46*), has received prominence without unreserved acceptance (*46*). The aggregation of synaptic vesicles in thickened regions of apposed synaptic membranes (possible transmission points) also has been observed (*37*). The continued release of acetylcholine for a short period following chronic

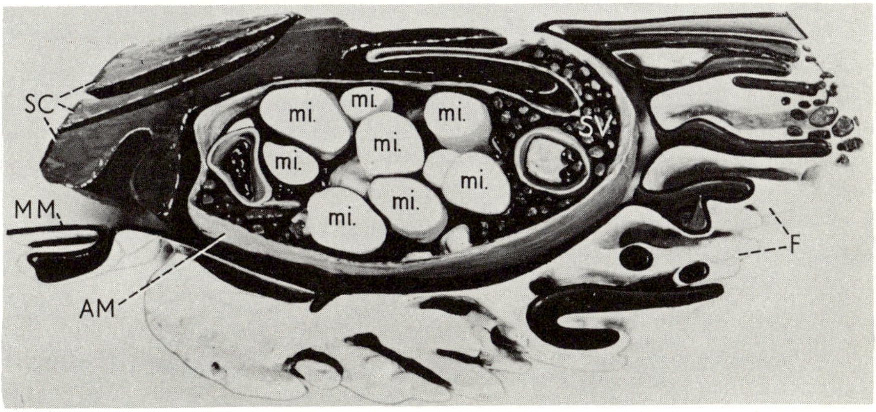

Fig. 5.1. Three-dimensional reconstruction of part of a motor end plate from electron micrographs of serial sections (*24*). AM, terminal axon membrane; F, folds of muscle-fiber membrane MM; SV, synaptic vesicles; Mi, mitochondria. From *J. Ultra Structure Res.*, Suppl. 1, 72 (1959).

denervation of the neuromuscular junction has been ascribed to the Schwann cell (*45*), although it may be due to the latter's ability to engulf the vesicles from which the transmitter is quantally liberated.

The enzyme responsible for the hydrolysis of acetylcholine, acetylcholinesterase, is localized in highest concentrations postsynaptically (*47*, *48*) in the lamellae of the postsynaptic junctional folds (*23*). A comparatively small amount of acetylcholinesterase also has been found within the nerve fiber in the endoplasmic reticulum, as evidenced by electron microscopy (*49*). The view that transmitter synthesis arises in mitochondria has now been rejected (*50*), largely on evidence from centrifugation studies, which have confirmed the close association of choline acetylase, the enzyme involved in the synthesis of acetylcholine, and the small granule or microsomal (rather than mitochondrial) fraction of homogenized nerve; see the reviews by Hebb (*51*) and Nachmansohn (*52*). The association of mitochondria with energy yielding mechanisms in transmitter synthesis remains confirmed.

Although the presence of a homogeneous material, probably hydrated mucopolysaccharide or mucoprotein (*53*), between the axolemma and sarcolemma may be important in neuromuscular transmission, its role as a potential diffusional barrier or in ion transfer must remain speculative (*29*).

B. Chemical Transmission

The classic experiments of Claude Bernard (*10*), demonstrating the peripheral site of action of curare, were responsible initially for indicating the specialized nature of the skeletal neuromuscular junction and for stimulating interest in its properties. Subsequent physiological and pharmacological investigations have established the participation in neuromuscular transmission of specific chemical substances liberated from motor nerve terminals (*39*, *54–59*). The earlier view was that transmission was a purely electrical process (*60–63*), but the essential role of acetylcholine at the neuromuscular junction has now been accepted (*52*, *64*, *65*), although chemical transmission has not been established at all synapses. Electrical transmission has been confirmed in the cray fish (*66*) and in the chicken ciliary ganglion (*67*). The specialized role of the end plate in neuromuscular transmission (*68*, *69*), the ease with which it becomes fatigued compared to either nerve or muscle (*52*, *68*, *69*), its high concentration of acetylcholinesterase compared to that of other tissues (*21*, *70*), and its high and specific sensitivity to acetylcholine (*71–73*) support this view. That the specific chemical concerned at the mammalian neuromuscular junction is acetylcholine rather than other cholinesters, such as propionylcholine (*74*), has been shown beyond reasonable doubt, although the observation that nervous tissue (in insects) can synthesize other choline analogues, at least in vitro (*75*), must be borne in mind.

C. Formation of Acetylcholine

Acetylcholine in animal tissues is synthesized from choline by a two-step acetylation procedure. In the first stage acetylcoenzyme A is formed from acetate in the presence of the "acetate-activating" enzyme acetylkinase (*76*). The second stage involves the transfer of the acetyl group from acetylcoenzyme A to choline, in which the specific catalyst is choline acetylase (*77*, *78*). The major energy source of these reactions is provided in the form of energy-rich bonds of adenosine triphosphate synthesized in carbohydrate metabolism (*76*, *79*). The occurrence of choline acetylase has thus been used for identifying sites of acetylcholine production. Its presence, associated with the microsomal or small-granule fraction of homogenized nerve tissue, has been confirmed in a variety of conducting tissues, including somatic nerve trunks (*51*, *80*). Although choline acetylase (and hence acetylcholine) may be present in all conducting tissues, concentrations in areas away from the junctional regions are relatively low. A marked divergence of opinion persists (*48*, *76*) as to whether these low concentrations can support a transmitter role in non-junctional areas.

The maintenance of adequate supplies of choline for acetylcholine synthesis, under all conditions of nervous activity may depend upon the presence of a specific "choline-carrier" mechanism located on or within the presynaptic nerve-terminal membrane (*81*). Stores of intracellular choline would thus be insufficient for adequate transmitter synthesis. By means of the carrier mechanism extracellular choline stores derived from acetylcholine breakdown may be transported to intracellular sites for acetylation.

D. Storage of Acetylcholine

Acetylcholine is stored in a protein-bound form probably associated with choline acetylase (*80*) but protected from cholinesterases (*82*) both within synaptic vesicles ("bound") and without ("surplus" or "free") (*83*). Bound acetylcholine, which is physiologically inactive, provides the store from which the transmitter is released.

E. Release of Acetylcholine

A spontaneous, intermittent release of acetylcholine persists at rest at the neuromuscular junction, eliciting minute potential changes in the post-junctional membrane, the so-called miniature end-plate potentials (*84*). These potentials, which are below the threshold necessary to excite the adjacent muscle membrane, have been attributed, mainly on pharmacological evidence, to the release of multimolecular quanta of acetylcholine from the synaptic vesicles (*71*, *84*).

Acetylcholine, released physiologically in response to nerve stimulation (*85*), elicits the end-plate potential that is derived from a simultaneous, transient acceleration of the resting random discharge of numerous miniature end-plate potentials (*86–88*). Thus, the end-plate potential represents an increased probability of obtaining multiple quanta of transmitter.

Attempts to quantitate the amount of acetylcholine released by a single nerve impulse have been made (*81*, *89*) by measuring the transmitter output from a relatively large number of electrically stimulated fibers. The discrepancies between the amount of transmitter recovered from nerve endings and that required to mimic, by injection, the neuronal response to stimulation have, to some extent, been remedied by the iontophoretic application of acetylcholine to the end plate (*90*). By this means end-plate potentials have been obtained in response to quantities of exogenous acetylcholine approximating those released by nerve stimulation (*91–93*).

Transmitter release may also be brought about by drugs that penetrate nerve membranes, such as cobra venom lecithinase (*94*, *95*), by freezing and thawing, by high concentrations of K^+, Rb^{++}, Cs^{++}, or $NH_4{}^+$, which attack storage particles (*82*, *96*), and by agents that exchange with acetylcholine in synaptic vesicles, such as carbachol and acetylcholine itself (*97*, *98*).

The physiological release of acetylcholine in quantities sufficient for chemical transmission is initiated by the nerve impulse. Conduction of the nerve impulse is an electrical phenomenon, and a coupling mechanism is implicated in the subsequent release of the chemical transmitter. Following observations of the effect of alterations in the external ionic environment, such as in the concentrations of Ca^{++}, K^+, Na^+, and Mg^{++} (*99–101*), tentative suggestions concerning the mechanism of acetylcholine release have been made. In this connection the entry of calcium into the presynaptic axoplasm during the action potential and its expulsion between action potentials (*102–105*) have implicated this ion in altering the "properties of the vesicles" and inducing the liberation of acetylcholine (*81*).

A mutually antagonistic reaction involving Ca^{++} and Mg^{++} and those receptors which control the amount of neurally released transmitter may also occur (*106*, *107*).

Although high exogenous concentrations of Mg^{++} and low concentrations of Ca^{++} may reduce the over-all amount of acetylcholine liberated (*108*, *109*), large concentrations of Ca^{++} have the opposite effect (*110*).

That the mechanism of spontaneous liberation of acetylcholine may differ from the liberation evoked by a nerve impulse has been suggested (*80*) by the observation that, although Mg^{++} may affect the amount of transmitter in each quantum, it does not affect the frequency of the miniature end-plate potentials (*86–88*). On the other hand, a highly significant correlation between the methods of release has been obtained (*85*). Carbon dioxide concentrations (*81*) and temperature fluctuations also affect transmitter release (*111*).

F. Transmitter Function

Acetylcholine reduces the potential difference across the membrane of the motor end plate whether it is released spontaneously, in response to motor nerve stimulation or after local application. The motor end plate is extremely sensitive to the transmitter, unlike the remainder of the muscle membrane (*70*, *71*, *84*, *112–114*). If sufficient acetylcholine is released, the ensuing quantal depolarization (end-plate potential) subsequently activates the adjacent muscle membrane, causing a propagated potential change, the action potential, which in turn gives rise to the mechanical response.

After the transmitter–receptor interaction there is, underlying the changes in membrane potential, a rapid increase in the permeability of the muscle cell membrane, an indiscriminate aqueous channel being opened to all small ions (such as Na^+, K^+, NH_4^+) on each side of the membrane (*39*, *64*, *68*, *69*, *99*, *100*). Acetylcholine-induced changes in the potential of the end plate differ from the specific and strictly separate changes in Na^+ and K^+ permeability that occur during the action potential (*100*, *115*). The increase in ionic permeability simulates short-circuiting of the end-plate membrane, producing a local current of high density (*99*) and enabling a transfer of the impulse from the very small nerve endings to the comparatively much larger surface of the muscle fiber. The local ionic currents at the end plate increase the permeability to Na^+ of the adjacent portions of the muscle membrane, so initiating the action potential. Conduction of the action potential is an energy-dissipating process, normal cellular sources restoring the internal ionic environment over a comparatively long period of rest.

The period of depolarization produced by prolonged application of acetylcholine to the motor end plate is brief, and the membrane becomes rapidly and completely repolarized (desensitized) to both neurally released and locally applied transmitter and to other depolarizing drugs acting on the cholinergic synapse (*116–120*).

Controversy persists concerning the precise role of acetylcholine in transmission. The proposal (*51*, *64*, *121*) that acetylcholine is secreted quantally only at the nerve terminals, reaching the postsynaptic membrane by diffusion across the synaptic space, has been rejected by Nachmansohn and his associates (*52*, *122*, *123*) in favor of a more general view such as was earlier suggested by Dale (*124*), that its action at the neuromuscular junction is merely a "local intensification of a general process for the propagation of impulses along the nerve fiber." The proposal has also been made that acetylcholine reacts initially with presynaptic terminals to effect the release of additional transmitter (*125*). This well-documented controversy, discussion of which is beyond the scope of this article, has been already adequately reviewed (*48*, *126*).

Conduction in nerve and muscle fibers caused by fish toxins may be inhibited by a specific block of the increase of permeability to Na^+ associated with excitation (*127*). Unlike the action of tubocurarine, local anesthetics, and other agents postulated (*128*) as blocking axonal conduction by inhibiting the transmitter, the action of marine toxins does not appear dependent upon the presence of acetylcholine. This had already been suggested by Nachmansohn and his associates (*128*).

G. Transmitter Destruction

The essential role of acetylcholinesterase (*129–132*) as the principal enzyme (*133*) in the rapid hydrolysis of the transmitter has been clearly established. Other means of removing acetylcholine, such as its diffusion from muscle (*134*) or ganglia (*89*, *135*) into the extracellular fluid and hence into the blood stream or its restitution to presynaptic terminals in a manner analogous to the uptake of choline (*136*), are probably of minor importance.

The high postsynaptic concentration of acetylcholinesterase at the neuromuscular junction, in contrast to its predominantly presynaptic localization at autonomic ganglia, may be explained in terms of its function at each site. Although cholinesterases in ganglia may support several functions on both sides of the synapse (*127*), its exclusive postsynaptic localization at the neuromuscular junction may indicate its specific role in terminating the action of the transmitter.

5.4. NEUROMUSCULAR BLOCKING AGENTS AND THE RECEPTOR

A. Theories of Drug–Receptor Interaction

Much of modern pharmacological theory rests upon the concept of the receptor, the assumed presence of which offers indeed the most satisfactory means of explaining the effects, following the combination of a neuromuscular blocking agent and structures upon the postsynaptic membrane.

Modern receptor theory originates from the studies of Ehrlich, who visualized cells as carrying side chains capable of combining not only with oxygen and nutrients but also with toxins and drug molecules (*137*). A similar view was inherent in the lock-and-key analogy of Fischer (*138*, *139*) and in the work of Langley (*140*) who, in order to explain pharmacological activity, conceived the idea of a "receptive substance." It was believed that this could be altered selectively by curarelike agents (*141*).

A direct consequence of the receptor theory is the principle of biological antagonism, which maintains that a drug competes for the receptor with a natural substrate, an essential metabolite, or some other drug. The concept of biological antagonism has been placed on a quantitative basis, and experimental observations have been given theoretical expression by the derivation of a number of equations from a variety of scientific disciplines, including those of physical adsorption laws, enzyme kinetics, and chemical reactions—all capable of being expressed in identical mathematical forms. The correlating of pharmacological activity with adsorption laws by Langmuir (*142–144*) and the early work of Clark (*145*) and Gaddum (*146*), modified and extended by Stephenson (*147*), Nickerson (*148*), Ariëns (*149*), Schild (*150*), and Van Maanen (*151*), represent the basis upon which our present-day understanding of the mode of action of neuromuscular blocking agents may be rationalized and expressed. The studies outlined above assume that the effect produced is dependent upon the occupation of receptors by the drug molecule and so are recognized as "occupation" studies.

In their application to neuromuscular blocking agents the theories of Ariëns and his colleagues (*149*) and of Stephenson (*147*) are particularly relevant. Ariëns had been led to a reconsideration of the accepted views of biological antagonism by the existence of apparent discrepancies encountered during a study of several homologous series, in which certain members possessed a dual mode of action while presumably acting on the same receptor. Drawing heavily upon enzyme kinetic analogies, Ariëns related drug–receptor interaction to the two basic constants of affinity and intrinsic activity, both of which vary with the chemical structure, molecular configuration, and physicochemical properties of the drug.

The affinity of a drug may be defined as its ability to enter into complex formation with a given receptor and may be conceived of as a product of a general interaction of electric fields of force originating in the drug molecule and the receptor. Intrinsic activity, on the other hand, is a measure of the power of the drug–receptor complex to evoke a positive biological response. Efficacy, a concept adopted by Stephenson (*147*), is closely allied to intrinsic activity and may be defined as the ability of a drug to bring about responses of similar magnitude while occupying widely different proportions of the total available receptors. Intrinsic activity (and efficacy) constants and affinity constants can be calculated and used for quantitatively evaluating neuromuscular blocking agents of different chemical structure, thus enabling a classification to be made. Moreover, this approach has offered a means of describing the mode of action of those compounds, hitherto unconsidered, whose activity falls somewhere between evoking a positive response (high intrinsic activity) and inducing receptor blockade (low intrinsic activity).

Contradicting the view that mere occupation of the receptor site was responsible for the observed biological response, Paton (*152*) proposed that excitation of a receptor can be effected only at the moment of impact with a drug and that activation is proportional to the total encounters in a given unit of time. It follows that differences in the actions of agonistic and antagonistic drugs will depend on differences in the ability of the molecules to dissociate from the receptor. Thus, a high dissociation rate enables subsequent drug–receptor encounters to proceed and leads to an agonistic response, whereas persistent occupation (slow dissociation rate) produces antagonism. Paton further proposed that cationic drug molecules exchange with receptor-bound K^+, which tends to move passively via its concentration gradient outward through cell membranes. This model of drug action is dependent, therefore, upon intracellular K^+, a reduction in the supply of which has been implicated in the phenomenon of desensitization. Belleau (*153*) recently attempted a theoretical physicochemical explanation of drug–receptor kinetics and certain structure–activity relationships pertaining to the cholinergic muscarinic receptor. The theory relies upon the analogy between drug–receptor interaction and enzyme kinetics and, in particular, upon the ability of enzymes to alter their conformation in response to substrate interaction. On the assumption that the muscarinic receptor is a protein, with the properties of regulatory enzymes, Belleau divided drugs interacting with it into two basic categories according to the nature of that part of the receptor with which "perturbation" (impact) is made. On the one hand, compounds whose interaction with the receptor involve only the nonpolar acetylcholine-binding portion of the latter's surface are regarded as inducing a "specific conformational perturbation." This type of drug–receptor combination is directly analogous to the classic, specific lock-and-key enzyme substrate relationship. Only those compounds capable of causing the specific conformational perturbation could cause a response analogous to a high intrinsic activity or high dissociation constant in terms of the Ariëns and Paton theories, respectively. All other compounds are believed to interact with adjoining hydrophobic areas of the receptor surface and would induce a "nonspecific conformational perturbation" leading to competitive antagonism with the transmitter. In the light of the Ariëns and Paton theories, such compounds would possess respectively a low intrinsic activity or a slow rate of dissociation from the receptor. Compounds inducing a partially agonistic effect are rationalized in terms of their ability to interact with both parts of the receptor, that is, with both acetylcholine and peripheral hydrophobic sites, and so give rise to equilibrium mixtures of specific and nonspecific perturbations.

Belleau also speculates that the muscarinic cholinergic receptor may be acetylated acetylcholinesterase formed from the continuous quantal discharge of the transmitter. The receptor would, it is suggested, be a self-regenerating system derived from a biochemical pool, such a process being analogous to the participation of enzymes in carbohydrate metabolism. No explanation of the mechanism of involvement of acetylcholine with the same enzyme in producing nicotinic effects is offered. Observations of conformational rearrangements at cholinergic sites, analogous to those seen by electron microscopy to be produced by insulin (*154*), also give pertinent support to the perturbation theory.

B. Chemical-Stereochemical Rationalization of the Nicotinic Cholinergic Receptor

The first intimation of the existence of a close association between muscle-relaxant activity and the quaternary ammonium function was the work of Crum-Brown and Fraser in 1869 (*155–157*). These workers demonstrated that, in contrast to the highly individual pharmacological properties exhibited by a number of chemically diverse alkaloids, the derived quaternary salts all showed a common property, that of paralyzing skeletal muscle. The importance of the quaternary ammonium function in muscle-relaxant activity subsequently has been amply verified (*158*, *159*).

It is now accepted generally that the initial step in the reaction between drug and receptor involves the formation of an ionic bond between the onium cation and an oppositely charged anionic receptor group. Additionally, secondary bonding may occur subsequently between other parts of the drug molecule and the receptor. Bonds formed by London and van der Waals dispersion forces are probably the most prominent in this connection, though hydrogen bonds and nondipole bonds also exist. The nature and extent of secondary bond formation will depend upon the physicochemical and mechanical properties of the structure that supports the onium ions.

The early demonstration (*15*, *16*) that tubocurarine contained two quaternary nitrogen centers at opposite ends of the molecule led to the view that the postsynaptic membrane might carry a lattice of regularly spaced anionic receptor sites (*159*). This postulate was reinforced by the high neuromuscular blocking activity of tubocurarine as compared with that of known monoquaternary derivatives and by the observation that, while not entirely rigid, tubocurarine is capable of only relatively small changes in configuration.

Attempts have been made at predicting the molecular shape and electrical characteristics of the receptor by considering similar features found in biologically active molecules, in the belief that the receptor would have properties complementary to those of the most active species (*160–163*). The high potency of bisquaternary agents, as compared with that of the corresponding monoquaternary agents (*164*, *165*), led to the postulate that activity of the former group could be rationalized by the interaction of optimally spaced onium centers approximately 13 to 15 A apart with equidistant coreactive receptor groups on the motor end plate. The complex so formed by the bivalent molecule (*166*), it was suggested, would be twice as stable as that formed by a corresponding monoquaternary compound. Although the so-called equidistance concept gained a measure of support from the fact that the most active member in each of several series of compounds possessed an interonium distance comparable to that of tubocurarine, 10 to 15 A (*167*, *168*), it soon became evident that a one-dimensional approach oversimplified the picture of drug–receptor interaction. Interonium distance in nonrigid molecules has no fixed value, on account of conformational isomerism arising from uninhibited rotations about single C—C bonds in the polymethylene chain (*169*). Moreover, in chemical media at least, pairing of a di-cation and an anion may occur, so that both onium centers of a bisquaternary compound may bond to a single anionic receptor (*159*). There is, therefore, no reason to assume that the thermodynamically most stable conformation of the molecule is that actually involved in receptor complex formation. The differences in the estimated interonium distance in tubocurarine, which has been reported as 13 to 15 A (*165*), although it may be only 9 to 12 A (*170*, *171*) because of molecular folding, would thus be accounted for. Differences between conductimetric values (*172*, *173*) and statistically calculated interonium distances (*174*) have underlined these difficulties. The equidistance concept was undermined further by the lack of uniformity in interonium distances among approximately equipotent derivatives (*175*) and by the high neuromuscular block in short-chained asymmetric bisquaternaries (*176*, *177*). The adumbration hypothesis (*175*) was developed from these criticisms and emphasized the need for a consideration of other factors than interonium distance, such as shape, geometry, and bonding potentialities of the molecule, in determining the degree of drug–receptor interaction. This hypothesis ascribed neuromuscular block to a spatial competition with acetylcholine, the adumbrating, or umbrellalike, structure of the molecule hindering access to the receptor site by steric interference. Similar views have been advanced by Wien (*178*) and are embodied in the pictorial representation of the nicotinic cholinergic receptor (*179*, *180*).

It is interesting to note that 14.5 A, the distance postulated as the ideal interonium distance in bisquaternary ammonium neuromuscular blocking agents (*164*, *165*), is 4×3.61 A, the "identity distance" between peptide bonds in a maximally extended peptide (*181*).

A necessary extension of studies with bisquaternary salts, in which the concept of a lattice surface of equally spaced anionic sites is assumed, was the examination of tris-, tetra-, and polyonium salts in the belief that a higher degree of activity than that found among bisquaternaries would be confirmed by virtue of their being reactants with respect to a polymeric hypothetical receptor system (*182–184*). Of these, gallamine (*182*, *185*) has been singularly successful and is now clinically established. Straight-chain tris-, tetra-, and polyonium compounds, in which the interonium chain length was varied, have been studied by the authors and their colleagues (*170*, *186–194*). Wide species variations in potency were observed, but compounds more potent than tubocurarine were found. Thus, in the cat, chick, mouse, and rabbit the hexamethylene hexaonium salt (**I**) (*190*) was almost four times as potent as tubocurarine. The increased neuromuscular blockade, which was associated in several species, especially in the cat, rabbit, and mouse, with an

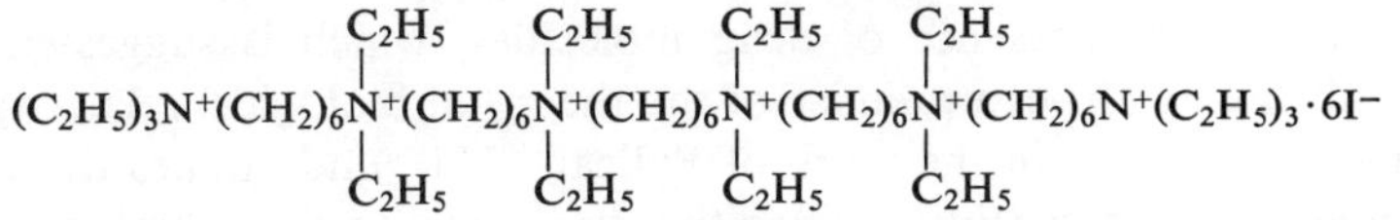

(I)

7,7,14,14,21,21,28,28-Octaethyl-7,14,21,28-tetrazoniatetratriacontylene bis(triethylammonium) hexaiodide

increase in the number of onium centers, supports the concept of a regularly occurring, anionic, receptor lattice and favors a multipoint attachment as a factor in increased potency. Many of the molecules concerned were extremely flexible, and numerous conformations are possible with the hypothetical receptor. The presence of multiple cationic centers in those compounds would extend the over-all chain length because of the repulsion of like charges on the nitrogen centers. In consequence, as in the case of the bisquaternary derivatives already discussed, the spatial features of the receptor cannot be outlined properly, and high potency may be attributed feasibly to other molecular features, especially to the ratio of lipophilic to hydrophilic groupings (*159*).

Criticism of the use of flexible molecules in assessing the spatial features of the receptor would appear, at first sight, capable of being overcome through the use of rigid molecules. Naturally occurring (*195–197*) and synthetic (*198–201*) steroidal derivatives of the pregnane and androstane types have been favored in this approach, and nondepolarizing compounds almost equipotent with tubocurarine have been produced. Several 3β- and 17β-bisquaternary ammonium androstane derivatives, in which the interonium distance can vary between 10.5 and 11.2 A, show potent short-acting neuromuscular blocking properties (*200*). However, perhaps the most important theoretical implication of the results with rigid molecules has arisen from the high activity (as high as that of tubocurarine) of 3α,17β-bistrimethylammonium-5α-androstane bismethiodide (*198, 199*), a short-acting nondepolarizing compound in which the quaternary heads lie on opposite sides of the plane of the steroid nucleus. The interonium distance in this compound is about 11 A, but on account of the planar separation and interposition of the steroidal moiety between the onium centers, it clearly is not an indication of interreceptor distance. Additionally, the potency of this compound is not comparable to that of *C*-toxiferine-1, a fully rigid calabash curare, in which the (optimal) interonium distance is 9.7 A (*180*). These observations have cast doubt upon the value of using rigid molecules in assessing interreceptor distance and have confirmed the view that a limited degree of flexibility is necessary for neuromuscular block (*174, 202*), as already evidenced by the ineffectiveness of *N,N,N,N′,N′,N′*-hexamethyl-*p*-phenylenediamine bisiodide (*203*).

Furthermore, acceptance of the view that receptor characteristics may alter in response to the presence of drug molecules, which is suggested in the induced-fit theory (*204*), a premise of the theory of biological relativity (*205*), and which is inherent in the work of Belleau (*153*), undermines the value of rigid molecules. Alternatively, since the discussion so far substantiates only the existence of numerous anionic sites, the interspacing of which is uncertain, interaction with one such receptor unit is not precluded. Indeed, *C*-toxiferine-1 may dissociate in solution into two monoquaternary-containing halves (*206*). However, although monoquaternary steroids are also known to possess neuromuscular blocking activity (*207–209*), this approach has not yielded highly active compounds.

Physicochemical studies have provided a certain amount of additional information, particularly with regard to the behavior of long-chain bisquaternary salts in solution. The value of extrapolating the behavior of molecules in purely chemical media to that in the biophase must, however, remain speculative. Many such studies (*210–214*) have stressed the ability of long-chain aliphatic compounds to curve, rather than remain maximally distended, in solution. Elworthy (*213*, *214*) suggests that this reduction in chain length represents an attempt made by the molecule to minimize interfacial energy between the water molecules and the hydrocarbon chain. On the basis of conductance measurements, Elworthy has speculated that 9.5 A may be the critical distance between anionic receptor sites, as found for decamethonium. If the anionic sites are regularly arranged—though this idea is not universally accepted (*174*)—each group of four will have a diagonal of 13.6 A, which could also be used for two-point attachment. Compounds having interonium distances of either 9.5 or 13.6 A might then be equipotent.

It is clear that interonium distance is not the sole determinant of potency. Many of the important stereochemical deductions concerning the nicotinic cholinergic receptor have been embodied in Waser's pictorial representation of the site (*179*, *180*); see Figure 5.2. This has been represented as a pore 12 to 14 A in diameter with anionic sites around the rim, the inner surface containing other reactive receptor groupings with which other regions of the drug molecule could combine. Under physiological circumstances acetylcholine reacts with the receptor sites, the initial attachment taking place through formation of an ionic bond at the pore rim and a secondary bond between the ether or carbonyl groups. This results in depolarization, which is accompanied by ion flux and conductance of Na^+ and K^+. Neuromuscular blocking agents may also form an initial bond at the pore rim, and the rest of the molecule, if bulky (as is tubocurarine), may occlude, with varying degrees of completeness, the orifice of the pore. Long slender molecules are visualized as bridging the pore along cords that correspond to the interonium distance. This picture accommodates the single, two-point, and multipoint views of

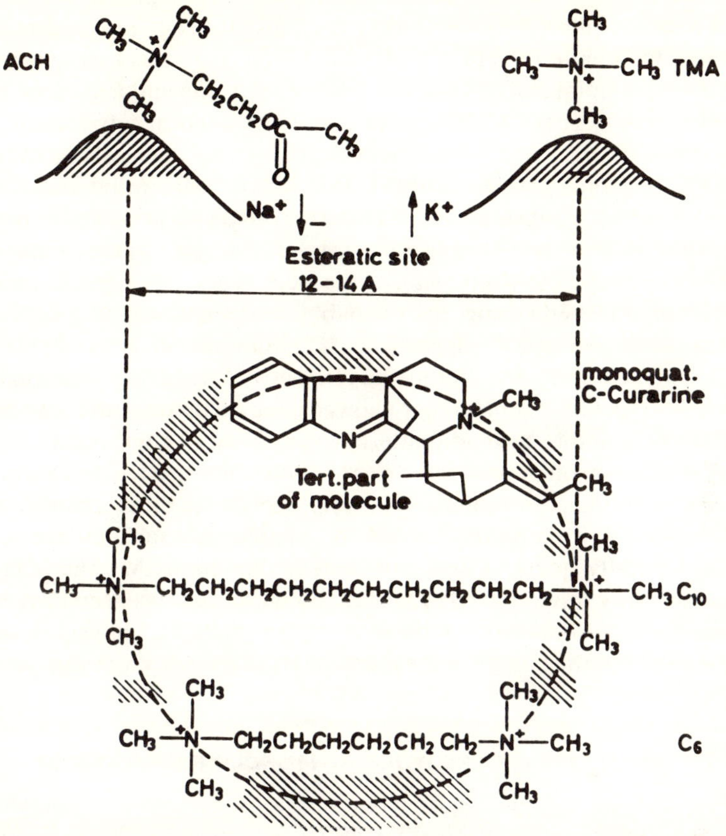

Fig. 5.2. Model of a receptor pore in section and from above. Anionic wall occupied by depolarizing ACh or TMA, at the bottom permeation of Na or K ions. The pore can be blocked by one bisquaternary or two monoquaternary curarine molecules, or by many smaller diamines such as hexamethonium (C_6). Depolarizing decamethonium (C_{10}) will leave enough room for ions to pass beside the molecule. From Waser, in Bovet, Bovet-Nitti, and Marini-Bettolo, *Curare and Curare-like Agents*, Elsevier, Amsterdam, 1959, p. 227.

drug–receptor attachment. The change from depolarizing to nondepolarizing activity, seen after the prolonged use of depolarizing agents, may be regarded as a gradual occlusion of the pore by an accumulation of slender molecules.

C. The Receptor Substance

Although the existence of a receptor was postulated over fifty years ago (*140*), evidence for its presence as a distinct cellular constituent has accrued only in recent years. Nachmansohn and his associates (*76*) observed that certain compounds, including acetylcholine and tubocurarine, blocked conduction without interfering with acetylcholinesterase activity, effects that were attributed to an interaction with the postulated receptor. From an examination of the uptake of radioactive muscle relaxants and neostigmine in mouse diaphragms Waser (*179*, *180*) confirmed the distinction between enzyme and receptor and formulated his concept of the latter's geometrical dimensions (see Section 5.4, B). Numerous attempts (*215–220*) at isolating and identifying chemically the receptor substance have also been made by means of complex formation with radioactive muscle relaxants and several animal and fish preparations, especially the electroplax of the electric eel. Initially, the experimental evidence indicated strong, but probably nonspecific, binding of radioactive gallamine to a mucopolysaccharide (*215*). Subsequent work (*216*) with a more refined fractionation technique has led, however, to the isolation and purification of a protein material that showed many characteristics of the in vivo receptor in its ability to bind quaternary ammonium compounds. However, the postulated protein material did not show the expected great avidity for such depolarizing compounds as acetylcholine and decamethonium whereas, conversely, its affinity for other compounds, such as procaine, appeared abnormally great. It was concluded, therefore, that the isolated protein was not the cholinergic receptor (*217*), a view that has been contested (*221*). Thus, the physiological significance of the protein that was isolated remains in doubt and the nature of the receptor substance as yet unknown (see Chapter 1).

5.5. MECHANISMS OF PRODUCING MUSCLE RELAXATION

It is clear that any agent affecting the synthesis, release, or removal of acetylcholine or interfering with the formation or destruction of the complex it forms with receptors will interrupt or modify the physiological process of neuromuscular transmission and merit inclusion as a muscle-relaxant. For the purposes of this review the term "neuromuscular blocking agent" will be reserved for those drugs interfering with the postsynaptic functioning of the transmitter rather than with its presynaptic synthesis or release or its enzymatic destruction.

A. Factors Modifying Transmitter Release

High-frequency tetanic stimulation of the motor nerve, associated with a gradual decrease in the size of the end-plate potentials [Wedensky inhibition, (*222*)], has been attributed to a diminution of transmitter output per nerve volley resulting from a block of conduction in the fine terminal branchlets of the motor nerve (*223–226*). Although Mg^{++} clearly reduces the amount of transmitter released per nerve volley (*108*, *109*), it has also been suggested that the effects of Mg^{++} in high concentrations (*227*) and of Ca^{++} in low concentrations (*81*) may be due to failure of conduction in the fine terminal branchlets. Conduction block may also explain the presynaptic action of procaine (*228*) and other local anesthetics, whose effects, demonstrable in entire nerve axons as decreasing the amount of transmitter released (*229*), may first be mediated at the fine motor nerve-terminal branchlets (*230*). Local anesthetics may inhibit the permeability changes necessary for the conduction of impulses and the release of acetylcholine by stabilizing the membrane (*231*), while procaine itself may also depress the sensitivity of the motor end plate to the transmitter (*228, 232, 233*).

On the other hand, the blocking of the release of acetylcholine by botulinum toxin (*234–237*), although reducing the frequency but not the amplitude of miniature end-plate potentials, does not affect either the nervous conduction or the ability of the muscle to respond to intra-arterially injected transmitter (*237*). These effects appear independent of any alteration in either the structure of the motor nerve terminals or the number or size of the presynaptic vesicles. The latter retain multimolecular quanta of acetylcholine even in the botulinum-treated muscle, a feature that is suggestive of a selective action of the toxin on the mechanisms responsible for transmitter release (*238*).

B. Inhibition of Transmitter Synthesis

Although no specific in vivo inhibitor of choline acetylase is available, synthesis of the transmitter may be inhibited by a series of compounds, collectively termed the hemicholiniums (*239, 240*). Of these the most active is α,α'-dimethylethanolamino-4,4′-bisacetophenone[H.C.3], which inhibits both central (*241*) and peripheral (*242*) autonomic and voluntary (*243–247*) transmission. The inhibiting of ACh synthesis by the hemicholiniums, it is believed, is achieved by means of their relatively specific combination with the postulated choline-carrier mechanism (see Section 5.3, C). In consequence, the nerve terminals become deficient in choline, and transmitter synthesis is impaired. Because of its mechanism of action hemicholinium-induced block is characteristically slow in onset and is dependent on exhausting the pre-existing stores of acetylcholine. Block is therefore accelerated by nerve stimulation and is related to its frequency.

Interference with acetylcholine synthesis may also account, at least in part, for the block produced by 3,6-bis(3-diethylaminopropoxy)pyridazine bismethiodide, Win-4981 (*246*) and during tick paralysis (*247*).

Block produced by triethylcholine may also be partly attributable to a mistaken uptaking of this substance by the nerve terminals and its acetylation by means of choline acetylase, with the consequent production of an inactive, false transmitter (*248–250*).

C. Factors Interfering with Postsynaptic Functioning of Acetylcholine: Neuromuscular Blocking Agents

Neuromuscular blocking agents have been divided conveniently into two main categories on the basis of their effects on transmitter function:

(1) Agents whose combination with the receptor of acetylcholine on the postsynaptic membrane leads to an inactive complex and a rise in the threshold of stimulation of the skeletal muscle; tubocurarine is the classic example.

(2) Agents that mimic the action of the transmitter and whose combination with the receptor of acetylcholine leads to an active complex and to a depolarization of the postsynaptic membrane; decamethonium and suxamethonium are the classic examples.

Whereas the response to depolarizing compounds is largely dependent on the species employed (*251–253*), that to nondepolarizing compounds is qualitatively uniform.

The terminology used in describing the mechanisms of action of neuromuscular blocking agents is often confusing and incorrect. Regrettably, the terms "curariform" or "curarizing" drugs continue to be employed (*254*, *255*), irrespective of whether or not their mode of action is identical with that of tubocurarine. Scant attention has been paid to the proper use of the term "competitive", which may be used to describe the action of both depolarizing and nondepolarizing agents, since both compete with acetylcholine for similar postsynaptic receptors. The biochemical and pharmacological criteria of a truly competitive antagonism (*256*) may not be met, however, by either the depolarizing compounds or by tubocurarine itself (*233*, *257*).

1. NONDEPOLARIZING NEUROMUSCULAR BLOCKING AGENTS

The majority opinion adheres to the classic view (*54*) that nondepolarizing blocking agents affect principally postsynaptic sites by occupying the receptors of acetylcholine. In consequence, the end-plate potential undergoes a progressive reduction in amplitude, duration, and rate of development, terminating in its complete disappearance (*32*, *39*, *63*, *69*, *258*). When the amplitude of the end-plate potential has fallen below the threshold necessary to trigger the action potential in the membrane of the muscle fiber, conduction ceases and block ensues (*114*). Conduction in the motor nerve and the response of the skeletal muscle to direct, ionic, and electrical stimulation remain unimpaired (*74*, *259*, *260*), the muscle being electrically normal (*254*) and there being no apparent alteration in either the membrane's resting potential or its ionic permeability. The output of acetylcholine is not reduced significantly by tubocurarine (*54*). The suggested combining of acetylcholine with the receptor in a two- or three-stage process (*261*) may be affected by tubocurarine in the initial stage of attachment without being involved in the subsequent changes in the physical properties of the membrane itself. The precise mechanism of the acetylcholine–tubocurarine antagonism may be competitive according to accepted biochemical and pharmacological criteria (*262*), but on account of the evanescent nature of acetylcholine the rate of hydrolysis by acetylcholinesterase may preclude a truly competitive effect (*257*).

On account of the antagonistic nature of the block induced by nondepolarizing agents, any effective local increase in the concentration of acetylcholine, such as due to repetitive stimulation of the motor nerve (*260*, *263*) or by the use of anticholinesterases (*264*), will antagonize their effects. Likewise, the locally induced depolarization, through the application of a cathodal current or potassium ions, will oppose nondepolarizing agents. Conversely, agents raising the membrane threshold, such as an anodal current, will intensify this type of block (*254*).

Contrary to the classic theory, which assumes tacitly an exclusive postsynaptic locus of action and which is based largely on experiments with single stimuli, an additional presynaptic site of action of tubocurarine and other compounds has been claimed (*265–270*). This hypothesis is based on the observed susceptibility of the motor nerve terminals to excitation due to acetylcholine and related compounds, as indicated by antidromic firing along the motor nerves following injection of these drugs (*271*, *272*). Proponents of this hypothesis (*273*, *274*) view the gradual decline in the size of end-plate potentials during tetanic stimulation as a presynaptic effect of tubocurarine on transmitter release rather than a physiological phenomenon (*226*, *275*). The ability of tubocurarine and other quaternary compounds to block the action potentials in motor nerve fibers (*276–279*) also has been used as circumstantial evidence for the hypothesis, being taken to indicate the presynaptic existence of free, unbound acetylcholine. On the other hand, results have confirmed that during tubocurarine block the transmitter release is not impaired (*54*, *89*, *280*) and that a reduction in end-plate potentials can take place in the absence of tubocurarine (*281*). Moreover, the observation that the supposed presynaptic effect of tubocurarine during neuromuscular depression required high-frequency stimulation (*270*) is irreconcilable with similar observations made with a frequency of 0.25/sec (*274*).

2. DEPOLARIZING NEUROMUSCULAR BLOCKING AGENTS

These achieve their effects primarily by a depolarization of the motor end plate analogous to that produced by acetylcholine, which itself, in high doses or in the presence of an anticholinesterase, produces block (*282*, *283*). Transmitter synthesis and release are probably unaffected (see, however, *284*), and direct stimulation of the muscle remains effective (*285*). Characteristically, depolarization block is preceded by manifestations of excitation of brief duration, during which muscular fasciculations or even sustained contracture may be observed. These phenomena may be associated with the activation of muscle spindles (*286*). After the initial increase in excitability, however, the depolarized area becomes impervious to direct electrical stimulation, and block ensues. The muscle membrane undergoes complete repolarization, although remaining insensitive to acetylcholine and other depolarizing agents. Blocks produced by depolarizing compounds have thus been described according to two distinct aspects. In one stage they produce a block of short duration by depolarizing the motor end plate; this has been called phase I block (*252*). It is followed by membrane repolarization, although transmission remains blocked and no end-plate potentials are evident. The second stage, phase II block, called desensitization (*117*), fade (*152*), or tachyphylaxis (*285*), is more prolonged, being limited in duration only by the removal of the drug, and resembles the block produced by nondepolarizing agents, with which it may be synergistic.

All quaternary ammonium, depolarizing drugs appear capable of producing what has been termed collectively biphasic (*252*), multiphasic (*253*), and dual or mixed (*251*) block in all types of voluntary muscle including that of man himself (*287*). The rate at which the change in the sequence of events occurs depends on both the chemical nature of the drug and the species under investigation, differences in the latter being manifested in the relative duration of each phase of activity. Thus, alteration from the initial phase of block of both decamethonium and suxamethonium occurs more readily in the rabbit, hare, dog, and monkey than in man or cat, while the component of depolarization in the last two is more prolonged than in the former (*288*, *289*).

Despite what has been said earlier concerning the qualitatively uniform mode of action of nondepolarizing agents it has been claimed (*289*) that tubocurarine can depolarize in the lizard (*290*) and that decamethonium may block by an apparently exclusive nondepolarizing mechanism in monkey (*291*). Recent investigations (*292–294*) have attempted to explain the mode of action of depolarizing and nondepolarizing drugs. It has been suggested that depolarizing drugs penetrate muscle fibers by enhancing the permeability of the end plate to ions (*295*) or by means of a specific carrier mechanism (*287*). There is, however, no evidence that the cholinergic transmitter functions in this way. Tubocurarine, on the other hand, does not penetrate, but it may prevent depolarizing agents from inducing a depolarization phase I block (*287*); conversely, it will enhance a phase II block already under way. The phenomena of desensitization and of increased sensitivity of denervated preparations have been related similarly to the penetration of muscle fibers by depolarizing drugs. The former may be an early manifestation of phase II block, the recovery of the biphasic response (return of sensitivity) being related to the slow elimination of the depolarizing agent. Tubocurarine block, on the other hand, is characterized by an increasing sensitivity to the same dose of drug (*296*). Following chronic denervation of voluntary skeletal muscle, the uptake of tritium-labeled decamethonium is greater in denervated voluntary muscle than in normal (*287*). Whatever will be the final explanation of biphasic block due to initially depolarizing compounds, problems of species and of muscle variation within one species (*297*) have restricted the choice of clinically valuable compounds to nondepolarizing, or very briefly acting depolarizing, agents.

5.6. CLASSIFICATION OF MUSCLE-RELAXANTS

Not all compounds relaxing skeletal muscle act by identical mechanisms, although it was a former practice to group all such drugs together, regardless of their site or mechanism of action. Thus, quaternary ammonium bases, pyridine, quinoline, aconitine, muscarine, and veratrine were classified as curarizing drugs, although the manner in which their effect is achieved varies greatly [Santesson, quoted by Bovet, (*298*)]. This practice has now been superseded by several attempts to subdivide muscle-relaxants into logical categories on the basis of their common chemical or pharmacological properties.

The first classification (*298*) distinguished two main categories. The "leptocurares," or long thin molecules, were assumed to exert a depolarizing action, while the "pachycurares," or bulky molecules, behaved like tubocurarine. This stereochemical, rather than pharmacological, classification is unsatisfactory owing to the absence of a demarcation between depolarizing and nondepolarizing agents and to the two quite different modes of action. Thus, nicotine, stereochemically a pachycurare, may depolarize in the cat (*299*), whereas tridecamethonium, a leptocurare, exerts a tubocurarinelike action in the chicken (*288*).

The classification proposed by Paton and Zaimis (*300*) assumes a specific and different mode of action for the two categories of competitive and noncompetitive blocking agents. This division, initially complicated by variation in the response of different species to depolarizing compounds, has been extended and modified by Zaimis (*288*) to accommodate substances inhibiting acetylcholinesterase activity and permitting transmitter accumulation (e.g., neostigmine), substances competing with acetylcholine (e.g., tubocurarine), substances mimicking acetylcholine (e.g., suxamethonium), and substances producing a dual effect (e.g., decamethonium).

After a consideration of both the chemical structures of the drugs and the protein nature of the receptor system (*301*), Foldes suggested dividing the quaternary ammonium blocking agents into depolarizing and antidepolarizing agents. By this means the use of defective terminology ("competitive" and "noncompetitive") has been avoided at the same time that the variation in species response to a particular drug is taken into account. This author has further proposed (*289*), in contrast to Zaimis, that no fundamental difference exists between depolarizing and antidepolarizing drugs, the species being the dominant factor in the qualitative responses observed (see Section 5.5, C, 2).

As a corollary to their theoretical treatment of drug–receptor interaction Ariëns and his colleagues (*302*) have considered three principal groups of substances: the depolarizers, or cholinomimetics, having a high intrinsic activity (e.g., decamethonium), the competitors, or cholinolytics, having a low intrinsic activity (e.g., tubocurarine), and the noncompetitors (e.g., prodeconium*) having an affinity for receptors other than those occupied by acetylcholine. The last group has been divided into compounds that block transmitter synthesis (e.g., the hemicholiniums), release (e.g., botulinum toxin), and destruction (e.g., neostigmine). Within the two concepts of affinity and intrinsic activity this classification is not rigid and recognizes that variations in dose level or molecular configuration may cause gradual changes in intrinsic activity and affinity and consequent alterations from one main category to another.

Similarly, the rate theory (*152*, *303*, *304*) permits neuromuscular blocking agents to be classified according to the dissociation constants of the complexes formed by the receptors. This classification also is not rigid and allows alterations in chemical structure to be reflected in changes from depolarizing (e.g., decamethonium) to nondepolarizing (e.g., tubocurarine) compounds via substances exhibiting the characteristics of either class, that is, an intermediate dissociation rate (e.g., nicotine).

The complex sequence of events associated with depolarizing compounds is not reflected in this classification.

The proposed perturbation theory of drug–receptor interaction (*153*) may also form a basis for classifying neuromuscular blocking agents. The categories implicit in the theory relate physicochemical molecular properties to perturbations produced in the receptor surface (see Section 5.4, A). On the one hand, the action of depolarizing agents such as suxamethonium could be derived from specific molecular perturbations and, on the other, that of nondepolarizing agents could involve a less specific binding with the hydrophobic nonacetylcholine portion of the receptor surface. Intermediate degrees of activity also are envisaged.

5.7. SPECIES VARIATION AND NEUROMUSCULAR BLOCK

The most important single factor in the investigation of neuromuscular block is the choice of animal species. Species variation concerns not only the choice of animal but also the strain and conditioning of it for the tests employed

* Prodeconium: 3,14-dioxohexadecane-1,16-bis(dimethylcarboproxymethylammonium bromide).

(*305*). On account of the supply and random nature of the source of many of the more useful animal species, such as the cat and dog, it is often difficult to ensure uniformity either of strain or of conditioning. In consequence, a qualitative and, especially, a quantitative correlation of results from different laboratories in which similar drugs and species were used is often difficult.

The pharmacological evaluation of neuromuscular block involves the use of a variety of animal species, including man. Because of the large quantitative and qualitative variation in the response of different species to the same agent (*288*) and of different muscles within the same species (*297*), it has been advocated repeatedly that the drugs be evaluated on the basis of human subjects. The necessity of animal experimentation, however, as a preliminary pharmacological investigation emphasizes the problem of choice of species and the care in assessing the results obtained.

Variations in potency among different species are more marked with depolarizing than with nondepolarizing agents. For instance, the potency of decamethonium in the least sensitive species [hen > cat > man > rabbit = dog > monkey > hare > rat, (*288*)] is approximately 1/100th that in the most sensitive. On the other hand, only a 5-fold range in potency separates the most from the least sensitive species with respect to tubocurarine (rat > hare = monkey > rabbit > man > dog > cat = hen).

A general, reciprocal sensitivity of a variety of species to each class of compound has also been confirmed; thus, although of all laboratory animals the rat is among the most insensitive to depolarizing agents, it is comparatively sensitive to nondepolarizing drugs, and the hen is relatively sensitive to depolarizing agents but insensitive to nondepolarizing ones. The difference in response to depolarizing agents between avian and mammalian species is particularly evident. The inhibition of twitch height, the contractural shortening of the muscle, and the development of a spastic paralysis in avia are in sharp contrast to the uniform flaccid effect and transient excitation prior to the reduction in twitch height that are observed in mammals (*300*, *306*, *307*).

Attempting to determine the optimal species for predicting the potency of neuromuscular blocking agents in man, Hoppe (*308*) reviewed the activities of a number of drugs, including gallamine, tubocurarine, and suxamethonium, in several species and correlated them with observed clinical effects. No single species could fulfill the function reliably, the most accurate estimate being obtained from the cat and dog, with the exception of suxamethonium, the potency of which in man appeared to be indicated best by the rabbit. Hoppe suggested that at best rodents and amphibia would serve to distinguish between active and inactive drugs. On the other hand, dipyrandium chloride,* a tubocurarinelike drug, showed a duration of action comparable to that of suxamethonium in rabbit, chicken, and cat, but only in the monkey and in man

* Dipyrandium chloride: 3β,17β-dipyrrolidin-1′-yl-5α-androstane bismethiodide.

did it exert a more prolonged effect, comparable to that of gallamine (*309*). Besides observed quantitative differences, the choice of species is at least partially responsible for the qualitative differences in depolarizing and nondepolarizing agents. Those who reject the concept of the individuality of a dual blocking mechanism (*289*) attribute the qualitative nature of the block observed with both depolarizing and nondepolarizing drugs to the choice of species.

Qualitative variation in the response of different muscles to the same drug has been correlated with the established existence in skeletal muscle of varying proportions of both the tonic, red, or slowly contracting fibers and the tetanic, white, or more rapidly contracting ones (*310*), each type possessing different physiological and anatomical features. Red and white muscles are divisible, according to their appearance in cross section on the electron microscope, into two morphological groups (*311*, *312*), *fibrellen struktur* (tetanic) and *felderstruktur* (tonic), the former being associated solely with end plates (*en plaque*) and the latter with clusterlike endings (*en grappe*) (*313–316*). *En grappe* endings may occur in man only in extraocular muscle (*317*).

That the contraction speed of each type of muscle in the cat is largely determined by neural influences has been demonstrated in the elegant experiments of Eccles and his co-workers (*318*), who transformed slow muscles into fast ones and vice versa by altering the nervous pathways involved. However, the structure of the individual human neuromuscular junction does not appear to be of great significance in its functional capacity (*319*), there being no clear distinction in structure or physiological properties between red and white muscles (*320*). The quantitative and qualitative discrepancies between red and white muscle fibers cannot be explained, therefore, on the basis of observed anatomical differences in the human. On the other hand, the well-known differences between mammalian and certain avian species in their responses to depolarizing agents may be explained at least in part by variations in the transmission process at each junction. In avian muscle the amount of transmitter released may be sufficient to excite only 75% of the muscle fibers, whereas in mammalian muscle the amount released by a single nerve impulse is believed generally to be in excess of that necessary to trigger the action potential (*321*, *322*). Thus, a single supramaximal stimulus will induce all mammalian muscle fibers to contract. In consequence, in avian species a drug-induced potentiation of the maximal twitch height may be related to the induction of contraction of otherwise dormant muscles while in the cat it may signify a positive ability to produce repetitive firing of the muscle (*323*, *324*).

Differences in the properties of avian and mammalian ChE also may exist. Observations of the comparative ineffectiveness in avian species of certain mammalian anticholinesterases, including benzoquinonium, ambenonium,*

* Ambenonium: [*N*,*N'*-bis(2-diethylaminoethyl) oxamide bis(2-chlorobenzyl chloride)].

and methoxybenonium,* (*323*, *325*, *326*), may indicate a difference in the affinity of the two enzymes for these drugs.

A variety of other factors influence the responses of neuromuscular blocking agents. These include physiological states, physical and physicochemical factors, and the presence of other drugs, discussion of which has been adequately covered in the excellent reviews of Foldes (*327*) and Cavallito and Gray (*159*).

5.8. STRUCTURE–ACTIVITY RELATIONSHIPS

Few aspects of pharmacology have witnessed so many endeavors to correlate chemical structure with biological function as has neuromuscular pharmacology. After the chemical identification of the tubocurarine molecule a large number of chemical compounds, both simple and complex, have been synthesized and tested for their ability to relax skeletal muscle. The outcome of many of these investigations has not been particularly rewarding, as evidenced both by the paucity of present-day clinically favored agents and by the incomplete and fragmentary state of pharmacological knowledge pertaining to the cholinergic receptor. Of the compounds involved comparatively few were designed for investigations of any particular aspect of the receptor problem, and because of the prevailing uncertainty about the underlying mechanisms the production of clinically useful derivatives has perforce remained haphazard. It is beyond the scope of this text to review all the compounds investigated, as well as quite unnecessary, considering the several excellent commentaries already available (*1–3*). In consequence, only those researches closely associated with the more important theoretical and clinical landmarks will be discussed.

A. Tubocurarine and Substituted Derivatives

(+)-Tubocurarine chloride [see **(II)**, where R is H] is a bistetrahydroisoquinoline derivative containing two quaternary nitrogen centers and two free phenolic groups (*15*, *16*). All four stereoisomers are known: (+)-tubocurarine, (−)-tubocurarine, (+)-*N*-dimethylcurine, and (−)-*N*-dimethylcurine. Curine is also known as bebeerine or chondodendrine. The potencies of the isomers differ (*328*), possibly as a result of the molecule's not being rigid and so permitting variation in both interquaternary distance and conformation (*170*).

Potency may be affected also by the position of the methoxyl substituents in the molecule. The isomeric (+)-chondocurarine **(III)** which differs from

* Methoxybenonium: [*N*,*N*′-bis(2-diethylaminoethyl) oxamide bis(2-*o*-methoxybenzyl chloride)].

tubocurarine solely in the position of the methoxyl and hydroxyl substituents, is some three times more potent than the latter in the rabbit. Tubocurarine dimethyl ether (*329*), in which the phenolic groups of tubocurarine are converted to methyl ethers [**(II)**, where R is CH_3], possesses qualitative properties similar to those of the parent compound and is more potent in several species, including man (*328*). With the exception of (+)-*N*-dimethylcurine, *O*-methylation in tubocurarine isomers is associated generally with an increase in activity.

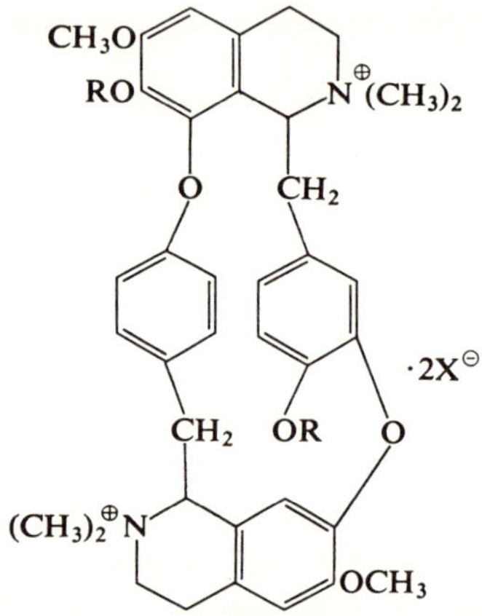

(II)
Tubocurarine (R=H); tubocurarine dimethyl ether: R=CH_3

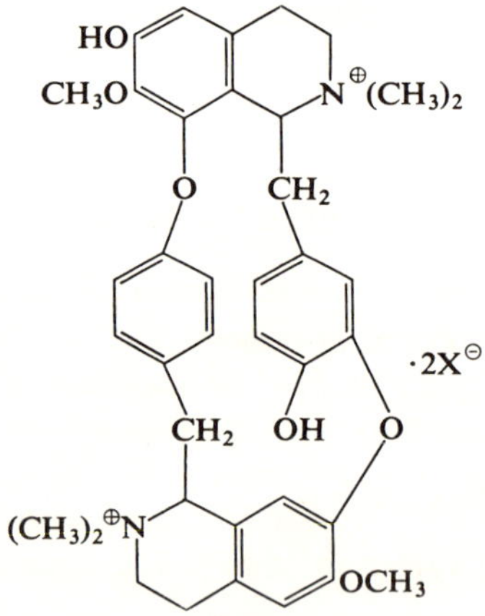

(III)
(+)-Chondocurarine

On the other hand, under conditions that reduce the ionization of the phenolic groups (low pH) tubocurarine is more potent than the dimethyl ether in the frog. This observation has been attributed (*330*) to zwitterion formation in tubocurarine as a result of the presence of the free phenolic groups. It may be argued similarly that the greater potency of chondocurarine than of tubocurarine is due to the further removal of one free phenolic group from the influence of the nitrogen center. It is interesting to note that (−)-coclaurine **(IV)**, which closely resembles half of the molecule of tubocurarine, possesses no neuromuscular blocking activity in the dog in doses up to 1 mg (*331*).

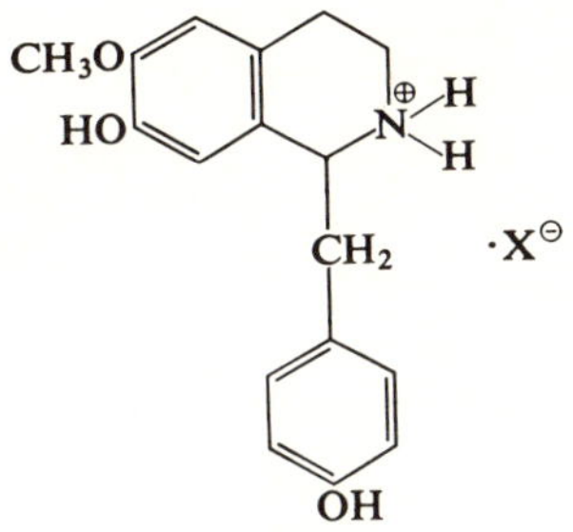

(IV)
Coclaurine

The marked differences in potency among compounds structurally related to tubocurarine suggests a fairly high degree of stereospecificity for the receptor, and Barlow (*166*) has speculated on the most favorable configuration for it. He has also suggested that in addition to the nitrogen centers the simple phenolic hydroxyl group and the ether oxygen between the aromatic rings may be important in receptor binding.

In general, an increase in the size of the ether-containing alkyl radical reduces potency, although in the rat the diethyl ether of tubocurarine is more potent than the parent compound. Di-*n*-butyl and dibenzyl tubocurarine are less active than tubocurarine. The potency of (+)-tubocurarine and the dimethyl ether may be enhanced dramatically by diethyl and other aliphatic ethers (*327*) and by a variety of other drugs, including barbiturates, sulfonamides, and antibiotics. For a discussion of the effects of these factors on tubocurarine activity reference should be made to the review by Foldes (*327*).

B. Other Synthetic Derivatives

1. GALLAMINE

The chemical identification of (+)-tubocurarine (*15, 16*) stimulated interest in bisquaternary compounds and led to the investigation of many structurally similar derivatives (*298*). Among the most important of the earlier compounds investigated was a series of β-hydroxyethyltriethylammonium ethers, from which gallamine, 1,2,3-tris(β-triethylammoniumethoxy)benzene triiodide **(V)**

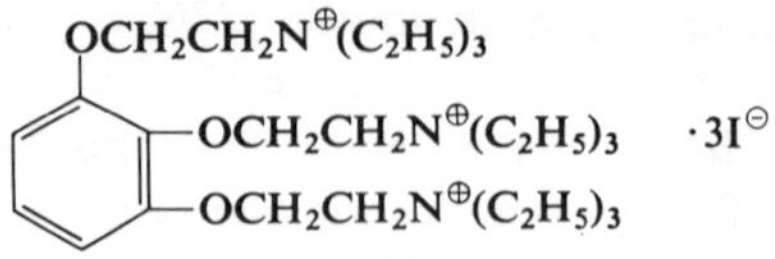

(V)

Gallamine triethiodide

has emerged as a potent tubocurarinelike relaxant of proved clinical value (*182, 185*). The presence of a third quaternary ammonium function in gallamine might, it has been suggested, modify the freedom of rotation of the other two side chains attached to the aromatic ring. In this way the two terminal nitrogen groups might be kept at an interatomic distance optimal for neuromuscular block (*185*).

2. DECAMETHONIUM

The almost simultaneous investigation of simpler bisonium derivatives based on the neuromuscular blocking potency of simple mono-onium salts (*161*), led to the synthesis and testing of a series of polymethylene bistrimethylammonium salts **(VI)** (*332, 333*); in which *n* is 2, 3, 4, 5, 6, 7, 8, 9, 10, 11, 12, and 13 (see also Chapter 4). Potency varies with chain length in the series, being very weak and nondepolarizing in the lower members ($n=2$, 3, 4, 5, and 6) and potent and depolarizing in the higher members ($n=9$ and 10). A further increase in chain length reveals a further decline in activity and the appearance of surface activity properties (*334*). The decamethylene member, decamethonium ($n=10$), initially achieved considerable importance as a clinically useful agent and, particularly from the theoretical point of view, on account of its mode of action (see Section 5.5, C, 2). Extensive modification of the molecule has been made, although the unsuitability of long-acting depolarizing drugs has limited the clinical application of the results (*335*). Oxydipentonium (*336*) and decamethonium itself (*337*) have been used successfully in certain surgical procedures.

3. SUXAMETHONIUM (SUCCINYLCHOLINE)

Modifying the decamethonium structure by introducing ester linkages led to the synthesis of suxamethonium **(VII)**, now used widely and clinically as a short-acting depolarizing compound that is readily hydrolyzed by plasma esterases. These enzymes split the molecule, creating first succinylmonocholine and then succinic acid and choline (*338, 339*), all of which exert negligible neuromuscular block. The action of suxamethonium may be prolonged and so cause apnea in cases of deficiency of plasma esterase as a result of liver disease or for other reasons (*340, 341*).

$$(CH_3)_3N^{\oplus}(CH_2)_nN^{\oplus}(CH_3)_3 \cdot 2X^{\ominus}$$

(VI)

Polymethylene bistrimethylammonium series: decamethonium, $n = 10$

$$(CH_3)_3N^{\oplus}CH_2CH_2\underset{\displaystyle \overset{\|}{O}}{C}OCH_2CH_2O\underset{\displaystyle \overset{\|}{O}}{C}CH_2CH_2N^{\oplus}(CH_3)_3 \cdot 2I^{\ominus}$$

(VII)

Suxamethonium iodide

Suxaethonium, in which one methyl radical on each quaternary nitrogen center has been replaced with an ethyl group, has also been used clinically (*342*). This compound has an even shorter duration of action than suxamethonium, but on a molar basis is only half as potent. It is hydrolyzed by plasma ChE more quickly than is suxamethonium (*340*). Several clinical advantages have been claimed for it, including a reduction in the incidence of muscle fasciculations and postoperative pain, and its very short duration of action is suitable to electro-shock therapy (*343*, *344*).

In yet another successful sphere of investigation tubocurarine and decamethoniumlike structures were combined. Whereas the combination of bisquinoline and isoquinoline nuclei with a decamethylene chain produced only feebly active molecules (*166*, *345*, *346*), the introduction of methoxyl radicals and the reduction of the heterocyclic ring system increased potency sharply. Of these compounds the salts of decamethylene-α-ω-bis-1-(3,4-dimethoxybenzyl)-1,2,3,4-tetrahydro-6,7-dimethoxy-2-methylisoquinoline, laudexium, has proved clinically useful (*347*) as a long-acting agent (*348*) with predominantly nondepolarizing properties.

An interesting variation and simplification of this type of structure introduced benzoquinonium chloride (*349*, *350*), which has been used clinically (*351–353*). This compound is tubocurarinelike (*354*) but is only feebly antagonized by neostigmine. It possesses fairly pronounced anticholinesterase activity in mammals (*355*) but not in avia (*323*). The latter property and its accompanying muscarinelike effects (such as marked increase in salivary and bronchial secretions) may be offset clinically by anticholinergic agents. It is not now widely used in surgical anesthesia. The related compound carbolonium (*356*, *357*) has been used in surgical anesthesia (*358*) and is approximately as potent as decamethonium. The accumulated evidence suggests that this compound exerts a depolarization block in man (*359*, *360*) with accompanying fasciculations even greater than those caused by suxamethonium (*361*).

5.9. CONCLUSION

Physiological events at the neuromuscular junction have been well clarified, and the therapeutic value of neuromuscular blocking agents in surgery and anesthetics has been established. However, the intimate mode of action of many of these drugs, particularly of depolarizing agents, at a cellular level, remains unclear, while attempts to construct an accurate picture of the receptor site on the basis of highly active molecules have failed to elaborate beyond the hypothesis that one onium or other center of charged intensity is necessary for activity.

Each of the three muscle-relaxant preparations in current clinical use (tubocurarine, gallamine, and suxamethonium) is capable of producing side effects. Gallamine may produce tachycardia (*185*), tubocurarine can cause both histamine release (*362*) and ganglionic blockade (*335*), and the occurrence of muscle pain and the irreversible nature of the paralysis produced by suxamethonium and other depolarizing drugs are disadvantageous to their use (*335*). The need for a neuromuscular blocking agent whose action is easily reversed, free from side effects and, preferably, tubocurarinelike persists and, together with the need for definite knowledge concerning the cholinergic receptor, remains the mandate for continued chemical and pharmacological research in this field.

REFERENCES

1. D. Bovet, F. Bovet-Nitti, and G. B. Marini-Bettolo, eds., *Curare and Curare-like Agents*, Elsevier, Amsterdam, 1959.
2. J. J. Lewis, *Rept. Progr. Appl. Chem. (Soc. Chem. Ind.)*, **45**, 220 (1960).
3. J. B. Stenlake, *Progr. Med. Chem.*, **3**, 1 (1963).
4. W. C. Bowman, *Progr. Med. Chem.*, **2**, 88 (1962).
5. S. Thesleff and D. M. J. Quastel, *Ann. Rev. Pharmacol.*, **5**, 263 (1965).
6. A. R. McIntyre, *Curare, its History, Nature and Clinical Use*, Chicago Univ. Press, Chicago, Ill., 1947.
7. K. Bryn Thomas, *Curare, its History and Usage*, Pitman, London, 1964.
8. M. de la Condamine, *Relation Abrégée d'un Voyage Fait dans l'intérieur de l'Amérique Méridionale*, Chez la veuve Pissot, Paris, 1745, p. 67, 208.
9. M. de la Condamine, *Journal du Voyage Fait par Ordre du Roi a l'Equateur Servant d'Introduction Historique à la Mésure des Trois Premiers Degrés du Méridien*, De L'imprimerie Royale, Paris, 1751, p. 189.
10. C. Bernard, *Compt. Rend.*, **43**, 825 (1856).
11. A. E. Bennett, *J. Am. Med. Assoc.*, **114**, 322 (1940).
12. A. E. Bennett, *Am. J. Psychiat.*, **97**, 1040 (1941).
13. A. E. Bennett, A. R. McIntyre, and A. L. Bennett, *J. Am. Med. Assoc.*, **114**, 1791 (1940).
14. O. Wintersteiner and J. D. Dutcher, *Science*, **97**, 467 (1943).
15. H. King, *J. Chem. Soc.*, **2**, 1381 (1935).
16. H. King, *Nature*, **135**, 469 (1935).
17. H. R. Griffith and G. E. Johnson, *Anesthesiology*, **3**, 418 (1942).
18. J. C. Hinsey, *Physiol. Rev.*, **14**, 514 (1934).
19. O. W. Tiegs, *Physiol. Rev.*, **33**, 90 (1953).
20. R. Couteaux, *Rev. Can. Biol.*, **6**, 563 (1947).
21. R. Couteaux, *Intern. Rev. Cytol.*, **4**, 335 (1955).

22. R. Couteaux, *Exptl. Cell Res., Suppl.*, **5**, 294 (1958).
23. J. D. Robertson, *J. Biophys. Biochem. Cytol.*, **2**, 369 (1956).
24. E. Andersson-Cedergren, *J. Ultrastruct. Res., Suppl.*, **1**, 1 (1959).
25. E. De Robertis, *Intern. Rev. Cytol.*, **8**, 61 (1959).
26. E. De Harven and C. Coërs, *J. Biophys. Biochem. Cytol.*, **6**, 7 (1959).
27. E. R. Bickerstaff, J. V. Evans, and A. L. Woolf, *Brain*, **83**, 638 (1960).
28. S. I. Zacks and J. M. Blumberg, *J. Biophys. Biochem. Cytol.*, **10**, 517 (1961).
29. S. I. Zacks, *The Motor End Plate*, Saunders, Philadelphia, 1964.
30. E. De Robertis and S. H. Bennett, *Federation Proc.*, **13**, 35 (1954).
31. E. De Robertis and S. H. Bennett, *J. Biophys. Biochem. Cytol.*, **1**, 47 (1955).
32. J. del Castillo and B. Katz, *Progr. Biophys. Biophys. Chem.*, **6**, 121 (1956).
33. J. F. Reger, *Exptl. Cell Res.*, **12**, 662 (1957).
34. J. F. Reger, *Anat. Record*, **130**, 7 (1958).
35. G. A. Edwards, H. Ruska, and E. De Harven, *J. Biophys. Biochem. Cytol.*, **4**, 107 (1958).
36. V. P. Whittaker, *Handbuch Exptl. Pharmakol.*, **15**, 1 (1963).
37. E. De Robertis, in *Bioelectrogenesis* (C. Chagas and A. P. de Carvalho, eds.), Elsevier, Amsterdam, 1961, p. 288.
38. J. C. Eccles, *The Physiology of Nerve Cells*, Johns Hopkins Press, Baltimore, Md., 1957.
39. J. C. Eccles, *The Physiology of Synapses*, Springer, Berlin, 1964.
40. B. Katz, *Bull. Johns Hopkins Hosp.*, **102**, 275 (1958).
41. V. L. Van Breemen, E. Anderson, and J. F. Reger, *Exptl. Cell. Res., Suppl.*, **5**, 153 (1958).
42. S. L. Palay, *J. Biophys. Biochem. Cytol., Suppl.*, **2**, 193 (1956).
43. R. Birks, H. E. Huxley, and B. Katz, *J. Physiol. (London)*, **150**, 134 (1960).
44. J. F. Reger, *J. Ultrastruct. Res.*, **2**, 269 (1959).
45. R. Birks, B. Katz, and R. Miledi, *J. Physiol. (London)*, **150**, 145 (1960).
46. C. O. Hebb, K. Krnjević, and A. Silver, *J. Physiol. (London)*, **171**, 504 (1964).
47. M. A. Gerebtzoff, *Cholinesterases*, Pergamon, New York, 1959.
48. G. Koelle, *Handbuch Exptl. Pharmakol.*, **15**, 187 (1963).
49. P. R. Lewis and C. C. D. Shute, *J. Physiol. (London)*, **180**, 8P (1965).
50. V. P. Whittaker and E. G. Gray, *Brit. Med. Bull.*, **18**, 223 (1962).
51. C. O. Hebb, *Physiol. Rev.*, **37**, 196 (1957).
52. D. Nachmansohn, *Chemical and Molecular Basis of Nerve Activity*, Academic Press, New York, 1959.
53. J. D. Robertson, *Am. J. Phys. Med.*, **39**, 1 (1960).
54. H. H. Dale, W. Feldberg, and M. Vogt, *J. Physiol. (London)*, **86**, 353 (1936).
55. H. H. Dale, *Harvey Lectures, Ser. 32*, **1936–37**, 229.
56. G. L. Brown, *Physiol. Rev.*, **17**, 485 (1937).
57. J. C. Eccles, *Ergeb. Physiol. Biol. Chem. Exptl. Pharmakol.*, **38**, 339 (1936).
58. J. C. Eccles, *Physiol. Rev.*, **17**, 538 (1937).
59. H. H. Dale, *J. Pharmacol. Exptl. Therap.*, **6**, 147 (1914).
60. J. Erlanger, *J. Neurophysiol.*, **2**, 370 (1939).
61. R. Lorente De Nó, *Am. J. Physiol.*, **121**, 331 (1938).
62. H. S. Gasser, *Physiol. Rev.*, **10**, 35 (1930).
63. J. C. Eccles, *Ann. N.Y. Acad. Sci.*, **47**, 429 (1946).
64. B. Katz, *Proc. Roy. Soc. (London)*, **155B**, 455 (1962).
65. J. C. Eccles, *Arch. Sci. Physiol.*, **3**, 567 (1949).
66. E. J. Furshpan and D. D. Potter, *Nature*, **180**, 342 (1957).
67. A. R. Martin and G. Pilar, *J. Physiol. (London)*, **168**, 443 (1963).
68. B. Katz, *Bull. Johns Hopkins Hosp.*, **102**, 275 (1958).
69. B. Katz, *Rev. Mod. Phys.*, **31**, 524 (1959).

70. R. Couteaux and D. Nachmansohn, *Proc. Soc. Exptl. Biol. Med.*, **43**, 177 (1940).
71. F. Buchthal and J. Lindhard, *Acta Physiol. Scand.*, **4**, 136 (1942).
72. S. W. Kuffler, *J. Neurophysiol.*, **6**, 99 (1943).
73. S. W. Kuffler, *J. Neurophysiol.*, **8**, 77 (1945).
74. W. D. M. Paton, *Can. J. Biochem. Physiol.*, **41**, 2637 (1963).
75. J. E. Gardiner and V. P. Whittaker, *Biochem. J.*, **58**, 24 (1954).
76. D. Nachmansohn, *Handbuch Exptl. Pharmakol.*, **15**, 701 (1963).
77. D. Nachmansohn and A. L. Machado, *J. Neurophysiol.*, **6**, 397 (1943).
78. F. Lipmann and N. O. Kaplan, *J. Biol. Chem.*, **162**, 743 (1946).
79. H. McIlwain, in *Biochemistry and the Central Nervous System*, Churchill, London, 1959, p. 210.
80. C. Hebb, *Handbuch Exptl. Pharmakol.*, **15**, 55 (1963).
81. F. C. MacIntosh, *Can. J. Biochem. Physiol.*, **37**, 343 (1959).
82. W. Feldberg, *Physiol. Rev.*, **25**, 596 (1945).
83. F. C. MacIntosh, *Can. J. Biochem. Physiol.*, **41**, 2555 (1963).
84. P. Fatt and B. Katz, *J. Physiol.* (*London*), **117**, 109 (1952).
85. J. C. Eccles and A. W. Liley, *Am. J. Phys. Med.*, **38**, 96 (1959).
86. I. A. Boyd and A. R. Martin, *J. Physiol.* (*London*), **132**, 74 (1956).
87. A. W. Liley, *J. Physiol.* (*London*), **132**, 650 (1956).
88. A. W. Liley, *J. Physiol.* (*London*), **133**, 571 (1956).
89. N. Emmelin and F. C. MacIntosh, *J. Physiol.* (*London*), **131**, 477 (1956).
90. D. W. Straughan, *Brit. J. Pharmacol.*, **15**, 417 (1960).
91. W. L. Nastuk, *Federation Proc.*, **12**, 102 (1953).
92. K. Krnjević and J. F. Mitchell, *Nature*, **186**, 241 (1960).
93. K. Krnjević and J. F. Mitchell, *J. Physiol.* (*London*), **155**, 246 (1961).
94. J. Gautrelet and E. Corteggiani, *Compt. Rend.*, **131**, 951 (1939).
95. B. M. Braganca and J. H. Quastel, *Nature*, **169**, 695 (1952).
96. G. L. Brown and W. Feldberg, *J. Physiol.* (*London*), **86**, 290 (1936).
97. R. R. Renshaw, D. Green, and M. Ziff, *J. Pharmacol. Exptl. Therap.*, **62**, 430 (1938).
98. D. N. McKinstry, E. Koenig, W. A. Koelle, and G. B. Koelle, *Can. J. Biochem. Physiol.*, **41**, 2599 (1963).
99. W. L. Nastuk, *Ann. N.Y. Acad. Sci.*, **81**, 317 (1959).
100. A. L. Hodgkin, *Biol. Rev. Cambridge Phil. Soc.*, **26**, 339 (1951).
101. R. I. Birks, *Can. J. Biochem. Physiol.*, **41**, 2573 (1963).
102. A. L. Hodgkin and R. D. Keynes, *J. Physiol.* (*London*), **138**, 253 (1957).
103. A. M. Harvey and F. C. MacIntosh, *J. Physiol.* (*London*), **97**, 408 (1940).
104. R. I. Birks and F. C. MacIntosh, *Brit. Med. Bull.*, **13**, 157 (1957).
105. O. Hutter and K. Kostial, *J. Physiol.* (*London*), **124**, 234 (1954).
106. D. H. Jenkinson, *J. Physiol.* (*London*), **138**, 434 (1957).
107. J. I. Hubbard, *J. Physiol.* (*London*), **159**, 507 (1961).
108. J. del Castillo and L. Engbaek, *J. Physiol.* (*London*), **120**, 54P (1953).
109. J. del Castillo and L. Engbaek, *J. Physiol.* (*London*), **124**, 370 (1954).
110. J. del Castillo and L. Stark, *J. Physiol.* (*London*), **116**, 507 (1952).
111. G. L. Brown, *J. Physiol.* (*London*), **124**, 26 (1954).
112. H. Göpfert and H. Schaefer, *Arch. Ges. Physiol.*, **239**, 597 (1938).
113. S. W. Kuffler, *Arch. Sci. Physiol.*, **3**, 585 (1949).
114. J. C. Eccles, B. Katz, and S. W. Kuffler, *J. Neurophysiol.*, **4**, 362 (1941).
115. J. del Castillo and B. Katz, *J. Physiol.* (*London*), **128**, 396 (1955).
116. B. Katz and S. Thesleff, *J. Physiol.* (*London*), **138**, 63 (1957).
117. J. Axelsson and S. Thesleff, *Acta Physiol. Scand.*, **43**, 15 (1958).

118. D. Elmquist and S. Thesleff, *Rev. Can. Biol.*, **21**, 229 (1962).
119. S. Thesleff, *Physiol. Rev.*, **40**, 734 (1960).
120. S. Thesleff, *Progr. Neurobiol. V, Neural Physiopathol.*, **1963**, 1.
121. W. Feldberg, *Brit. Med. J.*, **1**, 967 (1951).
122. D. Nachmansohn, *Ann. N.Y. Acad. Sci.*, **81**, 215 (1959).
123. D. Nachmansohn, *Anesthesiology*, **20**, 421 (1959).
124. H. H. Dale, *Pharmacol. Rev.*, **6**, 7 (1954).
125. G. B. Koelle, *J. Pharm. Pharmacol.*, **14**, 65 (1962).
126. S. Ehrenpreis, *Nature*, **201**, 887 (1964).
127. C. Y. Kao and A. Nishiyama, *J. Physiol.* (*London*), **180**, 50 (1965).
128. W. D. Dettbarn, H. Higman, P. Rosenberg, and D. Nachmansohn, *Science*, **132**, 300 (1960).
129. A. Marnay and D. Nachmansohn, *J. Physiol.* (*London*), **92**, 37 (1938).
130. D. Nachmansohn and M. A. Rothenberg, *J. Biol. Chem.*, **158**, 653 (1945).
131. E. Stedman, E. Stedman and L. H. Easson, *Biochem. J.*, **26**, 2056 (1932).
132. K. B. Augustinsson, *Acta Physiol. Scand.*, *Suppl.* **15**, 1 (1948).
133. G. B. Koelle, *J. Pharmacol. Exptl. Therap.*, **100**, 158 (1950).
134. G. L. Brown, H. H. Dale, and W. Feldberg, *J. Physiol.* (*London*), **87**, 394 (1936).
135. A. G. Ogston, *J. Physiol.* (*London*), **128**, 222 (1955).
136. W. L. M. Perry, *J. Physiol.* (*London*), **119**, 439 (1953).
137. P. Ehrlich, *Proc. Roy. Soc.* (*London*), **66**, 424 (1900).
138. E. Fischer, *Chem. Ber.*, **27**, 2985 (1894).
139. E. Fischer, *Chem. Ber.*, **28**, 1429 (1895).
140. J. N. Langley, *J. Physiol.* (*London*), **1**, 339 (1878).
141. K. Lucas, *J. Physiol.* (*London*), **36**, 113 (1907).
142. I. Langmuir, *J. Am. Chem. Soc.*, **38**, 2221 (1916).
143. I. Langmuir, *J. Am. Chem. Soc.*, **39**, 1848 (1917).
144. I. Langmuir, *J. Am. Chem. Soc.*, **40**, 1361 (1918).
145. A. J. Clark, *Handbuch Exptl. Pharmakol.*, **4**, 1 (1937).
146. J. H. Gaddum, *Proc. Roy. Soc.* (*London*), **121B**, 598 (1937).
147. R. P. Stephenson, *Brit. J. Pharmacol.*, **11**, 379 (1956).
148. M. Nickerson, *Nature*, **178**, 697 (1956).
149. E. Ariëns, ed., *Molecular Pharmacology. The Mode of Action of Biologically Active Compounds*, Academic Press, New York, 1964.
150. H. O. Schild, *Brit. J. Pharmacol.*, **2**, 189 (1947).
151. E. F. Van Maanen, *J. Pharmacol. Exptl. Therap.*, **99**, 255 (1950).
152. W. D. M. Paton, *Proc. Roy. Soc.* (*London*), **154B**, 21 (1961).
153. B. Belleau, *J. Med. Chem.*, **7**, 776 (1964).
154. M. E. Krahl, *The Action of Insulin on Cells*, Academic Press, New York, 1961, p. 180.
155. A. Crum-Brown and T. R. Fraser, *Trans. Roy. Soc. Edinburgh*, **25**, 151 (1869).
156. A. Crum-Brown and T. R. Fraser, *Trans. Roy. Soc. Edinburgh*, **25**, 693 (1869).
157. A. Crum-Brown and T. R. Fraser, *Proc. Roy. Soc. Edinburgh*, **7B**, 663 (1872).
158. H. R. Ing, *Progr. Drug. Res.*, **7**, 307 (1964).
159. C. J. Cavallito and A. P. Gray, *Progr. Drug Res.*, **2**, 135 (1960).
160. C. C. Pfeiffer, *Science*, **107**, 94 (1948).
161. H. R. Ing, *Physiol. Rev.*, **16**, 527 (1936).
162. K. K. Kimura, K. Unna, and C. C. Pfeiffer, *J. Pharmacol. Exptl. Therap.*, **95**, 149 (1949).
163. F. W. Schueler, *Arch. Intern. Pharmacodyn.*, **93**, 417 (1953).
164. R. B. Barlow and H. R. Ing, *Brit. J. Pharmacol.*, **3**, 298 (1948).
165. W. D. M. Paton and E. J. Zaimis, *Brit. J. Pharmacol.*, **4**, 381 (1949).

166. R. B. Barlow, *Introduction to Chemical Pharmacology*, Methuen, London, 1964, p. 87.
167. K. K. Kimura and K. R. Unna, *J. Pharmacol. Exptl. Therap.*, **98**, 286 (1950).
168. E. W. Pelikan and K. R. Unna, *J. Pharmacol. Exptl. Therap.*, **104**, 354 (1952).
169. C. J. Cavallito, A. P. Gray, and E. E. Spinner, *J. Am. Chem. Soc.*, **76**, 1862 (1954).
170. F. M. Carey, D. Edwards, J. J. Lewis, and J. B. Stenlake, *J. Pharm. Pharmacol., Suppl.*, **11**, 70T (1959).
171. C. G. Haining and R. G. Johnston, *Brit. J. Pharmacol.*, **18**, 275 (1962).
172. S. A. Rice, *J. Am. Chem. Soc.*, **78**, 5247 (1956).
173. S. A. Rice, *J. Am. Chem. Soc.*, **80**, 3207 (1958).
174. E. W. Gill, *Proc. Roy. Soc. (London)*, **150B**, 381 (1959).
175. S. Loewe and S. C. Harvey, *Arch. Exptl. Pathol. Pharmakol.*, **214**, 214 (1952).
176. H. O. J. Collier, J. M. Z. Gladych, B. Macauley, and E. P. Taylor, *Nature*, **182**, 1424 (1958).
177. F. J. Macri, *Proc. Soc. Exptl. Biol. Med.*, **85**, 603 (1954).
178. R. Wien, *Arch. Intern. Pharmacodyn.*, **97**, 395 (1954).
179. P. G. Waser in *Curare and Curare-like Agents* (D. Bovet, F. Bovet-Nitti, and G. B. Marini-Bettolo, eds.), Elsevier, Amsterdam, 1959, p. 219.
180. P. G. Waser, *J. Pharm. Pharmacol.*, **12**, 577 (1960).
181. J. P. Long and F. W. Schueler, *J. Am. Pharm. Assoc.*, **43**, 79 (1954).
182. D. Bovet, F. Depierre, S. Courvoisier, and Y. de Lestrange, *Arch. Intern. Pharmacodyn.*, **80**, 172 (1949).
183. C. J. Kensler, H. Langemann, and C. L. Zirkle, *J. Pharmacol. Exptl. Therap.*, **110**, 127 (1954).
184. C. J. Kensler, C. L. Zirkle, A. Matallana, and G. Condouris, *J. Pharmacol. Exptl. Therap.*, **112**, 210 (1954).
185. W. F. Riker and W. C. Wescoe, *Ann. N.Y. Acad. Sci.*, **54**, 373 (1951).
186. D. Edwards, J. J. Lewis, J. B. Stenlake, and M. S. Zoha, *J. Pharm. Pharmacol.*, **9**, 1004 (1957).
187. D. Edwards, J. J. Lewis, J. B. Stenlake, and M. S. Zoha, *J. Pharm. Pharmacol., Suppl.*, **10**, 106T (1958).
188. D. Edwards, J. J. Lewis, J. B. Stenlake, and F. Stothers, *J. Pharm. Pharmacol., Suppl.*, **11**, 87T (1959).
189. D. Edwards, J. B. Stenlake, J. J. Lewis, and F. Stothers, *J. Med. Chem.*, **3**, 369 (1961).
190. D. Edwards, J. J. Lewis, D. E. McPhail, T. C. Muir, and J. B. Stenlake, *J. Pharm. Pharmacol., Suppl.*, **12**, 137T (1960).
191. J. J. Lewis, D. E. McPhail, T. C. Muir, and J. B. Stenlake, *J. Pharm. Pharmacol.*, **13**, 543 (1961).
192. F. M. Carey, J. J. Lewis, J. B. Stenlake, and W. D. Williams, *J. Pharm. Pharmacol., Suppl.*, **13**, 103T (1961).
193. J. J Lewis, M. Martin-Smith, and T. C. Muir, *Brit. J. Pharmacol.*, **20**, 307 (1963).
194. F. M. Carey, C. I. Furst, J. J. Lewis, and J. B. Stenlake, *J. Pharm. Pharmacol., Suppl.*, **16**, 89T (1964).
195. M. M. Janot, F. Laine, and R. Goutarel, *Ann. Pharm. Franc.*, **18**, 673 (1960).
196. A. Quevauviller and F. Laine, *Ann. Pharm. Franc.*, **18**, 678 (1960).
197. F. Khuong Huu-Laine and W. Pinto-Scognamiglio, *Arch. Intern. Pharmacodyn*, **147**, 209 (1964).
198. May and Baker Ltd., South African Pat., 63,940 (1963).
199. May and Baker Ltd., South African Pat., 63,941 (1963).
200. R. S. Biggs, M. Davis, and R. Wien, *Experientia*, **20**, 119 (1964).
201. M. Martin-Smith and M. F. Sugrue, *J. Pharm. Pharmacol.*, **16**, 569 (1964).

202. E. W. Gill and H. R. Ing, *J. Chem. Soc.*, **4**, 4728 (1958).
203. R. Wien and D. F. J. Mason, *Brit. J. Pharmacol.*, **8**, 306 (1953).
204. D. E. Koshland, *Proc. Natl. Acad. Sci. U.S.*, **44**, 98 (1958).
205. G. J. Martin, *J. Chem. Educ.*, **33**, 204 (1956).
206. K. Bernauer, F. Berlage, W. von Philipsborn, H. Schmid, and P. Karrer, *Helv. Chim. Acta*, **41**, 2293 (1958).
207. O. Blanpin and J. Bretaudeau, *Compt. Rend. Soc. Biol.*, **155**, 878 (1961).
208. O. Blanpin and R. Pierre, *Therapie*, **16**, 179 (1961).
209. H. H. Ross and M. Martin-Smith, personal communication, 1965.
210. R. M. Fuoss and D. Edelson, *J. Am. Chem. Soc.*, **73**, 269 (1951).
211. R. M. Fuoss and V. F. H. Chu, *J. Am. Chem. Soc.*, **73**, 949 (1951).
212. F. E. Harris and S. A. Rice, *J. Chem. Phys.*, **24**, 326 (1956).
213. P. H. Elworthy, *J. Chem. Soc.*, **1**, 388 (1963).
214. P. H. Elworthy, *J. Pharm. Pharmacol., Suppl.*, **15**, 137T (1963).
215. C. Chagas in *Curare and Curare-like Agents* (D. Bovet, F. Bovet-Nitti, and G. B. Marini-Bettolo, eds.), Elsevier, Amsterdam, 1959, p. 327.
216. S. Ehrenpreis, *Biochim. Biophys. Acta*, **44**, 561 (1960).
217. S. Ehrenpreis in *Modern Concepts in the Relationship between Structure and Pharmacological Activity* (K. J. Brunings, and P. Lindgren, eds.), Pergamon, London, 1963, p. 119.
218. E. Schoffeniels, *Arch. Intern. Physiol. Biochim.*, **70**, 423 (1962).
219. K. E. Neet and S. L. Friess, *Arch. Biochem. Biophys.*, **99**, 484 (1962).
220. K. Kiyota, *J. Neurochem.*, **9**, 555 (1962).
221. D. Nachmansohn, *Science*, **136**, 177 (1962).
222. N. E. Wedensky, *Arch. Ges. Physiol.*, **100**, 1 (1903).
223. A. Rosenblueth and R. S. Morison, *Am. J. Physiol.*, **119**, 236 (1937).
224. A. W. Liley and K. A. K. North, *J. Neurophysiol.*, **16**, 509 (1953).
225. V. B. Brooks and R. E. Thies, *J. Physiol. (London)*, **162**, 298 (1962).
226. M. Otsuka, M. Endo, and Y. Nonomura, *Japan J. Physiol.*, **12**, 573 (1962).
227. J. del Castillo and B. Katz, *J. Physiol. (London)*, **124**, 553 (1954).
228. A. M. Harvey, *Bull. Johns Hopkins Hosp.*, **65**, 223 (1939).
229. P. J. Watson, *J. Pharm. Pharmacol.*, **12**, 257 (1960).
230. D. W. Straughan, *J. Pharm. Pharmacol.*, **13**, 49 (1961).
231. A. M. Shanes, *Pharmacol. Rev.*, **10**, 59 (1958).
232. J. G. Nicholls and J. P. Quilliam, *Brit. J. Pharmacol.*, **11**, 151 (1956).
233. J. del Castillo and B. Katz, *Proc. Roy. Soc. (London)*, **146B**, 339 (1957).
234. A. S. V. Burgen, F. Dickens, and L. J. Zatman, *J. Physiol. (London)*, **109**, 10 (1949).
235. V. B. Brooks, *J. Physiol. (London)*, **134**, 264 (1956).
236. V. B. Brooks, *J. Physiol. (London)*, **123**, 501 (1954).
237. A. C. Guyton and M. A. Macdonald, *AMA Arch. Neurol. Psychiat.*, **57**, 578 (1947).
238. S. Thesleff, *J. Physiol. (London)*, **151**, 598 (1960).
239. F. W. Schueler, *J. Pharmacol. Exptl. Therap.*, **115**, 127 (1955).
240. F. W. Schueler, *Intern. Rev. Neurobiol.*, **2**, 77 (1960).
241. J. E. Gardiner, *Biochem. J.*, **81**, 297 (1961).
242. K. C. Wong and J. P. Long, *J. Pharmacol. Exptl. Therap.*, **133**, 211 (1961).
243. V. G. Longo, *Arch. Intern. Pharmacodyn.*, **119**, 1 (1959).
244. H. Wilson and J. P. Long, *Arch. Intern. Pharmacodyn.*, **120**, 343 (1959).
245. E. R. Evans and H. Wilson, *J. Pharm. Pharmacol., Suppl.*, **14**, 34T (1962).
246. R. M. Gesler and J. O. Hoppe, *Federation Proc.*, **20**, 587 (1961).
247. P. Emmons and H. McLennan, *Nature*, **183**, 474 (1959).

248. W. C. Bowman and M. J. Rand, *Brit. J. Pharmacol.*, **17**, 176 (1961).
249. W. C. Bowman, B. A. Hemsworth, and M. J. Rand, *Brit. J. Pharmacol.*, **19**, 198 (1962).
250. D. V. Roberts, *J. Physiol.* (*London*), **160**, 94 (1962).
251. E. J. Zaimis, *J. Physiol.* (*London*), **122**, 238 (1953).
252. D. J. Jenden, K. Kamijo, and D. B. Taylor, *J. Pharmacol. Exptl. Therap.*, **103**, 348 (1951).
253. R. J. H. Hodges and F. F. Foldes, *Lancet*, **1**, 373 (1957).
254. W. D. M. Paton, *Ann. N.Y. Acad. Sci.*, **54**, 347 (1951).
255. C. C. Hunt and S. W. Kuffler, *Pharmacol. Rev.*, **2**, 96 (1950).
256. J. H. Gaddum, *Pharmacol. Rev.*, **9**, 211 (1957).
257. D. B. Taylor, *Anesthesiology*, **20**, 439 (1959).
258. S. Thesleff, *Acta Physiol. Scand.*, **34**, 218 (1955).
259. P. Fatt and B. Katz, *J. Physiol.* (*London*), **115**, 320 (1951).
260. J. I. Hubbard and R. F. Schmidt, *Nature*, **196**, 378 (1962).
261. J. del Castillo and B. Katz, *Proc. Roy. Soc.* (*London*), **146B**, 357 (1956–57).
262. W. D. M. Paton, *Anesthesia*, **8**, 151 (1953).
263. S. Thesleff, in *The Structure and Function of Muscle*, Vol. 3 (G. H. Bourne, ed.), Academic Press, New York, 1961, p. 1.
264. W. F. Riker, *Pharmacol. Rev.*, **5**, 1 (1953).
265. K. Naess, *Acta Pharmacol. Toxicol.*, **8**, 400 (1952).
266. K. Naess, *Acta Pharmacol. Toxicol.*, **9**, 196 (1953).
267. J. A. Barstad, *Experientia*, **18**, 579 (1962).
268. W. F. Riker, Jr., G. Werner, J. Roberts, and A. Kuperman, *J. Pharmacol. Exptl. Therap.* **125**, 150 (1959).
269. G. Lilleheil and K. Naess, *Experientia*, **16**, 550 (1960).
270. G. Lilleheil and K. Naess, *Acta Physiol. Scand.*, **52**, 120 (1961).
271. R. L. Masland and R. S. Wigton, *J. Neurophysiol.*, **3**, 269 (1940).
272. W. F. Riker, Jr., G. Werner, J. Roberts, and A. Kuperman, *Ann. N.Y. Acad. Sci.*, **81**, 328 (1959).
273. T. P. Feng, *Sheng Li Hsuch Pao*, **16**, 341 (1941).
274. A. Takeuchi, *Japan. J. Physiol.*, **8**, 102 (1958).
275. O. F. Hutter, *J. Physiol.* (*London*), **118**, 216 (1952).
276. H. Grundfest, D. Nachmansohn, C. Y. Kao, and R. Chambers, *Nature*, **169**, 190 (1952).
277. K. Koketsu, *Am. J. Physiol.*, **193**, 213 (1958).
278. J. Stovner, *Acta Pharmacol. Toxicol.*, **14**, 317 (1958).
279. W. D. Dettbarn, *Nature*, **186**, 891 (1960).
280. J. Cheymol, F. Bourillet, and Y. Ogura, *Arch. Intern. Pharmacodyn.*, **139**, 187 (1962).
281. J. del Castillo and B. Katz, *J. Physiol.* (*London*), **124**, 574 (1955).
282. E. Zaimis, *J. Physiol.* (*London*), **112**, 176 (1951).
283. Z. M. Bacq and G. L. Brown, *J. Physiol.* (*London*), **89**, 45 (1937).
284. L. Wislicki, *Arch. Intern. Pharmacodyn.*, **132**, 413 (1961).
285. B. D. Burns and W. D. M. Paton, *J. Physiol.* (*London*), **115**, 41 (1951).
286. W. D. M. Paton, *Anesthesiology*, **20**, 453 (1959).
287. D. B. Taylor and O. A. Nedergaard, *Physiol. Rev.*, **45**, 523 (1965).
288. E. Zaimis in *Curare and Curare-like Agents* (D. Bovet, F. Bovet-Nitti, and G. B. Marini-Bettolo, eds.), Elsevier, Amsterdam, 1959, p. 191.
289. F. F. Foldes in *Curare and Curare-like Agents* (D. Bovet, F. Bovet-Nitti, and G. B. Marini-Bettolo, eds.), Elsevier, Amsterdam, 1959, p. 425.
290. F. F. Foldes, R. D. Hunt, and A. J. Ceravolo, *Anesthesia Analgesia, Current Res.*, **31**, 185 (1952).
291. E. J. Zaimis, *J. Physiol.* (*London*), **122**, 238 (1953).

292. D. B. Taylor in *Curare and Curare-like Agents* (A. V. S. de Rueck, ed.), Churchill, London, 1962, p. 21.
293. R. Creese, D. B. Taylor, and B. Tilton, *J. Pharmacol. Exptl. Therap.*, **139**, 8 (1963).
294. D. MacKay, *Nature*, **197**, 1171 (1963).
295. W. D. M. Paton in *Curare and Curare-like Agents* (A. V. S. de Reuck, ed.), Churchill, London, 1962, p. 29.
296. P. E. B. Holmes, D. J. Jenden, and D. B. Taylor, *J. Pharmacol. Exptl. Therap.*, **103**, 382 (1951).
297. H. H. Su, F. T. Kao, and M. Karp, *Science*, **113**, 743 (1951).
298. D. Bovet, *Ann. N.Y. Acad. Sci.*, **54**, 407 (1951).
299. W. D. M. Paton and E. J. Zaimis, *J. Physiol. (London)*, **112**, 311 (1951).
300. W. D. M. Paton and E. J. Zaimis, *Pharmacol. Rev.*, **4**, 219 (1952).
301. F. F. Foldes, *Brit. J. Anaesthesia*, **26**, 394 (1954).
302. J. M. Van Rossum, E. J. Ariëns, and G. H. Linssen, *Biochem. Pharmacol.*, **1**, 193 (1958).
303. W. D. M. Paton and D. R. Waud, *Brit. J. Anaesthesia*, **34**, 251 (1962).
304. W. D. M. Paton and D. R. Waud in *Curare and Curare-like Agents* (A. V. S. de Reuck, ed.), Churchill, London, 1962, p. 34.
305. W. Lane-Petter, *J. Pharm. Pharmacol.*, **14**, 397 (1962).
306. G. A. H. Buttle and E. J. Zaimis, *J. Pharm. Pharmacol.*, **1**, 991 (1949).
307. A. Crema, W. Scognamiglio, and D. Bovet, *Arch. Intern. Pharmacodyn.*, **122**, 152 (1959).
308. J. O. Hoppe, *Anesthesiology*, **16**, 91 (1955).
309. W. W. Mushin and W. W. Mapleson, *Brit. J. Anaesthesia*, **36**, 761 (1964).
310. L. Ranvier, *Compt. Rend.*, **77**, 1030 (1873).
311. P. Krüger and P. G. Günther, *Z. Anat. Entwicklungsgeschichte*, **118**, 313 (1955).
312. P. Krüger and P. G. Günther, *Acta Anat.*, **33**, 325 (1958).
313. P. Krüger, *Anat. Anz.*, **97**, 169 (1949).
314. P. G. Günther, *Anat. Anz.*, **97**, 175 (1949).
315. A. Hess, *J. Cell. Comp. Physiol.*, **58**, 63 (1961).
316. A. Hess, *Rev. Can. Biol.*, **21**, 241 (1962).
317. C. Kupfer, *J. Physiol. (London)*, **153**, 522 (1960).
318. A. J. Buller, J. C. Eccles, and R. M. Eccles, *J. Physiol. (London)*, **150**, 399 (1960).
319. E. Gutmann and J. Z. Young, *J. Anat.*, **78**, 15 (1944).
320. C. Coërs and A. L. Woolf, *The Innervation of Muscle*, Blackwell, Oxford, 1959.
321. G. L. Brown and A. M. Harvey, *J. Physiol. (London)*, **93**, 285 (1938).
322. G. L. Brown and A. M. Harvey, *J. Physiol. (London)*, **94**, 101 (1938).
323. L. C. Blaber and W. C. Bowman, *Arch. Intern. Pharmacodyn.*, **138**, 90 (1962).
324. L. C. Blaber and W. C. Bowman, *Arch. Intern. Pharmacodyn.*, **138**, 185 (1962).
325. J. O. Hoppe, *Ann. N.Y. Acad. Sci.*, **54**, 395 (1951).
326. G. B. Koelle, *J. Pharmacol. Exptl. Therap.*, **120**, 488 (1957).
327. F. F. Foldes, *Anesthesiology*, **20**, 464 (1959).
328. O. Wintersteiner in *Curare and Curare-like Agents* (D. Bovet, F. Bovet-Nitti, and G. B. Marini-Bettolo, eds.), Elsevier, Amsterdam, 1959, p. 153.
329. H. O. J. Collier, S. K. Paris, and L. I. Woolf, *Nature*, **161**, 817 (1948).
330. W. Kalow, *J. Pharmacol. Exptl. Therap.*, **110**, 433 (1954).
331. J. Finkelstein, *J. Am. Chem. Soc.*, **73**, 550 (1951).
332. R. B. Barlow and H. R. Ing, *Nature*, **161**, 718 (1948).
333. W. D. M. Paton and E. J. Zaimis, *Nature*, **161**, 718 (1948).
334. W. D. M. Paton and E. J. Zaimis, *Brit. J. Pharmacol.*, **4**, 381 (1949).
335. F. F. Foldes, *Clin. Pharmacol. Therap.*, **1**, 345 (1960).
336. P. Mundaleer, *Acta Anesthesiol. Belg.*, **3**, 203 (1952).

337. J. I. M. Lawson, *Brit. J. Anaesthesia*, **30**, 240 (1958).
338. V. P. Whittaker and S. Wijesundera, *Biochem. J.*, **52**, 475 (1952).
339. F. F. Foldes and F. J. Tsuji, *Federation Proc.*, **12**, 321 (1953).
340. F. F. Foldes, *Muscle Relaxants in Anesthesiology*, Thomas, Springfield, Ill., 1957, p. 52.
341. H. C. Churchill-Davidson, *Anesthesiology*, **20**, 535 (1959).
342. P. Valdoni, *Rend. Ist. Super. Sanita*, **12**, 255 (1949).
343. A. Edridge, *Proc. Roy. Soc. Med.*, **45**, 869 (1952).
344. V. T. Stephen, *Med. J. Australia*, **1**, 372 (1953).
345. E. P. Taylor, *J. Chem. Soc.*, **2**, 1150 (1951).
346. H. O. J. Collier and E. P. Taylor, *Nature*, **164**, 491 (1949).
347. R. I. Bodman, *Brit. J. Pharmacol.*, **7**, 409 (1952).
348. H. O. J. Collier and B. Macauley, *Brit. J. Pharmacol.*, **7**, 398 (1952).
349. J. O. Hoppe, *J. Pharmacol. Exptl. Therap.*, **100**, 333 (1950).
350. E. Philippot and M. J. Dallemagne, *Arch. Intern. Pharmacodyn.*, **96**, 485 (1954).
351. J. G. Arrowood, *Anesthesiology*, **12**, 753 (1951).
352. F. F. Foldes, *Ann. N.Y. Acad. Sci.*, **54**, 503 (1951).
353. J. W. Dundee, T. C. Gray, and G. J. Rees, *Anaesthesia*, **7**, 134 (1952).
354. W. C. Bowman, *Brit. J. Pharmacol.*, **13**, 521 (1958).
355. J. W. Dundee, T. C. Gray, and J. E. Riding, *Brit. J. Anaesthesia*, **26**, 13 (1954).
356. H. Klupp, O. Kraupp, H. Stormann, and C. Stumpf, *Arch. Intern. Pharmacodyn.*, **96**, 161 (1953).
357. H. Klupp and O. Kraupp, *Arch. Intern. Pharmacodyn.*, **98**, 340 (1954).
358. K. Wiemers and W. Overbeck, *Brit. J. Anaesthesia*, **32**, 607 (1960).
359. F. F. Foldes, B. Wolfson, M. Torres-Kay, and A. Monte, *Anesthesiology*, **20**, 767 (1959).
360. T. H. Christie, R. P. Wise, and H. C. Churchill-Davidson, *Lancet*, **2**, 648 (1959).
361. W. C. Bowman, B. A. Callingham, and A. A. J. Goldberg, *Anesthesiology*, **22**, 573 (1961).
362. W. Sniper, *Brit. J. Anaesthesia*, **24**, 232 (1952).

CHAPTER 6

REVERSIBLE INHIBITORS OF CHOLINESTERASE*

J. P. LONG and C. J. EVANS

DEPARTMENT OF PHARMACOLOGY
COLLEGE OF MEDICINE
STATE UNIVERSITY OF IOWA
IOWA CITY, IOWA

Research into the structure–activity relationships of reversible inhibitors of cholinesterase illustrates the rewards, hazards, and frustrations of chemically oriented biologists. There is every indication that the challenges of such research, enumerated in the following questions, will be raised continually.

6.1. QUESTIONS ON STRUCTURE–ACTIVITY RELATIONSHIPS

(1) Are two compounds acting by the same mechanism? This question can be raised in every structure–activity study involving relative-potency bioassays. Unfortunately, there is no way of proving whether they do or do not, and undoubtedly many erroneous conclusions on similar sites of action have been drawn.

Assuming that a linear series of biochemical reactions is needed to produce a normal physiological response, as shown below,

$$S_1 \xrightarrow{E_1} S_2 \xrightarrow{E_2} S_3 \xrightarrow{E_3} S_4 \rightarrow \text{Physiological response}$$

a drug could act with any of the enzymes (E) or with any of the substrates (S); actions at any of these sites would produce the same physiological response. If compounds in a given series are obvious chemical analogues, they probably possess similar pharmacological actions. There are notable exceptions, such as

* This work was supported in part by USPHS Grant NB-1396.

biological antagonists, but even in their case it is probable that at least some of the points on the enzyme are complementary to those of the substrate. Experience in the pharmacology of the autonomic nervous system has shown that homologous series of compounds usually vary quantitatively and not qualitatively. Any biological evaluation should include a comparison of the activities of compounds in vivo as well as in vitro. If the compounds possessed the same relative activity, it would be suggestive of similar mechanisms of action and similar abilities to reach the sites of action. Further important information can be gained by checking the activities against various substrates or receptor systems.

(2) Is physiological response a measure of drug–receptor interaction? This question, too, is very difficult to answer experimentally. One compound may readily reach the site of action and another compound may not (because it may be bound to plasma protein or have difficulty in penetrating membranes, etc.). If we assume that mutual binding between a drug and a receptor involves multiple attachments, then we should consider the possibility of a balanced interaction between functional groups on a drug and those on a receptor surface. For example, let us assume the following. Compound A has three points with which it binds with the receptor. Presumably, these three points have different bond strengths. Compound B has the same general groups with which to bind on the receptor. Two of the points are more strongly bound than those of compound A. However, the third point of compound B is only weakly bound. In other words, a compound A may produce a stronger physiological response, even though certain moieties of a compound B are better subjects for interaction with the receptor.

(3) Is there proper statistical design in the experiments? In a literature review of relative activities of inhibitors of cholinesterase it becomes apparent that rarely have statistical designs been used that can result in statistical analysis of the data. Most workers have been content to express a single observation; this leaves the reader with no idea about the variations inherent in the experimental procedure. Everyone engaged in structure–activity work must be careful that their conclusions are based on actual and not apparent biological differences.

(4) Are the data collected by various investigators valid for comparison? The I_{50} values reported by various workers for physostigmine or neostigmine illustrate this point. It is always a dangerous procedure to compare data from one laboratory with those obtained in another.

The application of structure–activity relationships to the naturally occurring inhibitors of cholinesterase has yielded the essential structural features of the alkaloid; from these features synthetic analogues have been prepared that were superior for most therapeutic applications. Further synthesis and evaluation of compounds raised numerous, yet unresolved, problems concerning the normal function and metabolism of acetylcholine. Few workers have attempted to elucidate the type of inhibition involved. Various tests for competitive inhibition (*1*, *2*) have been described and should be applied to critical members in a given homologous series. These tests can provide good evidence that the substrate and inhibitor have at least some common points of interaction on the enzyme surface. Reasoning beyond this point is a bit hazardous.

For competitive inhibition of an enzyme at least two requirements must be fulfilled. First, the geometry of the inhibitor must be complementary to that of the enzyme surface and there will be no interference as the functional groups in the drug molecule approach the reactive sites on the receptor surface. These spatial aspects probably account for the quantitative differences in biological activity seen with stereoisomers (see Chapter 2). The field of stereoisomerism affords us good evidence both of drug–receptor interactions and of multiple-point attachments on the receptor surface (*3–5*).

Second, the inhibiting molecule must possess charges opposite (but not necessarily equal) to those of the receptor. The spacing of charges on the inhibitor should approximate closely the interatomic spacings of points for attachment on the receptor surface. This does not mean that one can measure interatomic distances on the inhibitor and have a space model of the receptor. If the substrate attaches at two or more points on the receptor and simultaneous association is essential for activity, the inhibitor could act by combining with one point on the receptor where the substrate attaches and with other points where it does not. The types of bonding occurring in a drug–receptor interaction are important with respect to inhibitors of cholinesterase. In the case of reversible inhibitors the types of polar (electrostatic) bonding involved in drug–receptor interactions in order of decreasing strength are ion–ion > ion–dipole > dipole–dipole > van der Waals' forces = induced-dipole–induced-dipole. The orientation of a molecule for proper (and perhaps simultaneous) contact between functional groups of the molecule and the receptor would be expected to involve the stronger and longer range forces. If the geometries of the inhibitor and receptor are highly complementary, then short-range forces, such as van der Waals and induced-dipole–induced-dipole forces, probably contribute much to the assocation energy of the interaction. To consider this point we are faced with the concept of a receptor. For a detailed discussion of cholinergic receptors and drug–receptor interactions the reader is referred to Chapter 1.

6.2. STRUCTURE–ACTIVITY RELATIONSHIPS

During the past three or four decades there have been marked advances in the study of structure–activity relationships of drugs that act on the autonomic nervous systems. The reasons for these advances are numerous, but the realization that certain functional-group moieties were associated with specific biological activity has served as an important stimulus. Concurrently, chemically oriented pharmacologists began applying interatomic distance measurements to biologically active compounds (*6*, *7*). Biologists then began to incorporate modern electronic organic chemistry into the emerging field of drug design. Most of the factors that should be considered in discussing and evaluating structure–activity relationships are illustrated by the reversible inhibitors of cholinesterase.

A. Physostigmine

Jobst and Hesse nearly one hundred years ago isolated physostigmine (eserine) **(I)** and unknowingly entered the field of reversible inhibitors of cholinesterase; The suggestion was not made for many years that the action of physostigmine on the heart was due to inhibition of acetylcholine destruction by an esterase normally present in the tissues. Engelhart and Loewi (*8*)

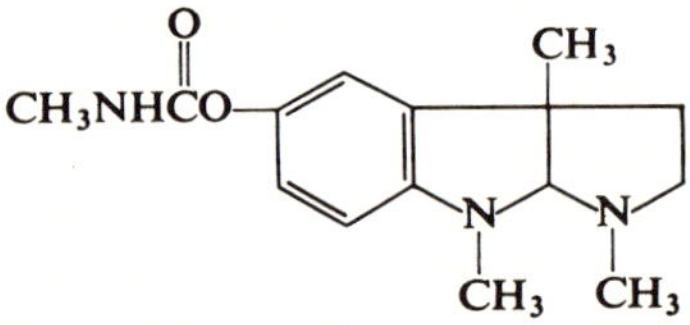

(I)
Physostigmine

and Matthes (*9*) demonstrated that the inactivation of acetylcholine was produced by an enzyme; physostigmine was highly active in its ability to inhibit the enzyme. Physostigmine is among the few compounds that are equally active as inhibitors of both acetylcholinesterase and *pseudo*-cholinesterase; a molar concentration between 10^{-6} and 10^{-8} M is required for 50% inhibition of either type. It is used by many investigators as a reference standard for evaluation of new inhibitors of cholinesterase. Apparently most if not all of the peripheral pharmacological properties reported for physostigmine are due to the inhibition of cholinesterase, and its pharmacology appears to be limited to this activity. Although many alkaloids other than physostigmine have been isolated from the Calabar bean, they have not been evaluated for anticholinesterase or pharmacological activity. Physostigmine readily undergoes oxidation, and the various oxidation products may be either inactive or no more than 1/100th as active as physostigmine (*10–12*). After its structural elucidation (*13*) there was rapid progress in the development of synthetic anticholinesterase compounds. Stedman and co-workers were pioneers in chemical pharmacology, the approach that has yielded so many active therapeutic agents for use in medicine. From the very earliest they reasoned that the two linked pyrrolidine rings in physostigmine may not be essential for activity and proceeded to investigate less complex molecules. The simplest analogues studied were the methylcarbamates of aminophenols **(II)**. Maximal

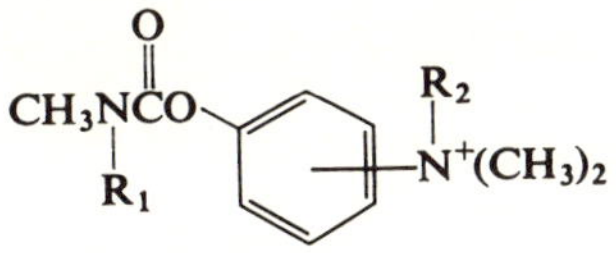

(II)
$R_1 = H, CH_3, C_2H_5$
$R_2 = H, R$

miotic activity in the rabbit was obtained when the carbamate and amino groups were *meta* or *para* to each other. The alkyl substitution on the amine was tertiary or quaternary, and the substitution on the carbamate was hydrogen, methyl, or ethyl. This work demonstrated that compounds related to structure **(II)** may be active agents; the carbamate group was essential for activity in this series. Quaternization of the *meta*-amino group intensified the activity.

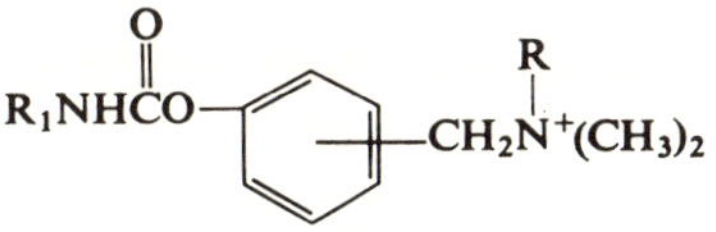

(III)
$R = H, CH_3$
$R_1 = CH_3, C_2H_5$

Compounds such as **(III)** were prepared for the purpose of evaluating the inductive effects of the amino group and producing compounds that were more stable in solution (*14*). In this series quaternization of the tertiary amine increased the activity of the *ortho*-substituted compounds, diminished that of the *meta*-substituted, and abolished the activity of the *para*-substituted. The observation that the quaternary derivatives of the *meta*-amino **(II)** and *ortho*-benzyl **(III)** compounds are the more active led to the postulation that activity is related to a formal charge and not to inductive effects on the quaternary nitrogen atom. The interatomic distance between the quaternary nitrogen and the carbonyl group is approximately the same in these two derivatives. The observation that the urethanes of choline or tropine are inactive indicated that the carbamate group by itself was not sufficient for activity and that activity was not related to a urethane decomposition product, but that the entire molecule, with proper substitution, was needed.

Continued synthesis in this series led to the development of the first useful

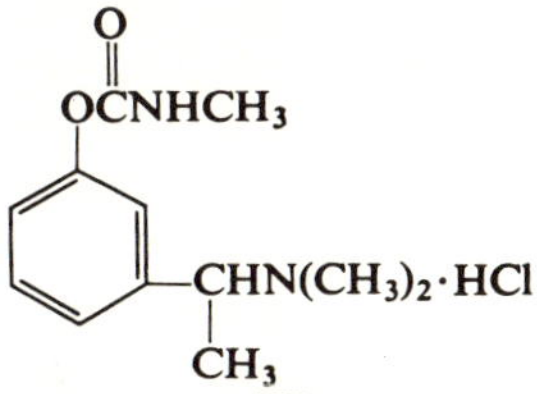

(IV)
Miotine

synthetic miotic agent, miotine **(IV)** (*14*). Early studies demonstrated that the pharmacological properties of *dl*-miotine resembled those of physostigmine both qualitatively and quantitatively. Later the optical isomers were separated (*15*), and studies indicated that the *l* isomer is the active component when evaluated on isolated intestinal strips (*16*). Dimethyl substitution on the benzyl carbon increases the miotic activity over that observed for *dl*-miotine. It is interesting to speculate that this dimethyl-substitution product has approximately the same activity as *l*-miotine; here asymmetry does not increase the activity. Substitution with a group larger than methyl appeared unfavorable for activity, and substitution on the ring, such as *para*-methoxy substitution (*17*), resulted in inactivation; quaternization of miotine decreased activity (*18*).

B. Neostigmine Analogues

In a classic paper Aeschlimann and Reinert (*17*) reported on various pharmacological properties of analogues of miotine **(IV)** and neostigmine **(V)** (Prostigmine). They did not perform esterase studies, but the marked ability of neostigmine to inhibit acetylcholinesterase has been confirmed repeatedly.

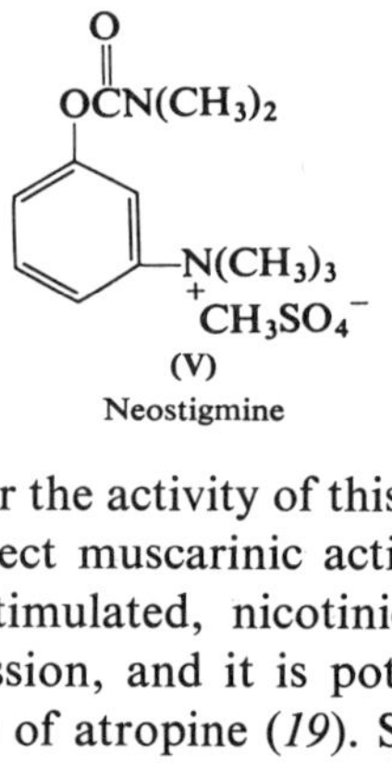

(V)
Neostigmine

The question remains whether the activity of this compound is due entirely to cholinesterase inhibition, direct muscarinic action or, as in the case of the rabbit intestine, which is stimulated, nicotinic action. Neostigmine does facilitate ganglionic transmission, and it is potentiated by hexamethonium and inhibited by small doses of atropine (*19*). Since arecoline, its analogues (*20*), and 3-hydroxypiperidine derivatives (*21*) are known muscarinic agents, neostigmine analogues may have this component of action. However, in all probability the analogues of miotine and neostigmine produce their pharmacological action primarily through inhibition of cholinesterase. The possibility that these compounds release acetylcholine from storage sites remains to be explored. Physostigminelike activity was strongest in the methyl, dimethyl, allyl, benzyl, and methylphenyl carbamates. The activity appeared weak in ethyl and phenyl and was absent in diethyl and diallyl analogues. The quaternary salts of the aromatic bases were more effective than the corresponding tertiary derivatives. Neostigmine possesses the advantage of being stable in solution, whereas miotine and physostigmine are quite unstable.

A number of analogues of neostigmine appear to be equally active as intestinal stimulants. After Aeschlimann and Reinert (*17*) demonstrated that neostigmine possessed pharmacological properties similar to those of physostigmine and that it was stable in solution, many workers have synthesized and still are synthesizing and evaluating its analogues. Possible structural modifications of neostigmine are almost without limit. The two most common points for structural alterations are the carbamate and the ammonium groups. Other alterations include the replacement of aromatic hydrogen atoms with various groups. Some of the conclusions drawn from the literature concerning the effect of specific substitutions on activity are given in the following paragraphs.

1. ROLE OF THE CARBAMATE GROUP

It has become obvious that the carbamate substitution is not essential for activity but that it may be a factor contributing to high anticholinesterase activity. The first observation to this effect was made with *m*-acetoxyphenyl-*N*,*N*,*N*-trimethylammonium, which was an effective miotic agent and stimulated the isolated rabbit intestine (*17*). Block (*22*) evaluated the activity of the acetoxy and isobutyroxy analogues against human and dog serum cholinesterase and established that inhibition of cholinesterase was the mechanism involved in the pharmacological actions. Although both analogues were less active than neostigmine in inhibiting human or dog serum butyrocholinesterase, this demonstrated that sterically similar groups could be interchanged in a molecule and still retain activity. Randall and Lehmann (*23*) found similar cholinesterase inhibition with the neostigmine analogues, in which the carbamate group was replaced with hydroxy and acetoxy groups. The acetyl derivative readily hydrolyzed at a slightly alkaline pH to the parent hydroxy compound. In this series the absence of the carbamate group leads to compounds no more than 1/100 as active as neostigmine. The low anticholinesterase activity is probably responsible for the relatively weak intestinal stimulant and miotic properties observed, but it was felt that the anticurare and direct stimulating action on striated muscle could not be explained entirely by the anticholinesterase properties. Wescoe et al. (*24*) evaluated the activity of the acetyl derivative of edrophonium and showed that the acetoxy and hydroxy derivatives are of the same order of activity. They also suggested that because of its low anticholinesterase activities the compound's physiological properties were due to some other mechanism of action. Other authors report that *meta*-hydroxyphenyltrialkylammonium compounds are about 1/10 as active as neostigmine (*25–27*). Hobbiger (*28*) evaluated the anticholinesterase activity of *m*-hydroxyphenyltrialkylammonium esters and concluded that, since the ester group was rapidly hydrolyzed by human serum cholinesterase, at least part of the pharmacological activity must be due to the corresponding hydroxy analogue. Burgen and Hobbiger (*29*) reported a series of compounds in which the carbamate group of neostigmine was replaced with various phosphates. The anticholinesterase activity of the dimethyl phosphate derivative was completely reversible, whereas larger alkyl substitutions on the phosphate produced very active compounds that were irreversible inhibitors of cholinesterase.

Substitutions on the carbamate portion have included aryl and alkyl groups. Most authors reported that the dimethylcarbamate, besides being more stable than the monomethyl derivative, is about twice as active. Papers by Lehmann (*30*) and Aeschlimann and Stempel (*31*) summarize much of the work these authors have done with analogues of neostigmine. Disubstituted carbamate analogues of neostigmine with aryl groups or aliphatic groups larger than methyl showed a sharp reduction in activity when compared with neostigmine (*31*).

2. SUBSTITUTION ON THE AMINO NITROGEN

In most analogues of neostigmine alkyl groups are substituted for nitrogen. Optimal activity was obtained with the dimethylethyl or diethylmethyl derivatives (*32*); higher homologues have not been extensively investigated. In some of their early work Stedman and Aeschlimann and Reinert studied various benzylamine derivatives. Similar effects have been reported for edrophonium (*26*, *27*) and its acetoxy analogues (*28*).

3. HETEROCYCLIC ANALOGUES

The incorporation of the nitrogen atom into a heterocyclic ring has long been considered a possible structural alteration for the production of active anticholinesterase agents. Stedman (*14*) prepared two derivatives of 8-hydroxyquinoline, but did not report the pharmacological activities. Aeschlimann and Reinert (*17*) reported that certain carbamate derivatives of 8-hydroxyquinoline were active intestinal stimulants. Wuest and Sakal (*35*) reported that carbamates of quaternized 3-pyridol exhibited cholinesterase inhibition and parasympathomimetic activity; the dimethylcarbamate derivatives were more active than the diethyl- or phenylcarbamates. Stempel and Aeschlimann (*36*) reported a series of 3-pyridol analogues with activities equal to that of neostigmine.

4. SUMMARY OF STRUCTURAL REQUIREMENTS OF NEOSTIGMINE ANALOGUES

Marked alterations of structure can be made and still retain significant cholinesterase inhibition. This suggests that it is a matter of an enzyme without stringent structural specificity toward inhibitors. The carbamate portion is not necessary for activity, but its incorporation probably increases the effectiveness. The ammonium group may be incorporated in a heterocyclic ring, be an aniline derivative, or be removed from the ring by one or even two methylene groups. Here, as with the anticholinergic agents (see Chapter 2), maximum blocking action is found when one or two ethyl groups are located on the quaternary nitrogen. Methyl, bromo, and chloro substituents in the *para* position appear to enhance activity. Structure **(VI)** indicates the requirements for anticholinesterase activity.

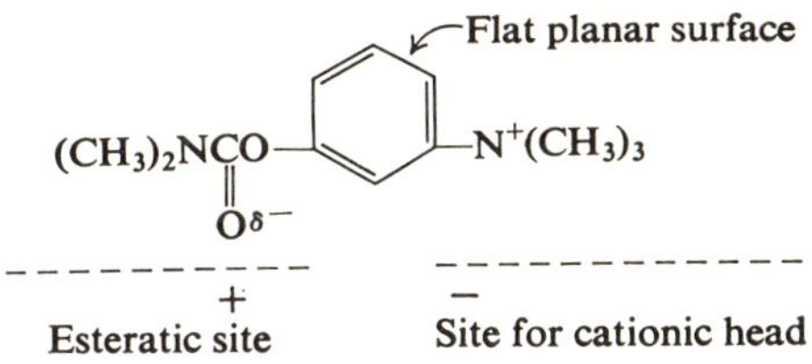

(VI)

Foldes et al. (*34*) studied the importance of the interatomic distance from N^+ to C=O and observed maximal activity at an interatomic distance of 4.7 A. The distance is most critical with acetylcholinesterase. This is further evidence that acetylcholinesterase contains two sites of attachment whereas *pseudo*-cholinesterase may have only one (*37*, *38*). Wilson and Quan (*39*) reported that the introduction of a *meta*-hydroxy group into phenyltrimethylammonium increased the binding strength by a factor of 120. This marked increase in binding strength is suggestive of strong hydrogen bonding. They noted that the distance from N^+ to OH was approximately 5 A. A sharp decrease in activity was noted with *para*-hydroxy. *Ortho* compounds were intermediate in activity and probably represented too short a distance between N^+ and OH.

C. Bisquaternary Inhibitors of Cholinesterase

Recent advances in the development of competitive cholinesterase inhibitors have resulted from the synthesis and pharmacological evaluation of bisquaternary compounds. It was hoped that compounds would be developed that would be more selective inhibitors of acetylcholinesterase (*40–43*, *47*, *48*, *50*, *51*, *58*, *59*). Assessment of the structural requirements is very difficult from one series to another. Most of the series do not have common groups or common interatomic distances between the cationic heads. Within the various series, however, there is high structural specificity.

An equally challenging question is, Why are two quaternary heads required for high activity in these apparently unrelated series? In most series the monoquaternary analogues are inactive. On a single cholinesterase molecule there may be as many as 48 different receptors of acetylcholine. The molecular weight of cholinesterase may be as high as 3×10^6; the monomer has a molecular weight of about 1.05×10^5. Any of several theoretical possibilities, given below, could explain the mechanism of action of these agents (*44*).

(1) The bisquaternary compounds may bracket the receptor on the cholinesterase molecule and shield this site from acetylcholine. A schematic outline, at least of those compounds whose cationic heads are separated by 14 A, can be visualized as shown in structure **(VII)**.

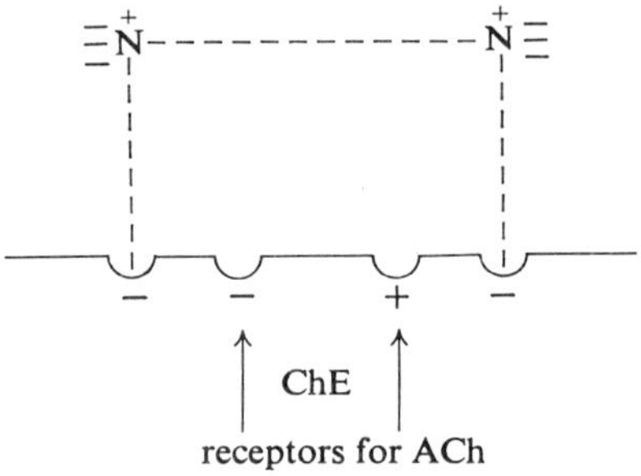

(VII)

(2) These agents may combine with the same cationic site as acetylcholine and some site other than one with which acetylcholine combines; see structure **(VIII)**.

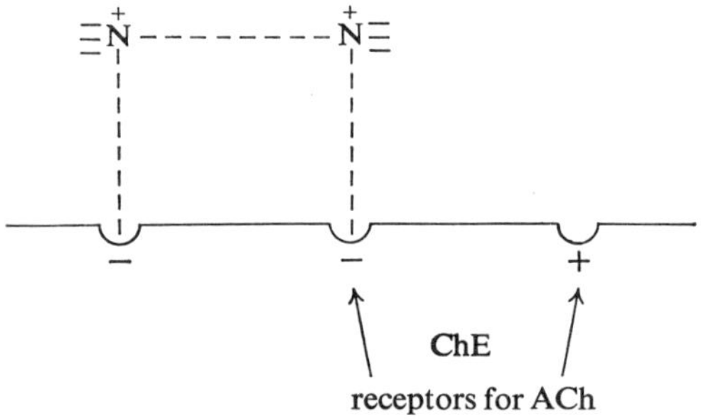

(VIII)

(3) There may be a repetition of the cationic site for acetylcholine on the cholinesterase molecule. This would allow attachment of the inhibitor at two cationic sites and subsequent shielding of the esteratic site; see structure **(IX)**. In this case the binding interatomic distance would be less than the extended distance of the inhibiting molecule. Since none of these compounds is a highly rigid structure, binding with sites less than their maximal distance is possible.

(4) The considerations outlined above involve only one cholinesterase molecule. An alternate suggestion is that the inhibitor is binding between two

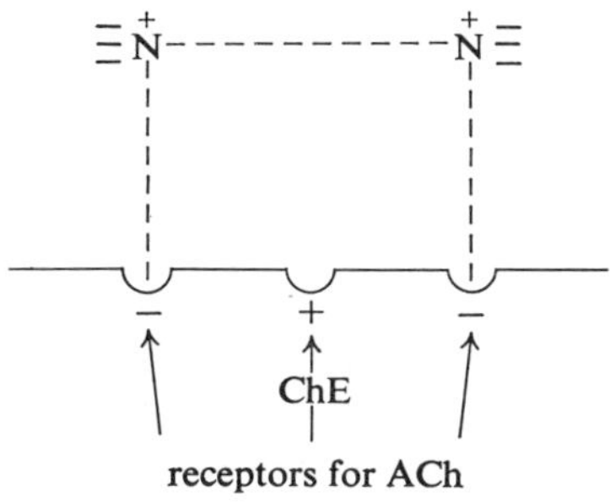

(IX)

molecules (*40*). If this were the mechanism, it would have to be postulated that the cholinesterase molecules are rigid in their relationship to each other; see structure **(X)**.

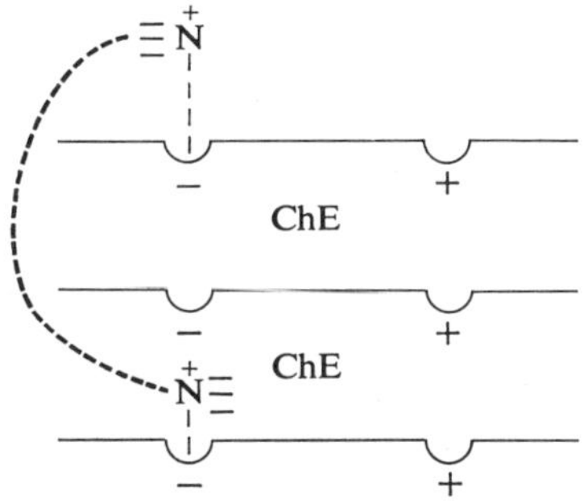

(X)
Cholinesterase

These theories cannot explain the binding of molecules with shorter interatomic distances. For an excellent discussion of other factors that may be involved with these "shorter" compounds, the reader is referred to the discussion of Cavallito and Gray (*45*).

In 1952 it was reported that bisneostigmine analogues linked together with 1,3-dihydroxypropane possessed extremely high activity when evaluated with the use of acetylcholinesterase obtained from dog red blood cells (*46*). Later studies indicated an activity not as high as originally reported but still equal to, or more active than, neostigmine and probably as much as that of any series of compounds that had yet been synthesized (*47*, *48*). Levin and Jandorf (*49*) re-evaluated critical members of this series with human red-cell acetylcholinesterase and found comparable activity. Linking bisneostigmine analogues together through the carbamate nitrogen (*50*, *51*) gives compounds which, when the interatomic distance between the carbamate nitrogens is approximately 14 A, are extremely active. Bisquaternary compounds structurally unrelated to neostigmine have been synthesized and also show high activity. In these analogues no particular structure–activity relationship can be discerned. Biquinolinium, bi-isoquinolinium (*52*), and bipyridinium (*53*) derivatives have been reported, but they appear to be considerably less active than neostigmine. Bisquaternary compounds based on phthalic acid isomers appear to be 1/10 to 1/100 as active as neostigmine (*54, 55*). A number of bisquaternary compounds based on biphenyl or diphenylmethane have been reported (*40, 42, 56, 57*). The dimethylaminoethanol quaternary with 2,2′-dibromo-4,4′-bisacetophenone (hemicholinium, HC-3) is inactive as an inhibitor of cholinesterase but interferes with cholinergic transmission at all cholinergic transmission sites (*40, 58*). A marked increase in activity appeared when the nitrogen was contained in a heterocyclic ring. Pyridyl derivatives possessed anticholinesterase activity equal to that of neostigmine and the 2- or 3-methylpyridyl derivatives were at least 10 times as active.

Potent cholinesterase inhibitors have been derived from oxamide (*59, 60*); see structure **(XI)**.

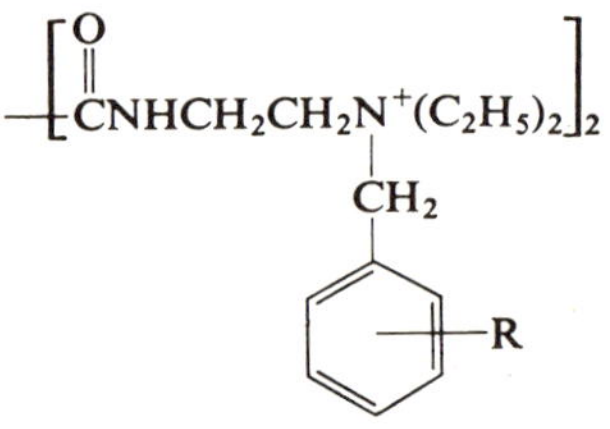

(XI)

Halogen-substituted benzyl derivatives were extremely potent compounds; the 2-bromobenzyl diethyl derivative was 41 times as active as neostigmine. Other 2-halobenzyl moieties also possessed high anticholinesterase activity. Movement of the halogens to the 3 or 4 position of the benzyl group resulted in a marked reduction in activity. In these compounds the optimal distance between the quaternary nitrogens was approximately 14.5 A. The order of activity for *o*-halobenzyl substituents (bromine > chlorine > iodine > fluorine) does not follow either the size of the halogen or the expected inductive effects of this substitution. This suggests that on the cholinesterase enzyme at 5 or 6 A from the site of attachment of the cationic head there is a positive center with which the halogen may interact. If this is the reason for increased activity, it would have to be postulated that this center is specific to size, that is, that the chloride ion is too small and the iodide too large.

D. Summary of Bisquaternary Compounds

No structural specificity between the bisquaternary compounds and their ability to inhibit cholinesterase appears to exist. The bisneostigmine analogues may exhibit higher activity than a single neostigmine molecule; this would be good evidence of a repeated receptor on the cholinesterase molecule. In such cases the total binding energy of the inhibitor merely may be increased by exposure of cholinesterase to a molecule that can attach at repeated receptor positions on the cholinesterase molecule. Other bisquaternary inhibitors apparently act like neostigmine and physostigmine: they have durations of action similar to neostigmine and they probably bind with some of the same receptor sites. These compounds would combine with one or all of the cationic sites with which acetylcholine normally combines. Ordinary kinetics studies cannot distinguish among the various possibilities. The additional sites of attachment may increase the stability of the drug–enzyme complex. The highest activity is observed with the nitrogen heterocycles and, particularly, pyridine derivatives with nuclear substitution. This again is suggestive of additional points of attachment. Because 2- or 3-pyridyl derivatives both markedly increase activity, the increased activity is not due to an alteration of charge on the pyridyl nitrogen. That other points of attachment may be involved is suggested by the oxamide derivatives (*59, 60*). In the oxamide series a marked increase in activity was noted with the *ortho*-halobenzyl group. This marked increase in cholinesterase inhibition of the benzylhalo derivatives is not found with the muscarinic activity of various halo derivatives of benzyltrimethylammonium (*61*).

E. Miscellaneous Compounds

Many other compounds have been synthesized and evaluated for anticholinesterase activity. Relating their pharmacological action to cholinesterase inhibition has been attempted frequently, but stronger evidence than has been presented thus far will be required before it is generally accepted. At one time or another a compound that demonstrated any cholinergic side effects was credited with an ability to inhibit cholinesterase. Most of the studies were based on anticholinesterase action evaluated in vitro, in which a concentration of 10^{-3} to 10^{-4} *M* was necessary before inhibition occurred; it is highly doubtful that in vivo concentration of this magnitude is ever attained with these agents. Thus, although the activities of many of these agents have been tabulated (*44*), to describe their structure–activity relationships would be rather hazardous.

REFERENCES

1. H. Lineweaver and D. Burk, *J. Am. Chem. Soc.*, **56**, 658 (1934).
2. A. Goldstein, *J. Gen. Physiol.*, **27**, 529 (1944).
3. A. H. Beckett, *J. Pharm. Pharmacol.*, **8**, 848 (1956).
4. J. P. Long, F. P. Luduena, B. F. Tullar, and A. M. Lands, *J. Pharmacol. Exptl. Therap.*, **117**, 29 (1956).

5. F. W. Schueler, *Chemobiodynamics and Drug Design*, McGraw-Hill, New York, 1960.
6. F. W. Schueler, *Science*, **103**, 221 (1946).
7. C. C. Pfeiffer, *Science*, **107**, 94 (1948).
8. E. Engelhart and O. Loewi, *Arch. Exptl. Pathol. Pharmakol.*, **150**, 1 (1930).
9. K. Matthes, *J. Physiol.* (*London*), **70**, 338 (1930).
10. S. Ellis, *J. Pharmacol. Exptl. Therap.*, **79**, 364 (1943).
11. S. Ellis, O. Krayer, and F. L. Plachte, *J. Pharmacol. Exptl. Therap.*, **79**, 295 (1943).
12. S. Ellis, O. Krayer, and F. L. Plachte, *J. Pharmacol. Exptl. Therap.*, **79**, 309 (1943).
13. E. Stedman and G. Barger, *J. Chem. Soc.*, **1925**, 247.
14. E. Stedman, *Biochem. J.*, **23**, 17 (1929).
15. J. M. MacDonald and E. Stedman, *J. Chem. Soc.*, **1932**, 2513.
16. L. H. Easson and E. Stedman, *Biochem. J.*, **27**, 1257 (1933).
17. J. A. Aeschlimann and M. Reinert, *J. Pharmacol. Exptl. Therap.*, **43**, 413 (1931).
18. A. Schweitzer, E. Stedman, and S. Wright, *J. Physiol.* (*London*), **96**, 302 (1939).
19. J. P. Long and J. W. Eckstein, *J. Pharmacol. Exptl. Therap.*, **133**, 216 (1961).
20. R. Hunt and R. R. Renshaw, *J. Pharmacol. Exptl. Therap.*, **35**, 75 (1929).
21. F. W. Schueler, *J. Pharm. Sci.*, **45**, 197 (1956).
22. H. Bloch, *Arch. Exptl. Pathol. Pharmakol.*, **193**, 292 (1939).
23. L. D. Randall and G. Lehmann, *J. Pharmacol. Exptl. Therap.*, **99**, 16 (1950).
24. W. C. Wescoe, W. F. Riker, and V. L. Beach, *J. Pharmacol. Exptl. Therap.*, **99**, 265 (1950).
25. D. W. MacFarlane, E. W. Pelikan, and K. R. Unna, *J. Pharmacol. Exptl. Therap.*, **100**, 382 (1950).
26. H. L. Cohen and K. R. Unna, *J. Pharmacol. Exptl. Therap.*, **103**, 340 (1951).
27. C. M. Smith, S. L. Cohen, E. W. Pelikan, and K. R. Unna, *J. Pharmacol. Exptl. Therap.*, **105**, 391 (1952).
28. F. Hobbiger, *Brit. J. Pharmacol.*, **7**, 223 (1952).
29. A. S. Burgen and F. Hobbiger, *Brit. J. Pharmacol.*, **6**, 593 (1951).
30. G. Lehmann, *Festschr. Emil Barell*, **1946**, 314.
31. J. A. Aeschlimann and A. Stempel, *Festchr. Emil Barell*, **1946**, 306.
32. H. Blaschko, E. Bulbring, and T. C. Chou, *Brit. J. Pharmacol.*, **4**, 29 (1949).
33. R. D. Hawkins and J. M. Gunter, *Biochem. J.*, **40**, 192 (1946).
34. F. F. Foldes, E. G. Erdos, N. Baart, J. Zwart, and E. K. Zsigmond, *Arch. Intern. Pharmacodyn.*, **120**, 286 (1959).
35. H. M. Wuest and E. H. Sakal, *J. Am. Chem. Soc.*, **73**, 1210 (1951).
36. A. Stempel and J. A. Aeschlimann, *J. Am. Chem. Soc.*, **74**, 3323 (1952).
37. F. Bergmann and R. Segal, *Biochem. J.*, **58**, 692 (1954).
38. F. Bergmann, *The Physical Chemistry of Enzymes*, Aberdeen Univ. Press, Scotland, 1956, p. 126.
39. I. B. Wilson and C. Quan, *Arch. Biochem. Biophys.*, **73**, 131 (1958).
40. J. P. Long and F. W. Schueler, *J. Pharm. Sci.*, **43**, 79 (1954).
41. F. W. Schueler, *J. Pharmacol. Exptl. Therap.*, **115**, 127 (1955).
42. F. N. Marshall and J. P. Long, *J. Pharmacol. Exptl. Therap.*, **127**, 236 (1959).
43. R. H. Adamson, D. L. Boatman, and J. P. Long, *Arch. Intern. Pharmacodyn.*, **141**, 22 (1963).
44. J. P. Long, in *Handbuch der Experimentellen Pharmakologie Erganzungswerk*, Vol. XV (O. Eichler and A. Farah, eds.), Springer-Verlag, Berlin, 1963, pp. 374–427.
45. C. J. Cavallito and A. P. Gray, *Progr. Drug Res.*, **2**, 135 (1960).
46. A. Funke, J. Bagot, and F. DePierre, *Compt. Rend.*, **239**, 329 (1954).
47. A. Funke, F. DePierre, and M. W. Krucker, *Compt. Rend.*, Nr. **7**, 762 (1952).
48. F. DePierre and A. Funke, *Compt. Rend.*, **239**, 370 (1954).

49. A. P. Levin and B. J. Jandorf, *J. Pharmacol. Exptl. Therap.*, **113**, 206 (1955).
50. O. Kraupp, C. Stumpf, E. Herzfeld, and B. Pillat, *Arch. Intern. Pharmacodyn.*, **102**, 281 (1955).
51. H. Klupp, O. Kraupp, H. G. Schwarzacher, and C. Stumpf, *Arch. Intern. Pharmacodyn.*, **101**, 205 (1955).
52. C. M. Smith, E. W. Pelikan, L. R. Maranba, and K. R. Unna, *J. Pharmacol. Exptl. Therap.*, **108**, 317 (1953).
53. R. Hazard, J. Cheymol, and E. Corteggiani, *Arch. Exptl. Pathol. Pharmakol.*, **220**, 62 (1953).
54. F. Bovet-Nitti and D. Bovet, *Arch. Exptl. Pathol. Pharmakol.*, **220**, 52 (1953).
55. J. A. B. Barstad, K. H. S. Kramstad, and S. Oksne, *Arch. Intern. Pharmacodyn.*, **121**, 395 (1959).
56. W. J. Fleming, J. P. Long, R. J. Wulf, and R. M. Featherstone, *J. Pharmacol. Exptl. Therap.*, **121**, 113 (1957).
57. R. G. Hermann and R. H. Tust, *J. Pharmacol. Exptl. Therap.*, **117**, 75 (1956).
58. H. Wilson and J. P. Long, *Arch. Intern. Pharmacodyn.*, **120**, 343 (1959).
59. J. O. Hoppe, J. E. Funnell, and H. Lape, *J. Pharmacol. Exptl. Therap.*, **115**, 106 (1955).
60. A. M. Lands, J. O. Hoppe, A. Arnold, and F. K. Kirchner, *J. Pharmacol. Exptl. Therap.*, **123**, 121 (1958).
61. K. C. Wong and J. P. Long, *J. Pharmacol. Exptl. Therap.*, **137**, 70 (1962).

CHAPTER 7

ACID-TRANSFERRING INHIBITORS OF ACETYLCHOLINESTERASE

IRWIN B. WILSON

DEPARTMENT OF CHEMISTRY
UNIVERSITY OF COLORADO
BOULDER, COLORADO

In this chapter I have endeavored to write only about newer aspects of the chemistry of acid-transferring inhibitors of cholinesterase and certain facets of the subject that have not been previously emphasized in reviews, and of older and well known material (*1*) I have included only what seemed necessary for an orderly presentation of the subject. I have tried to show that what originally was considered simply a group of organophosphates is, in principle and also in practice, a much larger group of inhibitors containing families of substances, including even substrates, that have a common mechanism of reaction with cholinesterase.

The term acid-transferring inhibitor has been applied to those substances, including diisopropyl fluorophosphate, prostigmine, and methanesulfonyl fluoride, which in their reaction with acetylcholinesterase transfer an acidic group, that is, a phosphoryl group (*2–7*), a carbamoyl group (*8*, *9*), or a methanesulfonyl group (*10–12*), to the active site of the enzyme, yielding a relatively stable enzyme derivative. Although they occur more slowly, these reactions are analogous to the reaction of acetylcholine with the enzyme, a reaction in which an acetyl group is transferred to the enzyme (*13*). The substances are inhibitors rather than substrates because, unlike the acetyl enzyme, which is derived from acetylcholine and reacts with water in 100 μsec (*14–17*), the enzymic derivatives of these substances may require several minutes or several days, or even longer, to react with water. The enzyme is therefore tied up in the form of the derivative.

Because these inhibitors in their reaction with the enzyme are analagous to the substrate, it is instructive to review briefly the catalytic mechanism of the enzyme. The active site of the enzyme contains two subsites, an anionic site (*4*, *18*), which serves to bind and orient the substrate, and an esteratic site, which contains the catalytic functional groups of the enzyme: a nucleophilic group thought to be the hydroxyl group of serine (*19–22*), probably an imidazole group (*23*, *24*), and possibly an acidic group (*25*). These groups

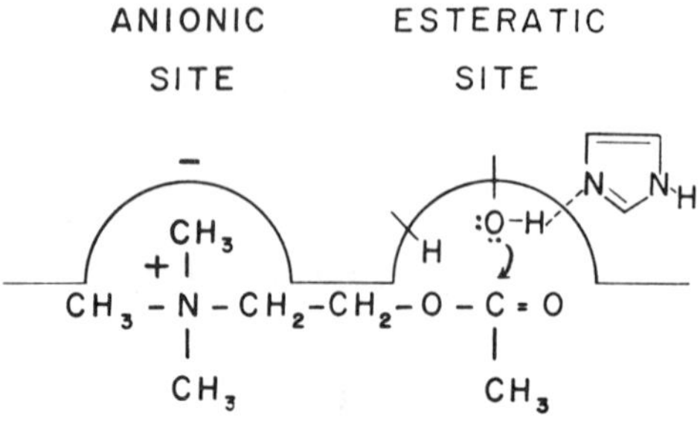

Fig. 7.1

together bring about the hydrolysis (*12*, *26*, *27*); see Figure 7.1. The hydrolysis is itself a multistep process (7.1). [Here E is the enzyme, E′ is the acetylenzyme, S is the substrate, P_1 and P_2 are choline and acetic acid.]

$$\text{Enzyme} + \text{acetylcholine} \rightleftharpoons \text{Michaelis complex} \rightarrow \text{acetyl enzyme} + \text{choline}$$
$$\downarrow$$
$$\text{enzyme} + \text{acetic acid}$$

$$E + S \underset{k_2}{\overset{k_1}{\rightleftharpoons}} E{\cdot}S \overset{k_3}{\rightleftharpoons} E' + P_1 \xrightarrow[k_4]{H_2O} E + P_2 \tag{7.1}$$

The anionic site, although not a catalytic site per se is a prominent feature of this enzyme. In general, substituted ammonium ions, tetraethylammonium, trimethylphenylammonium, etc., are reversible inhibitors. They inhibit by two mechanisms: first, by competing with the substrate for the free enzyme and, second, by combining with the still existing anionic site in the acetyl enzyme and thereby preventing it from reacting with water (*28*, *29*). Similarly, substrate inhibition is produced by the reversible binding of acetylcholine to the acetyl enzyme (*30*).

These observations suggest that there is a definite spatial order in the catalytic configuration and that a water molecule must approach from the direction of the anionic site.

The anionic site may incorrectly align a potential substrate. Although ethyl acetate is a substrate, esters containing a quaternary ammonium function in the acidic moiety rather than in the alcohol residue, as in ethyltrimethylammonioproprionate, for example, are not substrates but reversible inhibitors (*29*). Ethyl acetate, lacking the charge and nonpolar substituents of a quaternary ammonium function, has a 5×10^3 times higher K_m than acetylcholine (*31*). The V_{max} is 1/7 as great, but the acylation step is probably only 1/40 as rapid as in the case of acetylcholine. It is easy to understand that the anionic site might contribute to the catalytic process by binding and orienting the substrate. Is it possible that the binding of ammonium ions also promotes the activity of the enzyme in some more active but less understandable way? This question will be taken up later.

The kinetic consequences of the enzymic steps given above are that the rate of hydrolysis follows the Michaelis-Menten equation (7.2) (*30*):

$$v = \frac{kE^0 S}{S+K_m} \tag{7.2}$$

where

$$k = k_3 \Big/ \left(1+\frac{k_3}{k_4}\right)$$

$$K_m = \frac{k_2+k_3}{k_1} \Big/ \left(1+\frac{k_3}{k_4}\right)$$

At $[S] \ll K_m$, the velocity approaches second order, $v = k'[E][S]$, where $k' = k/K_m$ (independent of k_4) is the second-order rate constant for acetylation of the enzyme. The values for eel acetylcholinesterase and acetylcholine are $k = 8.3 \times 10^5$ min^{-1} and $K_m = 1 \times 10^{-4}$ M. The value of k_3 is probably larger than k_4, perhaps about 6 times larger (*30*). A high ratio of k_3 to k_4 tends to make K_m small.

As mentioned above, substituted ammonium ions are bound at the anionic site of acetylcholinesterase. In general, such complexes play a prominent part in the reactions of this enzyme. Are these complexes loose or well defined? That is, are there numerous, more or less equally stable, relative orientations of the ammonium ion and the enzyme, or are there but one or two preferred configurations? Clearly, this must depend upon the ion, and gradations between the extremes of numerous orientations and a single configuration should be expected.

Considering the reversible inhibitors $(CH_3)_4N^+$, $(CH_3)_3N^+C_6H_5$, and m-$HOC_6H_4N^+(CH_3)_3$, in which the binding constants increase by a factor of 100 from compound to compound (*32*), it is reasonable to suppose that 3-hydroxyphenyltrimethylammonium ion may form an ordered complex, even though tetramethylammonium ion may form a very loose one.

The second-order rate constant for acetylcholine is about 8×10^9 liter mole^{-1} min^{-1}; for ethyl acetate it is about 10^5 liter mole^{-1} min^{-1} (*31*). As has been seen, this large difference arises mainly from the large difference in Michaelis constants. There are numerous organophosphate inhibitors, and some carbamate inhibitors with second-order rate constants of 10^5 to 10^9 liter mole^{-1} min^{-1} in the reaction with acetylcholinesterase.

The reaction of acid-transferring inhibitors with acetylcholinesterase is formally identical with the reaction of acetylcholine and the enzyme and can

$$\begin{array}{c} \mathrm{HE+I} \underset{k_2}{\overset{k_1}{\rightleftharpoons}} \mathrm{HE \cdot I} \underset{k_{-3}}{\overset{k_3}{\rightleftharpoons}} \mathrm{E'+HX} \\ \qquad\qquad\qquad\qquad\qquad \downarrow k_4\,(\mathrm{H_2O}) \\ \qquad\qquad\qquad\qquad\qquad \mathrm{E+P_2} \end{array} \tag{7.3}$$

be written as (7.3) where E′ is a phosphoryl enzyme, carbamoyl enzyme, or methanesulfonyl enzyme, according as the inhibitor is an organophosphate, carbamate, or methanesulfonate ester, and where X is a labile group in the inhibitor I:

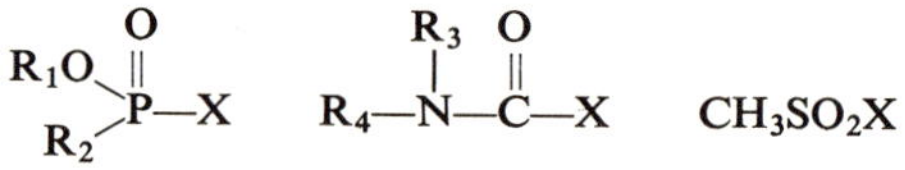

(7.4)

Here R_1 is an alkyl or aryl group, R_2 is an alkyl, alkoxy, aryloxy, or amino group, R_3 and R_4 are hydrogens, alkyl groups, or aryl groups. The group X is usually such that HX is distinctly acidic: for example, fluoro, chloro, *p*-nitrophenyl, phosphato, cyano, trimethylammoniophenoxy, etc.

Not only is there a large variety of X groups, but there is also a large selection of R groups, depending to some extent upon X, so that there are a very large number or organophosphate and carbamate inhibitors. Although thiophosphates are also potent inhibitors, thionophosphates are not, but they are poisonous because in tissues they are oxidized to the oxo compounds.

There is far more than a formal identity between the reaction of acid-transferring inhibitors and that of substrates with the enzyme. Not only is the same site "acylated," but in general essentially the same mechanism is believed to be involved, although the detailed mechanisms may not be precisely the same in all cases of inhibition and reactivation. The pH dependence of tetraethylpyrophosphate inhibition is similar to the pH dependence of the hydrolysis of acetylcholine (*3*), and there is an excellent correlation with the hydrolysis of ethyl bromoacetate (*33*). Acid-transferring inhibitors are very poor substrates; they are inherently poor, because "deacylation" is slow. Carbamates were recognized as competitive substrates by Goldstein (*34*). In the usual experiment with organophosphates and methanesulfonates the reaction goes to completion and follows pseudo first-order kinetics, $[\mathrm{I}] \gg [\mathrm{HE}]$, the pseudo first-order rate constant being given by

$$k_1o = \frac{k_3}{1+(K_I)/[\mathrm{I}]} \qquad K_I = k_2/k_1 \tag{7.5}$$

Usually $[\mathrm{I}] \ll K_I$ in experiments with organophosphates, for otherwise the reaction would be too fast, and the reaction is generally second-order with the rate constant $k_{2o} = k_3/K_I$. The reaction can usually, but not always, be run as a pseudo first-order reaction at different inhibitor concentrations and the second-order rate constant calculated. In order to demonstrate kinetically the formation of an addition complex, [I] must be comparable to K_I and, therefore, with ordinary equipment k_3 must be of the order of one per minute or less, which means either that K_I must be quite small or that the substance must be a relatively poor inhibitor. The formation of complexes is easily demonstrated with methanesulfonates containing quaternary groups in X.

As may be deduced from the scheme, the reaction should proceed to a steady state, in which the rate of inhibition of the enzyme equals its rate of recovery through reaction with water and in which

$$([E']/[E])_{ss} = k_3[I]/K_I k_4 \tag{7.6}$$

where the subscript *ss* indicates the steady state. In the case of organophosphates, with the exception of dimethyl phosphoryl esters, and in the case of methanesulfonates the k_4 of the corresponding enzyme derivative is so small that the reaction of the enzyme with even low concentrations of any reasonably potent inhibitor will go to completion. Suppose the half-time for recovery of an enzyme derivative is of the order of one day, or $k_4 \approx 10^{-3}$ min^{-1}. For a convenient rate of inhibition $k_{2o}[I] = 10^{-2}$ to 10^{-1} min^{-1}, so that for a reasonably potent inhibitor ($k_{2o} = 10^6$ liter mole^{-1} min^{-1}) the concentration of I would be about 10^{-7} *M*. Under these conditions

$$([E']/[E])_{ss} = 10^1 \text{ to } 10^2$$

That is, the reaction goes pretty much to completion. On the other hand, if the half-time for recovery is of the order of one hour, or $k_4 = 10^{-2}$, then

$$([E']/[E])_{ss} = 1 \text{ to } 10$$

and the reaction does not go to completion.

In the case of dimethyl phosphoryl esters, carbamates, *N,N*-dimethylcarbamates, and *N*-methylcarbamates, but not in the case of *N*-phenylcarbamates, the k_4 for the corresponding enzyme derivative is fairly large, so that steady states corresponding to various degrees of inhibition are readily obtained. If a solution containing a carbamate and enzyme in such a steady state is extensively diluted, the rate of carbamoylation will be greatly diminished, but the rate of decarbamoylation will remain the same, and the return of enzymic activity can be observed. This step is analogous to the hydrolysis of the acetyl enzyme and, like it, is slowed by substituted ammonium ions. Because the binding of these ions with the enzyme is almost always greater than with the carbamoyl enzyme (*29*), adding them to the solution displaces the steady state in the direction of less inhibition.

Experiments with acid-transferring inhibitors are usually best done in the absence of substrate; the enzyme solution is added to the substrate solution for only a brief period, enough to assay the amount of active enzyme. However, experiments with carbamates have often been carried out in the presence of acetylcholine, and in this case the rate of hydrolysis of substrate in the steady state is

$$\frac{1}{v} = \frac{1}{kE^0} + \frac{K_m}{kE^0}\left[1 + \frac{[\mathrm{I}]}{K_I}\left(1 + \frac{k_3'}{k_4'}\right)\right]\frac{1}{[\mathrm{S}]} \tag{7.7}$$

where the primed constants refer to the acid-transferring inhibitor (not to the substrate). It is assumed here that neither S nor I combines significantly with the acetyl enzyme at the concentrations used. This equation is the same as that for the hydrolysis of one substrate in the presence of another. In that case $K_I/[1+(k_3'/k_4')]$ is the Michaelis-Menten constant for the second substrate.

This equation also is formally the same as that for competitive reversible inhibition. If acid-transfer inhibition occurs, however, some time usually is required to reach the steady state.

These equations apply in principle also to organophosphates and methanesulfonates but, as already noted, the k_4 for nearly all phosphorylacetylcholinesterases and for methanesulfonylacetylcholinesterase is so small that the steady state usually corresponds to complete inhibition.

Thus, although the mechanisms of inhibition caused by carbamates and organophosphates are the same, the expression of the inhibition is sensitive to the values of the kinetic constants and the "usual" character of the inhibition for a particular group of inhibitors, that is, whether or not the inhibition appears to be reversible depends largely upon the value of k_4. Thus, organophosphate inhibitors were considered to be irreversible and carbamates reversible. Although these terms may be appropriate in describing the state of inhibition as a distinct quality independent of the chemistry of inhibition, they are not at all appropriate in describing the chemical reactions involved.

The most important carbamates are *N*-methyl- and *N*,*N*-dimethylcarbamates. The *N*-methyl- and *N*,*N*-dimethylcarbamoyl enzymes hydrolyze with a half-time of about 30 min and the unsubstituted carbamoyl enzyme recovers in 2 min (*9*, *35*). These relatively rapid rates make carbamate inhibitors of this type appear to be reversible, and the faster hydrolysis of the unsubstituted carbamoyl enzyme tends to make unsubstituted carbamates weaker inhibitors than *N*-methyl compounds. On the other hand, *N*,*N*-methylphenyl- and *N*,*N*-diphenylcarbamoyl enzyme derivatives hydrolyze very slowly, and therefore phenylcarbamate inhibitors act more like the usual organophosphates. Again, since dimethylphosphorylacetylcholinesterase, in contrast to other phosphoryl enzyme derivatives, reacts relatively fast with water (*6*, *7*), dimethylorganophosphate inhibitors behave like the "usual" carbamates.

The rate of inhibition ought to depend in part upon the intrinsic ease with which the inhibitor can serve as an acid-transferring agent or the extent to which it can be considered an anhydride. Evidently, the pK_a of HX should be an important factor in determining activity, although relationships of this kind in organic chemistry can in general be demonstrated only under such favorable circumstances that other factors do not obscure the correspondence. The rate of inhibition of the enzyme would be expected to bear a closer relationship to the rate of base-catalyzed hydrolysis of the inhibitor; a linear relationship between the logarithms of the rate constants for inhibition and hydrolysis was found with a series of mostly closely related diethyl phosphate esters (*6, 7*). A relationship also holds for the pK_a of HX, but the rate of inhibition falls off rapidly for pK_a>9. In general, it is quite clear that anhydride character is very important in the organophosphates and in the methanesulfonates, but is decidedly less important in the carbamates. Because of the chemical similarity of the carbamate esters to carboxylic esters, it is not unexpected that anhydride character does not play a dominant role in reactivity and that structural features are relatively more important. This kind of relationship between the different groups of inhibitors is illustrated by the failure of diethyl phosphorylcholine and methanesulfonylcholine to react with the enzyme, even though N-substituted and unsubstituted carbamoyl derivatives of choline are active. On the other hand, diethyl phosphorylthiocholine is a very potent inhibitor (*36*), presumably in part because thiocholine is a million times more acidic than choline.

The difference in the relative importances of anhydride character and molecular complementarity in the three series of inhibitors is again illustrated by the diethyl phosphoryl and methanesulfonyl esters of 1-methyl-3-hydroxypyridinium, pK_a=5, which are much more potent than the corresponding esters of 3-hydroxyphenyltrimethylammonium ion, pK_a=8.1 (*37, 38*), whereas the potency of the carbamate esters is, by a large margin, in the reverse order (*39*).

It would seem that lowering K_I, that is, increasing the binding of an inhibitor, would increase the second-order rate constant, but changes that affect K_I are likely to change k_3. The rate of phosphorylation, $E \cdot I \xrightarrow{k'} E' + HX$, is determined by the difference in stability between E·I and the transition state. The electronic instability of the transition state in enzymes can be partially offset by an increase in binding relative to the Michaelis complex. A change in structure, which increases the binding in E·I, may increase or decrease k_3, depending upon how much it increases or decreases the binding in the transition state.

Thus, we cannot predict how a decrease in K_I may affect k_3. An increase in binding that is partially lost in the transition state would lower k_3, but the net effect would be to increase the second-order rate constant. This could be the situation with the introduction of a positive charge. Even if not optimally located, the relatively long range of coulombic forces could contribute to the stability of the transition state. In fact, numerous diethyl phosphates containing quaternary ammonium functional groups (*N*-methylpyridines, *N*-methylquinolines and isoquinolines, choline derivatives, and aryltrimethylammonium derivatives) are very potent inhibitors having second-order rate constants between 10^6 and 10^8 liter mole^{-1} min^{-1} (*36*, *37*, *38*). Although the conjugate phenols of a number of these compounds have pK_a's between 6 and 7, the inhibitors are far more active than diethyl phosphoryl fluoride and tetraethyl pyrophosphate ($k = 2.3 \times 10^5$ and 2×10^6 liter mole^{-1} min^{-1}, respectively). They are 100 to 1000 times more active than would be expected from the acidity constants [on the basis of the relationship obtained by Aldridge (*6*, *7*)]. Diethyl fluorophosphate, not examined by Aldridge, fits this relationship. It appears, therefore, that binding can contribute to the activity of organophosphorus inhibitors.

To sum up: whereas in the case of the carbamates the importance of molecular complementarity in determining the rates of inhibition is easily discerned, in the case of the organophosphates the greater importance of anhydride character tends to obscure other effects, although binding is none the less important.

Many of the phosphoryl enzyme derivatives can be dephosphorylated and the catalytic activity of the enzyme restored by reaction with nucleophilic agents such as water, hydroxylamine, imidazole, pyridine, choline, thiocholine, amine oxides, hydroxamic acids, and oximes (*5*, *40*). It is thought that most, if not all, of these reactivators function as nucleophiles toward phosphorus rather than as general base catalysts for the hydrolysis of the phosphoryl enzyme, and some of them may use the catalytic machinery of the enzyme. This surely seems to be true of choline which, although a reactivator, is hardly a nucleophilic agent. But the structure of choline is especially suited for the catalytic machinery of this particular enzyme, and the analogous reaction of choline with the acetylenzyme is certainly one in which the enzymic mechanism is involved.

Since the phosphorylation of the enzyme is in principle a reversible reaction, the product HX or its conjugate base X^- must be a reactivator. Similarly, if a reactivator acts as a nucleophile toward phosphorus, the resulting product must be an inhibitor. The relative strengths of an inhibitor and its conjugate reactivator are determined by the equilibrium constant for the reaction. Thiocholine and fluoride (*41*) are examples of products of the inhibition reaction that are fairly active reactivators.

The product of the inhibition reaction must be capable of acting as a nucleophile toward the phosphoryl enzyme, but this does not bar it from acting as a general base also, and it is at least possible that a particular substance will act more rapidly as a general base in reactivating the enzyme.

As in the case of inhibition, reactivation may involve the initial formation of a Michaelis complex between the phosphoryl enzyme and the reactivator, especially when the reactivator contains a substituted ammonium function:

$$E' + R \underset{}{\overset{K_R}{\rightleftharpoons}} E' \cdot R \xrightarrow{k_r'} E + I$$

where R is the reactivator (HX or X^-). The pseudo first-order rate constant is given by

$$k_r' \Big/ \left(1 + \frac{K_R}{[R]}\right)$$

and the second-order rate constant, when $[R] \ll K_R$, by

$$k_r = k_r'/K_R$$

The equilibrium constant for reaction (7.7),

$$(EtO)_2P(O){-}F + HE \underset{k_r}{\overset{k_i}{\rightleftharpoons}} (EtO)_2P(O){-}E + HF \qquad (7.7)$$

was determined by measuring the second-order rate constants for inhibition, k_i, and reactivation, k_r (*42*). The values in terms of total concentrations of reactants, without distinguishing between HF and F^- or the different prototropic forms of the enzyme, are 2.3×10^5 and 10 liter $mole^{-1}$ min^{-1}, yielding the equilibrium constant

$$k_i/k_r = 2.3 \times 10^4$$

at pH 7.0; this constant is in terms of total concentrations and therefore depends upon pH.

The equilibrium constant K_2 for the hydrolysis of the diethyl phosphoryl

$$(EtO)_2P(O){-}E + H_2O \rightleftharpoons HE + (EtO)_2P(O){-}OH \qquad (7.8)$$

enzyme, (7.8) is related to the equilibrium constant K_1 for the hydrolysis of diethyl fluorophosphate by

$$K_2 = K_1 k_r/k_i$$

The value of K_1 was taken to be the same as the value for fluorophosphoric acid, which is 3, when the equilibrium expression is written in terms of the undissociated acids (*43*). The value of K_1 becomes 5×10^9 for total concentrations at pH 7.0, and K_2 is therefore 2×10^5 for total concentrations, or 0.5 if diethyl phosphoric acid is written in undissociated form. This value is typical of low-energy phosphates.

The fact that the acid hydrolysis of phosphoryl enzymes yield derivatives of *O*-phosphoryl serine is strong evidence that the hydroxyl group of serine is the enzymic nucleophile (*19*, *20–22*). It is not quite conclusive evidence, because there is the possibility that the phosphoryl group is transferred to serine during acid digestion (*44*) or even during tryptic digestion, especially since the enzyme can be reactivated by amino acid derivatives, including serine methyl ester and serine amide (*40*). It is therefore reassuring to find that the free energy of hydrolysis of the diethyl phosphoryl enzyme, as evaluated from kinetic measurements, is in agreement with an *O*-phosphoryl serine bond and not with a phosphorylimidazole bond. In making this comparison it is assumed that in the formation of the phosphoryl enzyme there are no concomitant changes or interactions that very greatly stabilize what would otherwise be an unstable phosphorus–enzyme linkage.

If without the support of these data it is accepted that serine is the site of phosphorylation and is the enzymic nucleophile, the interesting conclusion can be drawn that, although the serine nucleophile of the active site is, in its chemical reactivity, a remarkably abnormal serine, the resulting *O*-phosphoryl derivative has the normal free-energy value.

Returning to reactivation, there is, then, a thermodynamic relationship between the potency of a reactivator and its conjugate inhibitor. The inhibitor is the more potent relative to the conjugate reactivator, the greater its equilibrium constant for hydrolysis. This constant will tend to be larger for the stronger acids HX. It is also apparent that changes in the structure of X that have little effect on the equilibrium constant in the hydrolysis of an inhibitor must affect inhibition and reactivation to the same extents. This being the case, if molecular complementarity is involved in the reaction of an inhibitor and the enzyme, it must be involved in the reaction of the conjugate reactivator and the inhibited enzyme, and it is a fact that, like the more potent inhibitors, the more potent reactivators contain a quaternary ammonium function.

One might question whether a reactivator forms a loose or a well-defined complex. It would seem reasonable to seek an explanation of very high activity in terms of a well-defined complex whose nucleophilic atom is placed at a proper distance and is directed toward the phosphorus atom in the phosphoryl enzyme. Such an explanation has been offered and it ties together the molecular complementarity of carbamates and the high reactivating capacity of pyridine-2-aldoxime methiodide, 2-PAM, and pyridine-4-aldoxime methiodide, 4-PAM (*45*, *46*) on the assumption that these reactivators had the *anti* configuration (*47*). Since that time the synthesis of the geometric isomer of the existing 4-PAM enabled it to be shown that the older compound has the *syn* configuration and the newer compound the *anti* (*48*). There is relatively little difference in the activity of the two isomers (*48*), and this is also true in the phenyl ketoxime series (*49*); in both cases the *syn* compound is a few times more active. Those results, if they do not completely invalidate the theory, leave it in an uncertain position. Because the 4-PAM isomers are both active, it must be considered that they form loosely ordered complexes. It is still possible, of course, that 2-PAM, being 70 times more active than 4-PAM, does form a well-ordered complex.

It is generally considered that the reactant species are the conjugate bases of the reactivators, because they are far more nucleophilic than the acids. The pH dependence of the reactivation can be accounted for by assuming that a specific acidic group is required in the phosphoryl enzyme. Of course, the acid form of the reactivator and a specific basic group in the enzyme would give the identical pH dependence, and it is possible that in some cases this is the actual mechanism. Suppose that in the acetylation of the enzyme by means of acetylcholine there is a hydrogen ion transfer from the enzyme to the departing choline residue; there is some evidence to support this possibility. Then, in the reverse direction choline should supply a hydrogen ion to a basic group in the acetyl enzyme. If this is the mechanism, and if in its reactivation reactions choline utilized the enzymic machinery, choline rather than its conjugate base would be the reactant.

The spontaneous reactivation of the dimethyl phosphoryl enzyme has a bell-shaped pH dependence. This can be rationalized by assuming that both an acidic and a basic group in the enzyme are necessary and that the reactant is water. If the reactant species is not water but hydroxide ion, it is necessary to assume that two acidic groups in the enzyme are required.

Evidently, various possibilities are available. In accordance with present views on enzymic hydrolysis it appears that in "deacylations" an acidic imidazolium group is involved and functions so as to transfer a hydrogen ion to the leaving serine oxygen. The participation of another group in its acidic or basic form may depend upon the particular reactivator (Figure 7.2).

Introducing a second quaternary group into 4-PAM as in 1,1′-trimethylene-bis(pyridinium-4-dialdoxime), TMB-4, increases the activity of the reactivator

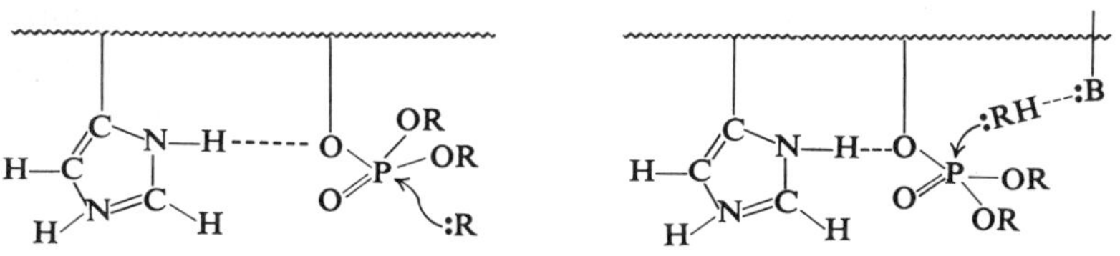

Reactant species: conjugate base of reactivator
Acidic group (imidazolium ion)

Reactant species: acidic form of reactivator
Acidic group (imidazolium ion)
Basic group

Fig. 7.2

400 times (*50–52*). The effect is even more pronounced in the phenyl ketoxime derivatives, where the activity increases 2000 times (*49*).

The greater activity of the diquaternary compounds can be rationalized by the greater binding that generally occurs between diquaternary ions and this enzyme (*53*), but it has not been shown that the binding of the reactivator with the phosphoryl enzyme increases to the required extent.

A small increase is in some cases obtained by introducing a second quaternary group in 2-PAM (an increase of 3 to 4 times, 2 times being expected from merely doubling the concentration of functional groups), but many diquaternary derivatives are less active. The large changes obtained by introducing a second quaternary group in 4-PAM and the phenyl ketoximes are relatively insensitive to the actual structure. The activities of both the *syn* and *anti* compounds are increased, the length of the bridge and its structure seem to be of little importance, and the nature of the second quaternary group is not critically important.

The permissive nature of the requirements for the diquaternary effect does testify to the formation of loose rather than well-ordered complexes, but in the absence of data concerning the binding of these compounds it is problematical whether the anticipated increase in binding would be sufficient to account for the increases in activity.

Increasing the quaternary chain length in monoquaternary compounds, from methyl to pentyl to dodecyl, markedly increases the activity of 4-PAM but decreases the activity of 2-PAM. This effect and the diquaternary effect could be rationalized by assuming that a loose complex is formed with 4-PAM, so that increases in binding tend to increase the second-order rate constants, but that a well-ordered complex is formed with 2-PAM, so that indiscriminate increases in binding tend to spoil the complex.

Evidently, our knowledge in this area is scant. From the relationship between the activity of a reactivator and its conjugate inhibitor we might expect the phosphoryl derivatives of 2-PAM and 4-PAM to be potent inhibitors. Only isopropyl methyl phosphoryl–4-PAM has been described (*54*), and its second-order rate constant for inhibiting eel enzyme is 6×10^7 liter mole^{-1} min^{-1}. This value, which is about the same as for the corresponding fluoride, is consistent with a quaternary structure and a leaving group with a pK_a of about 8.

It certainly appears that the free energy of hydrolysis of a phosphoryl oxime would be little different whether the compound were a quaternary or a diquaternary. Therefore, the diquaternary effect should hold for the conjugate inhibitors of 4-PAM. In the case of the isopropyl methyl phosphoryl enzyme the diquaternary effect for reactivation is only about 50 times. Therefore, the expected second-order rate constant for inhibition by a diquaternary bis compound of isopropyl methyl phosphoryl–4-PAM is about 3×10^9 liter mole^{-1} min^{-1}. The diquaternary effect is larger for diethyl phosphoryl enzyme but, since diethyl phosphoryl inhibitors are usually weaker than isopropyl methyl phosphoryl inhibitors, the two changes tend to offset each other, and the rate constant for the unknown diethyl phosphoryl–4-PAM is probably on the order of 10^9 liter mole^{-1} min^{-1}. Many workers have noticed what seemed to be a "back inhibition" during reactivation with potent reactivators. This effect can be very pronounced with TMB-4; the second-order rate constant for reactivation is about 3×10^5 liter mole^{-1} min^{-1}. The highest concentration of TMB-4 that might be used is about 3×10^{-6} *M*, corresponding to a half-time of 0.7 min. If the phosphoryl enzyme concentration is about 10^{-8} *M*, a convenient concentration, it is apparent that, after 30% of the enzyme is reactivated, there will be about 3×10^{-9} *M* of conjugate inhibitor and, assuming a k_i of 3×10^8, the reactivation will be at equilibrium and no further reactivation will occur (unless the inhibitor decomposes). This is, in fact, what happens, and it appears that k_i for diethyl phosphoryl-bis–4-PAM is about 3×10^8 liter mole^{-1} min^{-1}.

The diquaternary effect is not restricted to oximes. The diethyl phosphoryl esters of some diquaternary phenols are about 20 times more potent than the monoquaternary compounds. Within the assumption that the free energy of hydrolysis of a diquaternary phosphate ester is about the same as for a monoquaternary, provided the second cationic group is well removed from the phenolic functional group, a diquaternary effect in the conjugate reactivators might be expected but, since now extrapolation is being made from a relatively small observed effect, the predicted effect may turn out to be quite small. The smallness of the effect in these cases raises the question whether it is quite the same kind of phenomenon as has been under discussion. This relatively small effect can be accounted for by increased binding.

The extent to which an enzyme inhibited by an organophosphate can be reactivated depends upon the time interval between the inhibition and the addition of the reactivator (*55–58*). The explanation of this aging effect lies in the progressive dealkylation of the phosphoryl enzyme, which yields a new enzyme derivative,

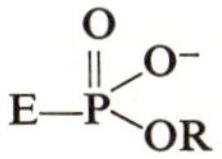

which cannot be reactivated (*59, 60*). This relationship of the two enzyme derivatives resembles the relative reactivity of tertiary and secondary phosphate esters. The former react readily with hydroxide ion; the latter, hardly at all.

Aging occurs more rapidly with enzyme inhibited by isopropyl phosphates than with enzyme inhibited by ethyl phosphates, and it occurs extremely rapidly with enzyme inhibited by pinacolyl methyl phosphonofluoridate (*60*).

Since dealkylation does not occur rapidly with simple compounds nor with the phosphoryl derivatives of other enzymes, it is evident that the enzyme plays some important part in the process.

The order of the alkyl groups with respect to rapidity of dealkylation is opposite to what it would be if the mechanism involved a nucleophilic attack on phosphorus or on carbon. The order corresponds to the stability of the carbonium ions. One might speculate, then, that the mechanism involves an electrophilic attack on the phosphoryl oxygen made by an acidic group in the enzyme:

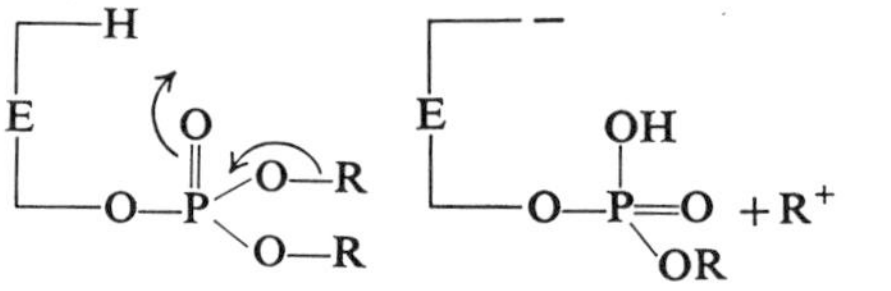

Fig. 7.3

It has been thought that chlorophosphates are inactive as inhibitors, but since diethyl chlorophosphate hydrolyzes "immediately" in water, it is doubtful that a proper experiment has ever been conducted. Diphenyl carbamoyl chloride and phenyl methyl carbamoyl chloride are relatively stable in water, and methanesulfonyl chloride is sufficiently stable in water for the rates of inhibition of acetylcholinesterase to be easily measured. The chlorides are all active inhibitors (*25*). In the carbamates the fluorides are far more active than the chlorides, and in the sulfonates the fluoride is one half as active as the chloride. The activities of the fluorides as compared with the chlorides even in the sulfonate are far greater than would be expected from the comparative chemical reactivities of the compounds. This may be explained by assuming that a hydrogen ion transfer from the enzyme to the halogen is involved. The greater basicity of fluorine and its greater ability to form hydrogen bonds would then account for the much greater reactivity of the fluorides than of the chlorides. This explanation is supported by the fact that some reactions involving fluorides, such as the hydrolysis of benzoyl fluoride, are acid-catalyzed, whereas the reactions involving the chlorides are not.

An alternative explanation is that a tetrahedral intermediate involving the serine oxygen is first formed in the reaction with carbamates. If the formation of the intermediate is rate-controlling—and this is equivalent to saying that in the intermediate the halogen is a better leaving group than the enzyme—then the greater electropositivity of carbon (sulfur) joined to fluorine than of carbon (sulfur) joined to chlorine would make the fluorides the faster reactants.

The reactions of acid-transferring inhibitors and the enzyme can themselves be inhibited by simple reversible inhibitors, such as tetramethylammonium ion. The simplest picture of this inhibition is that the ammonium ion is bound at the anionic site and merely because of its bulkiness prevents the proper approach of the attacking acid-transferring inhibitor. One might question whether there would be interference if the acid-transferring inhibitor contained a small X group such as fluoride. The reaction of diethyl fluorophosphate is completely inhibited by tetramethylammonium ion. However, the reactions of the enzyme and dimethyl carbamoyl fluoride and methanesulfonyl fluoride (*61*, *62*), far from being inhibited, are accelerated by many substituted ammonium ions, quaternary or not. The maximum acceleration is about 100 times. This is an exciting result, because it quite obviously suggests that acetylcholine contains its own built-in accelerator and that the anionic site plays a dynamic role in catalysis. As required for binding at a specific site, the acceleration does show saturation at high concentrations, and the binding constants of the ammonium ions derived from the concentration dependence are the same as those obtained from the inhibition of acetylcholine hydrolysis. The inhibited enzyme derived from the accelerated reaction is reactivated at the same rate as the inhibited enzyme derived from the normal reaction.

There are, however, problems. Tetraethylammonium ion is one of the most potent of the reactivators studied, and tetramethylammonium ion is not more active than trimethyl- or dimethylammonium ion; this order is quite different from the order of the activity of the corresponding substrates. The change from accelerator to inhibitor with increasing size does not occur with compounds smaller in size than tetrabutylammonium ion.

Acceleration occurs also with human serum cholinesterase and with chlorides, such as methanesulfonyl chloride. It does not occur with diphenyl carbamoyl fluoride, possibly because of the large size of the carbamoyl group. It does not occur with diethyl fluorophosphate, but it might occur with a smaller phospho group.

Acceleration of the reactions of carbamoylation and sulfonylation of cholinesterase caused by substituted ammonium ions appears to be evidence that acetylcholine carries its own accelerator and that interaction between a substrate and an enzyme leads to a greatly altered protein configuration, as proposed by Thoma and Koshland (*63*).

REFERENCES

1. The whole subject of "cholinesterase" including chemical, physiological and pharmacological information has been excellently reviewed by several leading workers in these fields in "Cholinesterase and Anticholinesterase Agents," *Handbuch Der Experimentellen Pharmakologie*, Ergänzungswerk XV (G. B. Koelle, ed.), Springer-Verlag, Berlin, 1963. This book contains extensive references.

2. E. F. Jansen, M. D. F. Nutting, R. Jang, and A. K. Balls, *J. Biol. Chem.*, **185**, 209 (1950).

3. E. F. Jansen, M. D. F. Nutting, and A. K. Balls, *J. Biol. Chem.*, **179**, 201 (1949).

4. I. B. Wilson and F. Bergmann, *J. Biol. Chem.*, **185**, 479 (1950).
5. I. B. Wilson, *J. Biol. Chem.*, **190**, 111 (1951).
6. W. N. Aldridge and A. N. Davison, *Biochem. J.*, **55**, 763 (1953).
7. W. N. Aldridge, *Chem. & Ind.* (*London*), **1954**, 473.
8. I. B. Wilson, M. A. Hatch, and S. Ginsburg, *J. Biol. Chem.*, **235**, 2312 (1960).
9. I. B. Wilson, M. A. Harrison, and S. Ginsburg, *J. Biol. Chem.*, **236**, 1498 (1961).
10. R. Kitz and I. B. Wilson, *J. Biol. Chem.*, **237**, 3245 (1962).
11. J. Alexander, I. B. Wilson, and R. Kitz, *J. Biol. Chem.*, **238**, 741 (1963).
12. D. E. Fahrney and A. M. Gold, *J. Am. Chem. Soc.*, **85**, 997 (1963).
13. I. B. Wilson, F. Bergmann, and D. Nachmansohn, *J. Biol. Chem.*, **186**, 781 (1950).
14. H. O. Michel and S. Krop, *J. Biol. Chem.*, **190**, 119 (1951).
15. J. Cohen and M. G. P. J. Warringa, *Biochim. Biophys. Acta*, **11**, 52 (1953).
16. H. C. Lawler, *J. Biol. Chem.*, **236**, 2296 (1961).
17. I. B. Wilson and M. A. Harrison, *J. Biol. Chem.*, **236**, 2292 (1961).
18. D. H. Adams and V. P. Whittaker, *Biochim. Biophys. Acta*, **4**, 543 (1950).
19. N. K. Schaffer, S. C. May, Jr., and W. Summerson, *J. Biol. Chem.*, **202**, 67 (1953).
20. N. K. Schaffer, S. C. May, Jr., and W. H. Summerson, *J. Biol. Chem.*, **206**, 201 (1954).
21. J. A. Cohen, R. A. Oosterbaan, M. G. P. J. Warringa, and H. S. Jansz, *Discussions Faraday Soc.*, **20**, 114 (1955).
22. H. S. Jansz, C. H. Posthumus, and J. A. Cohen, *Biochim. Biophys. Acta*, **33**, 387 (1959).
23. I. B. Wilson and F. Bergmann, *J. Biol. Chem.*, **186**, 683 (1950).
24. L. Weil, S. James, and A. R. Buchert, *Arch. Biochem. Biophys.*, **46**, 266 (1953).
25. H. P. Metzger and I. B. Wilson, *Biochemistry*, **3**, 926 (1964).
26. L. W. Cunningham, *Science*, **125**, 1145 (1957).
27. F. H. Westheimer, *Proc. Natl. Acad. Sci. U.S.*, **43**, 969 (1957).
28. R. M. Krupka and K. J. Laidler, *J. Am. Chem. Soc.*, **83**, 1445 (1961).
29. I. B. Wilson and J. Alexander, *J. Biol. Chem.*, **237**, 1323 (1962).
30. I. B. Wilson and E. Cabib, *J. Am. Chem. Soc.*, **78**, 202 (1956).
31. I. B. Wilson, *J. Biol. Chem.*, **197**, 215 (1952).
32. I. B. Wilson and C. Quan, *Arch. Biochem. Biophys.*, **73**, 131 (1958).
33. D. F. Heath, *Organophosphorus Poisoning*, Pergamon, New York, 1961. This book is also an excellent source of information of organophosphorus anticholinesterases.
34. A. Goldstein and R. E. Hamlisch, *Arch. Biochem. Biophys.* **35**, 12 (1952).
35. R. J. Kitz, *Biochem. Pharmacol.*, **13**, 1275 (1964).
36. L. E. Tammelin, *Acta Chem. Scand.*, **11**, 1340 (1957).
37. A. S. V. Burgen and F. Hobbiger, *Brit. J. Pharmacol.*, **6**, 593 (1951).
38. F. Hobbiger, *Brit. J. Pharmacol.*, **9**, 159 (1954).
39. H. Blashko, E. Bulbring, and T. C. Chow, *Brit. J. Pharmacol.*, **4**, 29 (1949).
40. I. B. Wilson, *J. Biol. Chem.*, **199**, 113 (1952).
41. E. Heilbronn, *Acta Chem. Scand.*, **18**, 2410 (1964).
42. I. B. Wilson and R. Rio, *J. Mol. Pharmacol.*, **1**, 60 (1965).
43. W. Lange, *Z. Anorg. Allgem. Chem.*, **214**, 44 (1933).
44. R. E. Plapinger and T. Wagner-Jauregg, *J. Am. Chem. Soc.*, **75**, 5757 (1953).
45. D. R. Davies and A. L. Green, *Discussions Faraday Soc.*, **20**, 269 (1955).
46. I. B. Wilson and S. Ginsburg, *Biochim. Biophys. Acta*, **18**, 168 (1955).
47. I. B. Wilson, S. Ginsburg, and C. Quan, *Arch. Biochem. Biophys.*, **77**, 286 (1958).
48. E. J. Poziomek and D. N. Kramer, *J. Org. Chem.*, **26**, 423 (1961).
49. R. J. Kitz, S. Ginsburg, and I. B. Wilson, *Biochem. Pharmacol.*, **14**, 1471 (1965).
50. E. J. Poziomek, B. E. Hackley, and G. M. Steinberg, *J. Org. Chem.*, **23**, 714 (1958).
51. F. Hobbiger, D. G. O'Sullivan, and P. W. Sadler, *Nature*, **182**, 1672 (1958).

52. I. B. Wilson and S. Ginsburg, *Biochem. Pharmacol.*, **1**, 200 (1959).
53. F. Bergmann and E. Shimoni, *Biochem. J.*, **55**, 50 (1953).
54. B. E. Hackley, G. H. Steinberg, and J. C. Lamb, *Arch. Biochem. Biophys.*, **80**, 169 (1959).
55. F. Hobbiger, *Brit. J. Pharmacol.*, **10**, 356 (1955).
56. I. B. Wilson, S. Ginsburg, and E. K. Meislich, *J. Am. Chem. Soc.*, **77**, 4286 (1955).
57. D. R. Davies and A. L. Green, *Biochem. J.*, **63**, 529 (1956).
58. B. J. Jandorf, H. O. Michel, N. K. Schaffer, R. Egan, and W. H. Summerson, *Discussions Faraday Soc.*, **20**, 134 (1955).
59. F. Berends, C. H. Posthumus, I. van der Sluys, and F. A. Deierkauf, *Biochim. Biophys. Acta*, **34**, 576 (1959).
60. J. H. Fleischer and L. W. Harris, *Biochem. Pharmacol.*, **14**, 641 (1965).
61. R. J. Kitz and I. B. Wilson, *J. Biol. Chem.*, **238**, 745 (1963).
62. H. P. Metzger and I. B. Wilson, *J. Biol. Chem.*, **238**, 3432 (1963).
63. J. A. Thoma and D. E. Koshland, Jr., *J. Am. Chem. Soc.*, **82**, 3329 (1960).

CHAPTER 8

SYMPATHOMIMETIC (ADRENERGIC) STIMULANTS

A. M. LANDS and THEODORE G. BROWN, Jr.

STERLING-WINTHROP RESEARCH INSTITUTE
RENSSELAER, NEW YORK

8.1. INTRODUCTORY REMARKS

The term "sympathomimetic" was introduced in 1910 by H. H. Dale to describe the actions of various amines which had engaged his interest and that of his chemist colleague, G. Barger (*1*). The years since have produced a vast literature describing these actions and concerning many additional amines. Much of this literature has been presented in reviews (*2–7*), and it would not be useful for us to repeat this coverage here. We shall, instead, present some concepts and structure–activity correlations that appear to be a direct extension of those investigations.

The scope of our presentation may be adequately described by a direct quotation from the summary given by Barger and Dale (*1*):

An action simulating that of the true sympathetic nervous system is not peculiar to adrenine, but is possessed by a larger series of amines, the simplest being primary fatty amines. We describe all such amines and their action as "sympathomimetic".

Approximation to adrenine in structure is, on the whole, attended with increasing intensity of sympathomimetic activity, and with increasing specificity of action.

All the substances producing this action in characteristic manner are primary and secondary amines. The quaternary amines corresponding to the aromatic members of the series have an action closely similar to that of nicotine.

The optimum carbon-skeleton for sympathomimetic activity consists of a benzene ring with a side-chain of two carbon-atoms, the terminal one bearing the amino group. Another optimum condition is the presence of two phenolic hydroxyls in the 3:4 position relative to the side-chain: when these are present, an alcoholic hydroxyl still further intensifies the activity. A phenolic hydroxyl in the 1 position does not increase the activity.

Motor and inhibitor sympathomimetic activity vary to some extent independently. Of the catechol bases those with a methylamino group, including adrenine, reproduce inhibitor sympathetic effects more powerfully than motor effects; the opposite is true of the primary amines of the same series.

The authors in discussing the theoretical implications of their results with various amines state that Elliott (*8*) considered that the parallelism between the actions of epinephrine and sympathetic nerve stimulation may be due to the fact that the latter produce their effects by liberating epinephrine at their endings. This idea was extended by Dixon and Hamill (*9*), who proposed that not only the nerve impulse but also drugs may cause the release of this hormone and produce a sympathetic effect.

The subsequent investigations of Tainter and associates (*10–15*) into a variety of sympathomimetic amines led to the observation that cocaine antagonized tyramine, ephedrine, amphetamine, and various other amines but that it increased the response to epinephrine, norepinephrine, phenylephrine, and related compounds. Tainter (*11*) proposed a classification on the basis of this observation, the potentiated drugs being called "sympathicotropic" (truly sympathomimetic) and the tyraminelike drugs "pseudosympathicotropic." Burn and Tainter (*16*) showed that similar effects followed sympathetic denervation. Later Fleckenstein and Burn (*17*) and Fleckenstein and others (*18*, *19*) provided structure–activity data with regard to the importance of structural variation for these effects and added that the presence of a hydroxyl on the β carbon resulted in compounds that exerted both actions.

The use of reserpine for releasing catecholamines provided Burn and Rand (*20*) with additional support for the concept that tyramine and related substances act through an indirect mechanism. The importance of molecular structure for this action has been described by Maxwell et al. (*21*). These investigators reported three classes of sympathomimetic amines based upon pressor action in dogs after reserpinization, in which a group with mixed actions, as indicated above, is described (Table 8.1). A detailed review of the phenomenon would carry us beyond the purpose of the present mission; however, the reader is directed to the review by Trendelenburg (*22*), which presents a careful analysis of the data on supersensitivity and subsensitivity to sympathomimetic amines.

The "motor" and "inhibitor" sympathomimetic activity described by Barger and Dale (*1*) were the subject of detailed investigations by Youmans and associates (*23–25*), who evaluated the importance of the structural groups of

TABLE 8.1

Effect of Reserpine on the Pressor Response to Sympathomimetic Amines (*21*)

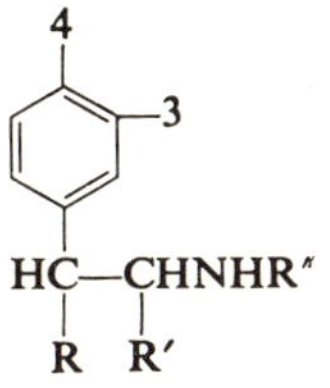

Compound	Structure 4	3	R	R′	R″	Group classification	Reserpine-pretreated pressor response, % untreated response[a]
Norepinephrine	OH	OH	OH	H	H	1	+64
Epinephrine	OH	OH	OH	H	CH_3	1	+10
Nordefrine	OH	OH	OH	CH_3	H	1	+78
Epinine	OH	OH	H	H	CH_3	1	+47
Phenylephrine	H	OH	OH	H	CH_3	1	+15
Synephrine (Sympatol)	OH	H	OH	H	CH_3	1	+69
Phenylpropanolamine	H	H	OH	CH_3	H	2	−50
Ephedrine	H	H	OH	CH_3	CH_3	2	−48
Tyramine	OH	H	H	H	H	3	−71
Hydroxyamphetamine	OH	H	H	CH_3	H	3	−84
Hydroxymethamphetamine	OH	H	H	CH_3	CH_3	3	−87
Amphetamine	H	H	H	CH_3	H	3	−74
Methamphetamine	H	H	H	CH_3	CH_3	3	−60
Phenylpropylmethylamine	H	H	CH_3	H	CH_3	3	−46
Phenethylamine	H	H	H	H	H	3	−64

[a] Increased, +; decreased, −. Group 2 compounds were reported to have mixed actions.

the epinephrine molecule for these actions. They suggested that a possible difference in the reception of epinephrine by adrenergically innervated effector cells could be explained by assuming that certain groups of the epinephrine molecule are necessary for the effective union with the receptive mechanism in one type of effector, while one or more different groups unite with the receptive mechanism in another type; they pointed out the necessity for postulating two or more receptor mechanisms (*23*). Some structure–activity relationships are outlined in Table 8.2, including those reported by Youmans.

The demonstration that both norepinephrine and epinephrine are formed in the animal body (*26–30*) and that the substance elicited those effects which Cannon and Rosenblueth (*31*) identified with Sympathin E stimulated efforts at identifying the substance which has the properties of Sympathin I. Epinephrine has mixed properties and may cause opposite effects in the same organ,

TABLE 8.2

Relation of the Groups of the Epinephrine Molecule for Sympathomimetic Activity

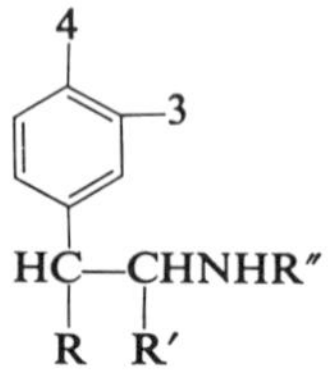

Compound	Structure 4	3	R	R′	R″	Relative activity: Intestinal motility[a]	Heart rate[a]	Blood pressure[b]	Nictitating membrane
Epinephrine	OH	OH	OH	H	CH_3	1000	1000	1000	1000
dl-Norepinephrine	OH	OH	OH	H	H	250–670	500–1330	1000–1600	33–100[c]
Epinine	OH	OH	H	H	CH_3	40–100	20	140	50[c]
Kephrine	OH	OH	O	H	CH_3	10–40		20	13[c]
Nordefrine	OH	OH	OH	CH_3	H	100–400		500	
Phenylephrine	H	OH	OH	H	CH_3	10–40	20–40	140	250–330[c]
Synephrine	OH	H	OH	H	CH_3	<1	<1	<1	8–33[c]
Tyramine	OH	H	H	H	H		17	21	1[d]
Ephedrine	H	H	OH	CH_3	CH_3		20	10–20	50[d]

[a] Youmans et al. (*23, 24*); heart denervated.
[b] Lands (*6*).
[c] Bacq (1936, 1938), quoted by Youmans (*23*).
[d] Trendelenburg et al. (*22a*).

depending upon dosage and physiological state. The availability of isoproterenol and related compounds provided new tools for the evaluation of the actions (*32*). Lands et al. (*33–36*) reported that structural requirements for sympathomimetic vasodepression are as specific as those for vasoconstriction and, in organs other than the heart, usually have actions opposing those of norepinephrine, that is, mimic Sympathin I. Ahlquist (*37*) carried out an analysis of the pattern of action of six sympathomimetic amines and suggested the convenient classification of receptors into alpha (α) and beta (β) types according to the norepinephrine-sensitive and isoproterenol-sensitive mechanisms. A precise statement of the meaning of these terms has been provided in a more recent communication (*38*). The receptors are further differentiated by blocking agents, in that phenoxybenzamine or phentolamine block the α receptor but are without important effect on the β receptor. The observations of Coret and van Dyke (*39*), confirmed by Butterworth (*40*), also indicated that specific blockade of the β receptor was possible by administering large amounts of isoproterenol. This concept was extended by Powell and Slater (*41*) in the demonstration of blockade of β receptors with dichloroisoproterenol (DCI).

Results obtained in our investigations with various sympathomimetic amines have shown that the response of the heart is somewhat different from what would be expected if sympathomimetic action were mediated by a β receptor. Relative effectiveness of sympathetic amines at other receptive sites cannot be predicted from results obtained with this organ (*42*). However, the cardiac effects of isoproterenol are blocked by DCI (*43*). Illustrative data are shown later in Table 8.13. Some of the implications of these findings will be discussed in another portion of this chapter.

The data referred to above have established that sympathomimetic amines may act at either of two distinct receptor sites and that each site has specific molecular requirements for optimal activation or blockade. Norepinephrine is an effective activator at the α receptor and only a weak activator at the β receptor, whereas isoproterenol is a most effective activator of the β receptor. Both compounds have some activating potential at both receptor sites (*44, 45*). Structural modifications, as represented by many active sympathomimetic amines, may activate one or both of these receptor mechanisms to a greater or lesser degree or may indirectly stimulate by causing the release of an activator substance. A detailed description of the pharmacological actions of norepinephrine and isoproterenol would be useful for the subsequent evaluation of other sympathomimetic amines.

8.2. NOREPINEPHRINE

Norepinephrine was synthesized by Stolz and Flacher in 1904 and was very soon recognized to be of high biological activity (*49–52*). The careful experimentation of Euler demonstrated that it is released by adrenergic nerve stimulation and plays an important role in sympathetic nervous activity (reviewed *29*, *53*). A vast and growing literature describes the role of this agent and the conditions influencing its storage and release. The reader may wish to consult the review by Trendelenburg (*22*).

Norepinephrine is found in organs from many invertebrates and vertebrates (*54–56*). Although it is difficult to generalize with regard to the specific action of this substance in each species, there are many species in which comparable responses are elicited (*54, 57*). The potency of norepinephrine relative to that of epinephrine is quite variable among species. Some of the differences are shown in Table 8.3. The data do not correlate well with the organ content of amine. Östlund (*54*) has pointed out that the hagfish heart is rich in both amines but is totally insensitive to them when administered by perfusion.

TABLE 8.3

Comparison of the Actions of Epinephrine and Norepinephrine in Various Animal Species

Species	Experimental preparation	Relative potency, epi./norepi.	Ref.
Squid (*Eledone cirossa*)	Perfused heart	1/1	*54*
Hagfish (*Myxine glutinosa*)	Perfused heart	0/0	*54*
Dogfish (*Squalus acanthias*)	Perfused heart	1/50–100	*54*
Ray (*Raja batis*)	Perfused heart	1/4–10	*54*
Codfish (*Gadus callarias*)	Perfused heart	1/10–20	*54*
Frog (*Rana temp.* and *R. pipiens*)	Perfused heart	1/10–20, 1/7–8	*54, 58*
Sand dab (*Scopthalamus aquosis*)	Chromatophore aggregation	1/1	*59*
Turtle (*Graptymys geographica*)	Heart, in situ; diastolic pressure	1/4, 1/1.5	*57*
Alligator (*Alligator mississipiensis*)	Heart, in situ; diastolic pressure	1/1[a]	*57*
Chicken	Heart, in situ; diastolic pressure	0/0, 1/2	*57, 73*
Opossum (*Didedphis virginianis*)	Heart, in situ; diastolic pressure	1/2, 1/1.2	*57*
Dog, heart: chronic denervated		2/1	*185*
Man, heart: contractile force		1/1	*106*

[a] A dose of 3 μg/kg of epinephrine caused a marked elevation, whereas this amount of norepinephrine was without effect.

Further, the dogfish is relatively insensitive to norepinephrine, yet the heart tissue contains somewhat more of it than of epinephrine. The frog (*Rana temp.*) contains very little norepinephrine (*60*). Further evidence that norepinephrine is less important than epinephrine in the frog has been obtained by Clark et al. (*61*). The release of spermatozoa was induced by the lymphatic administration of epinephrine in doses 1/5 to 1/10 of those required for norepinephrine.

The data establish the importance of both norepinephrine and epinephrine in invertebrate and lower vertebrate species. However, it is not possible to generalize on the role played by each of these agents. Possibly, the evolutionary process leading to mammalia also evolved specific functional roles for the two amines. This thought will be pursued in subsequent portions of the chapter.

Euler (*53*) has reviewed the occurrence of norepinephrine and epinephrine in the suprarenal medulla and chromaffin cells. As of the data presented above, a generalization regarding the functional significance of these amines in various species based on adrenal content is not readily apparent. The norepinephrine content of primate adrenal glands is low (none found in the baboon, 7 to 24% in man) and in rodents (0 to 39%), somewhat more in ungulates and carnivores, and most in whales. With regard to the effect of age, the evidence suggests that norepinephrine predominates before birth and then diminishes rapidly to the adult amount subsequent to birth. Norepinephrine constitutes 90% of the total catecholamine in man at twenty-two weeks before birth, 70% at birth, and somewhat less at two or more years of age (*62*).

These findings emphasize the importance of both norepinephrine and epinephrine but does not permit a generalization with regard to the over-all action of either. Norepinephrine is found at sympathetic nerve endings and is generally considered to play a major role in transmitting the adrenergic nerve impulse (*29*, *63–65*). However, low bronchodilator potency suggests that epinephrine, rather than norepinephrine, is involved in the lung. In the heart the relative effectiveness varies with species, but in the dog, cat, and man the amines appear to be equiactive.

The formation and metabolism of norepinephrine and epinephrine have been reviewed (*5*, *29*, *66*, *67*), but no evidence was given that would distinguish between the two amines. Probably the primary amine is formed first and the secondary is obtained by *N*-methylation. The results obtained by Butterworth and Mann (*40*a) from the cat support this view. After adrenal depletion norepinephrine is replaced first and then epinephrine with a concomitant reduction in total norepinephrine content. Catechol-*O*-methyl transferase converts both amines to the corresponding metanephrine, and this appears to be the principal inactivation process in man and rodents. Monoamine oxidase is mainly concerned with deamination of these metabolites rather than of the catecholamines (*66*).

A. Cardiovascular Actions of Norepinephrine and Related Compounds

The intravenous injection or infusion of norepinephrine causes an elevation of mean arterial blood pressure associated with a contraction of vascular smooth muscle, particularly that of the arterioles. The vasoconstrictor profile has been carefully detailed by Green and associates (reviewed *68*). Norepinephrine vasoconstriction equals, or is somewhat less than, that induced by the same dose of epinephrine, but it is not associated with secondary vasodilatation (*68–70*).

Response in man after intramuscular injection causes elevations of systolic and diastolic pressures and an increase in peripheral and elastic resistance (*71*). Analysis of norepinephrine-induced vasoconstriction in the various organs of the dog after intra-arterial injection has been described by Green (*72*). The changes in conductance (flow divided by pressure) are compared with those of epinephrine in Table 8.4. It is interesting to note the secondary dilator responses to norepinephrine in skeletal muscle and mesenteric and splenic arterial beds. The investigators state that the responses are not significantly related to reactive hyperemia. This stimulation of β receptors at some dose

TABLE 8.4

Response in Various Vascular Beds to Intra-arterial Injections of *l*-Norepinephrine in Percent Control Conductance (*68*)

Organ	Primary response[a] (vasoconstr.)	Action relative to epinephrine[b]	Secondary response[a] (vasodilat.)	Action relative to epinephrine[b]
Muscle	75	1.08	40	0.36
Mesenteric artery	84	1.10	25	1.00
Hepatic artery	55	0.84	0	
Portal vein	40	0.89	0	
Spleen	58	0.93	17	1.00
Skin	80	0.94	0	
Heart	0		8	
Total	75	1.07	0	

[a] Conductance: flow in millimeters per minute divided by pressure in millimeters of mercury. Estimate of difference from control value.

[b] Comparison with response to intra-arterial injection of 1 μg of epinephrine.

levels resembles the results obtained in the lung perfusion experiments described by Luduena et al. (*44*), in which it was found that the bronchodilator action of *l*-norepinephrine was 1/58 that of epinephrine.

Modifying the structure of norepinephrine can bring about important changes in the vascular profile and potency, as we have seen. The replacement of an H on the α carbon (α to the N) with an alkyl group causes a distinct reduction in pressor potency (Table 8.5). The results obtained with cats and dogs indicate a pressor potency of nordefrine (or the *l* isomer) of 1/4 to 1/2 that of epinephrine (*47, 74, 75, 79*). The replacement of one H on the N with a methyl group, giving the corresponding secondary amine, caused a reduction in potency, and there was evident a large depressor component of action. Increasing the size of the substituent on the carbon α to ethyl or propyl also resulted in a marked reduction in pressor potency and a concomitant increase in depressor action. There is a large degree of structural specificity for α-receptor activation with catechol-C(OH)—C—N= molecules. Increase in the size of the side chain at the α carbon or increase in the size of the N substituent reduced the potency.

Replacement of the hydroxyl group at the β carbon with H or O greatly reduced the pressor potency (Table 8.5). Epinine with 14% (7% in terms of *l*-epinephrine), is the most potent of this group of compounds. The corresponding ketones are less active. These results emphasize the importance of

TABLE 8.5

Effect of Modification of Norepinephrine Side Chain on Vasopressor Potency

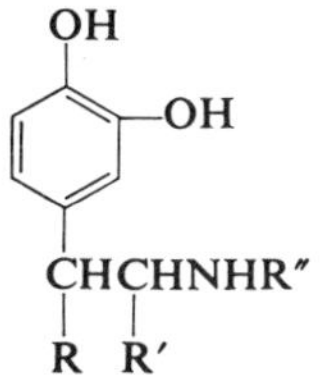

Structure

Compound	R	R′	R″	Relative vasopressor potency	Ref.
Epinephrine	OH	OH	CH_3	1000	
Norepinephrine[a]	OH	H	H		
l				1700; dog	*69*
				1300; dog	*77*
dl				830; cat	*13*
				1430; cat	
				2000; cat	*75*
d				60; dog	*69*
Nordefrine	OH	CH_3	H		
l				430; dog	*47*
				800; dog	*74*
dl				250; cat	*74*
				420; cat	*75*
d				3; dog	*47*
l	OH	CH_3	CH_3	710; cat	*75*
				Depressor; dog, cat, and rabbit	*79*
				Pressor/depressor[b] dog	*80*
Ethylnorepinephrine	OH	C_2H_5	H	Pressor/depressor, cat	*81, 82*
2	OH	C_3H_7	H	<0.1; dog	*80, 83*
3	OH	H	C_2H_5	Pressor/depressor;[b] dog	*84*
4	OH	H	Cyclopentyl	Depressor; dog	*83*
5	OH	H	*n*-Propyl	Depressor; dog	*83*
Dopamine	H	H	H	30;[c] cat	*1, 109*
				20; dog	*85*
Epinine	H	H	CH_3	140;[c] cat	*1*
				60; dog	*86*
6	H	H	C_2H_5	60;[c] cat	*1*
7	O	H	H	40;[c] cat	*1*
Kephrine (adrenalone)	O	H	CH_3	<40;[c] cat	*1*
				10; dog	*86*
8	O	H	C_2H_5	60;[c] cat	*1*
9	O	H	C_3H_7	<10; cat	*1*

[a] Vasoconstrictor action in cutaneous, hepatic, and portal circulations less than with epinephrine (*66, 67*); *l*-norepinephrine is levarterenol.

[b] Combined with local anesthetic and injected intradermally, estimated to have 1/5 epinephrine vasoconstrictor potency.

[c] Value relative to *dl*-epinephrine.

the β hydroxyl for α-receptor activation and are in agreement with the ideas advanced by Easson and Stedman (*87*) and by Luduena and Tullar (*88*). In the case of the *d* isomers of epinephrine and norepinephrine the hydroxyl appears to play little or no part in the binding to, or action on, the sympathetic receptor. Substitution on the phenyl ring of a hydroxyl in the 3 position is more effective in providing vasopressor action than substitution at the 4 position (Table 8.6). Compounds of the latter type are no more effective than the

TABLE 8.6

Effect of Modification of the Norepinephrine Phenyl Ring Hydroxyls on Vasopressor Potency

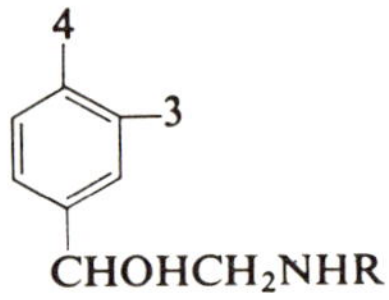

Compound	Structure			Relative vasopressor potency	Ref.
	4	3	R		
Epinephrine	OH	OH	CH_3	1000	
10	H	H	H	8 to 10; cat, dog	*75, 90*
11	H	H	CH_3	4; dog	*35, 90*
12	H	H	C_2H_5	Depressor	*88*
13	H	H	$CH(CH_3)_2$	Depressor; dog	*35, 90*
14	OH	H	H	5 to 10; cat, dog	*22a, 35, 106*
Synephrine (Sympatol)	OH	H	CH_3	2.5 to 5.0; dog, cat	*22a, 35, 91, 92, 105, 106*
15	OH	H	C_2H_5	Depressor; dog, cat	*35, 91, 92*
16	OH	H	n-C_4H_9	Depressor; dog	*33, 91*
dl-17	H	OH	H	30 to 70; cat, dog	*35, 106*
l-17				140; dog	*22a, 36*
Phenylephrine	H	OH	CH_3		
l				100 to 140; cat, dog	*22a, 36, 106*
dl				70; dog	*35, 106*
18	H	OH	C_2H_5	10; cat	*92*
19	H	F	H	5	*93*
20	H	F	CH_3	3	*93*
21	H	F	C_2H_5	Depressor	*93*
22	H	F	$CH(CH_3)_2$	Depressor	*93*
23	H	NH_2	H	10	*95*
24	H	NH_2	CH_3	8	*95*
25	H	NH_2	C_2H_5	4	*95*
26	H	NH_2	$CH(CH_3)_2$	Depressor	*95*
27	OH	OCH_3	H	Weak or inactive	*80*
28	OH	OCH_3	CH_3	Weak or inactive	*80, 179*

corresponding unsubstituted compounds (Nos. 10 and 11). Substitution on the nitrogen of groups larger than methyl greatly reduces (No. 18) or abolishes pressor action (Nos. 12, 13, 15, and 16 are depressor). Ring substitution at position 3 with fluorine, NH_2, or OCH_3 does not favor vasopressor action. Again, compounds with N substituents larger than methyl were vasodepressor.

A hydroxyl group at the β carbon is important for the highest levels of vasopressor action (Table 8.7). Ring hydroxyl substitution in the absence of this group is important only in the case of the *N*-methyl compound (Epinine). In the presence of ring hydroxyls at positions 3 and 4, the addition of the alcoholic hydroxyl provides potent vasopressor compounds (epinephrine and norepinephrine).

Vasopressor action is greatest when the phenethylamine nucleus has been modified by substitution of the ring with hydroxyls at the 3 and 4 positions and by addition of an alcoholic hydroxyl at the β carbon. Vasoconstrictor action in some vascular beds (skin and splanchnic areas) is further increased by replacement of one hydrogen of the amine with a methyl group. Substitution of larger groups on the amine or on the carbon adjacent to the amine reduces

TABLE 8.7

Effect of Modification of Norepinephrine "Alcoholic Hydroxyl" on Vasopressor Potency

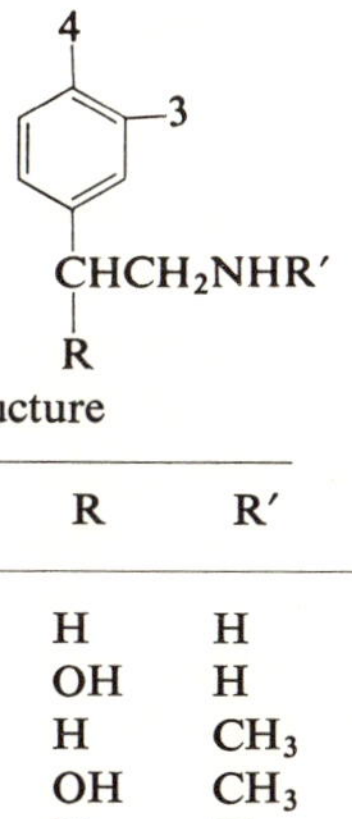

Compound	Structure 4	3	R	R′	Relative vasopress. potency	Ref.
Phenethylamine	H	H	H	H	5 to 23; cat	*75*
10	H	H	OH	H	8 to 10; cat, dog	*75, 90*
29	H	H	H	CH_3	2 to 3; cat	*1*
11	H	H	OH	CH_3	4	*35, 90*
Tyramine	OH	H	H	H	8 to 20; cat	*1, 22a, 75*
14	OH	H	OH	H	5 to 10; cat, dog	*22a, 35*
m-Tyramine	H	OH	H	H	10; cat	*1, 22a*
17	H	OH	OH	H	45 to 60; cat, dog	*22a, 35*
Dopamine	OH	OH	H	H	20 to 100; cat, dog	*1, 85*
l-Norepinephrine	OH	OH	OH	H	1420	*22a*
dl-Norepinephrine					830 to 2000; cat, dog	*1, 69, 75*
Epinine	OH	OH	H	CH_3	60 to 140; cat, dog	*1, 86*
Epinephrine	OH	OH	OH	CH_3	1000	

vasopressor action and, in most instances, vasodepression is the dominant effect. Replacement of the ring hydroxyl at the 3 position with fluorine, chlorine, NH_2, or OCH_3 did not provide potent vasopressor agents.

The vasopressor action of sympathomimetic amines has been described by Tainter and Chang (*10, 11*) as sympathicotropic (increased response after cocainization) and pseudosympathicotropic (tyraminelike: response reduced after cocainization). Subsequent investigations by Burn and Tainter (*16*) showed that sympathetic denervation of the cat iris, like cocainization, increased sensitivity to epinephrine and decreased sensitivity to tyramine and ephedrine. More recently catecholamine depletion with reserpine has permitted further extension of these pioneer studies and has provided a means of classifying the mechanism of action into direct, indirect, and mixed types (*20–22, 94, 96, 97*). There is strong evidence that tyramine and related substances cause vasoconstriction secondary to the release of norepinephrine.

A classification of sympathomimetic amines of interest reported by Trendelenburg (*22*) is shown in Table 8.8. Mixed actions are noted in a group of relatively weak sympathomimetic compounds regarding which there is the suggestion that large doses cause catecholamine release in addition to direct action on the adrenergic receptor. The release may be induced by a considerable number of structurally diverse compounds (reviewed, *97*). The data in Table 8.8 suggest that direct (sympathicotropic) action is favored by the presence of the alcoholic hydroxyl (except for dopamine and Epinine) and is absent for the most part when this group is absent. Amphetamine and related compounds induce vasopressor responses secondary to the release of the biogenic amines.

Norepinephrine is found in the mammalian heart along with a smaller amount of epinephrine (reviewed *53, 98*). Analysis of five different regions of the dog heart disclosed the highest concentration in the right atrium and the lowest in the left ventricle (*99*). Essentially similar results have been reported by Shore et al. (*100*). Intravenous administration of norepinephrine causes an increase in the force of myocardial contraction with or without some increase in the rate of contraction (*101–103, 259*). These changes are similar to those following sympathetic nerve stimulation of this organ (*53*).

Youmans et al. (*24*) evaluated the relation of the groups of the epinephrine molecule to cardioaccelerator action in unanesthetized dogs after cardiac denervation. They found that removal of the methyl group (norepinephrine) did not significantly affect potency but that removal of any one of the three hydroxyl groups resulted in a compound 1/25 to 1/2500 as potent as epinephrine. The most important of the four groups was found to be the 3-hydroxyl on the phenyl ring. Results obtained with various sympathomimetic amines in the rabbit perfused heart preparation are shown in Table 8.9. Youmans et al. (*24*) used *dl*-norepinephrine in their comparison with epinephrine (*l* isomer), so their observed potency of 50 to 130% indicates an equal or slightly greater

TABLE 8.8

Effect of Molecular Structure of Sympathomimetic Amines on Mechanism of Action[a]

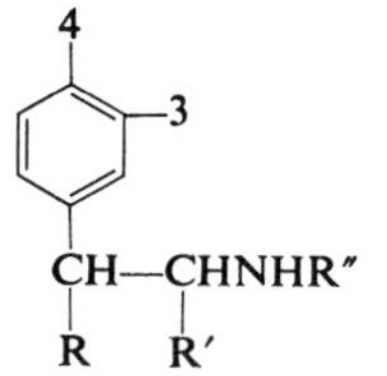

Compound	Structure 4	3	R	R′	R″	Mechanism of action[b]
Norepinephrine	OH	OH	OH	H	H	1
Epinephrine	OH	OH	OH	H	CH_3	1
Norphenylephrine	H	OH	OH	H	H	1
Phenylephrine	H	OH	OH	H	CH_3	1
Synephrine	OH	H	OH	H	CH_3	1–(?)2
Dopamine	OH	OH	H	H	H	1
Epinine	OH	OH	H	H	CH_3	1
Kephrine	OH	OH	O	H	CH_3	2
Nordefrine	OH	OH	OH	CH_3	H	1
1	OH	OH	OH	CH_3	CH_3	1
m-Tyramine	H	OH	H	H	H	2–3
30	H	OH	OH	CH_3	H	2
31	OH	H	OH	CH_3	H	2
32	H	OH	OH	CH_3	CH_3	2
Metaraminol	H	OH	OH	CH_3	H	2
33	OH	H	OH	CH_3	CH_3	2
Phenylpropanolamine	H	H	OH	CH_3	H	2
Ephedrine	H	H	OH	CH_3	CH_3	2–3
Tyramine	OH	H	H	H	H	3
34	OH	H	H	CH_3	H	3
35	OH	H	H	CH_3	CH_3	3
Amphetamine	H	H	H	CH_3	H	3
Methamphetamine	H	H	H	CH_3	CH_3	3
Phenethylamine	H	H	H	H	H	3
l-10	H	H	OH	H	H	1–2

[a] Based on classification of Trendelenburg (*22*).
[b] 1, direct action; 2, mixed action; 3, indirect action.

effect of the former. The results obtained with the rabbit perfused heart, isolated atrial appendage, and spinal cat heart have been compared with vasopressor action in dogs and spinal cats (*22a*, *80*, *255*); see Table 8.10. Norepinephrine and epinephrine are the most potent and show no certain difference

TABLE 8.9

Effect of Modification of Norepinephrine Molecule on Cardiac Stimulation (Rabbit Isolated Perfused Heart)

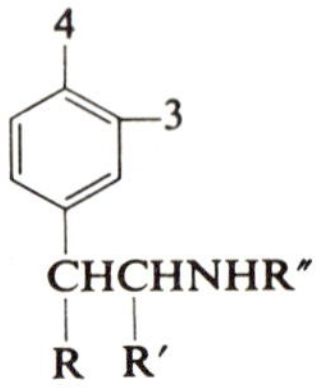

Compound	Structure					Cardiac stimulating dose,[a] μg/heart	
	4	3	R	R′	R″	Force	Rate
l-Norepinephrine	OH	OH	OH	H	H	0.029	0.029
Epinephrine	OH	OH	OH	H	CH_3	0.025	0.05
Dopamine[b]	OH	OH	H	H	H	0.5	1.0
Epinine	OH	OH	H	H	CH_3	2.0	20.0
l-Nordefrine	OH	OH	OH	CH_3	H	0.02	0.04
l-Ethylnorepinephrine	OH	OH	OH	C_2H_5	H	1.0	1.5
l-17	H	OH	OH	H	H	1.0	10.0
l-Phenylephrine	H	OH	OH	H	CH_3	50.0	100.0
14	OH	H	OH	H	H	16.0	16.0
dl-Synephrine	OH	H	OH	H	CH_3	50.0	50.0
l-Metaraminol	H	OH	OH	CH_3	H	2.7	5.0
m-Tyramine	H	OH	H	H	H	8.0	<8.0
Tyramine	H	OH	H	H	H	8.0	8.0
Phenethylamine	H	H	H	H	H	Depress.	128.0

[a] Dose required to produce a 20% increase.

[b] Gurd (*109*) reported a potency of 1/14.5 that of epinephrine on the cat perfused heart.

between them. Structural modification reduces potency. Interpretation of the effects of structural modification on receptor activation is complicated by the release of catecholamines, which characterizes many of these substances. A more exact judgment can be formed from the reserpinized preparation with which direct action predominates. Some results so obtained are shown in Table 8.11. Again, we find differences between vasopressor and cardiac accelerator actions. Phenylephrine is more effective as a vasopressor agent than as a cardiac accelerator, whereas with ephedrine and the corresponding primary amine, phenylpropanolamine, the relationship is reversed. Ephedrine is more effective than *m*-tyramine in inducing cardiac acceleration, whereas it

TABLE 8.10

Effects of Structural Modification of Norepinephrine Molecule on Vasopressor and Cardiac Accelerator Actions

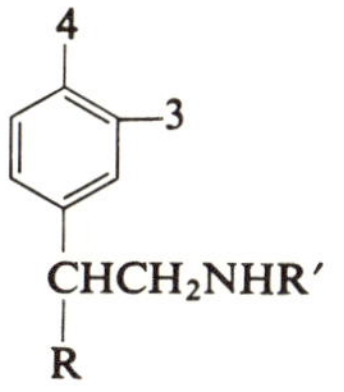

Compound	Structure				Order of potency (1 = most potent)				
					Vasopressor		Cardiac action		
	4	3	R	R′	([a])	([b])	([a])	([b])	([c])
Norepinephrine	OH	OH	OH	H	1	1	1	2	1–2
Epinephrine	OH	OH	OH	CH_3	2	2	2	1	2–1
Phenylephrine	H	OH	OH	CH_3	3	3	10	7	5
l-17	H	OH	OH	H	3	3	6	3	
Epinine	OH	OH	H	CH_3	4		8		4–3
Dopamine	OH	OH	H	H	5		3		3–4
Tyramine	OH	H	H	H	6	4	5	5	3–4
m-Tyramine	H	OH	H	H	7	5	4	4	
Phenethylamine	H	H	H	H	8		11		7
14	OH	H	OH	H	9	6	7	6	
Synephrine	OH	H	OH	CH_3	10	7	9	8	6

[a] Anesthetized dog.
[b] Spinal cat; Trendelenburg et al. (*22 a*).
[c] Amplitude, rabbit atrial preparation (*255*).

is less effective as a vasopressor agent. Epinine and dopamine follow as vasopressor agents, but for cardiac acceleration there is a difference (Table 8.10), although both compounds are reported to act directly.

The data indicate a complex relationship between molecular structure, vasopressor, and cardiac accelerator actions. The importance of each group of the epinephrine molecule is influenced to some degree by all other groups. Epinine, with two ring hydroxyls (at the 3 and 4 positions) has a vasopressor potency comparable to that of phenylephrine with hydroxyls at the ring 3 position and on the β carbon. When the ring hydroxyl is at the 4 position, the pressor potency is of a low order. The substitution of a methyl group at the nitrogen atom has a variable effect. Epinephrine may or may not be more

TABLE 8.11

Relative Effectiveness of Selected Sympathomimetic Amines in Reserpinized Cat Preparation ("Direct" Action) (*22a*)

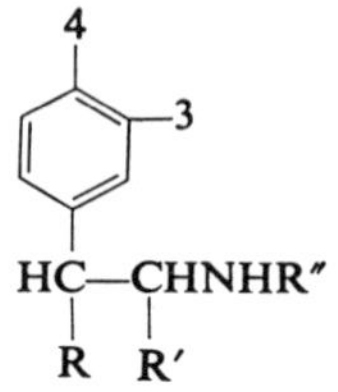

Compound[a]	Structure					Relative effectiveness[a]	
	4	3	R	R′	R″	Blood press.	Heart rate
Norepinephrine	OH	OH	OH	H	H	1000.0	1000.0
Epinephrine	OH	OH	OH	H	CH_3	144.0	1700.0
l-17	H	OH	OH	H	H	29.0	12.0
Phenylephrine	H	OH	OH	H	CH_3	49.0	8.6
l-14	OH	H	OH	H	H	0.2	5.6
Synephrine	OH	H	OH	H	CH_3	3.0	2.8
Metaraminol	H	OH	OH	CH_3	H	10	2.4
Phenylpropanolamine	H	H	OH	CH_3	H	1.8	0.8
Ephedrine	H	H	OH	CH_3	CH_3	0.6	5.0
m-Tyramine	H	OH	H	H	H	1.0	2.5
Tyramine	OH	H	H	H	H	NA	NA

[a] Value for the racemates expressed in terms of the *l* isomers.

vasoconstrictive than norepinephrine but, on balance, is a little less vasopressive. Epinine is more vasopressive than dopamine; phenylephrine is equal in potency to the corresponding primary amine (No. 17); synephrine is less potent than the primary amine (No. 14; Table 8.10).

Epinephrine and norepinephrine have comparable cardiac accelerator potencies, varying somewhat among mammalian species. In the absence of the β hydroxyl the most potent compound is dopamine. Methyl substitution of the nitrogen (Epinine) markedly reduces potency. A ring hydroxyl at the 3 or 4 position alone (tyramine, *m*-tyramine) is more effective than when it is present with the β hydroxyl (No. 17, No. 14). Addition of the *N*-methyl group (phenylephrine, synephrine) further reduces cardiac accelerator potency.

Effects on the force of myocardial contraction are influenced by these molecular changes, and in many instances an effect is obtained with smaller doses than those required for acceleration (*42*). Some results obtained with the rabbit isolated perfused heart are shown in Table 8.9. The stimulation thresholds for force changes clearly were smaller than those for rate in the case of epinephrine, Epinine and No. 17. These compounds appear to have no structural component that would distinguish them from other structures in which the threshold values are near or equal to those for cardiac accelerator action. The most potent compounds are the catecholamines, norepinephrine, epinephrine, nordefrine, ethylnorepinephrine, and dopamine; these are followed by No. 17 (the primary amine analogue of phenylephrine), Epinine, and metaraminol. There is a suggestion that the receptor mechanism for force change differs from that of cardiac acceleration, inasmuch as the order of relative potency differs along each parameter.

B. Action of Norepinephrine and Related Compounds on Smooth Muscle of Various Organs

The preceding sections have presented data with regard to the importance of the molecular structure of sympathomimetic amines for vasopressor and cardiac actions. The analysis has been extended to include effects on the response of the small intestine, nictitating membrane, uterus (rabbit), and vas deferens (rat). Some of the results are presented in Tables 8.12 and 8.13. Arranged in order of decreasing potency they are epinephrine > norepinephrine > phenylephrine. A replacement of one hydrogen of the α carbon with a methyl group causes some reduction in potency. A replacement of the *N*-methyl with hydrogen (primary amine) reduces potency, as indicated by the following changes: epinephrine > norepinephrine, Epinine > dopamine, phenylephrine > *l*-17 (norphenylephrine), synephrine > 14 (norsynephrine). Although the data on it are less complete, a similar relationship appears to exist between ephedrine and norephedrine (phenylpropanolamine). In the absence of a ring hydroxyl at the 3 position, the effectiveness is quite low. A hydroxyl at the β carbon is essential for high potency. Epinine and dopamine are somewhat less effective than phenylephrine and its nor analogue.

An assessment of the relative importance of the groups of the epinephrine molecule is difficult, because there is a complex interrelationship between them and the responsive receptors. However, concerning the effects shown in Table 8.12 it appears that the relative importances are: a ring hydroxyl at the 3 position > alcoholic OH at the β carbon > a methyl group on the nitrogen. The similarity in relative potencies indicates that there is a single variety of receptor involved. However, the detailed study of Van Rossum (*254*) led to the conclusion that there are different types of α receptors. His correlation has been extended to include a variety of adrenergic α-receptor responses, the sympathomimetic amines being arranged in order of decreasing potency (Table 8.13). Results obtained with the heart are different and suggest that the receptor has structural requirements differing from those in the vascular bed, small intestine, nictitating membrane, and uterus. Similarly, the effect on

TABLE 8.12

Action of Norepinephrine and Related Compounds on Smooth Muscle of Various Organs

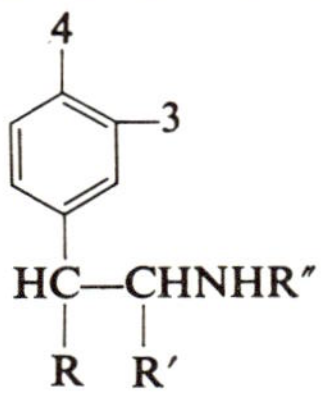

Compound	Structure: 4	3	R	R′	R″	Relative effectiveness[a]: Nict. memb., cat	Uterus, rabbit	Small intest., rabbit
Epinephrine	OH	OH	OH	H	CH_3	1000	1000	1000
Norepinephrine	OH	OH	OH	H	H	200 (*22a*)	200–500 (*111*)	500 (*110*), 330 (*254*)
							1000 (*162*)	
Nordefrine	OH	OH	OH	CH_3	H	130	50 (*112*)	500 (*112*)
						100 (*37*)	33 (*162*)	
Epinine	OH	OH	H	H	CH_3	50 (*111*)	280	25–100[b] (*23*), 1 (*254*)
Dopamine	OH	OH	H	H	H		11	20–50 (*109*), <1 (*254*)
Phenylephrine	H	OH	OH	H	CH_3	200 (*111*)		250[b] (*23*), 72 (*254*)
						143 (*22a*)	200 (*110*)	120 (*110*), 167–250 (*115*)
l-17	H	OH	OH	H	H	37 (*22a*)	40–100 (*110*)	60–120 (*110*), 300–500 (*115*)
Synephrine	OH	H	OH	H	CH_3	17 (*22a*)	2 (*110*)	2 (*110*), <1 (*254*)
14	OH	H	OH	H	H	11 (*22a*)	0.2–1 (*110*)	0.4–1.5[b] (*23*)
								2 (*110*)
Ephedrine	H	H	OH	CH_3	CH_3	57 (*22a*)	<1 (*113*)[c]	<1 (*113*)[c]
Phenylpropanolamine	H	H	OH	CH_3	H	19 (*22a*)	<1 (*113*)[c]	<1 (*113*)[c]

[a] Activity relative to epinephrine; numbers in parentheses, references.
[b] Thirey-Vella dogs.
[c] Variable, either contraction or relaxation.

TABLE 8.13

Effectiveness of Norepinephrinelike Compounds on Various Adrenergically Innervated Organs[a]

Order	Blood pressure[b]	Small intestine[c]	Nict. memb.[d]	Uterus[e]	Symp. gang.[f]	Heart: Rabbit[g]	Heart: Cat[h]	Blood sugar[i]
1	Norepinephrine	Epinephrine	Epinephrine	Epinephrine	Epinephrine	Norepinephrine	Epinephrine	Epinephrine
2	Epinephrine	Norepinephrine	Norepinephrine	Norepinephrine	Norepinephrine	Epinephrine	Norepinephrine	Nordefrine
3	Nordefrine	Nordefrine	Phenylephrine	Phenylephrine	Epinine	Nordefrine		Norepinephrine
4	Phenylephrine	Phenylephrine	Ephedrine	Epinine	Nordefrine	Dopamine	*l*-17	Phenylephrine
5	*l*-17	*l*-17	Epinine	*l*-17	Phenylephrine	*l*-17	Phenylephrine	Synephrine
6	Epinine	Epinine	*l*-17	Nordefrine		14	Ephedrine	
7	Dopamine	Dopamine				Epinine	14	
8	Synephrine	Synephrine	Synephrine	Synephrine	Synephrine	Synephrine	Synephrine	Dopamine
9	14	14	14	14	Ephedrine	Phenylephrine		Epinine
10	Ephedrine	Ephedrine		Ephedrine		Ephedrine		14
								Ephedrine

[a] Some results for the dog retractor penis and for the rat vas deferens are, for the former, epinephrine > norepinephrine > nordefrine > Epinine > dopamine (*116*) and, for the latter, epinephrine > norepinephrine > dopamine = phenylephrine = *l*-14 (*116*, *254*). Results obtained with the rabbit aortic strip give *l*-norepinephrine > epinephrine > phenylephrine > epinine > dopamine > synephrine > tyramine > *l*-ephedrine (*78*).

[b] From Tables 8.5–8.7.

[c] From Tables 8.12 and 8.26.

[d] Spinal cat (*22a*).

[e] Rabbit isolated uterus.

[f] Cat superior cervical ganglion (*108*).

[g] From Table 8.9.

[h] Reserpinized spinal cat (*22a*).

[i] Hyperglycemia (*7*).

blood sugar, as summarized by Ellis (*7*), suggests that the receptor involved here differs in affinity from both of the previous two.

The results obtained with α-adrenolytic drugs are useful in characterizing the receptors. Coret (*114*) has examined a number of sympathomimetic amines for vasopressor blockade and reversal. He found little reversal (after *N*-benzyl-*N*-β-chloroethyl-β-phenylisopropylamine · HCl) with norepinephrine and nordefrine, less than epinephrine with Epinine and Kephrine (epinephrine ketone), none with phenylephrine, and little or none with synephrine. Assuming validity for the quantitative aspects of the data upon which Table 8.13 is based, there are differences in activity ratios and orders of potency in various test organs that suggest that the α receptor is not a single entity but is made up of a population with somewhat different chemical affinities in the various species and organs.

The recent observations of Ciuchita and Gautieri (*174*) obtained with perfused full-term human placentas are of interest. Isoproterenol caused powerful vasodilation of long duration, whereas serotonin caused vasoconstriction. It had been reported previously that epinephrine constricted placental blood vessels (*136*). Inasmuch as these vessels are devoid of innervation (*141*), it would appear that adrenergic receptors of both the α and β types play a role in homeostatic adjustment beyond the regulating actions of the autonomic nervous system.

8.3. ISOPROTERENOL

Dale (*1*) noted, as pointed out previously in this chapter, that "motor and inhibitor sympathomimetic activity vary to some extent independently. Of the catechol bases those with a methylamino group, including adrenine, reproduce inhibitor sympathetic effects more powerfully than motor effects: The opposite is true of the primary amines of the same series." Commenting on this finding in his *Adventures in Physiology*, Dale states that upon finding that the *N*-*n*-propyl member of the homologous series examined had weaker action than the *N*-methyl and ethyl compounds the investigators did not study the *N*-isopropyl analogue of norepinephrine (*117*).

This omission was corrected by Konzett (*32*, *118*) and Rossler (*119*) in 1940–1941. Konzett (*32*) described the pharmacological results obtained with the *N*-ethyl, *N*-propyl, *N*-isopropyl, *N*-butyl, and *N*-isobutyl analogues of norepinephrine, synthesized by Scheuing in the laboratories of C. H. Boehringer Sohn, Ingelheim. The results showed clearly that the inhibitor sympathomimetic activity was increased by ethyl and isopropyl substitution of the nitrogen, and Konzett stated further that the molecular arrangement was more important than the size of this group. Bronchodilator action of the *N*-isopropyl analogue (isoproterenol) was reported to be 10 times greater than that of epinephrine and *N*-propylarterenol. Additional compounds were synthesized by Corrigan et al. (*120*) and these, along with those previously described by Konzett, were evaluated by Lands and associates (*33–36*, *86*, *121*, *122*).

Lockett (*123*, *124*) has made the interesting suggestion that isoproterenol is released into the pulmonary circulation of cats upon stimulation of the sympathetic nerve supply. This, however, awaits confirmation by other investigators.

A. Cardiovascular Actions of Isoproterenol and Related Compounds

1. VASCULAR RESPONSE

Previously we discussed the role of norepinephrine in the transmission of the sympathetic nerve impulse. The control of peripheral resistance does not appear to involve "adrenergic" vasodilator nerves. Uvnäs and associates (*125–127*) and Celander and Folkow (*128*) found no experimental evidence of the existence of such fibers. They reported that the vasodilator fibers serving the muscle are cholinergic and are blocked by atropine. The nervous regulation of blood flow is considered to result largely from variation in vasoconstrictor tonus. Epinephrine may cause vasodilatation in some vascular beds when in low concentration, and it frequently causes vasodilatation and a fall in blood pressure (epinephrine reversal) after adrenergic blockade. Isoproterenol either causes vasodilatation or has no important effect (Table 8.14). Vasoconstriction

TABLE 8.14

Response in Various Vascular Beds to Intra-arterial or Intravenous Injections of Epinephrine and Isoproterenol (*72*)[a]

	Response to epinephrine		
Organ	Primary response	After α-blockade	Response to isoproterenol
Muscle	v.d. or v.c./v.d.	v.d.	v.d.
Mesenteric artery	v.c./v.d.	v.d.	v.d.
Hepatic artery	v.c.	n.a.	n.a.
Portal vein	v.c.	n.a.	n.a.
Spleen	v.c./v.d.	v.d.	v.d.
Skin	v.c.	weak v.d.	weak v.d.
Heart	v.d./v.c.	?	v.d.

[a] V.d., vasodilatation; v.c., vasoconstriction; n.a., no important effect; v.c./v.d., vasoconstriction followed by vasodilatation. Coronary flow changes may be secondary to increased myocardial metabolic activity.

with a rise in blood pressure can be obtained with relatively large amounts of *l*-isoproterenol administered intravenously to anesthetized dogs (*45*). Aortic strips also may be contracted (*138*). No such effect was obtained with the *d* isomer, and it has been suggested that the vasopressor effect obtained with the *l* isomer, as with epinephrine, is due to stimulation of the α receptor.

Konzett (*32*) observed a progressive decrease in pressor potency, as the N substituent was increased from methyl to ethyl and propyl, and an increase in depressor action, which was most prominent with isopropyl. Lands and associates (*34*, *86*, *131*) extended these observations and reported vasodepressor potency with a series of *N*-alkylarterenols in the order *t*-butyl ⩾ isopropyl > *sec*-butyl > ethyl > butyl. The results obtained by us and others are summarized in Table 8.15. The most potent vasodepressor compounds are No. 43 > No. 36 > isoproterenol. The vasodepressor action of epinephrine after α-receptor blockade is about one third that of the *N*-ethyl analogue and about one sixth that of isoproterenol. The presence of a second methyl group near the nitrogen of the secondary amine appears to be important, judging from the greater potency of *N*-ethyl than of propyl and of *N*-*sec*-butyl than of *n*-butyl or isobutyl. The *N*-cyclopentyl analogue is approximately equal to the *N*-ethyl and clearly more vasodepressive than the *N*-cyclohexyl compound. Quite large groups may be substituted on the nitrogen and retain high levels of potency, if the N—$CH(CH_3)$— arrangement is present (for example, No. 43, No. 44, and protokylol).

TABLE 8.15

Vasodepressor Action of Various *N*-Alkylarterenols

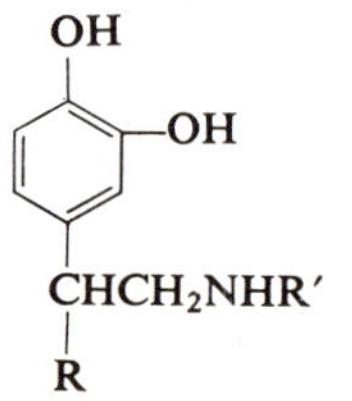

Compound	Structure: R	Structure: R′	Relative vasodepressor potency	Ref.
Isoproterenol	OH	$CH(CH_3)_2$	1000	
Epinephrine	OH	CH_3	165	*130*
3	OH	C_2H_5	500[a]	*83*
36	OH	$C(CH_3)_3$	1300	*131*
37	OH	$CH(CH_3)CH_2CH_3$	500	*83, 133*
38	OH	$CH_2CH(CH_3)_2$	77	*83*

TABLE 8.15—*continued*

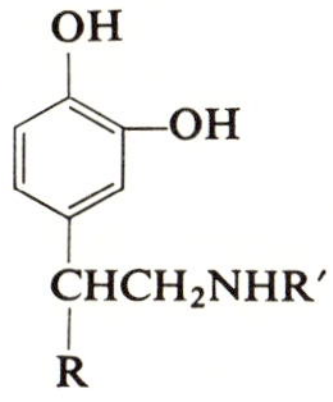

Compound	Structure: R	Structure: R′	Relative vasodepressor potency	Ref.
39	OH	$CH(C_2H_5)_2$	40	*83*
40	OH	$CH(CH_3)CH(CH_3)_2$	40	*83*
41	OH	$CH(CH_3)CH_2CH(CH_3)_2$	< 300	*80*
42	OH	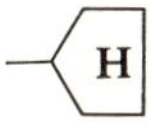	250	*83*
43	OH	$CH(CH_3)CH_2$— 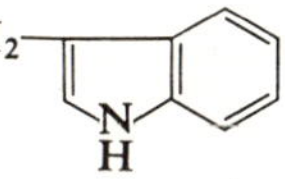	1660	*132*
Protokylol	OH	$CH(CH_3)CH_2$— 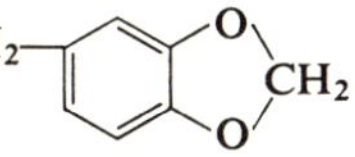	340	*132*
44	OH	$CH(CH_3)CH_2CH_2$— 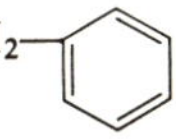	150[b]	*133*
45	OH	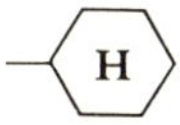	33	*83*
46	OH	n-C_3H_7	200	*83*
47	OH	n-C_4H_9	20–100[a]	*83, 133*
48	OH	n-C_5H_{11}	20–100[a]	*83*
49	OH	CH_2CH_2OH	100[b]	*133*
50	OH	$CH(OCH_3)CH_3$	100[b]	*133*
51	OH	n-C_8H_{17}	< 1[b]	*133*
52	O	$CH(CH_3)_2$	< 1	*86, 135*
53	O	CH_2CH_2OH	40	*135*
54	O	$CH_2CH_2CH_2$— 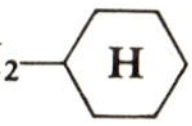	4	*135*
55	H	$CH(CH_3)_2$	1	*86*

[a] Pressor followed by depressor.
[b] Estimated from published values of Wiemers (*133*).

Modification of the side chain between the phenyl ring and the nitrogen reduces vasodepressor potency (Table 8.16). Substitution of a methyl group at the α carbon of isoproterenol (No. 56) causes a marked reduction in vasodepressor potency (9 to 28 % isoproterenol). Substitution of either an ethyl or a

TABLE 8.16

Effect of Modifying the Side Chain of Isoproterenol on Vasodepressor Action

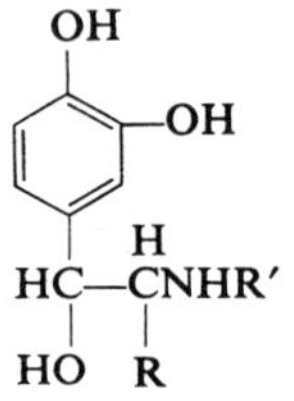

Compound	Structure: R	Structure: R′	Relative vasodepressor potency	Ref.
Isoproterenol	H	$CH(CH_3)_2$	1000	
1	CH_3	CH_3	1[a]	*79*
56	CH_3	$CH(CH_3)_2$	90, 280	*131, 135*
57	$(CH_3)_2$[b]	$CH(CH_3)_2$	5	*80*
Isoetharine	C_2H_5	$CH(CH_3)_2$	174	*131*
58	C_2H_5	$C(CH_3)_3$	±10	*80*
59	CH_3	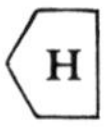	61	*80*
60	C_2H_5	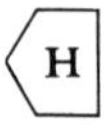	80, 140	*46, 80*
61	C_2H_5	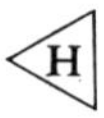	100	*80*
62	C_3H_7	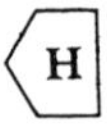	<1	*80*
Ethylnorepinephrine	C_2H_5	H	<1[a]	*80*
63	CH_3	CH_2CH_2— 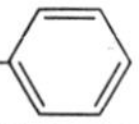	45[c]	*133*
64	CH_3	$CH_2CH_2CH_2C_6H_5$	100	*133*
65	CH_3	$CH(CH_3)CH_2CH_2C_6H_5$	70[c]	*133*
66	CH_3	$CH(CH_3)CH_2CH_2CH_2C_6H_5$	9[c]	*133*

[a] Pressor followed by depressor.
[b] α,α-dimethyl.
[c] Estimated from published values by Wiemers (*133*).

TABLE 8.17

Effect on Vasodepressor Action of Modifying Substituents on the Phenyl Ring of Various Isoproterenollike Compounds

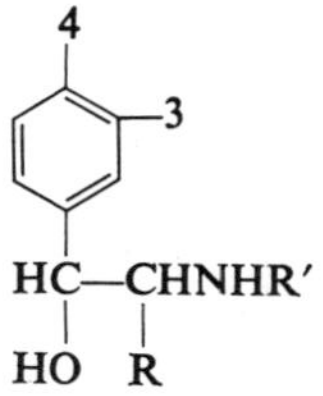

Compound	Structure: 4	Structure: 3	Structure: R	Structure: R′	Depressor dosage,[a] mg/kg	Relative vasodepressor potency	Ref.
Isoproterenol	OH	OH	H	$CH(CH_3)_2$		1000	
67	H	OH	H	C_2H_5		Pressor	*92*
68	H	OH	H	C_3H_7		Inactive	*92*
69	H	OH	H	C_4H_9		<1	*92*
70	H	OH	H	$CH(CH_3)_2$	0.3–0.5	13	*33, 83*
71	H	OH	CH_3	$CH(CH_3)_2$	>1.0	<1	*80*
72	H	OH	C_2H_5	$CH(CH_3)_2$		<1	*80*
73	H	OH	C_2H_5	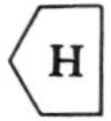 H	>1.0	<1	*80*
74	H	OH	C_2H_5	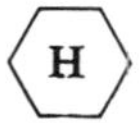 H		<1	*80*
75	OH	H	H	C_2H_5	0.5–1.0	<1	*80*
76	OH	H	H	C_3H_7		<1	*80*
77	OH	H	H	$CH(CH_3)_2$	0.2–0.5	1–2[b]	*33, 91*
78	OH	H	H	$C(CH_3)_3$	0.2	1–2	*91*

TABLE 8.17—*continued*

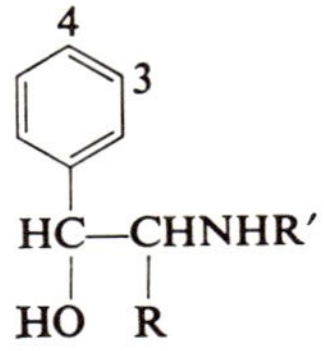

Compound	Structure: 4	3	R	R′	Depressor dosage,[a] mg/kg	Relative vasodepressor potency	Ref.
79	OH	H	H	C_4H_9	> 0.5	< 1	*137, 91*
80	OH	H	H	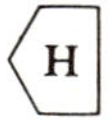	1.0–2.0	< 1	*80*
81	OH	H	CH_3	$CH(CH_3)_2$		< 1	*80*
82	OH	H	C_2H_5	$CH(CH_3)_2$	> 2.0	Weak	*80*
83	H	H	H	$CH(CH_3)_2$	0.5	< 1[c]	*33*
84	H	H	C_2H_5	$CH(CH_3)_2$	> 2.0	Weak	*80*
85	OH	CH_3O	H	$CH(CH_3)_2$		Pressor/depressor	*135*
86	CH_3O	CH_3O	H	$CH(CH_3)_2$		Inactive	*135*
87	OH	H	CH_3	$CH(CH_3)CH_2OC_6H_5$	0.02–0.05	6–15	*137*
88	Br	Br	H	$C(CH)_3$		Weak[d]	*139*
89	Cl	Cl	H	$C(CH_3)_3$		Weak[d]	*139*
90	5-OH	OH	H	$CH(CH_3)_2$		75	*140*
Isoprophenamine		2-Cl	H	$CH(CH_3)_2$		Weak	*256*

[a] Intravenous dose required for 30 to 40 mm. Hg fall in blood pressure.
[b] An intravenous injection of 0.2 mg/kg in the anesthetized dog caused a 35 mm. Hg mean fall in blood pressure.
[c] An intravenous injection of 0.5 mg/kg caused a 50 mm. Hg fall in blood pressure.
[d] Stimulating action less than dichloroisoproterenol.

propyl group at the α carbon causes a further reduction in potency. A cyclopropyl substitution of the nitrogen (No. 61) appears to be equivalent in action to the corresponding cyclopentyl (No. 60).

The presence of a hydroxyl on the β carbon of the side chain is important for vasodepressor action. When the hydroxyl is changed to keto oxygen (No. 52) or reduced to H (No. 55), vasodepressor potency is 40% or less that of isoproterenol. Wiemers (*133*) reported similar reductions in vasodepressor potency of the nordefrine analogue (No. 65) when the hydroxyl on the β carbon was reduced to hydrogen.

TABLE 8.18

Effect of Modifying Structure of Phenyl Ring and Side Chain of β-Phenethanolamine on Vasodepressor Activity

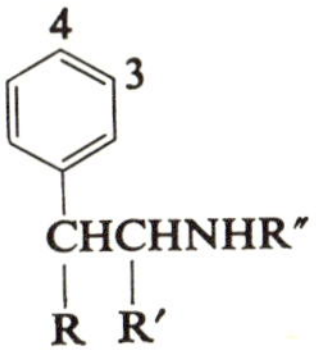

Compound	Structure 4	3	R	R′	R″	Relative vasodepressor potency[a]	Ref.
77	OH	H	OH	H	$CH(CH_3)_2$	1000	
76	OH	H	OH	H	n-C_3H_7	300	*33*
91	CH_3O	H	OH	H	$CH(CH_3)_2$	60	*80*
70	H	OH	OH	H	$CH(CH_3)_2$	700	*33*
81	OH	H	OH	CH_3	$CH(CH_3)_2$	200	*80*
82	OH	H	OH	C_2H_5	$CH(CH_3)_2$	50	*80*
71	H	OH	OH	CH_3	$CH(CH_3)_2$	Pressor/depressor	*80*
72	H	OH	OH	C_2H_5	$CH(CH_3)_2$	200	*80*
92	OH	H	H	H	$CH(CH_3)_2$	Inactive/weak pressor	*80*
93	H	OH	H	H	$CH(CH_3)_2$	Pressor/depressor	*80*
80	OH	H	OH	H	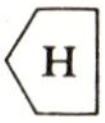 H	100–200	*80*
94	H	OH	OH	H	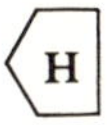 H	100–200	*80*
83	H	H	OH	H	$CH(CH_3)_2$	500	*33*
26	H	NH_2	OH	H	$CH(CH_3)_2$	160	*95*
22	H	F	OH	H	$CH(CH_3)_2$	660	*93*
83a	H	F	OH	H	$C(CH_3)_3$	460	*93*
83b	H	F	OH	H	C_3H_7	150	*93*
83c	H	F	OH	H	C_4H_9	140	*93*

[a] Potency expressed in terms of potency of No. 77.

Vasodepressor potency is modified importantly by modification of the substituents on the phenyl ring. The number and position of the hydroxyls influences potency, as shown by the data in Table 8.17. Although depressor action is obtained with compounds with one or no ring hydroxyl, they are much weaker than the corresponding catecholamine. It is interesting to note that replacement of 3-OH with —OCH_3 leads to a great loss of activity. Epinephrine and norepinephrine are inactivated by conversion to the 3-methoxy analogues through the action of *O*-methyl transferase (reviewed, *66*, *67*). It is probable that isoproterenol shares this metabolic pathway (*260*, *261*).

The importance of structural modification for vasodepressor action is illustrated better in the case of these weak compounds by a comparison of effectiveness with a less potent compound than isoproterenol. For this purpose *N*-isopropyl synephrine (No. 77) was used; the activity ratios are shown in Table 8.18. An isopropyl group at the nitrogen is more favorable than cyclopentyl or *n*-butyl; an alcoholic hydroxyl favors vasodepressor action (No. 77 > No. 92 and No. 70 > No. 93); a ring hydroxyl at the 3 or 4 position appears to be more favorable than a no-ring hydroxyl; substitution of the α carbon with a methyl or ethyl group reduces vasodepressor potency.

2. CARDIAC RESPONSE

Konzett (*32*) in his early study of epinephrinelike substances reported the marked stimulating action of isoproterenol on the dog heart of the Starling heart-lung preparation. This was characterized by an increase in rate and minute volume, an increase in stroke volume, and a reduction in right-auricular pressure. Effects on the heart, of which both force (or amplitude) and rate changes have been determined, have shown that the stimulating action of isoproterenol is distinctly greater than that of epinephrine or norepinephrine (*34*, *42*, *58*).

Experimental results obtained with the rabbit isolated auricle preparation demonstrated that isoproterenol caused a reduction in the refractory period, indicated by the maximal rate of response to an artificial pacemaker (*58*). The effect was greater than obtained with either epinephrine or norepinephrine. Similarly, Boyer and Chisholm (*105*) found isoproterenol more effective than the other two drugs in increasing the ventricular rate of dogs with surgically induced heart block (7 to 16 times more effective than norepinephrine and 10 to 16 times more than epinephrine). Roberts et al. (*149*) also reported that isoproterenol was about 10 times more effective in stimulating atrioventricular rhythms in cats and dogs. Comparable results have been obtained by Nathanson and Miller (*150*) both with patients showing idioventricular rhythms and after vagal inhibition induced by pressure on the carotid sinus.

Lands and Brown (*42*) have determined the dose–response relationship of

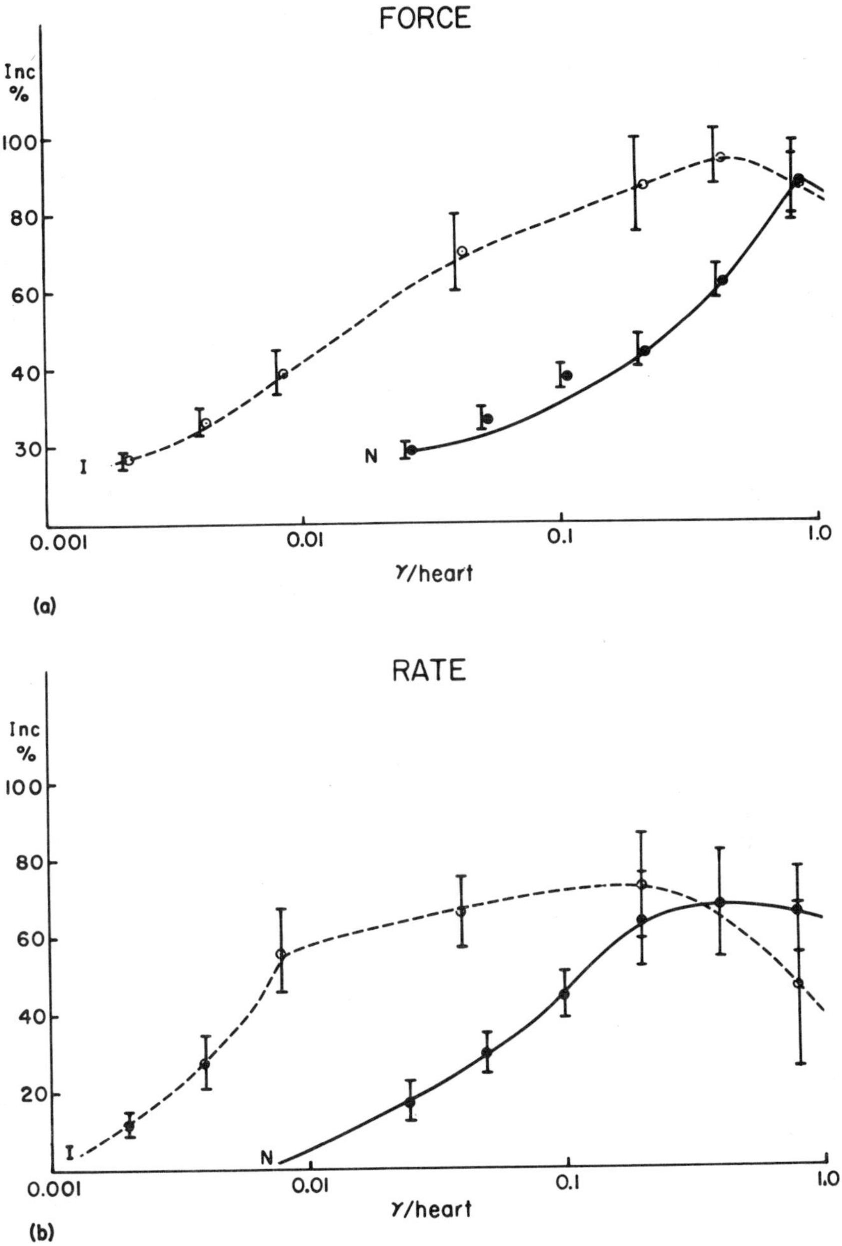

Fig. 8.1. The effect of isoproterenol (I) and norepinephrine (Levarterenol N) on the force and rate of contraction of the rabbit isolated perfused heart. Mean ±s.e. is shown for each dose. Method of Brown and Lands (*76*).

TABLE 8.19

Effect of Modification of Isoproterenol Molecule on Cardiac Stimulation (Rabbit Isolated Perfused Heart)

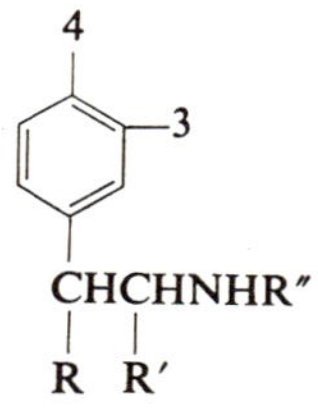

Compound	Structure					Cardiac stimulating dose,[a] μg/heart	
	4	3	R	R′	R″	Force	Rate
Isoproterenol	OH	OH	OH	H	$CH(CH_3)_2$	0.0025	0.003
Levarterenol	OH	OH	OH	H	H	0.029	0.029
Epinephrine	OH	OH	OH	H	CH_3	0.025	0.05
l-3	OH	OH	OH	H	C_2H_5	0.005	0.005
36	OH	OH	OH	H	$C(CH_3)_3$	0.027	0.032
37	OH	OH	OH	H	$CH(CH_3)CH_2CH_3$	0.0075	0.0056
42	OH	OH	OH	H	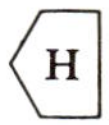	0.004	0.005
56	OH	OH	OH	CH_3	$CH(CH_3)_2$	0.120	8.000
59	OH	OH	OH	CH_3	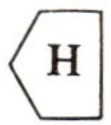	0.04	0.110
Ethylnorepinephrine	OH	OH	OH	C_2H_5	H	1.0	1.5
Isoetharine	OH	OH	OH	C_2H_5	$CH(CH_3)_2$	0.4	2.500

60	OH	OH	OH	C_2H_5	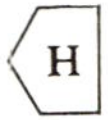	0.5–4.0	6.500
61	OH	OH	OH	C_2H_5	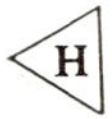	0.5–4.0[b]	8.000
57	OH	OH	OH	$(CH_3)_2$	$CH(CH_3)_2$	80.0	240.0
62	OH	OH	OH	C_3H_7	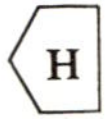	>400.0	>400.0
77	OH	H	OH	H	$CH(CH_3)_2$	0.4	0.4
80	OH	H	OH	H	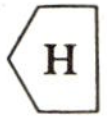	10.0	20.0
70	H	OH	OH	H	$CH(CH_3)_2$	0.3	2.1
94	H	OH	OH	H	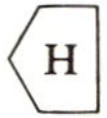	5.0	11.0
71	H	OH	OH	CH_3	$CH(CH_3)_2$	>200.0	>200.0
72	H	OH	OH	C_2H_5	$CH(CH_3)_2$	>200.0	>200.0
73	H	OH	OH	C_2H_5	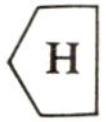	>200.0	>200.0
82	OH	H	OH	C_2H_5	$CH(CH_3)_2$	>200.0	>200.0
87	OH	H	OH	CH_3	$CH(CH_3)_2$	>200.0	>200.0
90	5-OH	OH	OH	H	$CH(CH_3)_2$	1/41 Iso.[c]	1/13 Iso.[c]
110	OH	OH	O	H	$CH(CH_3)_2$	>200.0	>200.0
13	H	H	OH	H	$CH(CH_3)_2$	30.0	20.0

[a] Dose required for an increase of 20%.
[b] Irregular response.
[c] Cat right auricle preparation, reported by Engelhardt et al. (*140*). ED_{20} for an increase in force, 1.30 ± 0.69 ng/ml; ED_{20} for change in rate, 1.10 ± 0.092 ng/ml.

isoproterenol and related amines in the rabbit isolated perfused heart. The response to the former is shown in Figure 1 and compared with norepinephrine. The threshold stimulating dose of norepinephrine is about 10 times greater than that of isoproterenol. With isoproterenol and many related amines a depressant action is noted at high dosage; this has been reported also by other investigators (*22*, *43*, *151*).

A structural modification of the basic phenethylamine nucleus causes important changes in the cardiac stimulating potency of the resultant molecules. Changes in the structure and position of the substituents on the ring or side chain markedly alter potency (Table 8.19). The substitution of a methyl or ethyl group at the α carbon causes a large reduction in effectiveness for force and rate. The chronotropic mechanism appears to be more sensitive to molecular structure than does the inotropic. The threshold stimulating doses for rate changes provide the following sequence: isoproterenol, 0.003 μg, and α-ethyl (isoetharine) and α-methyl (No. 56), 2.5 to 8.0 μg, with a poor dose–response relationship. For a change in force of contraction we find the following: isoproterenol, 0.0025 μg; α-methyl, 0.120 μg; and α-ethyl, 0.4 μg. A similar sequence is found with compounds in which the N substituent is cyclopentyl. Substitution at the α carbon of two methyl groups (No. 57) or a propyl group (No. 62) is not favorable to cardiac stimulation.

The number and position of the hydroxyl groups on the phenyl ring is important for cardiac stimulating action; the isoproterenol analogue in which the hydroxyls are in the 3,5 positions has a much lower potency (*140*). When there is only one hydroxyl on the ring in the 3 position (No. 70) or the 4 position (No. 77), the latter exerts the more chronotropic effect. The inotropic effects of the two compounds are quite similar (Table 8.19). The difference is seen also with the *N*-methylamines, phenylephrine, and synephrine (Table 8.9). The importance of the 4-hydroxy group for this action was recognized by Youmans et al. (*24*) in their 1940 evaluation of the effects of groups of the epinephrine molecule. Further, they stated that removal of the 4-hydroxyl group reduces the cardioaccelerator potency more than the reduction in pressor potency.

The isopropyl substituent on the amino group of isoproterenol can be changed considerably without a large loss of cardiac stimulating potency. Activity of a comparable order is found when the *N* substituent is ethyl (No. 3), *sec*-butyl (No. 37), or cyclopentyl (No. 42). Less potency is found with *t*-butyl (No. 36), methyl (epinephrine), and hydrogen (norepinephrine), as shown in Table 8.19.

A comparison of these data with the data of Tables 8.15 to 8.19 suggests that the optimal molecular structure for cardiac stimulation differs somewhat from that for vasodepressor action. Compound No. 36 equals or exceeds isoproterenol in its vasodepressor action but has less cardiac stimulating action; No. 42 is about one fourth as vasodepressive but three fifths as stimulant on the heart; Nos. 57 and 59 induce cardioaccelerator action at relatively larger doses than those needed for vasodepressor action. The differences in receptor affinity are also suggested by a comparison of the effects on rate and the effect on force of myocardial contraction. Other differences will be pointed out in the section that follows, in which bronchodilator action is described.

B. Action of Isoproterenol and Related Compounds on Smooth Muscle of Various Organs

1. BRONCHODILATOR ACTION

The existence of bronchodilator nerve fibers and their origin in the sympathetic division of the autonomic nervous system was demonstrated in the first decade of this century by the investigations of Prevost and Saloz (*152*),

TABLE 8.20

Effect of Structural Modification of the *N*-Alkyl Group of Isoproterenol on Bronchodilator Activity (Guinea Pig)

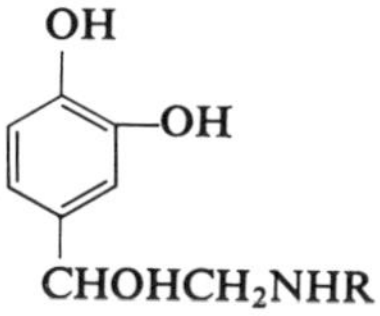

Compound	R	Relative bronchodilator activity	Ref.
Isoproterenol	$CH(CH_3)_2$	1000	
Norepinephrine	H		
dl		3–30	*46, 142, 143, 148*
l		6–10	*42, 44*
Epinephrine	CH_3	330–500	*44, 143, 144*
3	C_2H_5		
dl		250–300	*83, 143, 148*
l		1000	*116*
46	n-C_3H_7	40–170	*83, 143, 147, 148*
47	n-C_4H_9	50–100	*83, 143, 147*
94	n-C_5H_{11}	250	*83*
36	$C(CH_3)_3$	1500–2000	*83, 142–144, 148*
37	$CH(CH_3)CH_2CH_3$	300–1000	*80, 86, 148*
42	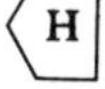	700	*42*
45	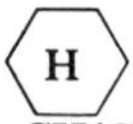	40–120	*83, 147*
95	$CH(CH_3)CH_2C(CH_3)_2CH_3$	20	*143*
96	$CH_2CH_2C_6H_5$	50–170	*143, 144, 147*
97	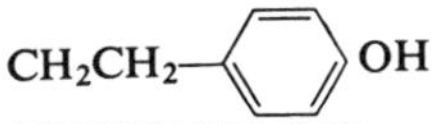	500	*143*
98	$CH(CH_3)CH_2C_6H_5$	1000	*143*

TABLE 8.20—*continued*

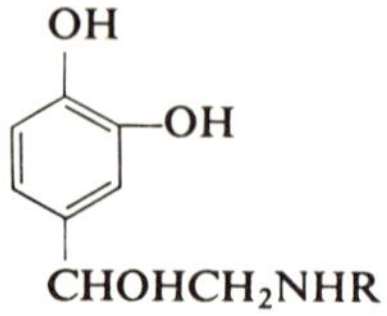

Compound	R	Relative bronchodilator activity	Ref.
99	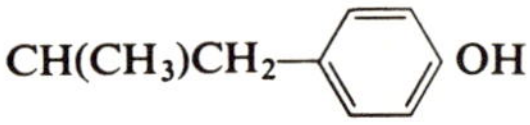	8000	*143*
100	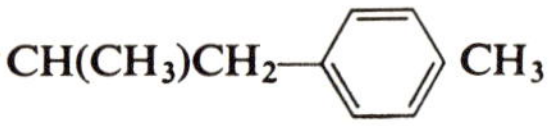	500	*143*
44	CH(CH$_3$)CH$_2$CH$_2$C$_6$H$_5$	1000	*143, 144*
102	CH$_2$CH$_2$CH$_2$C$_6$H$_5$	330–1000	*144, 147*
103	C(CH$_3$)$_2$CH$_2$C$_6$H$_5$	200–1000	*143, 147*
104	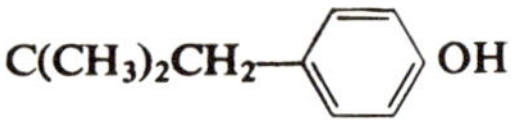	8000	*143*
105	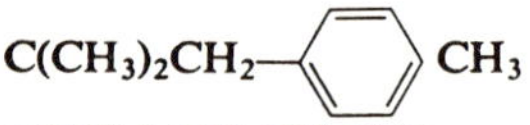	100	*143*
106	C(CH$_3$)$_2$CH$_2$CH$_2$C$_6$H$_5$	1000	*143*
107	C(C$_2$H$_5$)(CH$_3$)CH$_2$C$_6$H$_5$	30	*143*
108	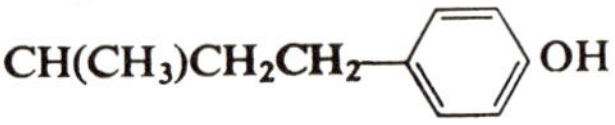	250	*143*
109	CH$_2$CH(CH$_3$)C$_6$H$_5$	10	*143*
Protokylol	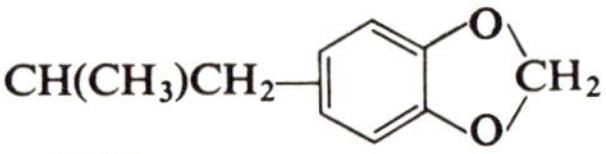	1000	*147*
111	*n*-C$_6$H$_{13}$	120	*147*
112	*n*-C$_7$H$_{15}$	100	*147*
113	*n*-C$_9$H$_{19}$	70	*147*
114	CH$_2$CH$_2$OH	100	*147*
115	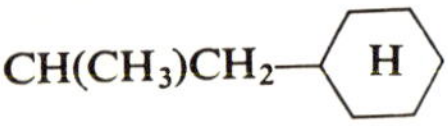	170	*147*
116	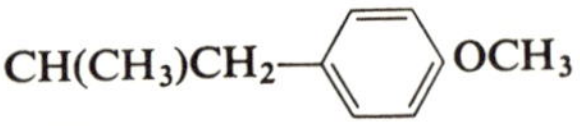	2000	*147*
117	CH(C$_2$H$_5$)CH$_2$C$_6$H$_5$	1000	*147*
43	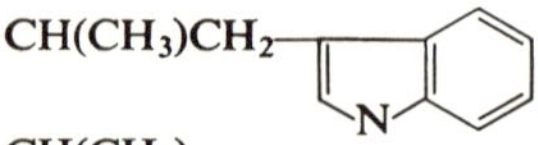	5000–10,000	*132*
90 (3,5-dihydroxy)	CH(CH$_3$)$_2$	27	*140*

Möllgaard (*153*), and Dixon and Ransom (*154*). Januschke and Pollak (*155*) and Dixon and Ransom (*154*) established a similarity between the action of epinephrine and the stimulation of these nerves. Trendelenburg (*156*) found that pilocarpine and epinephrine caused opposing actions in the smooth muscle of beef lungs, and Swanson and Webster (*157*) found similar effects in perfused rabbit, cat, and dog lungs.

TABLE 8.21

Effect of Structural Modification of the *N*-Alkyl Group of Isoproterenol on Protective Action in Guinea Pigs Exposed to a Histamine Aerosol

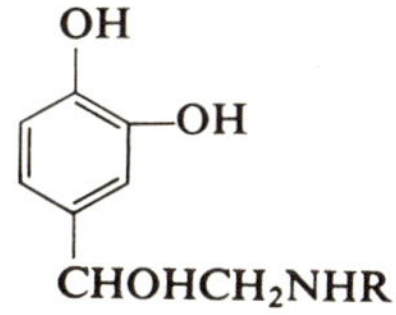

Compound	R	Relative protective action	Ref.
Isoproterenol	$CH(CH_3)_2$	1000	
Norepinephrine	H		
dl		350, 63	*121, 135*
l		125	*145*
Epinephrine	CH_3	500, 685, 124	*121, 145, 135*
3	C_2H_5	650, >250, <500, 1000	*121, 145, 135*
36	$C(CH_3)_3$	500–1000	*145*
37	$CH(CH_3)CH_2CH_3$	420, 500	*121, 145*
42	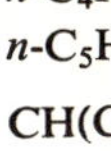	50–65	*146*
45		83	*146*
38	$CH_2CH(CH_3)_2$	<60, 23	*145, 146*
46	$n\text{-}C_3H_7$	100	*146*
47	$n\text{-}C_4H_9$	250, 400, 32	*135, 145, 146*
94	$n\text{-}C_5H_{11}$	100	*146*
43	$CH(CH_3)CH_2$ 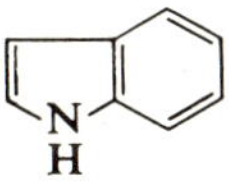	1000	*132*
Protokylol	$CH(CH_3)CH_2$– 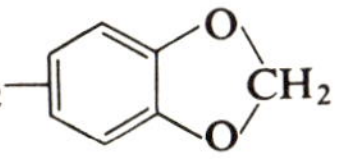	100	*132*
90 (3,5-dihydroxy)	$CH(CH_3)_2$	70	*140*

TABLE 8.22

Effect of Structural Modification of Side Chain of Various Isoproterenollike Compounds

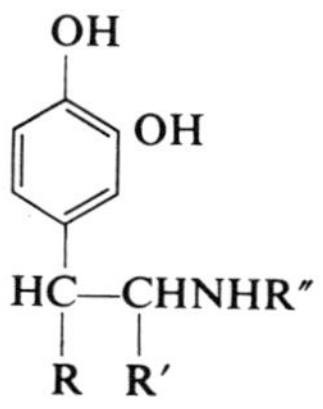

Compound	Structure			Relative bronchodilator activity	Ref.
	R	R′	R″		
Isoproterenol	OH	H	$CH(CH_3)_2$	1000	
59	OH	CH_3	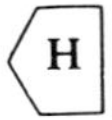	330	*42*
60	OH	C_2H_5	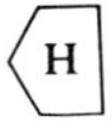	450	*42*
Ethylnorepinephrine	OH	C_2H_5	H	5	*48*
118	OH	C_2H_5	$CH_2CH_2C_6H_5$	60–85	*147*
119	OH	C_2H_5	$CH_2CH_2CH_2C_6H_5$	330–500	*147*
120	OH	C_2H_5	$CH(CH_3)CH_2$— 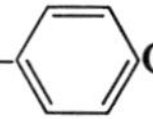 OCH_3	65–100	*147*
120a[a]	OH	C_2H_5	$CH(CH_3)CH_2CH_2C_6H_5$	17	*144*

121[a]	OH	CH_3	$CH_2CH_2CH_2C_6H_5$	250	*144*
52	O	H	$CH(CH_3)_2$	<0.5[b]	*143*
122	O	H	n-C_4H_9		*143*
123	O	H	$C(CH_3)_2CH_3$	<0.5	*143*
124	O	H	$CH_2CH_2C_6H_5$	<0.5	*143*
125	O	H	$CH(CH_3)CH_2C_6H_5$	<0.5	*143*
126	O	H	$CH(CH_3)CH_2$— 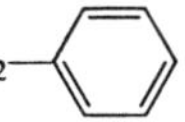 OH	<1	*143*
127	O	H	$CH(CH_3)CH_2$— 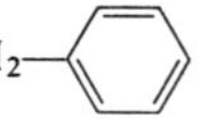 CH_3	<1	*143*
128	O	H	$CH(CH_3)CH_2CH_2$— 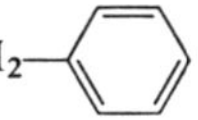 CH_3	<0.2	*143*
129	O	H	$C(CH_3)_2CH_2C_6H_5$	<0.5	*143*
130	O	H	$C(CH_3)_3$	Weak	*80*
151[a]	OH	H	$CH(CH_3)CH_2CH_2C_6H_5$	1000	*144*
152[a]	O	H	$CH(CH_3)CH_2CH_2C_6H_5$	<5	*144*
153[a]	OH	CH_3	$CH(CH_3)CH_2CH_2C_6H_5$	60	*144*
154[a]	O	CH_3	$CH(CH_3)CH_2CH_2C_6H_5$	7	*144*
55	H	H	$CH(CH_3)_2$	5	*86*
56	OH	CH_3	$CH(CH_3)_2$	330	*80*
57	OH	$(CH_3)_2$	$CH(CH_3)_2$	0.8	*80*
Isoetharine	OH	C_2H_5	$CH(CH_3)_2$	330	*42*
83	OH	$CH(CH_3)_2$	$CH(CH_3)_2$	Weak	*80*
Nordefrine	OH	CH_3	H	10	*44*

[a] Dog; method of Konzett and Rössler (*160*).
[b] Langecker and Friebel (*135*) reported less than 1% potency with the aerosol technique.

Bronchodilator action of epinephrine and other sympathomimetic amines has been described and compared in some detail by Tainter and associates (*48*, *158*). They reported a greater potency for epinephrine than for the corresponding primary amine, norepinephrine, and considerably more potency than for the analogue without the β-hydroxyl group (Epinine). Konzett (*32*) examined several *N*-alkylarterenols and found that the *N*-isopropyl compound was 10 times better as a bronchodilator than epinephrine. The *N*-ethyl analogue was found to be 3 times more active than epinephrine, and the *N*-propyl and *N*-butyl analogues were about equal to it. These observations were confirmed and extended by Lands and associates (*33*, *34*, *86*) and by Marsh and Herring (*91*).

Subsequent synthetic research has provided many modifications of the skeletal phenethylamine that showed important bronchodilator action. The effects of some modifications of the N substituent are shown in Tables 8.20 and 8.21. An examination of these data provides support for the generalization of Lands et al. (*33*), that the greatest bronchodilator potency is obtained when the structure of the *N*-alkyl substituent is —$CH(CH_3)R$. The R group need not be CH_3 as in isoproterenol. Significantly greater potency is obtained with compounds in which this group is aralkyl; the greatest potency was reported for *p*-hydroxybenzyl (No. 99) and 3-indolylmethylene (No. 43), the bronchodilator action being 8 to 10 times greater than that of isoproterenol. The corresponding unbranched chain (No. 97) or a chain branched by means of methyl substitution at another carbon (Nos. 109 and 98) is not favorable to this action. Unbranched normal alkyl substitution does not provide effective bronchodilator compounds (Nos. 46, 47, 94, 111, 112, and 113).

The effect of side-chain modification of catecholethylamine is shown in Tables 8.22 and 8.23. Replacement of the OH at the β carbon with H or O results in compounds with little or no bronchodilator action. Substitution at the α carbon for a CH_3 or C_2H_5 group reduces the potency from that of the corresponding unsubstituted compound (No. 56, isoetharine, and Nos. 118 and 120). The hydroxyl at the β carbon appears to be essential to effective bronchodilator action.

Hydroxyl substitution at the phenyl ring influences bronchodilator action importantly. The removal of either hydroxyl provides compounds with little or no bronchodilator action (Table 8.24). This is particularly apparent in a comparison of isoproterenol with Nos. 70 and 77, of No. 151 with Nos. 140 and 147, and of No. 120a with No. 150.

These data indicate that the structural requirements for bronchodilator action are quite as specific as those for cardiac stimulation or effect on blood pressure. There is some agreement between bronchodilator and vasodepressor actions (*262*). There is apparent agreement in a comparison of Nos. 36, 37, and 43; vasodepressor action appears to be somewhat less than broncho-

TABLE 8.23

Effect of Structural Modification of Isoproterenol Molecule on Protective Action in Guinea Pigs Exposed to a Histamine Aerosol

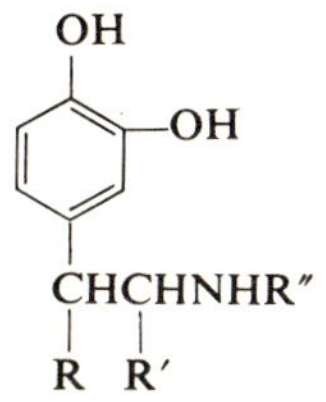

Compound	Structure: R	Structure: R′	Structure: R″	Relative bronchodilator activity[a]	Ref.
131	OH	CH_3	$CH_2CH_2OCH_3$	125	*135*
52	O	H	$CH(CH_3)_2$	0	*135*
54	O	H	$CH_2CH_2CH_2$— 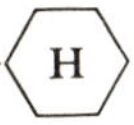	0	*135*
132	O	H	C_2H_5	0	*135*
133	O	CH_3	$CH(CH_3)_2$	30	*135*
134	O	CH_3	$CH_2CH_2OCH_3$	62	*135*
135	O	C_2H_5	$CH(CH_3)_2$	0	*135*
136	O	H	$C(CH_3)_3$	0	*80*
56	OH	CH_3	$CH(CH_3)_2$	250	*80*
61	OH	C_2H_5	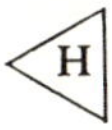	200	*80*
59	OH	CH_3	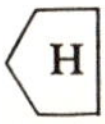	140	*80*
Isoetharine	OH	C_2H_5	$CH(CH_3)_2$	500	*46*
60	OH	C_2H_5	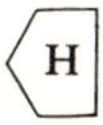	200	*46*
57	OH	$(CH_3)_2$	$CH(CH_3)_2$	0	*80*

[a] Isoproterenol, 1,000.

dilator action when some *N*-alkyl groups are used (Nos. 42 and 44 and protokylol), and there is less agreement with the molecular modifications illustrated by Nos. 59, 60, and 61 and isoetharine. The requirements for effective cardiac stimulation differ somewhat from the requirements of these parameters. Epinephrine and norepinephrine have comparable cardiac stimulating potency, but the latter is a weak bronchodilator agent (cf. Table 8.3). This is illustrated further by results obtained with nordefrine, a potent cardiac

TABLE 8.24

Effect on Bronchodilator Activity of Modifying Substituents on Phenyl Ring of Various Isoproterenollike Compounds

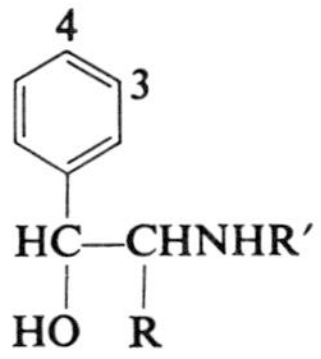

Compound	Structure: 4	Structure: 3	Structure: R	Structure: R′	Relative bronchodilator activity	Ref.
Isoproterenol	OH	OH	H	$CH(CH_3)_2$	1000	
70	H	OH	H	$CH(CH_3)_2$	12	*83*
77	OH	H	H	$CH(CH_3)_2$	Weak	*33*
80	OH	H	H	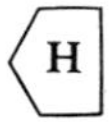	2	*80*
73	H	OH	C_2H_5	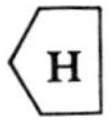	1	*83*

82	OH	H	C_2H_5	$CH(CH_3)_2$	4	*80*
83	H	H	H	$CH(CH_3)_2$	<2	*33*
137[a]	H	OH	CH_3	$CH(CH_3)_2$	0	*144*
138[a]	H	OH	CH_3	$CH_2C_6H_5$	0[b]	*144*
139[a]	H	OH	CH_3	$CH(CH_3)C_6H_5$	0	*144*
140[a]	H	OH	CH_3	$CH(CH_3)CH_2CH_2C_6H_5$	10	*144*
141	OH	H	CH_3	$CH(CH_3)_2$	0[b]	*144*
142	OH	H	CH_3	$CH_2C_6H_5$	0[b]	*144*
143	OH	H	CH_3	$CH(CH_3)C_6H_5$	0[b]	*144*
144	OH	H	CH_3	$CH_2CH_2C_6H_5$	<5	*144*
145	OH	H	CH_3	$CH(CH_3)CH_2C_6H_5$	<5	*144*
146	OH	H	CH_3	$CH_2CH_2CH_2C_6H_5$	<5	*144*
147	OH	H	CH_3	$CH(CH_3)CH_2CH_2C_6H_5$	60	*144*
148	OH	H	CH_3	$CH(CH_3)CH_2CH_2CH_2C_6H_5$	<5	*144*
149	OH	H	CH_3	$CH(CH_3)CH_2CH_2$— 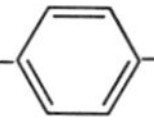 —OCH_3	<5	*144*
150	OH	H	C_2H_5	$CH(CH_3)CH_2CH_2C_6H_5$	7	*144*
Isoprophenamine	2-Cl		H	$CH(CH_3)_2$	Weak	*256*
Isoxsuprine	OH	H	CH_3	$CH(CH_3)CH_2OC_6H_5$	6–20	*257*

[a] Dog; method of Konzett and Rössler (*160*).
[b] Bronchoconstriction.

stimulating agent with weak bronchodilator action (*42*, *71*). Effective bronchodilator drugs may produce little direct cardiac stimulation (isoetharine and Nos. 56, 59, 60, and 61) or may be effective on all three systems (isoproterenol, epinephrine, and Nos. 3, 36, 37, and 42).

2. ACTION ON THE SMOOTH MUSCLE OF OTHER ORGANS

We have discussed the effects of norepinephrine and related compounds on the smooth muscle of various organs (cf. Table 8.13) and shall now discuss the effects of other compounds on the uterus; see Table 8.25. This organ is relaxed most effectively by isoproterenol and the *N*-ethyl analogue (No. 3). Epinephrine may be somewhat less potent than isoproterenol but more effective than phenylephrine, Kephrine, or dopamine. Little effect is noted in the absence of the alcoholic hydroxyl at the β carbon (Nos. 52 and 55, dopamine, Epinine, Kephrine). Replacement of hydrogen by a methyl or ethyl group at the α carbon reduces the uterine effect (Tables 8.13 and 8.25). The data obtained with the cat uterus are rather incomplete, but the results appear to support these generalizations. The nongravid rabbit uterus may contract or relax when exposed to sympathomimetic amines. The relaxing action, however, is greatest with those compounds most effective in relaxing the rat and cat uteri.

Experimentation with the small intestine, both isolated and in situ, have provided such discrepant results that any generalization is difficult. This is particularly notable with the data provided by McDougal and West (*166*) and Schmidt and Fleming (*167*). The peristaltic reflex preparation in the guinea pig, as used by McDougal and West, possibly involves receptor systems different from those involved in the pendular activity of the isolated intestinal segments. Isoproterenol appears to be less potent than epinephrine or norepinephrine in the hands of most investigators (Table 8.26). The *N*-ethyl analogue (No. 3) is somewhat more potent, and the indolylalkyl-substituted compound (No. 43) much more potent, than isoproterenol. A hydroxyl substitution at the β carbon of the side chain is necessary for important relaxing action. Epinine, Kephrine, dopamine, No. 52, and No. 55 have only weak inhibitory action on the uterus. Substitution of a methyl or ethyl group for one of the hydrogens at the α carbon of the side chain does not favor this action (isoetharine, ethylnorepinephrine, No. 60). The relaxing activity is diminished by the absence of either of the ring hydroxyls. There is some evidence that the 3-hydroxy position is more important than the 4 position for inhibitory action (*23*).

The stimulating action of various amines on the nictitating membrane is shown in Table 8.12. *N*-Ethylarterenol (No. 3) has 1/20 to 1/45 the potency of epinephrine, whereas isoproterenol, *N*-butyl, and *N*-propylarterenol are not

TABLE 8.25

Action of Isoproterenol and Related Compounds on Uterus

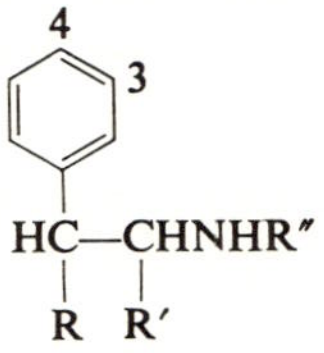

Compound	Structure 4	3	R	R′	R″	Relative effectiveness[a] Rabbit	Rat	Cat
Isoproterenol[d]	OH	OH	OH	H	$CH(CH_3)_2$	1000	1000	1000
55	OH	OH	H	H	$CH(CH_3)_2$	Weak/0 (*84*)	20 (*162*)	<1 (*161*)
52	OH	OH	O	H	$CH(CH_3)_2$	0 (*84*)		
3[d]	OH	OH	OH	H	C_2H_5	C (*84*)	500–1000 (*163*)	
Epinephrine[d]	OH	OH	OH	H	CH_3	C (*84*)	1000 (*163*)	100 (*172*)[b]
							200 (*162*)	10 (*165*)
Norepinephrine	OH	OH	OH	H	H	C	20 (*162*)	<10–10 (*172*)
							3–13 (*163*)	
Epinine	OH	OH	H	H	CH_3	C (*84*)	10 (*162*)	
							80 (*163*)	
Kephrine	OH	OH	O	H	CH_3	C (*84*)	100 (*162*)	
							40 (*163*)	
36	OH	OH	OH	H	$C(CH_3)_3$	250 (*84*)		1400 (*131*)
37	OH	OH	OH	H	$CH(CH_3)CH_2CH_3$	500 (*84*)		400 (*131*)
47	OH	OH	OH	H	n-C_4H_9	25 (*84*)		
Isoetharine	OH	OH	OH	C_2H_5	$CH(CH_3)_2$		5 (*116*)	
Ethylnorepinephrine	OH	OH	OH	C_2H_5	H		34 (*116*)	
							20 (*163*)	

TABLE 8.25—*continued*

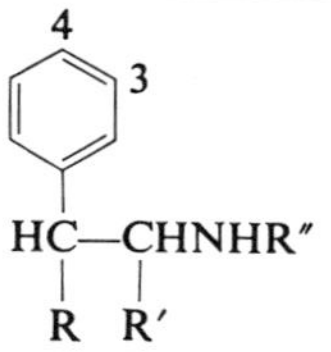

Compound	4	3	R	R′	R″	Rabbit	Rat	Cat
	Structure					Relative effectiveness[a]		
Nordefrine	OH	OH	OH	CH_3	H		13 (*47*)[c]	
							100 (*163*)	
Dopamine	OH	OH	H	H	H	< 1	110 (*109*)	
							< 1 (*163*)	
Phenylephrine	H	OH	OH	H	CH_3	200 (*106*)	100 (*164*)	
Synephrine	OH	H	OH	H	CH_3			10 (*164*)
14	OH	H	OH	H	H	40–100 (*106*)	< 1 (*116*)	
70	H	OH	OH	H	$CH(CH_3)_2$	< 1 (*78*)	20 (*80*)	
77	OH	H	OH	H	$CH(CH_3)_2$	< 1 (*33*)	Weak (*33*)	
72	H	OH	OH	C_2H_5	$CH(CH_3)_2$		< 1 (*80*)	
73	H	OH	OH	C_2H_5	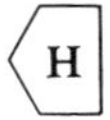		< 1 (*80*)	
Isoxsuprine	OH	H	OH	CH_3	$CH(CH_3)CH_2$—O— 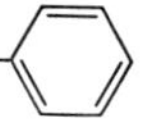		5 (*257*)	

[a] Numbers in parentheses indicate references: C, contraction. Oxytocin-induced milk ejection in New Zealand white lactating rabbits is inhibited by isoproterenol > epinephrine > norepinephrine > phenylephrine > dextroamphetamine > ephedrine. This effect is not influenced by α-(phenoxybenzamine) or β-(pronethalol) blockade (*107*).

[b] Estrogen–progesterone treatment favors stimulation with epinephrine > *l*-norepinephrine > isoproterenol (1/1000 epinephrine).

[c] *l*-Nordefrine reported to cause relaxation at 1/15 concentration of epinephrine.

[d] Epinephrine is the *l*-isomer. Others shown are racemic mixtures.

TABLE 8.26

Action of Isoproterenol and Related Compounds on Small Intestine

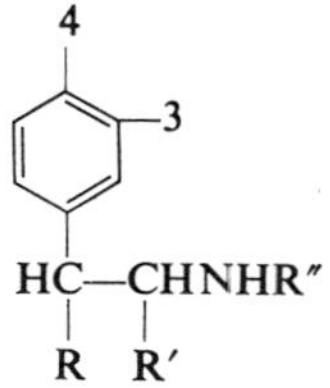

Compound	Structure					Relative effectiveness[a]		
	4	3	R	R′	R″	Rabbit	Guinea pig	Dog
Isoproterenol	OH	OH	OH	H	$CH(CH_3)_2$	1/20 epi.[b] (*166*) < epi. (*32*) 5 × epi. (*167*)	1/200 epi. (*166*) 1/1 epi. (*162*)	1/1 epi. (*46*) < epi. (*168*)
55	OH	OH	H	H	$CH(CH_3)_2$		1/100 epi. (*86*, *162*)	
52	OH	OH	O	H	$CH(CH_3)_2$		Weak (*86*)	
3	OH	OH	OH	H	C_2H_5	1/10 epi. (*166*)	1/20 epi. (*166*)	
43	OH	OH	OH	H	$CH(CH_3)CH_2$– 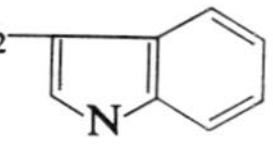	25 × iso. (*167*)	10 × epi. (*132*)	
Epinephrine	OH	OH	OH	H	CH_3	> iso. (*32*, *166*)	200 × iso. (*166*)	
Norepinephrine	OH	OH	OH	H	H	1/2 epi. (*166*) 1/1 epi. (*69*)	1/4 epi. (*166*) 1/2 epi. (*162*) ≥ epi. (*69*)	1/1 epi. (*46*, *168*) 1/3 epi. (*23*)
Epinine	OH	OH	H	H	CH_3	1/25 epi. (*166*) 1/20 iso. (*167*)	1/17 epi. (*166*) 1/16 iso. (*162*)	1/10 to 1/25 epi. (*23*)
Kephrine	OH	OH	O	H	CH_3	1/40 epi. (*166*) Weak (*167*)	1/28 epi. (*166*)	
36	OH	OH	OH	H	$C(CH_3)_3$		1/40 iso. (*86*)	

TABLE 8.26—*continued*

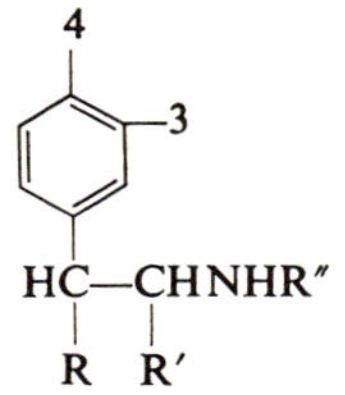

Compound	Structure: 4	3	R	R′	R″	Relative effectiveness[a]: Rabbit	Guinea pig	Dog
37	OH	OH	OH	H	$CH(CH_3)CH_2CH_3$		1/5 iso. (*86*)	
47	OH	OH	OH	H	C_4H_9	< iso. (*32*)	1/40 iso. (*86*)	
Isoetharine	OH	OH	OH	C_2H_5	$CH(CH_3)_2$		1/1000 iso. (*46*)	1/5 iso. (*46*)
60	OH	OH	OH	C_2H_5	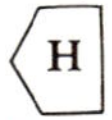		< 1/1000 iso. (*46*)	1/10 iso. (*46*)
Ethylnorepinephrine	OH	OH	OH	C_2H_5	H	1/100 epi. (*166*)	1/86 epi. (*166*)	Weak (*46*)
Nordefrine	OH	OH	OH	CH_3	H	1/10 epi. (*166*)	1/10 epi. (*166*)	1/6 epi. (*23*)
Dopamine	OH	OH	H	H	H	1/200 epi. (*166*)	1/250 epi. (*166*)	
Phenylephrine	H	OH	OH	H	CH_3	1/4 iso. (*167*)	1/5000 epi. (*166*)	1/25 to 1/100 epi. (*23*)
70	H	OH	OH	H	$CH(CH_3)_2$		< 1/500 iso. (*35*)	
Synephrine	OH	H	OH	H	CH_3		1/6000 epi. (*166*)	1/660 to 1/2500 epi. (*23*)
14	OH	H	OH	H	H	Weak (*91*)	1/7500 epi. (*166*)	
77	OH	H	OH	H	$CH(CH_3)_2$	Weak (*91*)	1/200 iso. (*35*)	
Phenylpropanolamine	H	H	OH	CH_3	H		1/3000 epi. (*166*)	
Isoxsuprine	OH	H	OH	CH_3	$CH(CH_3)CH_2O$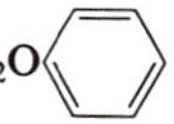	1/330 iso. (*257*)		

[a] Numbers in parentheses indicate references.
[b] Inhibition of peristaltic reflex (*166*).

stimulating (*32, 163*). Gaddum et al. (*163*) reported relaxation with isoproterenol.

The retractor penis preparation in the dog is contracted by epinephrine more powerfully than by the *N*-ethyl and *N*-propyl analogues and norepinephrine (*1*). Nordefrine, the α-methyl analogue of norepinephrine, is less effective than epinephrine, and this difference is noted also when equal pressor doses are administered intravenously (*47*). The stimulating potency is approximately that of norepinephrine, which has been reported to be 1/4 to 1/5 that of epinephrine (*69*). The cocaine-stimulated retractor is relaxed by isoproterenol and isoetharine, the former being about 10 times more effective than the latter. Too few data are available to permit a structure–activity analysis. Contraction is induced by epinephrine, and those modifications which reduce excitatory effects on smooth muscle of other organs also reduce the effects here. Isoproterenol induces relaxation, and this effect is diminished by side-chain modification, which reduces inhibitory action in other organs.

An analysis of the action of some sympathomimetic amines on the iris has been provided by Bennett et al. (*170*). Intraocular injection into albino rabbits produced an equal degree and duration of mydriasis, when compared on a molar basis, in the ratio of epinephrine to levarterenol to *l*-isoproterenol of 1:2.75:55. Bennett et al. reported further that the *d* isomers of epinephrine and norepinephrine were approximately as potent as *l*-isoproterenol. These investigators found only α-type receptors in this organ.

The rat vas deferens preparation responds to epinephrine by contraction. Luduena (*116*) has compared the potency of a few amines in this organ and found the sequence epinephrine > norepinephrine = phenylephrine > dopamine > Epinine. Similar results have been reported by Van Rossum (*254*). This pattern of response suggests an α-type receptor. Ariëns et al. (*171*) found the order epinephrine and norepinephrine > *N*-ethylarterenol > isoproterenol, which also suggests an α-type receptor.

Sympathetic innervation is not essential for adrenergic inhibitory action. Evans and Schild (*173*) have reported that both epinephrine and isoproterenol cause a relaxation of smooth muscle in the chick amniotic membrane, the latter being the more potent. Similar findings regarding the human placental vascular bed, as previously described, were reported by Ciuchita and Gautieri (*174*).

8.4. EFFECTS OF VARIOUS SYMPATHOMIMETIC AMINES ON VOLUNTARY MUSCLE

Epinephrine has been shown to increase the maximal twitch tension of skeletal muscle in various mammalian species (reviewed *175*). This action is shared by isoproterenol and other amines. Results obtained by Bowman et al. (*176–179*) are summarized in Table 8.27. These investigators have

TABLE 8.27

Effect of Various Sympathomimetic Amines on Twitch Tension of Voluntary Muscle

	Effect on twitch tension[a]		
Compound	Rat diaphragm,[b] μg/ml	Cat tibialis anterior,[c] μg/kg	Cat soleus,[c] μg/kg
Isoproterenol	2–10[d]	+, 2–8 (*176*) +, <3–5 (*177*)	−, 0.06–0.4 (*176*) −, <0.05 (*177*)
l-Norepinephrine	80–400[d]	+, 5–15 (*176*)	−, 5–20 (*176*)
d-Norepinephrine	10–20		
l-Epinephrine	3–10[d]	+, 3–10 (*176*) +, 3–5 (*177*)	−, 0.06–0.5 (*176*) −, 0.05 (*177*)
d-Epinephrine	10–20		
N-Ethylarterenol (No. 3)	200–400[d]		
Dopamine	2–4		
N-Isopropyldopamine (No. 55)	0.4–2		
Tyramine	40–200		
Ephedrine	10–30		
Methoxamine	Blocks		
N-Isopropylmethoxamine	Blocks		

[a] Numbers in parentheses indicate references.

[b] Phrenic nerve and hemidiaphragm preparation partially depressed by KCl. Concentration (base) required to produce 100% potentiation (*178*).

[c] Effect on maximal twitch tension: +, increase; −, decrease. See also Bowman and Raper (*179*). Paterson (*180*) reported *l*-isoproterenol 8 times more effective than the *d* isomer on the rat diaphragm.

[d] In nanograms per milliliter.

described two specific actions of epinephrine, an anticurare action, which is demonstrable with both the tibialis anterior and soleus muscles and which can be prevented by α-blocking agents, and an effect on twitch tension, which is prevented by β-blocking agents. The latter effect may involve a site of action at some stage after membrane depolarization in the series of events leading to contraction. Evidence is presented that an increase in the intracellular hexose-phosphate levels is involved. Isoproterenol does not possess anticurare action but is slightly more active than epinephrine on the muscle fibers themselves. As in the case of effects on involuntary muscle, the molecular structure of the amine is important for this action. The *l* isomer is more active than its corresponding *d* form, dopamine is less potent than norepinephrine, and isoproterenol is clearly more potent than *N*-isopropyldopamine (No. 55, Table 8.27). The results are similar to those obtained by Paterson (*180*). The rat denervated diaphragm responds to epinephrine with a transient contracture, which may be prevented by treatment with phenoxybenzamine and piperoxan. Drugs that block β receptors are less effective. Contracture induction is obtained with epinephrine = levarterenol > *d*-epinephrine = Epinine (1/10 epinephrine) > isoproterenol (almost inactive). Twitch potentiation with the potassium-depressed preparation confirms the results obtained by other investigators.

8.5. ACUTE TOXICITY OF SELECTED SYMPATHOMIMETIC AMINES

Acute intravenous toxicity of epinephrine and norepinephrine differs with the species of animal used (*181*), and this is particularly noted in comparisons

TABLE 8.28

Acute Toxicity in Mice of Several Sympathomimetic Amines

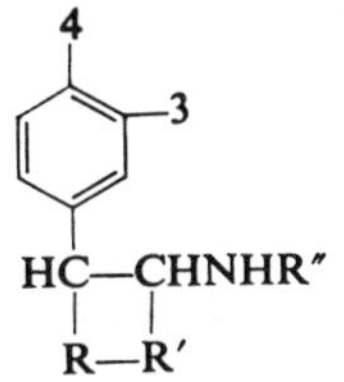

Compound	Structure					Acute toxicity, intravenous, $LD_{50} \pm$ s.e., mg/kg[a]
	4	3	R	R′	R″	
l-Norepinephrine	OH	OH	OH	H	H	5.0 ± 1.0
dl						7.5 ± 2.0
d						60.0 ± 20.0
Epinephrine	OH	OH	OH	H	CH_3	2.7 ± 0.2
d						50.0 ± 9.0
l-Nordefrine	OH	OH	OH	CH_3	H	12.6 ± 2.7
Dopamine	OH	OH	H	H	H	128.0 ± 21.0
17	H	OH	OH	H	H	90.4 ± 10.5
Phenylephrine	H	OH	OH	H	CH_3	19.0 ± 7.0
14	OH	H	OH	H	H	61.5 ± 1.3
Synephrine	OH	H	OH	H	CH_3	220.0 ± 9.7
Tyramine	OH	H	H	H	H	235.0 ± 17.8
Isoproterenol	OH	OH	OH	H	$CH(CH_3)_2$	61.7 ± 2.2
l						57.0 ± 2.0
d						100.0 ± 7.0
N-Ethylarterenol (No. 3)	OH	OH	OH	H	C_2H_5	12.6 ± 0.8
Isoetharine	OH	OH	OH	C_2H_5	$CH(CH_3)_2$	50.0 ± 4.0
60	OH	OH	OH	C_2H_5	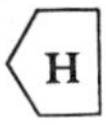	71.0 ± 5.8
Ethylnorepinephrine	OH	OH	OH	C_2H_5	H	78.5 ± 0.7
70	H	OH	OH	H	$CH(CH_3)_2$	104.0 ± 6.4
77	OH	H	OH	H	$CH(CH_3)_2$	121.0 ± 8.4

[a] Values expressed in terms of the base.

of the effects in the mouse and rat, the latter being much the more susceptible. The investigations of Nickerson et al. (*182*) and Luduena et al. (*183*) indicate that vasopressor action is an important etiological factor; this is supported by the observation that vasodepressor sympathomimetic amines have relatively little toxicity (*86*, *122*). Protection against the toxicity arising from pressor action could be obtained by blockade of α receptors. This has been demonstrated (*182*, *183*) with compounds including isoproterenol in large doses (*45*).

The acute toxicities (24 hours) of several compounds in mice, obtained in our laboratory, are shown in Table 8.28. The results are like those of others and suggest that differences among the most toxic compounds reflect their effectiveness on the vascular α-receptor system. Arranged in order of decreasing toxicity, we find epinephrine > norepinephrine > *l*-nordefrine = *N*-ethylarterenol > phenylephrine > norphenylephrine (No. 17) > dopamine. Isoproterenol and other vasodepressor compounds are not very toxic in mice. Their LD_{50} values are about the same as those of the *d* isomers of epinephrine and norepinephrine, compounds with little vasopressor action.

8.6. METABOLIC EFFECTS OF SYMPATHOMIMETIC AMINES

In the introductory portion of this chapter we reviewed the early studies of Barger and Dale (*1*) on the structure–activity concepts of the adrenergic amines. It was pointed out that many of the original ideas of Dale concerning the adrenergic receptor are still tenable today. In an early study Barcroft and Dixon (*184*) made equally tenable comments concerning the effects of epinephrine on the isolated and metabolically supported dog heart. They demonstrated increases in heart rate, contractile force, and myocardial oxygen consumption following epinephrine administration. Evans and Ogawa (*185*) demonstrated that increases in myocardial oxygen consumption following administration of epinephrine were approximately proportional to increases in heart rate, and Patterson and Starling (*186*) showed that the increase was partially dependent on arterial glucose concentration and was associated with depletion of myocardial glycogen, unless glucose was administered with the epinephrine. Some years later Bogue et al. (*187*) presented additional evidence that in the isolated heart, which was stimulated by either epinephrine or increased work loads, the utilization of both glucose and lactate was increased. This observation was followed by that of Braun-Menendez et al. (*189*), who reported that epinephrine stimulation did not affect the utilization of pyruvate. Prior to these two studies, Visscher and Mulder (*190*) had reported that increased work loads in the heart-lung preparation resulted in no change in myocardial glycogen content when the arterial glucose concentrations were maintained.

Since these early studies many tissues have been shown to exhibit alterations in metabolism after exposure to catecholamines, especially an increased glycogenolysis in liver and skeletal muscle. The number of such studies has been growing fast and appears to have a direct relationship to the availability of sophisticated biochemical techniques and procedures. In many respects the biochemist has moved ahead of the pharmacologist in providing biochemical and metabolic insight into the reactions involved in the control of glycogen breakdown as it is related to the actions of epinephrine and related amines. With this massive growth of biochemical and pharmacological literature have come many interesting and comprehensive reviews. It does not seem appropriate here to list all aspects of the metabolic and biochemical history of the adrenergic amines, and the reader is referred to the reviews (*7*, *159*, *169*, *175*, *191–194*). It is of interest, though, to point out that a casual review of the studies demonstrates a singular lack of uniformity in animal species or in biochemical and pharmacological techniques. Many of the variations or inconsistencies in results may be attributable to this multiplicity of experimental procedures. We shall attempt to draw some general conclusions concerning the structure–activity relationships of the metabolic actions of the adrenergic stimulants and to point out those areas of study which seem to us most promising.

There is general agreement that when epinephrine is given intravenously to man and animals the blood glucose concentration increases owing to hepatic glycogenolysis. Recent studies have shown that in the control of glycogen breakdown an early biochemical result of the interaction of epinephrine and the receptor is the formation of adenosine-3′,5′-phosphate (commonly referred to as cyclic 3′,5′-AMP and called here cyclic AMP). The effect of catecholamines on the formation of cyclic AMP in various tissues has been studied in some detail. Of particular interest are the studies of the nucleotide formation in heart preparations because of the possibility that the effect of catecholamines in stimulating cyclic AMP is associated with their inotropic effects. Since the studies have been extensively reviewed by Sutherland and Rall (*192*) and Haugaard and Hess (*258*), our purpose here will be to provide only a summary.

It is generally agreed, because of demonstrations in a number of tissues, including the dog heart (*195*), that cyclic AMP promotes the accumulation of active phosphorylase from inactive phosphorylase. The exact mechanism of this action of the nucleotide on the activation of phosphorylase is not known. Cyclic AMP may have further properties. One of the secondary actions is the formation of ketone bodies from acetate (*196*). Epinephrine and glucagon also cause an increase in lactone bodies (*197*), and because of this and other actions Sutherland and Rall (*192*) feel that the action of cyclic AMP on ketone body formation is of considerable interest, since it may represent an action of the nucleotide other than that leading to glycogenolysis. Epinephrine has been shown to increase glucose utilization in the fat pad (*198*) and in rat diaphragm

(*199*) under certain conditions. Although such changes in glucose utilization may be unrelated to cyclic AMP action, it is possible that the nucleotide plays a role in glucose utilization, because the adrenergic amines are able to stimulate its formation in the tissues. Finally, the ability of many diverse tissues to form cyclic AMP is an important consideration, since many cases of hormonal control have not been demonstrated and it is not clear whether changes in glycogenolysis are involved in the control mechanisms of all cells.

The original studies of Cori in the 1940's that led to the crystallization of phosphorylase were carried out with skeletal muscle. In the middle 1950's Cori (*200*) reinvestigated the results of his earlier studies of phosphorylase activity. He reported that phosphorylase *a*, the active form, is relatively low during rest and increases rapidly during contraction. Epinephrine, when injected into rats, increases markedly the phosphorylase *a* content of skeletal muscle, and the increase occurred within one minute after intravenous administration. Subcutaneous administration, on the other hand, caused a sustained increase in the phosphorylase *a* content of muscle. Epinephrine also caused an increase in the phosphorylase *a* content of isolated frog muscle (*201*). Owing to these investigations the following occurrences are generally acknowledged. Resting skeletal muscle contains inactive phosphorylase *b*, and upon stimulation the active phosphorylase *a* content rises rapidly. The active phosphorylase *a* of skeletal muscle decreases with prolonged stimulation, resulting in fatigue. The addition of epinephrine to muscle in vitro and in vivo produces an increase in phosphorylase *a*.

Recent studies from the laboratory of Cori (*202*) have reported that during a short tetanus applied to frog sartorius muscle the rate of glycogenolysis increased several hundred times and on relaxation returned to the resting rate. These changes in rate parallel a similar rise and fall in phosphorylase *a* content. It is postulated that glycogenolysis is actually regulated by the phosphorylase *b* kinase system, which is rapidly activated and deactivated during and after contraction. There is a much slower rise and fall in phosphorylase *a* during and after epinephrine administration. Furthermore, epinephrine and norepinephrine action on the contraction of muscle and the formation of phosphorylase *a* is inhibited by DCI, although DCI has no effect on the increase in phosphorylase *a* produced by muscle work. Thus it appears that two different mechanisms are involved in the activation.

Recently Morgan and Parmeggiani (*203*, *204*) reported that muscle phosphorylase activity appears to be regulated by a number of factors, including the portion of the enzyme in the *a* form and the intracellular concentrations of high-energy phosphate molecules. They believe that the regulation of glycogenolysis occurs not only by conversion of phosphorylase *b* to *a* but also by regulation of the activity of phosphorylase *b* through changes in concentration of glucose-6-phosphate, AMP, and adenosine triphosphate.

Ellis (*175*) in his recent review of the biochemical effects of epinephrine on muscle suggested that the activation of glycogenolysis, although perhaps important for the action of epinephrine on muscle, is not clearly established. Muscle contraction is a complex process that is not well understood. Nevertheless Ellis and his associates (*205*) showed that the relative potencies of the adrenergic amines in producing inotropic actions in rat diaphragm correlated with the relative potencies in producing glycogenolysis. In studies with the perfused isolated guinea pig hearts Ellis and Vincent (*206*) reported that acetylcholine inhibited the glycogenolytic action and also the inotropic and chronotropic action of epinephrine. Similarly, DCI blocks all three actions of epinephrine. Ellis proposes that there is a metabolic role of acetylcholine in the control of the utilization of cardiac glycogen and, possibly, a biochemical basis in the control of cardiac function by means of acetylcholine.

As pointed out in the introduction to this section, it has been known for some time that administering epinephrine to various animal species causes a decrease in cardiac glycogen (*186*). Ellis (*175*) recently reported that epinephrine reduced glycogen content and increased phosphorylase *a* activity in rabbit ventricle slices. Winterscheid et al. (*207*) studied the action of isoproterenol infused into the isolated, metabolically supported dog heart. The oxidative metabolism increased significantly and in proportion to the heart rate. The glucose utilization remained unchanged, pyruvate utilization increased slightly, and lactate was excreted. They conclude that the augmented oxidative metabolism cannot be accounted for by the observed changes in carbohydrate substrates. Moreover, the myocardial glycogen concentrations were insignificantly changed during the inotropic stimulation. This study, while demonstrating a similarity to epinephrine (increased myocardial oxygen consumption), also demonstrated that the changes in glucose and lactate utilization differ from those of epinephrine. Bogue et al. (*187*) had shown that epinephrine produces a rise in glucose and lactate utilization, while Winterscheid et al. (*207*) had shown isoproterenol produced no increase. These authors showed that isoproterenol increases the oxidative metabolism and heart rate by almost 40% yet did not increase the utilization of carbohydrate metabolites. In the absence of significant changes in tissue glucose concentration it is unlikely that significant anaerobic glycolysis will occur, and this fact suggests that other metabolites are involved in the increased oxidative metabolism, possibly fatty acids.

The metabolic actions of isoproterenol on various tissues indicate that they differ significantly from those of other amines. For example, Sutherland and Rall (*192*) reported that the formation of cyclic AMP is increased nearly 4 times in the presence of maximal inotropic-producing doses of the adrenergic amines. *l*-Isoproterenol was the most potent agent and was 5 to 10 times more active than *l*-epinephrine or *l*-norepinephrine, the latter two compounds being about equally active. *d*-Epinephrine was found to be about 1/20 as active as its *l* isomer or as *l*-norepinephrine. In liver tissue studies *l*-norepinephrine was reported to be considerably less active than *l*-epinephrine and essentially as active as *d*-epinephrine. Thus, Murad et al. (*208*) report that, although the potencies of the catecholamines in heart are similar with respect to the formation of cyclic AMP, in contrast to inotropic potencies, there is a considerable difference between the liver and the heart preparations from the same animals. Other studies point to a differential tissue order. Ali et al. (*209*) have shown that the stimulation of phosphorylase produced by epinephrine in skeletal muscle is effectively blocked by the β-blocking agents DCI and nethalide, whereas the α-blocking agent phentolamine had no effect. In liver tissue, however, the behavior is quite different, because all the adrenergic blocking agents are active inhibitors of the effect of epinephrine on phosphorylase activity. The authors feel that the receptors responsible for the metabolic action of epinephrine in skeletal muscle may be classified as β receptors in contrast to the receptors in liver, which have properties common to both the α and β adrenergic receptors.

As was reported by Sutherland and Rall (*192*), there have been many attempts to relate the inotropic action of epinephrine to its metabolic actions. There seems to be some evidence of a correlation between the inotropic action of epinephrine and other amines and the level of phosphorylase *a* content in cardiac tissue. Hess and Haugaard (*210*) reported that epinephrine increased the phosphorylase *a* content of perfused rat hearts. Kukovits et al. (*211*) reported a close correlation between the increased force of contraction and the increased phosphorylase *a* content in the isolated perfused rat heart after administration of *dl*-isoproterenol, *l*-norepinephrine, and *l*-epinephrine (in order of decreasing potency). They also report that Epinine, synephrine, and phenylephrine at high dose levels, capable of producing only a minimal increase in the force of contraction, likewise produce minimal increases in phosphorylase *a* activity. These general observations have been supported by Mayer and Moran (*212*) with epinephrine, norepinephrine, and isoproterenol in open-chest dogs, by Belford and Feinleib (*213*) with epinephrine on isolated rat auricles, and by Lacroix and Leusen (*214*). In contrast to these supporting data are some instances in which the administration of epinephrine at doses sufficient to produce an inotropic action failed to produce an increase in phosphorylase *a* activity. Mayer et al. (*215*) have shown that epinephrine in doses of less than 0.5 μg/kg given intravenously to the anesthetized dog failed to increase phosphorylase *a* activity, although it simultaneously produced a significant increase in the contractile force of the heart. Drummond et al. (*216*) have reported results similar to those of Mayer and co-workers. They have shown that small doses of epinephrine causing significant increases in the contractile force of perfused rat hearts and in situ dog hearts did not produce any raising of phosphorylase *a* levels. Somewhat similar results have been obtained by us with the administration of *l*-isoproterenol in isolated, perfused rabbit hearts. In these studies doses of *l*-isoproterenol sufficient to produce a 100 to 200% increase in the force of contraction failed to elicit significant increases in phosphorylase *a* activity (Lands and Brown, unpublished data). Hess et al. (*217*) have replied to the study of Mayer et al. (*215*) and maintain that the activation of phosphorylase *a* plays an important role in the action of adrenergic amines on heart function. They point out that differences in technique, the possible role of cardiovascular reflexes, and humoral factors may influence the action of epinephrine on heart phosphorylase. Finally, they state that small increases in phosphorylase *a* activity produced by low doses of epinephrine are difficult to measure, and this fact also may contribute to the differences in the reports from the two laboratories.

Inasmuch as epinephrine possesses metabolic properties similar to those of insulin and glucagon, it is not surprising that these hormones have been the subject of studies aimed at correlating the regulation of glycogenolysis in muscle with other metabolic activities. One of the first definitive studies was that reported by Farah and Tuttle (*218*), in which they studied the pharmacology of glucagon, and more recently Regan et al. (*219*) and Cornblath et al. (*220*) studied the same. Cornblath and his associates have shown that glucagon and anoxia accelerate glycogen breakdown, increase the output of lactate, and increase phosphorylase activity in the perfused rat heart. Regan et al. compared the effects of glucagon and epinephrine in the anesthetized dog; both compounds infused into the coronary circulation produced an increase in heart contractile force and a rise in heart rate, and both decreased the free fatty acid uptake in the heart. Glucagon produced a substantial increase in glucose utilized by the heart, whereas epinephrine produced a decrease in glucose extraction. The latter observation is at variance with the earlier studies of Bogue et al. (*187*), but similar results have recently been reported by others (*221*, *222*). Regan also stated that reserpine pretreatment did not modify the activity of glucagon, although DCI did not produce inhibition of the inotropic action; this suggests that glucagon acts directly on the β adrenergic receptor.

Cornblath and his group (*220*) report that anoxia is a greater stimulator of glycogenolysis and lactate production than glucagon but produces a smaller increase in phosphorylase *a* activity than glucagon. It is of particular interest that both anoxia and glucagon produce increased rates of glycogenolysis and lactate production and elevated levels of phosphorylase *a* in hearts from reserpinized animals. This observation is in agreement with that of Regan et al. (*219*).

Kreisberg and Williamson (*223*), using the perfused rat heart, observed that glucagon stimulates glucose transport and causes increased substrate utiliza-

TABLE 8.29

Effect of Sympathomimetic Amines on Blood Sugar[a]

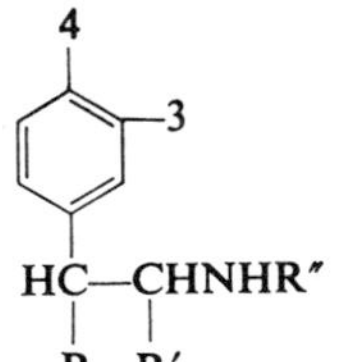

Compound	Structure: 4	3	R	R′	R″	Effect on blood sugar: Animal	Admin.[b]	Dose/kg	Increase, mg/100 ml	Ref.	Relative effect (7)
Isoproterenol	OH	OH	OH	H	$CH(CH_3)_2$	Rabbit	s.c.	25 mg	18	*247*	> 1/10 epi.
						Rat	s.c.	10 μg	112	*145*	Inactive
						Dog	i.v.	1.5 μg/min for 15 min	96	*248*	
						Dog	i.v.	1.4 μg/min for 15 min	102	*243*	
Epinephrine	OH	OH	OH	H	CH_3	Rabbit	s.c.	0.15 mg	106	*247*	
						Rat	s.c.	0.10 mg	110	*145*	
						Dog	i.v.	1.5 μg/min for 15 min	109	*248*	
						Dog	i.v.	1.0 μg/min for 15 min	106	*243*	
d isomer											1/20 epi.
Norepinephrine	OH	OH	OH	H	H	Rabbit	s.c.	1.0 mg	96	*247*	1/4 to 1/20 epi.
						Dog	i.v.	0.46 μg/min for 15 min	14	*243*	

d isomer:											1/20 *l* isomer
3	OH	OH	OH	H	C_2H_5	Rat	s.c.	1.0 mg	120	*145*	
36	OH	OH	OH	H	$C(CH_3)_3$	Rat	s.c.	40 μg	103	*145*	
Dopamine	OH	OH	H	H	H						1/5 Epinine
Isoetharine	OH	OH	OH	C_2H_5	$CH(CH_3)_2$	Rabbit	s.c.	5 mg	52	*247*	
								10 mg	84		
						Dog	i.v.	15 μg/min for 15 min	148	*248*	
60	OH	OH	OH	C_2H_5	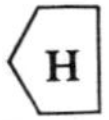	Rabbit	s.c.	10 mg	61	*247*	
								20 mg	83		
Ethylnorepinephrine	OH	OH	OH	C_2H_5	H	Rabbit	s.c.	5 mg	50	*247*	
								10 mg	76		
						Dog	i.v.	15 μg/min for 15 min	120	*248*	
43	OH	OH	OH	H	$CHCH_3$ – CH_2 – 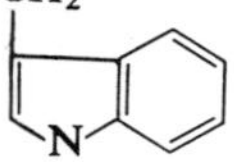	Dog	i.v.	2 μg/total (est. 50 × epi.)		*132*	
						Cat	i.v.	20 μg	87		
Nordefrine	OH	OH	OH	CH_3	H						1/10 epi.
Phenylephrine	H	OH	OH	H	CH_3						1/20 epi.
17	H	OH	OH	H	H						1/200 epi.
14	OH	H	OH	H	H						< Synephrine
13	H	H	OH	H	$CH(CH_3)_2$						Inactive
Tyramine	OH	H	H	H	H						Inactive
Ephedrine	H	H	OH	CH_3	CH_3						Inactive
Propadrine	H	H	OH	CH_3	H						Inactive

[a] Ellis et al. (*205*) reported glycogenolytic potencies with the rat diaphragm as follows: isoproterenol 10 times epinephrine, which in turn is > 10 times levarterenol, and levarterenol, phenylephrine, and ephedrine approximately equal.
[b] S.c., subcutaneous; i.v., intravenous.

tion. The latter was shown to be dissociated from the glycogenolytic effect and is believed to be due to the increased work of the heart. In general, though, the effects of glucagon on the perfused rat heart are like those of epinephrine. This is somewhat at variance with the data given by Regan et al. (*219*).

Williamson (*224*) has attempted to resolve these conflicting reports. His observations indicate that the effect of epinephrine on glucose uptake in muscle may be determined by the ability of the tissue to respond to the inotropic stimulus. Thus, he found that epinephrine increased glucose uptake in the perfused rat heart 3 to 4 times during a 30-minute period. Lactate increased 8 times and glycogen decreased by 45% during the first 5 minutes. DCI abolished the glycogenolytic action of epinephrine and inhibited the stimulation of glucose uptake. Norepinephrine is just as active as epinephrine in producing the metabolic changes, and isoproterenol is more active. Phosphorylase *a* activity increased from approximately 10% to 70% of total phosphorylase within 20 seconds of epinephrine addition, and decreased to 25% after 10 minutes. Glycogenolysis and lactate production approximately parallel phosphorylase *a* activity. These studies, Williamson believes, show that epinephrine causes an increased energy utilization, both when no glycogen change is demonstrable and when glycogen breakdown has ceased. The results suggest a dual action of epinephrine: an initial transient stimulation of glycogenolysis and, following it, a more prolonged increase in oxidative metabolism, which is a direct consequence of increased mechanical activity.

It is of great interest to speculate on the results reported by Williamson (*224*). The basis of the inotropic action of the adrenergic amines is not known, although Sutherland and Rall (*192*) suggest that there is evidence that cyclic AMP is involved. It would be of considerable interest also to know whether tissue levels of the nucleotide after epinephrine stimulation follow the relatively transient pattern of phosphorylase activation or the more prolonged time course of the increased mechanical activity and energy utilization. Williamson (*224*) suggests that if cyclic AMP is the mediator of both the glycogenolytic and inotropic actions of epinephrine, the contractile elements of the myocardium are probably more sensitive than the phosphorylase-activating system. Certainly, the similarity between the actions of glucagon (*218*, *220*, *223*) on the heart and those of epinephrine supports the idea that the agents act by a common pathway.

Some of the data given above have been tabulated (Tables 8.29 to 8.31) for effects on blood glucose, lactic acid, and phosphorylase activation in relation to molecular structure. They show important species differences. Results obtained with dogs and rats, however, indicate that isoproterenol influences these parameters importantly and to a greater degree than comparable doses of epinephrine and norepinephrine. The results obtained by McChesney et al. (*247*) disclose additional important differences in the rabbit.

TABLE 8.30

Effect of Various Sympathomimetic Amines on Lactacidemia

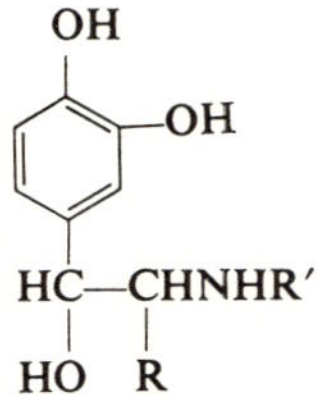

Compound	Structure: R	Structure: R′	Effect on lactic acid: Animal	Admin.[a]	Dose/kg	Lactic acid increase, %	Ref.
Isoproterenol	H	$CH(CH_3)_2$	Rat	s.c.	20 μg	68	*145*
			Dog	i.v.	1.5 μg/min for 15 min	150	*248*
Epinephrine	H	CH_3	Rat	s.c.	0.2 mg	90	*145*
			Dog	i.v.	1.5 μg/min for 15 min	122	*248*
Levarterenol	H	H	Rat	s.c.	0.5 mg	43	*145*
3	H	C_2H_5	Rat	s.c.	20 μg	67	*145*
36	H	$C(CH_3)_3$	Rat	s.c.	10 μg	65	*145*
Isoetharine	C_2H_5	$CH(CH_3)_2$	Dog	i.v.	15 μg/min for 15 min	136	*248*
Ethylnorepinephrine	C_2H_5	H	Dog	i.v.	15 μg/min for 15 min	129	*248*

[a] S.c., subcutaneous; i.v., intravenous.

TABLE 8.31

Effect of Various Sympathomimetic Amines on Phosphorylase *a* Activity of the Rat Isolated Perfused Heart (*211*)[a]

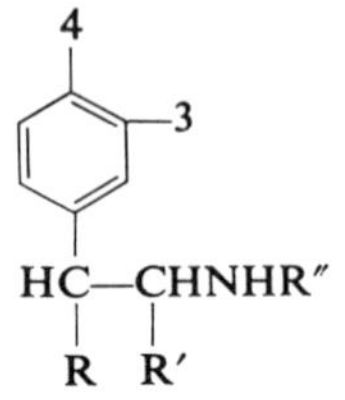

Compound	Structure					Approx. dose for 75% phosphorylase *a*, μg/heart
	4	3	R	R′	R″	
Isoproterenol	OH	OH	OH	H	$CH(CH_3)_2$	0.3
Levarterenol	OH	OH	OH	H	H	1.0
Epinephrine	OH	OH	OH	H	CH_3	4.0
Epinine	OH	OH	H	H	CH_3	50.0
Synephrine	OH	H	OH	H	CH_3	> 500–1000 (max. 67.5%)
Phenylephrine	H	OH	OH	H	CH_3	> 500–1000 (max. 66.0%)
Methoxamine	2,5	Methoxy	OH	CH_3	H	> 500 (max. 58.8%)
Metanephrine	OH	CH_3O	OH	H	CH_3	> 500 (max. 63.5%)

[a] Phosphorylase calculated in percent of total phosphorylase activity.

One extremely interesting aspect of the metabolic action of epinephrine activity is given by the work of Lundholm (*225*) and Mohme-Lundholm (*226*), who have proposed that the relaxing effect of epinephrine is caused by an increased tissue production of lactic acid. They have obtained significant correlations between lactic acid production and skeletal-muscle relaxation. The studies have been reviewed (*194*).

The vasodilator action of epinephrine is envisioned as being located principally in skeletal muscle, where epinephrine acts as a dilator after both intra-arterial and intravenous administration in low concentration. Administered in high concentration, epinephrine produces vasoconstriction. Lundholm and Mohme-Lundholm (*194*) have also shown that the intra-arterial administration of lactic acid in amounts equal to those of epinephrine produced vasodilation equal to that induced by epinephrine. They report that, when the production of lactic acid was inhibited, the vasodilator effect of epinephrine was converted to vasoconstriction. The ability of epinephrine to dilate skeletal-muscle vessels at low concentrations, but to constrict at high concentrations, is attributed to a lower threshold response for lactic acid production than for the separate and distinct constrictor action of epinephrine on the muscle. Thus, in high doses the constrictor action predominates. The typical action of epinephrine in low doses is to raise the cardiac output and decrease the mean blood pressure and total peripheral resistance. This cardiovascular action could be duplicated by the intravenous infusion of lactic acid.

Mohme-Lundholm (*226*) and Lundholm (*227*) also stated that norepinephrine causes a much smaller lactic acid production than does epinephrine and that this may account for its predominantly vasoconstrictive action. Isoproterenol is reported by Lundholm and Svedmyr (*229*) and Lundholm and Mohme-Lundholm (*194*) to stimulate lactic acid production in doses that are vasodepressive. They were unable to demonstrate in man, however, a significant increase in lactic acid production when isoproterenol was infused into the circulation of the forearm in doses causing increased circulation. This observation is in agreement with that made by Cobbold et al. (*230*), who also demonstrated that *dl*-isoproterenol in man caused an increase in oxygen consumption and blood glucose but no change in blood lactate levels. Recently Lundholm and Svedmyr (*231*) demonstrated that DCI simultaneously blocked the calorigenic action and lactic acid production caused by *l*-epinephrine and *dl*-isoproterenol.

Furchgott (*138*) has raised several points that oppose the theory that the relaxing action of epinephrine is mediated by an increased production of lactic acid. Ellis, in his review of the biochemical effects of epinephrine, (*175*), does not agree that Furchgott's objections are completely valid. It seems obvious that further studies are needed.

The early studies of the influence of epinephrine on fat metabolism and transport have been reviewed by Ellis (*7*). After these investigations, which gave diverse and often inconsistent changes in blood lipid levels, there was more interest in the nature and mechanism of the lipid mobilization. It has been shown, for example, that the administration of depot preparations of epinephrine in oil caused a rise in serum cholesterol, phospholipids, and triglycerides in dogs and rabbits (*232*, *233*). Epinephrine in aqueous solution was demonstrated to produce a marked rise in the blood level of free fatty acids in man (*234*, *235*) and to mobilize these acids from rat adipose tissue in vitro (*236*). Carlson and Orö (*237*) have shown that norepinephrine administration increases the free fatty acids and glycerol, whereas glucose administration decreases both. They report that in the dog norepinephrine increases, whereas glucose and insulin decrease, the adipose-tissue arterial-venous concentration gradient of these acids and the glycerol. Shafrir et al. (*238*) have demonstrated that depot epinephrine produces a prompt but transient rise in serum free fatty acids and a delayed 24-hour elevation in serum lipoproteins. If glucose is administered prior to, or at the same time as, the epinephrine, the elevation in free fatty acids can be prevented. Insulin alone was able to block the epinephrine-induced response of these acids without a parallel hyperglycemia, indicating that the availability of glucose for effective tissue utilization, rather than hyperglycemia per se, controls their release. Despite the block, whether it is caused by glucose or by insulin, there is still a definite rise in serum cholesterol and phospholipids 24 hours after administration of the drug. This suggests at least a partial, independent, lipoprotein-mobilizing action of epinephrine.

Havel and Goldfien (*239*) have shown that both epinephrine and norepinephrine increase the circulating levels of free fatty acids in man and in the dog. Steinberg et al. (*240*) report that not only does norepinephrine increase the rate of the mobilization of these acids but that the calorigenic action of norepinephrine is causally related to its ability to increase that mobilization. During norepinephrine infusion the increase in free fatty acids is sustained, whereas during epinephrine infusion the elevation is transient but the blood glucose levels remain. Havel and Goldfien (*239*) have shown that a greater depth of pentobarbital anesthesia in the dog is accompanied by a rise in free fatty acid concentration, whereas ganglionic blockade with hexamethonium is accompanied by a prompt and sustained fall. Norepinephrine and epinephrine administration during ganglionic blockade produce a rise in the concentration, whereas α adrenergic blockade with Dibenamine inhibits the response of both amines. Havel and Goldfien also reported that in the adrenalectomized dog maintained on corticosterone both epinephrine and norepinephrine induce a diminished response of free fatty acids. They believe that the sympathetic nervous system exerts a control over the mobilization of these acids from adipose tissue, a control that may be altered by stimulation of the central nervous system or by hormonal factors, that is, endogenous catecholamines. These general concepts of the role of the sympathetic nervous system in the control of the mobilization of free fatty acids have been recorded also by other investigators (*238*, *241*, *242*).

Continuing studies of the metabolic responses of the adrenergic stimulants have led inevitably to the increased use of the adrenergic blocking agents as a means of evaluating receptor mechanisms. It is becoming increasingly evident that glycogenolysis, lipid metabolism, lactic acid production, and activation of liver and muscle phosphorylase are intimately interrelated. Several examples of investigations in which the blocking agents were used for the study of adrenergic actions have recently appeared in the literature. Mayer et al. (*243*) have reported studies with adrenergic blockers of β receptors (DCI) and α receptors (phenoxybenzamine) and a drug with, possibly, mixed action (ergotamine). These studies show that DCI completely abolishes the increase in blood glucose and free fatty acid produced by epinephrine, norepinephrine, and isoproterenol in the dog, but that it does not block hyperglycemia in mice and only partially blocks epinephrine-induced hyperlactacidemia. Phenoxybenzamine, unlike DCI, does not block hyperglycemia, nor does it block increases in blood lactic acid produced by epinephrine in the dog. Ergotamine antagonizes the hyperglycemia but not the lactic acid increase. These data are of interest in light of the well-established action of phenoxybenzamine in blocking the vasopressive action of norepinephrine and epinephrine but not the inotropic action.

Both DCI and phenoxybenzamine in themselves produce an increase in blood glucose and lactic acid, whereas large doses of DCI antagonize the hyperglycemia produced by low doses of DCI and the hyperglycemia and hyperlactacidemia produced by phenoxybenzamine. DCI also produces a large and sustained increase in free fatty acids even with doses that do not block this action when it is caused by norepinephrine. Mayer et al. (*243*) agree with Furchgott (*138*) that another receptor, distinct from the α and β receptors of Ahlquist, is probably involved in the hyperglycemic action of the adrenergic amines. Their statement is a guarded one, however, in that they feel a final decision must await further experimental evidence.

Similar studies of the metabolic actions of adrenergic blocking agents have been reported by Salvador et al. (*244*), Burns et al. (*245*) and Maling et al. (*246*). In two of these studies (*244*, *245*) are described the use of *N*-isopropylmethoxamine for blocking the metabolic effects of adrenergic amines and for inhibiting lipid mobilization. This amine markedly lowers the plasma free fatty acids in the dog and in man, prevents the epinephrine-induced rise in blood glucose and lactic acid, and prevents the elevation of plasma free fatty acids produced by epinephrine and norepinephrine. Such results provide additional evidence that the sympathetic nervous system plays an important role in the mobilization of free fatty acids. *N*-Isopropylmethoxamine also should prove useful in investigating the possible routes of adrenergic control of carbohydrate metabolism.

8.7. GENERAL SUMMARY

The remarks introducing this chapter presented an outline of the conceptual history of the sympathomimetic amines and the receptors with which they interact. The investigations of Dale provided insight into the nature of this action and at the same time outlined some of the fundamental problems that have engaged the attention of many investigators since the first decade of this century. In his publication of 1910 he states, "The relation of the receptive mechanism to the base may well be one of solid solution or adsorption, and therefore more analogous to that of an enzyme to its substrate, as the widely different activities of optical isomers suggests." With the concept of Elliot before him, the concept that activation takes place through interaction with a "myoneural junction," Dale pointed out the necessity for postulating that "the myoneural junction, or parts of myoneural junctions, concerned with inhibition are not identical, in their affinities for chemical substances, with those which are concerned with motor effects."

Youmans et al. (*23–25*) obtained results that supported this concept of two or more receptive substances. They noted that a comparison of the actions of sympathomimetic compounds must be made with regard to a single type of effector, since the removal of each group of the epinephrine molecule may interfere with reception to a greater degree in one type of effector than in another. The correctness of this concept is amply illustrated by the data tabulated in this chapter. The results support the concept of different receptor types and indicate, further, that these constitute a population with somewhat different affinities for structurally varied sympathomimetic amines.

The available evidence suggests that sympathetic activity in mammals is mediated by epinephrine and norepinephrine. No other neurohumoral agents have been shown to play important roles in this action. These two substances can account for most of the actions observed on stimulation of adrenergic nerves (reviewed *53*, *55*). Epinephrine, with minor exceptions, is the more potent compound. However, unlike norepinephrine, it has a dual action, activating both α and β receptors whereas norepinephrine has a weak action on β receptors. The numerous investigations carried out by Cannon and associates (reviewed *249*) established the relationship between the secretion of epinephrine and strong emotional states involving anxiety and pain, and they observed that the administration of this neurohumoral agent would produce many of the bodily changes associated with the emotions. Activations of both α and β receptors play a role in responses to situations involving the expenditure of large amounts of energy. The preceding sections of this chapter have outlined these actions. A recent brief communication (*188*) describes the responses to fear and anger induced by hypnosis. The investigators observed an increase in cardiac output and heart rate, a decrease in stroke volume, an increase in mean arterial pressure, and a decrease in peripheral resistance, and they noted that right-atrial pressure often fell "rapidly and dramatically." Mean plasma hydrocortisone levels doubled, and plasma nonesterified fatty acids increased. Pronethalol (β-receptor) blockade did not prevent these emotionally induced changes.

The available evidence suggests that α receptors are important for the transmission of sympathetic nerve impulses, are probably located at or near the cell surface, and play a role in ion transport across the cell membrane (*250*). The β receptors appear to have a more general distribution and are importantly associated with those metabolic actions which make more energy available for the support of motor activity. This separation of effects has been demonstrated with a *Taenia coli* preparation exposed to a glucose-free medium for several hours, to reduce the glycogen stores. In this state epinephrine no longer causes a rise in membrane potential but, instead, often produces depolarization and may initiate spontaneous activity (*251*).

The dual role of epinephrine may be demonstrated also with voluntary muscle. A partially curarized muscle (cat tibialis anterior) treated with epinephrine gives an enhanced response, and this effect can be abolished by the α-blocking agents (*178*). Isoproterenol does not decurarize, and the effects of this drug and epinephrine on twitch amplitude are not altered by α-blocking, but are decreased or abolished by the β-blocking agents. Many investigators have described important and complex effects on carbohydrate and fat metabolism, as previously presented in this review, in which isoproterenol equals or exceeds the potency of epinephrine and which can be prevented or diminished by β-blocking agents.

Assessing the role of this dual receptor system in various organs and from one species to another presents many complex problems. The same organ may vary in response to epinephrine, norepinephrine, and isoproterenol, when compared in different species or in the same organ (uterus, sphincters along the gastrointestinal tract), depending upon the functional state. The effect on the heart of various species has been presented in Table 8.3. It will be noted that the activity of norepinephrine relative to epinephrine, which is weak in the frog, increases from the tortoise and the chicken to the mammalian heart. One may suppose that the evolutionary development of autonomic functions has provided for structural variations consistent with the needs for survival. A selection of random mutations has taken place during the long racial history of each species and subspecies. An activating of the receptor by these amines does not necessarily mean that the receptor is built of the same components in each organ or species, and the mass of available data actually suggests considerable variation when evaluated in terms of structure–activity relationships.* This is illustrated by the data shown in Table 8.13. Epinine, an "incomplete" sympathomimetic amine, occupies different relative positions when potency is determined in various organ systems. It is more effective than nordefrine on the rabbit uterus but less effective on blood pressure and the small intestine (α-receptor system). Similarly, dopamine is a moderately effective cardiac stimulant but has little effect on blood sugar (suggested β-receptor system).

Several compounds have been arranged in order of potency for several β-receptor systems in Table 8.32. There is good agreement in the position for isoproterenol and the two lower homologues, *N*-ethyl- and *N*-methylepinephrine. Other structures show much variation in relative effectiveness. Norepinephrine is quite effective on the heart and voluntary muscle, weak on the bronchioles, and ineffective in inducing vasodepression. Other metabolic effects, described by Pratesi et al. (*145*), on glycemia, lactic acid production, and calorigenic effects in rats also show considerable scatter for norepinephrine relative to epinephrine, *N*-ethylarterenol, and isoproterenol. For

* Investigations directed to other objectives have shown that enzymes (or receptor proteins) are much more varied than the substances with which they react (*252*, *253*).

TABLE 8.32

Potency of Isoproterenollike Compounds on Various Organ Systems

Order of potency	Heart (rabbit)	Bronchioles (guinea pig)	Blood pressure (dog, vasodil.)	Voluntary muscle (*178*) (rat, twitch pot.)
1	Isoproterenol	Isoproterenol	Isoproterenol	Isoproterenol
2	*N*-Ethylnorepinephrine	*N*-Ethylnorepinephrine	*N*-Ethylnorepinephrine	Epinephrine
3	Norepinephrine	Epinephrine	Epinephrine	Norepinephrine
4	Epinephrine	Phenylephrine		*N*-Ethylnorepinephrine
5	Nordefrine	Epinine	*N*-Isopropyldopamine	
6	Dopamine	Ethylnorepinephrine		*N*-Isopropyldopamine
7	Ethylnorepinephrine	Dopamine	Phenylephrine[a]	Dopamine
8	Epinine	*N*-Isopropyldopamine	Epinine[a]	
9	Tyramine	Nordefrine	Dopamine[a]	
10	Phenylephrine	Norepinephrine	Norepinephrine[a]	
11	*N*-Isopropyldopamine	Tyramine	Nordefrine	
			Tyramine	

[a] Inactive.

calorigenic effect, isoproterenol > *N*-ethylnorepinephrine > epinephrine = norepinephrine; for glycemia, isoproterenol > epinephrine > *N*-ethylnorepinephrine (approximately 1/500 isoproterenol); for lactic acid production, isoproterenol > *N*-ethylnorepinephrine > epinephrine > norepinephrine; and for adrenal cortex stimulation, isoproterenol = epinephrine > *N*-ethylnorepinephrine > norepinephrine.

The classification of adrenotropic receptors as motor-inhibiting or as α or β types afford only very broad generalizations. Structure–activity relationships obtained with a large number of structurally varied sympathomimetic amines indicate wide differences in receptor activation potential—so great that a more precise grouping of receptor types would be desirable. The pharmacology of adrenergic blocking agents will be presented in a subsequent chapter. It is sufficient to point out here that agents such as phentolamine, piperoxan, dichloroisoproterenol, or pronethalol administered in doses sufficiently large to produce receptor blockade can identify receptor systems primarily associated with the excitatory process and another system that plays a major role in supporting the excitatory process.

REFERENCES

1. G. Barger and H. H. Dale, *J. Physiol. (London)*, **41**, 19 (1910).
2. D. Bovet and F. Bovet-Nitti, *Medicaments du Systeme Nerveux Vegtatif*, Editions S. Karger S.A., Basle, 1948.
3. W. H. Hartung, *Chem. Rev.*, **9**, 389 (1931).
4. P. Trendelenburg, "Adrenalin und adrenalinverwandte Substanzen." *Handbuch der Experimentellen Pharmakologie*, Heffter, *2.2*: 1130 (1924).
5. A. M. Lands, *Pharmacol. Rev.*, **1**, 279 (1949).
6. A. M. Lands, First Symposium on Chemical and Biological Correlation, 1951, p. 73.
7. S. Ellis, *Pharmacol. Rev.*, **8**, 485 (1956).
8. T. R. Elliot, *J. Physiol. (London)*, **32**, 401 (1905); *ibid., Proceedings*, **31**, XX (1904).
9. W. E. Dixon and P. Hamill, *J. Physiol. (London)*, **38**, 314 (1909).
10. M. L. Tainter and D. K. Chang, *J. Pharmacol. Exptl. Therap.*, **30**, 193 (1927).
11. M. L. Tainter, *J. Pharmacol. Exptl. Therap.*, **36**, 569 (1929).
12. M. L. Tainter, *J. Pharmacol. Exptl. Therap.*, **40**, 43 (1930).
13. M. L. Tainter, *Arch. Intern. Pharmacodyn.*, **41**, 365 (1931).
14. M. L. Tainter, *Arch. Intern. Pharmacodyn.*, **46**, 192 (1933).
15. M. C. Morton and M. L. Tainter, *J. Physiol. (London)*, **98**, 263 (1940).
16. J. H. Burn and M. L. Tainter, *J. Physiol. (London)*, **71**, 169 (1931).
17. A. Fleckenstein and J. H. Burn, *Brit. J. Pharmacol.*, **8**, 69 (1953).
18. A. Fleckenstein and H. Bass, *Arch. Exptl. Pathol. Pharmakol.*, **220**, 143 (1953).
19. A. Fleckenstein and D. Stöckle, *Arch. Exptl. Pathol. Pharmakol.*, **224**, 401 (1955).
20. J. H. Burn and M. J. Rand, *J. Physiol. (London)*, **144**, 314 (1958).
21. R. A. Maxwell, H. Povalski, and A. J. Plummer, *J. Pharmacol. Exptl. Therap.*, **125**, 178 (1959).

22. U. Trendelenburg, *Pharmacol. Rev.*, **15**, 225 (1963).

22a. U. Trendelenburg, A. Muskus, W. W. Fleming, and B. G. Alonso de la Sierra, *J. Pharmacol. Exptl. Therap.*, **138**, 170 (1962).

23. W. B. Youmans, K. W. Aumann, and H. F. Haney, *Am. J. Physiol.*, **126**, 237 (1939)·

24. W. B. Youmans, H. F. Haney, and K. W. Aumann, *Am. J. Physiol.*, **130**, 190 (1940).

25. W. B. Youmans, A. I. Karstens, and K. W. Aumann, *Am. J. Physiol.*, **137**, 87 (1942).

26. P. Holtz, K. Credner, and G. Kroneberg, *Arch. Exptl. Pathol. Pharmakol.*, **204**, 228 (1947).

27. U. S. v. Euler, *Arch. Intern. Pharmacodyn.*, **77**, 477 (1948).

28. U. S. v. Euler, *Ergeb. Physiol. Biol. Chem. Exptl. Pharmakol.*, **46**, 261 (1950).

29. U. S. v. Euler, *Pharmacol. Rev.*, **6**, 15 (1954).

30. B. F. Tullar, *Science*, **109**, 536 (1949).

31. W. B. Cannon and A. Rosenblueth, *Am. J. Physiol.*, **104**, 557 (1933).

32. H. Konzett, *Arch. Exptl. Pathol. Pharmakol.*, **197**, 27 (1940); **197**, 41 (1940).

33. A. M. Lands, E. E. Rickards, V. L. Nash, and K. Z. Hooper, *J. Pharmacol. Exptl. Therap.*, **89**, 297 (1947).

34. A. M. Lands, V. L. Nash, H. M. McCarthy, H. R. Granger, and B. L. Dertinger, *J. Pharmacol. Exptl. Therap.*, **90**, 110 (1947).

35. A. M. Lands, *Am. J. Physiol.*, **169**, 11 (1952).

36. A. M. Lands, V. L. Nash, H. R. Granger, and B. L. Dertinger, *J. Pharmacol. Exptl. Therap.*, **89**, 382 (1947).

37. R. P. Ahlquist, *Am. J. Physiol.*, **153**, 586 (1948).

38. R. P. Ahlquist, *Arch. Intern. Pharmacodyn.*, **139**, 38 (1962).

39. I. A. Coret and H. B. van Dyke, *J. Pharmacol. Exptl. Therap.*, **95**, 415 (1949).

40. K. R. Butterworth, *Biochem. Pharmacol., Suppl.*, **12**, 86 (1963).

40a. K. R. Butterworth and M. Mann, *Brit. J. Pharmacol.*, **12**, 415 (1957).

41. C. E. Powell and I. H. Slater, *J. Pharmacol. Exptl. Therap.*, **122**, 480 (1958).

42. A. M. Lands and T. G. Brown, Jr., *Proc. Soc. Exptl. Biol. Med.*, **116**, 331 (1964).

43. N. C. Moran and M. E. Perkins, *J. Pharmacol. Exptl. Therap.*, **124**, 223 (1958).

44. F. P. Luduena, L. v. Euler, B. F. Tullar, and A. M. Lands, *Arch. Intern. Pharmacodyn.*, **111**, 392 (1957).

45. F. P. Luduena, *Arch. Intern. Pharmacodyn*, **137**, 155 (1962).

46. A. M. Lands, F. P. Luduena, J. I. Grant, and E. Ananenko, *J. Pharmacol. Exptl. Therap*, **99**, 45 (1950).

47. F. P. Luduena, J. O. Hoppe, I. H. Oyen, and G. D. Wessinger, *J. Dental Res.*, **37**. 206 (1958).

48. M. L. Tainter, J. R. Pedden, and M. James, *J. Pharmacol. Exptl. Therap.*, **51**, 371 (1934).

49. F. Stolz and F. Flacher, D.R.P., 157,300 (*Frdl.*, **7**, 689); U.S. Pat. 862,675.

50. F. Stolz, *Chem. Ber.*, **37**, 4149 (1904).

51. H. D. Dakin, *J. Physiol.* (*London*), **32**, 24 (1905).

52. J. Biberfield, *Mediklin.*, **1906**, 1177.

53. U. S. v. Euler, *Pharmacol. Rev.*, **3**, 247 (1951).

54. E. Östlund, *Acta Physiol. Scand., Suppl.*, **112**, 1 (1954).

55. U. S. v. Euler, *Noradrenaline*, Thomas, Springfield, Ill., 1956.

56. G. F. Wassermann and J. H. Tramezzani, *Proc. Intern. Union Physiol. Sci.* (XXII Intern. Congr.) Vol. II, 1962, p. 826.

57. T. K. Akers and C. N. Peiss, *Proc. Soc. Exptl. Biol. Med.*, **112**, 396 (1963).

58. A. M. Lands and J. W. Howard, *J. Pharmacol. Exptl. Therap.*, **106**, 65 (1952).

59. G. T. Scott, R. L. Clard, and J. C. Hickman, *Biol. Bull.*, **123**, 511 (1962).
60. U. S. v. Euler, *Acta Physiol. Scand.*, **12**, 73 (1946).
61. S. L. Clark, R. B. Greenblatt, and R. M. West, *Endocrinology*, **49**, 200 (1951).
62. B. Hokfelt, *Acta Physiol. Scand. Suppl.*, **25**, 92 (1951).
63. J. H. Burn, *Irish J. Med. Sci.*, **308**, 345 (1951).
64. J. H. Burn and M. J. Rand, *Brit. Med. J.*, **1958–1**, 137.
65. H. J. Schümann, *Arch. Exptl. Pathol. Pharmakol.*, **234**, 17 (1958).
66. J. Axelrod, *Physiol. Rev.*, **39**, 751 (1959).
67. M. C. Goodall, *Pharmacol. Rev.*, **11**, 416 (1959).
68. H. D. Green and J. H. Kepchar, *Physiol. Rev.*, **39**, 617 (1959).
69. F. P. Luduena, E. Ananenko, O. H. Sigmund, and L. C. Miller, *J. Pharmacol. Exptl. Therap.*, **95**, 155 (1949).
70. K. Matthes, *Kreislaufuntersuchungen am Menschen mit fortlanfend registrierenden Methoden*, Thieme, Stuttgart, 1951.
71. O. Bayer, K. Blumberger, and S. Effert, *Cardiologia*, **16**, 145 (1950).
72. H. D. Green, *Minn. Med.*, **41**, 241 (1958).
73. A. J. Kaufmann, *Arch. Intern. Pharmacodyn.*, **146**, 579 (1963).
74. O. Schaumann, *Med. Chemie, Abhandl. Med. Chem. Forschungsstaetten Farbwerke Hoechst A.G.*, **3**, 383 (1936).
75. C. A. Crismon and M. L. Tainter, *J. Pharmacol. Exptl. Therap.*, **66**, 146 (1939).
76. T. G. Brown, Jr. and A. M. Lands in *Screening for Drug Action: Pharmacometrics* (D. R. Laurence and A. L. Bacharach, eds.), Academic, New York, 1964.
77. A. M. Lands and J. I. Grant, *J. Pharmacol. Exptl. Therap.*, **106**, 341 (1952).
78. T. P. Pruss, G. D. Maengwyn-Davies, and M. Wierzel, *J. Pharmacol. Exptl. Therap.*, **147**, 76 (1965).
79. O. Schaumann, *Arch. Exptl. Pathol. Pharmakol.*, **160**, 127 (1931).
80. A. M. Lands, unpublished data, 1965.
81. W. M. Cameron, J. M. Crismon, L. J. Whitsell, and M. L. Tainter, *J. Pharmacol. Exptl. Therap.*, **62**, 318 (1938).
82. W. M. Cameron, L. J. Whitsell, J. M. Crismon, and M. L. Tainter, *J. Pharmacol. Exptl. Therap.*, **63**, 340 (1938).
83. A. M. Lands and M. L. Tainter, *Arch. Exptl. Pathol. Pharmakol.*, **219**, 76 (1953).
84. F. P. Luduena and T. G. Brown, Jr., unpublished data, 1965.
85. G. A. Alles, *J. Pharmacol. Exptl. Therap.*, **47**, 339 (1933).
86. A. M. Lands, V. L. Nash, B. L. Dertinger, H. R. Granger, and H. M. McCarthy. *J. Pharmacol. Exptl. Therap.*, **92**, 369 (1948).
87. L. H. Easson and E. Stedman, *Biochem. J.*, **27**, 1257 (1933).
88. F. P. Luduena and B. F. Tullar, *Perspectives in Biology* (C. F. Cori, V. G. Foglia, L. F. Leloir, and S. Ochoa eds.), Elsevier, Amsterdam, 1963, p. 85.
89. M. L. Tainter, *J. Pharmacol. Exptl. Therap.*, **36**, 29 (1929).
90. W. Osten, *Arzneimittel-Forsch.*, **5**, 84 (1955).
91. D. F. Marsh and D. A. Herring, *Arch. Intern. Pharmacodyn.*, **78**, 489 (1949).
92. K. Unna, *Arch. Exptl. Pathol. Pharmakol.*, **213**, 207 (1951).
93. A. M. Lands, *J. Pharmacol. Exptl. Therap.*, **106**, 440 (1952).
94. W. W. Fleming and U. Trendelenburg, *J. Pharmacol. Exptl. Therap.*, **133**, 41 (1961).
95. A. M. Lands, *J. Pharmacol. Exptl. Therap.*, **104**, 474 (1952).
96. U. Trendelenburg, *J. Pharmacol. Exptl. Therap.*, **134**, 8 (1961).
97. P. A. Shore, *Pharmacol. Rev.*, **14**, 531 (1962).
98. E. Zaimis, *Ann. Rev. Pharmacol.*, **4**, 365 (1964).
99. M. A. Klouda, *Proc. Soc. Exptl. Biol. Med.*, **112**, 728 (1963).

100. P. A. Shore, V. H. Cohn, Jr., B. Highman, and H. M. Malling, *Nature*, **181**, 848 (1958).
101. M. Goldenberg, K. L. Pines, E. de F. Baldwin, D. G. Greene, and C. E. Roh, *Am. J. Med.*, **5**, 792 (1948).
102. H. Barcroft and H. Konzett, *J. Physiol.* (*London*), **110**, 194 (1949).
103. K. G. Wakim and H. E. Essex, *Circulation*, **5**, 370 (1952).
104. M. De V. Cotten and S. Pincus, *J. Pharmacol. Exptl. Therap.*, **114**, 110 (1955).
105. S. H. Boyer, IV., and A. W. Chisholm, *Bull. Johns Hopkins Hosp.*, **103**, 47 (1958).
106. L. Goldberg, R. D. Bloodwell, E. Braunwald, and A. G. Morrow, *Circulation*, **22**, 1125 (1960).
107. W. Y. Chan, *J. Pharmacol. Exptl. Therap.*, **147**, 48 (1965).
108. A. S. Marrazzi, *Science*, **104**, 6 (1946).
109. M. R. Gurd, *Quart. J. Pharm.*, **10**, 188 (1937).
110. A. Engelhardt and H. J. Schümann, *Arzneimittel-Forsch.*, **3**, 205 (1953).
111. Z. M. Bacq, *Arch. Intern. Pharmacodyn.*, **60**, 456 (1938).
112. O. Schaumann, *Arch. Exptl. Pathol. Pharmakol.*, **157**, 114 (1930).
113. P. Patek and C. H. Thienes, *Arch. Intern. Pharmacodyn.*, **49**, 432 (1935); **50**, 15 (1935).
114. I. A. Coret, *Proc. Soc. Exptl. Biol. Med.*, **68**, 553 (1948).
115. N. Klapproth, *Proc. Soc. Exptl. Biol. Med.*, **100**, 786 (1959).
116. F. P. Luduena, personal communication, 1965.
117. H. H. Dale, *Adventures in Physiology*, Pergamon, New York, 1953, pp. 97–98.
118. H. Konzett, *Klin. Wochschr.*, **19**, 1303 (1940).
119. R. Rössler, *Wien Klin. Wochschr.*, **54**, 239 (1941).
120. J. R. Corrigan, M. J. Langerman, and M. L. Moore, *J. Am. Chem. Soc.*, **67**, 1894 (1945).
121. O. H. Siegmund, H. R. Granger, and A. M. Lands, *J. Pharmacol. Exptl. Therap.*, **90**, 254 (1947).
122. B. L. Dertinger, D. C. Beaver, and A. M. Lands, *Proc. Soc. Exptl. Biol. Med.*, **68**, 501 (1948).
123. M. F. Lockett, *J. Physiol.* (*London*), **133**, 73p (1956).
124. M. F. Lockett, *Brit. J. Pharmacol.*, **12**, 86 (1957).
125. S. Eliasson, P. Lindgren, and B. Uvnäs, *Acta Physiol. Scand.*, **27**, 18 (1952).
126. P. Lindgren and B. Uvnäs, *Circulation Res.*, **1**, 479 (1953).
127. P. Lindgren and B. Uvnäs, *Am. J. Physiol.*, **176**, 68 (1954).
128. O. Celander and B. Folkow, *Acta Physiol. Scand.*, **23**, 64 (1951).
129. B. Folkow and B. E. Gernandt, *Am. J. Physiol.*, **169**, 622 (1952).
130. T. G. Brown, Jr., and T. J. Green, *Am. Heart J.*, **63**, 545 (1962).
131. A. M. Lands, G. E. Groblewski, and T. G. Brown, Jr., *Arch. Intern. Pharmacodyn.*, **161**, 68 (1966).
132. C. G. Van Arman, L. M. Miller, and M. P. O'Malley, *J. Pharmacol. Exptl. Therap.*, **133**, 90 (1961).
133. K. Wiemers, *Arch. Exptl. Pathol. Pharmakol.*, **213**, 283 (1951); *ibid.*, **213**, 335 (1951).
134. A. M. Lands, F. P. Luduena, J. O. Hoppe, and I. H. Oyen, *J. Pharm. Sci.*, **47**, 744 (1958).
135. H. Langecker and H. Friebel, *Arch. Exptl. Pathol. Pharmakol.*, **226**, 493 (1955).
136. U. S. v. Euler, *J. Physiol.* (*London*), **93**, 129 (1938).
137. F. Bruck, G. Hertting, A. Lindner, and M. Landon, *Wien. Klin. Wochschr.*, **68**, 183 (1956).
138. R. F. Furchgott, *Pharmacol. Rev.*, **11**, 429 (1959).
139. D. Krciková, S. Hynie, D. Schusterová, and E. Muhlbachova, *Biochem. Pharmacol.*, *Supp.*, **12**, 86 (1963).
140. A. Engelhardt, W. Hoetke, and H. Wick, *Arzneimittel-Forsch.*, **11**, 521 (1961).
141. W. Schmitt, *Z. Biol.*, **75**, 19 (1922).

142. P. Siderius, *Acta Physiol. Pharmacol. Neerl.*, **2**, 546 (1951–52).
143. H. D. Moed, J. Van Dijk, and H. Niewind, *Rec. Trav. Chim.*, **74**, 919 (1955).
144. N. Ludwigs and M. Schneider, *Arch. Exptl. Pathol. Pharmakol.*, **218**, 432 (1953).
145. P. Pratesi, E. Grana, L. Lilla, A. LaManna, and L. Villa, *Farmaco, Ed. Sci.*, **18**, 920 (1963).
146. O. H. Siegmund, N. Beglin, and A. M. Lands, *J. Pharmacol. Exptl. Therap.*, **97**, 14 (1949).
147. P. A. Nuhfer, cited by J. H. Biel, E. G. Schwarz, E. P. Sprengleor, H. A. Leiser, and H. L. Friedman, *J. Am. Chem. Soc.*, **76**, 3149 (1954).
148. D. F. Marsh, M. H. Pelletier, and C. A. Ross, *J. Pharmacol. Exptl. Therap.*, **92**, 108 (1948).
149. J. Roberts, F. Standaert, Y. I. Kim, and W. F. Riker, Jr., *J. Pharmacol. Exptl. Therap.*, **117**, 375 (1956).
150. M. H. Nathanson and H. Miller, *Proc. Soc. Exptl. Biol. Med.*, **70**, 633 (1949); *Circulation*, **6**, 238 (1952).
151. F. Serin, *Acta Physiol. Scand.*, **26**, 291 (1952).
152. J. L. Prevost and J. Saloz, *Arch. Intern. Physiol. Biochim.*, **8**, 329 (1909); cited in Ref. *154.*
153. H. Mollgaard, *Skan. Arch. Physiol.*, **26**, 315 (1912); cited in Ref. *154.*
154. W. E. Dixon and F. Ransom, *J. Physiol. (London)*, **45**, 413 (1912–13).
155. H. Januschke and L. Pollack, *Arch. Exptl. Pathol. Pharmakol.*, **66**, 205 (1911).
156. P. Trendelenburg, *Arch. Exptl. Pathol. Pharmakol.*, **69**, 79 (1912).
157. E. E. Swanson and R. B. Webster, *J. Pharmacol. Exptl. Therap.*, **38**, 327 (1930).
158. J. R. Pedden, M. L. Tainter, and W. M. Cameron, *J. Pharmacol. Exptl. Therap.*, **55**, 242 (1935).
159. N. Haugaard and M. E. Hess, *Pharmacol. Rev.*, **17**, 27 (1965).
160. H. Konzett and R. Rössler, *Arch. Exptl. Pathol. Pharmakol.*, **195**, 71 (1940).
161. A. M. Lands, F. P. Luduena, and B. F. Tullar, *J. Pharmacol. Exptl. Therap.*, **111**, 469 (1954).
162. A. M. Lands, F. P. Luduena, E. Ananenko, and J. I. Grant, *Arch. Intern. Pharmacodyn.*, **83**, 602 (1950).
163. J. H. Gaddum, W. S. Pert, and M. Vogt, *J. Physiol. (London)*, **108**, 467 (1949).
164. G. Kuschinsky and K. Oberdisse, *Arch. Exptl. Pathol. Pharmakol.*, **162**, 46 (1931).
165. G. B. West, *J. Physiol. (London)*, **106**, 418 (1947).
166. M. D. McDougal and G. B. West, *Brit. J. Pharmacol.*, **9**, 131 (1954).
167. J. L. Schmidt and W. W. Fleming, *J. Pharmacol. Exptl. Therap.*, **139**, 230 (1963).
168. C. M. Gruber and R. J. Mathews, Jr., *Arch. Exptl. Pathol. Pharmakol.*, **219**, 1 (1953).
169. J. H. Hagen and P. B. Hagen, in *Actions of Hormones on Molecular Processes* (G. Litwack and D. R. Ritchevsky, eds.), Wiley, New York, 1964, p. 268.
170. D. R. Bennett, D. A. Reinke, E. Alpert, T. Baum, and H. Vasquez-Leon, *J. Pharmacol. Exptl. Therap.*, **134**, 190 (1961).
171. E. J. Ariëns, M. F. G. A. Waelen, P. F. Sonneville, and A. M. Simonis, *Arzneimittel-Forsch.*, **13**, 541 (1963).
172. T. H. Tsai and W. W. Fleming, *J. Pharmacol. Exptl. Therap.*, **143**, 268 (1964).
173. D. H. L. Evans and H. O. Schild, *J. Physiol. (London)*, **122**, 63p (1953).
174. H. P. Ciuchita and R. F. Gautieri, *J. Pharm. Sci.*, **52**, 974 (1963).
175. S. Ellis, *Pharmacol. Rev.*, **11**, 469 (1959).
176. W. C. Bowman and E. Zaimis, *J. Physiol. (London)*, **144**, 92 (1958).
177. W. C. Bowman, A. A. J. Goldberg, and C. Raper, *Brit. J. Pharmacol.*, **19**, 464 (1962).
178. W. C. Bowman and C. Raper, *Brit. J. Pharmacol.*, **23**, 184 (1964).

179. W. C. Bowman and C. Raper, *Brit. J. Pharmacol.*, **24**, 98 (1965).
180. G. Paterson, *Biochem. Pharmacol.*, **12**, Suppl., 85 (1963).
181. J. O. Hoppe, D. K. Seppelin, and A. M. Lands, *J. Pharmacol. Exptl. Therap.*, **95**, 502 (1949).
182. M. Nickerson, J. Berghout, and R. N. Hammerstrom, *Am. J. Physiol.*, **160**, 479 (1950).
183. F. P. Luduena, E. O'Malley, and I. H. Oyen, *Arch. Intern. Pharmacodyn.*, **122**, 111 (1959).
184. J. Barcroft and W. E. Dixon, *J. Physiol.* (*London*), **35**, 182 (1910).
185. C. L. Evans and S. Ogawa, *J. Physiol.* (*London*), **47**, 446 (1914).
186. S. W. Patterson and E. H. Starling, *J. Physiol.* (*London*), **47**, 137 (1914).
187. J. Y. Bogue, C. L. Evans, F. Grande, and F. Y. Hsu, *Quart. J. Exptl. Physiol.*, **25**, 213 (1935).
188. C. D. Schoenfeld, P. H. Gwynne, A. M. Weissler, and J. V. Warren, *J. Lab. Clin. Med.*, **64**, 867 (1964).
189. E. Braun-Menendez, A. L. Chute, and R. A. Gregory, *Quart. J. Exptl. Physiol.*, **29**, 91 (1939).
190. M. B. Visscher and A. G. Mulder, *Am. J. Physiol.*, **94**, 630 (1930).
191. F. R. Griffith, Jr., *Physiol. Rev.*, **31**, 151 (1951).
192. E. W. Sutherland and T. W. Rall, *Pharmacol. Rev.*, **12**, 265 (1960).
193. J. Tepperman and H. M. Tepperman, *Pharmacol. Rev.*, **12**, 301 (1960).
194. L. Lundholm and E. Mohme-Lundholm in "*Adrenergic Mechanisms*," Little, Brown, Boston, 1960, p. 305.
195. T. W. Rall and E. W. Sutherland, *J. Biol. Chem.*, **232**, 1005 (1958).
196. J. Berthet, *Proc. Intern. Congr. Biochem., 4th, Vienna*, **17**, 107 (1958).
197. E. S. Haugaard and N. Haugaard, *J. Biol. Chem.*, **206**, 641 (1954).
198. C. F. Cahill, Jr., B. Leboeuf, and R. Flinn, The Endocrine Society, 41st Meeting, June 1959, Abstract, p. 62.
199. E. W. Sutherland in *Phosphorus Metabolism*, Vol. 2 (W. D. McElroy and B. Glass, eds.), Johns Hopkins Press, Baltimore, 1952, p. 577.
200. C. Cori in *Enzymes; Units of Biological Structure and Function* (O. H. Gaebler, ed.), Academic Press, New York, 1956, p. 573.
201. G. T. Cori and B. Illingworth, *Biochim. Biophys. Acta.* **21**, 105 (1950).
202. W. H. Danforth, E. Helmreich, and C. F. Cori, *Proc. Natl. Acad. Sci. U.S.*, **48**, 1191, (1962).
203. H. E. Morgan and A. Parmeggiani, *J. Biol. Chem.*, **239**, 2435 (1964).
204. H. E. Morgan and A. Parmeggiani, *J. Biol. Chem.*, **239**, 2440 (1964).
205. S. Ellis, A. H. Davis, and H. L. Anderson, *J. Pharmacol. Exptl. Therap.*, **115**, 120 (1955).
206. S. Ellis and N. H. Vincent, *Biochem. Pharmacol.*, **8**, 133 (1961).
207. L. C. Winterscheid, R. A. Bruce, J. B. Blumberg, and K. A. Merendino, *Circulation Res.*, **12**, 76 (1963).
208. F. Murad, Y. M. Chi, T. W. Rall, and E. W. Sutherland, *J. Biol. Chem.*, **237**, 1233 (1962).
209. H. I. E. S. Ali, A. Antonio, and N. Haugaard, *J. Pharmacol. Exptl. Therap.*, **145**, 142 (1964).
210. M. E. Hess and N. Haugaard, *J. Pharmacol. Exptl. Therap.*, **122**, 169 (1958).
211. W. R. Kukovitz, M. E. Hess, J. Shanefeld, and N. Haugaard, *J. Pharmacol. Exptl. Therap.*, **127**, 122 (1959).
212. S. E. Mayer and N. C. Moran, *J. Pharmacol. Exptl. Therap.*, **129**, 271 (1960).
213. J. Belford and M. R. Feinleib, *J. Pharmacol. Exptl. Therap.*, **127**, 257 (1959).
214. E. Lacroix and I. Leusen, *Arch. Intern. Pharmacodyn.*, **133**, 89 (1961).
215. S. E. Mayer, M. D. V. Cotten, and N. C. Moran, *Biochem. Pharmacol.*, **8**, 133 (1961).

216. G. I. Drummond, J. R. E. Valadares, and L. Duncan, *Proc. Soc. Exptl. Biol. Med.*, **117**, 307 (1964).
217. M. E. Hess, J. Shanfeld, and N. Haugaard, *Biochem. Pharmacol.*, **11**, 1031 (1962).
218. A. Farah and R. Tuttle, *J. Pharmacol. Exptl. Therap.*, **129**, 49 (1960).
219. T. J. Regan, P. H. Lehan, D. H. Hanneman, A. Behar, and H. K. Hellems, *J. Lab. Clin. Med.*, **63**, 638 (1964).
220. M. Cornblath, P. J. Randle, A. Parmeggiani, and H. E. Morgan, *J. Biol. Chem.*, **238**, 1592 (1903).
221. S. E. Mayer, *Biochem. Pharmacol.*, **12**, 193 (1963).
222. S. Hupka and J. E. Dumont, *Biochem. Pharmacol.*, **12**, 1023 (1963).
223. R. A. Kreisberg and J. R. Williamson, *Am. J. Physiol.*, **207**, 721 (1964).
224. J. R. Williamson, *J. Biol. Chem.*, **239**, 2721 (1964).
225. L. Lundholm, *Acta Physiol. Scand., Suppl.*, **39**, 133 (1956).
226. E. Mohme-Lundholm, *Acta Physiol. Scand., Suppl.*, **29**, 108 (1953).
227. L. Lundholm, *Acta Physiol. Scand.*, **40**, 344 (1957).
228. L. Lundholm, *Acta Physiol. Scand.*, **43**, 27 (1958).
229. L. Lundholm and N. Svedmyr, *Acta Physiol. Scand.*, **62**, 67 (1964).
230. A. F. Cobbold, J. Ginsburg, and A. Paton, *J. Physiol. (London)*, **151**, 539 (1960).
231. L. Lundholm and N. Svedmyr, *Acta Pharmacol. Toxicol.*, **20**, 303 (1963).
232. A. Koplin, S. Jacques, and M. Gant, *Am. J. Physiol.*, **191**, 8 (1957).
233. A. Dury, *Circulation Res.*, **5**, 47 (1957).
234. R. S. Gordon, Jr., and A. Cherkes, *J. Clin. Invest.*, **3**, 206 (1956).
235. V. P. Dole, *J. Clin. Invest.*, **35**, 150 (1950).
236. R. S. Gordon, Jr., and A. Cherkes, *Proc. Soc. Exptl. Biol. Med.*, **97**, 150 (1958).
237. L. A. Carlson and L. Orö, *Metab. Clin. Exptl.*, 12, 132 (1963).
238. E. Shafrir, K. E. Sussman, and D. Steinberg, *J. Lipid Res.*, **1**, 109 (1959).
239. R. J. Havel and A. Goldfien, *J. Lipid Res.*, **1**, 102 (1959).
240. D. Steinberg, P. J. Nestel, E. R. Buskirk, and R. H. Thompson, *J. Clin. Invest.*, **43**, 167 (1964).
241. M. C. Shotz and I. H. Page, *J. Lipid Res.*, **1**, 466 (1960).
242. A. Gilgen, R. P. Maickel, O. Nikodijevic, and B. B. Brodie, *Life Sci.*, No. 12, 709 (1962).
243. S. Mayer, N. C. Moran, and J. Fain, *J. Pharmacol. Exptl. Therap.*, **134**, 18 (1961).
244. R. A. Salvador, K. I. Colville, S. A. April, and J. J. Burns, *J. Pharmacol. Exptl. Therap.*, **144**, 172 (1964).
245. J. J. Burns, K. I. Colville, L. A. Lindsay, and R. A. Salvador, *J. Pharmacol. Exptl. Therap.*, **144**, 163 (1964).
246. H. M. Maling, M. A. Williams, B. Highman, J. Garbus, and J. Hunter, *Arch. Exptl. Pathol. Pharmakol.*, **248**, 54 (1964).
247. E. W. McChesney, J. P. McAuliff, and H. Blumberg, *Proc. Soc. Exptl. Biol. Med.*, **71**, 220 (1949).
248. R. S. McCutcheon, *J. Pharmacol. Exptl. Therap.*, **136**, 209 (1962).
249. W. B. Cannon, *Bodily Changes in Pain, Hunger, Fear and Rage*, Charles T. Branford, Boston, 1953.
250. E. Bulbring in *Adrenergic Mechanisms* (J. R. Vane, G. E. Wolstenholme, and M. O'Connor, eds.), Churchill, London, 1960, p. 275.
251. J. Axelsson and E. Bulbring, *J. Physiol. (London)*, **153**, 30 P (1960).
252. R. L. Hill and J. Buethner-Janusch, *Federation Proc.*, **23**, 1236 (1964).
253. A. C. Wilson, N. O. Kaplan, L. Levine, A. Pesce, M. Reichlin, and W. S. Allison, *Federation Proc.*, **23**, 1258 (1964).
254. J. M. Van Rossum, *J. Pharm. Pharmacol.*, **17**, 202 (1965).

255. W. C. Lee and C. S. Yoo, *Arch. Intern. Pharmacodyn.*, **151**, 93 (1964).
256. C. E. Powell, W. R. Gibson, and E. E. Swanson, *J. Am. Pharm. Assoc.*, **45**, 785 (1956).
257. P. M. Lish, K. W. Dungan, and E. L. Peters, *J. Pharmacol. Exptl. Therap.*, **129**, 191 (1960).
258. N. Haugaard and M. E. Hess, *Pharmacol. Rev.*, **17**, 27 (1965).
259. L. I. Goldberg, M. de V. Cotten, T. D. Darby, and E. V. Howell, *J. Pharmacol. Exptl. Therap.*, **108**, 177 (1953).
260. W. D. Conway, *Federation Proc.*, **25**, 623 (1966).
261. H. Minatoya, *Federation Proc.*, **25**, 623 (1966).
262. A. Arnold, J. P. McAuliff, F. P. Luduena, T. G. Brown, Jr., and A. M. Lands, *Federation Proc.*, **25**, 500 (1966).

CHAPTER 9

SYNTHETIC POSTGANGLIONIC SYMPATHETIC DEPRESSANTS

N. B. CHAPMAN

DEPARTMENT OF CHEMISTRY
THE UNIVERSITY OF HULL
HULL, ENGLAND

JAMES D. P. GRAHAM

PHARMACOLOGY DEPARTMENT
THE WELSH NATIONAL SCHOOL OF MEDICINE
THE PARADE, CARDIFF, WALES

9.1. INTRODUCTION

The subject matter of this chapter is synthetic drugs that reduce or abolish the effects of administered catecholamines and of stimulating the postganglionic nerves of the sympathetic nervous system, in so far as these are mediated by the release of a catecholamine transmitter. Excluded from discussion, for example, are such drugs as atropine, which abolish the effects of stimulating the fibers of the sympathetic supply to the sweat glands in the pad of the cat, which have long been recognized as cholinergic.

A. Morphology of Sites of Action

The terminal parts of the adrenergic fiber have been found (*1*) to consist of bundles of unmyelinated axons covered by Schwann cells. In places there are axon surfaces naked of Schwann covering, which are separated from the surface of smooth-muscle cells by a narrow interval lined with basement membrane. If this is indeed the synapse of the adrenergic fiber, it is not less than 100 mμ in width. The nerve substance in this region contains a number of microvesicles of various sizes, which contain electron-dense material. More of these vesicles are in contact with the presumed synaptic surface than with surfaces of the nerve covered by Schwann cells, and administration of reserpine significantly diminishes the number of vesicles seen. No chromaffin cells in close proximity to this region are visible.

B. Synthesis of Transmitter

The stimulation of adrenergic nerves causes a release of norepinephrine, but it is noteworthy that some organs contain high concentrations of dopamine and that a small amount of epinephrine is released with the norepinephrine when certain sympathetic nerves are stimulated; see structures **(III)** to **(V)**. The pathway of synthesis of the transmitter which is generally accepted is

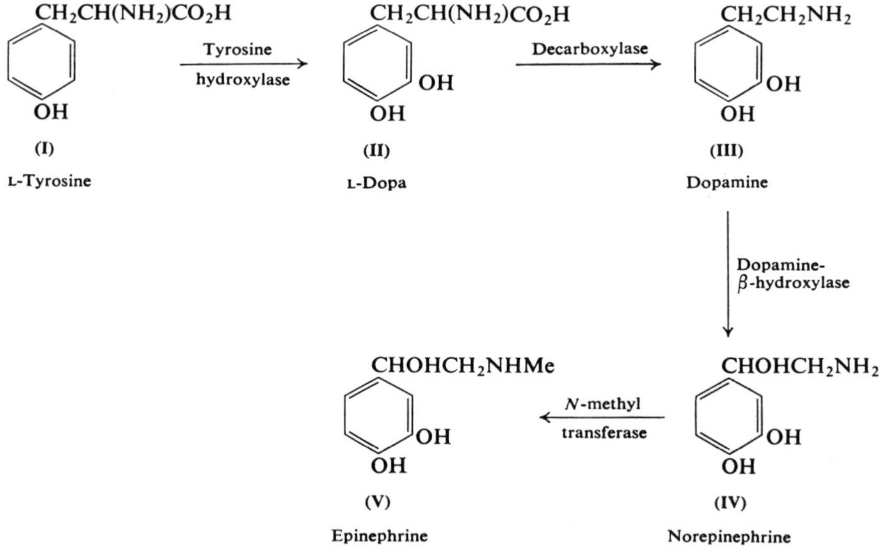

(I) L-Tyrosine

(II) L-Dopa

(III) Dopamine

(IV) Norepinephrine

(V) Epinephrine

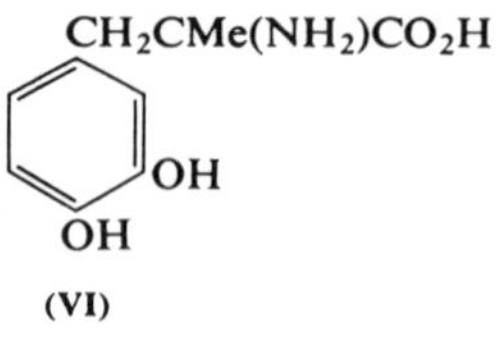

(VI) α-Methyldopa

indicated above. It has been elucidated by the administration to animals of isotopically labeled compounds which had been proposed as precursors and by the subsequent separation, largely chromatographic, and identification of the labeled end products. L-Tyrosine (4-hydroxyphenylalanine) **(I)**, which may be synthesized from phenylalanine (*2*), reaches the adrenergic nerve from the extracellular fluid and is converted into L-dopa (3,4-dihydroxyphenylalanine) **(II)** by a highly specific oxidative enzyme, tyrosine hydroxylase.* L-Dopa is then decarboxylated, forming dopamine (3,4-dihydroxyphenylethylamine or 3-hydroxytyramine) **(III)**. The enzyme responsible, a decarboxylase linked with pyridoxal phosphate, is not specific, as it can act upon L-5-hydroxytryptophan to form 5-hydroxytryptamine (5-HT) and upon other aromatic amino acids (*3*); it is, nevertheless, known colloquially as dopa decarboxylase. A number of other compounds, including α-methyldopa (AMD) **(VI)**, are known to be substrates for this system and are in clinical use for the relief of hypertension. The dopamine is stored in cytoplasmic granules or converted into norepinephrine. This step is catalyzed by dopamine-β-hydroxylase,† an enzyme which may be inhibited by adrenergic blocking agents such as xylocholine (TM-10).‡ The norepinephrine may be stored in granules in the adrenergic nerve, or it may exist free in the cytoplasm. In further stages methylation of the amino group in the side chain of norepinephrine, resulting in epinephrine or in *N*-methylepinephrine (*4*), is carried out in the adrenal medulla by *N*-methyltransferases. This is unimportant here. The rate of synthesis of norepinephrine is increased by stimulation of the adrenergic nerve, which is difficult to exhaust by physiological means, and there is no convincing evidence that dopamine is released from the nerve at any stage. The main transmitter is, therefore, norepinephrine.

C. Release of Transmitter

It is very difficult to determine whether or not physiologically released transmitter has emanated from the same source as norepinephrine which can be extracted from tissues or subcellular fractions or be released by the action of reserpine or some other drug. More is known about morphology and conditions in the adrenal medulla (*5*) and the brain (*6*) than about terminal

* According to M. S. Levitt and associates (*J. Pharmacol. Exptl. Therap.*, **148**, 1, 1965), this hydroxylation is the rate-limiting step in the biosynthesis of norepinephrine. See also T. Nagatsu et al., *J. Biol. Chem.*, **239**, 2910 (1964), S. Spector et al., *J. Pharmacol. Exptl. Therap.*, **157**, 86 (1965), and L. Maitre, *Life Sciences*, **4**, 2249 (1965), for studies of the isolation and inhibition of tyrosine hydroxylase and the blockade of the biosynthesis at the step catalyzed by it. For a review, see S. Udenfriend, *Pharmacol. Rev.*, **18**, 43 (1966).

† For reviews, see S. Kaufman, and S. Friedman, *Pharmacol. Rev.*, **17**, 71 (1965), and S. Kaufman, *Pharmacol. Rev.*, **18**, 61 (1966).

‡ *N*-2-(2,6-Dimethylphenoxyethyl)-*N*,*N*,*N*-trimethylammonium bromide.

adrenergic nerves (*7*). There is a widespread scatter of chromaffin cells throughout tissues (*8*), and it is the main contention of Burn (*9*) that so-called adrenergic nerves are, in fact, cholinergic, in that they release acetylcholine as their neurotransmitter, and that this acts upon chromaffin cells and brings about a release of catecholamine from them or from granules in the nerve.

D. Subsynaptic Receptors

Whatever the source of the norepinephrine, it diffuses across the synaptic gap and acts upon the subsynaptic membrane of the effector cell. The difficulties of interpreting various phenomena in terms of the classification of its receptors (*10*) which are named according to the relative potencies of sundry catecholamines, the nature of the response to them, and the efficacy of antagonists, are too well known to merit review here. Stimulation of the α receptor is followed by a depolarization phenomenon and a contraction of smooth-muscle cells. The receptor must, therefore, be on or in the cell membrane, and ion flux must follow its activation. Ion flux may involve a linked adenosine triphosphate complex resembling that of the so-called β receptor, but with essential differences. Monovalent and divalent cations will profoundly affect its action. The β receptor is now known to be a system of adenyl cyclase enzymes which promotes the formation of other nucleotides from adenosine triphosphate (*11*) and which is Mg^{++}-linked (*12*). Catecholamines have a hormonal function here as activators.

E. Depletion of Transmitter

If an abnormal precursor of catecholamine is present as a result of the administration of an unnatural compound, such as AMD, and is taken into the chain of reactions, an abnormal transmitter will be produced, such as α-methylnorepinephrine. If such a substance is less effective than the natural transmitter, the function of the nerve will be more or less inhibited.

The two main channels of inactivation of the released norepinephrine are storage and degradation, the latter being certainly enzyme-catalyzed. It is certain that norepinephrine in the extracellular fluid, whether it gets there as a result of injection into the bloodstream or release from functioning adrenergic nerves, can be taken up by tissues and held firmly in an inactive form. The site of this binding is not necessarily the same as the source of the norepinephrine released on stimulation of adrenergic nerve, but the interplay between the various stores will affect the functioning of the nerve, and drugs which block it may act, at least in part, on this storage site or pool. Thus, reserpine, bretylium, guanethidine, and cocaine may preferentially occupy various binding sites.

The enzymes which play a part in degradation are catechol *ortho*-methyl transferase, COMT (*13*),* and monoamine oxidase, MAO (*14*). Their action is illustrated by the conversion of **(III)** into **(VII)** or **(VIII)**. Similarly, if

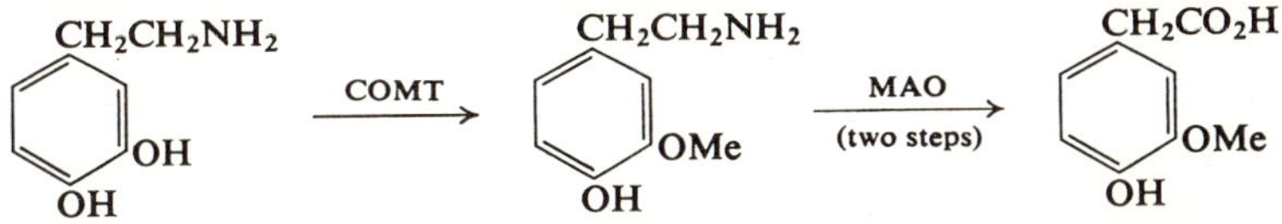

(III) Dopamine

(VII) 3-Methoxytyramine

(VIII) Homovanillic acid

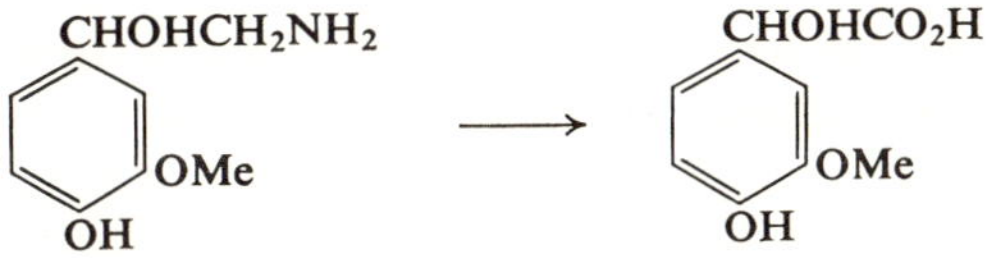

(IX) Normetanephrine

4-Hydroxy-3-methoxymandelic acid

norepinephrine is the substrate, normetanephrine **(IX)** and 4-hydroxy-3-methoxymandelic acid are the products. These are excreted in the urine unchanged, conjugated, or further metabolized. Many drugs are able to inhibit these enzymes.

F. Site of Action of Postganglionic Sympathetic Depressants

Synthetic drugs which reduce the activity of adrenergic nerves may act at any of the following places in the following ways. It is becoming clear, however, that the boundaries between them are less well defined than was previously believed.

(1) The drugs may act on the postganglionic neuronal axon so as to prevent conduction of the nerve impulse (local anesthesia). The classic local anesthetics will not be discussed here, but it may be mentioned that the undoubted local anesthetic action of bretylium and related drugs could play an important part in their activity as blockers of adrenergic neurones.

(2) The drugs may act on the synthesis of the transmitter by the following mechanisms:

inhibition of the transport of tyrosine into neurones (nothing is known of this mechanism),
inhibition of tyrosine hydroxylase,†

* See J. Axelrod, *Pharmacol. Rev.*, **18**, 95 (1966).
† See footnote, Section 9.1, B.

inhibition of dopa decarboxylase (AMD and its congeners are substrates and competitive inhibitors),
formation of an ineffective end product (AMD does this), and
inhibition of dopamine-β-hydroxylase (bretylium may be active, but a more potent and specific inhibitor should be obtainable).*

(3) The drugs may act on the release of the transmitter. Drugs which cause release of norepinephrine from its stores include reserpine, bretylium, guanethidine, phenoxybenzamine, and sympathomimetic amines. The last do not bring about failure of nerve function. The norepinephrine pools which these drugs drain are at different sites (*15*) and have different physiological significances.

(4) The drugs (for example, bretylium) may act as inhibitors of a cholinergic mechanism with unique properties—that is, if the nerve fibers are in fact cholinergic.

(5) The drugs may act on the enzymic degradation. Drugs which increase the rate of enzymic degradation caused by catechol *ortho*-methyl transferase or the action of MAO have not as yet been reported. The inhibitors of these enzymes enhance the effects of nerve stimulation.

(6) The drugs may act on the storage of precursor or transmitter. Drugs which prevent the re-entry of discharged catecholamine into the stores allow it to remain in a form vulnerable to degradation and thus may reduce subsynaptic receptor occupancy, and they enhance the effect due to injection of catecholamine or stimulation of the adrenergic nerve (as with cocaine); or they may reduce the availability of transmitter and block the nerve (guanethidine does this). These actions depend on the site of the store concerned. There is an overlap in the mechanism of action of such drugs which is still confusing.

(7) The drugs may act on the subsynaptic membrane or beyond. They may block the α or β receptor or both. A wide range of compounds, alkaloids and synthetics, can do this.

9.2. PRESYNAPTIC BLOCKADE OF ADRENERGIC NERVE

A. Synthetic Substances Interfering with the Synthesis of Norepinephrine

A stable preparation of hog kidney may be made (*16*) which contains active decarboxylase. Studies with this preparation (*16*, *17*) revealed that 3,4-dihydroxy-2′-methyl-(AMD) **(VI)**, 3,4-dihydroxy-6-methyl-phenylalanine, and *erythro*-3-hydroxyphenylserine are good substrates for the enzyme and, in sufficient concentration, completely inhibit its action on dopa. In the main, inhibitors of this enzyme system have structure **(X)**. Generally, activity is

* See M. Goldstein, *Pharmacol. Rev.*, **18**, 77 (1966).

greater when $R = R_1 = OH$ than when $R_1 = H$ and $R = OH$, and greatest when $R_2 = OH$, alkoxyl, alkyl, or aryl. Caffeic acid (3,4-dihydroxycinnamic acid), where $R = R_1 = R_2 = OH$ and $R_3 = R_4 = H$, is active, and substitution of a 3-mercapto group for the 3-hydroxyl increases activity. Esters of cinnamic

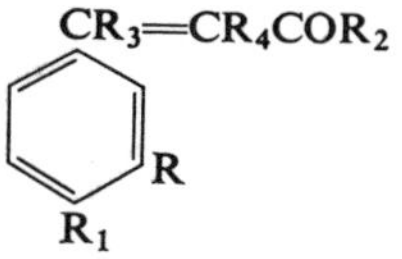

(X)

acids are as good inhibitors as the acids themselves. An α-methyl or an α-ethyl group substituted into the side chain does not alter activity relative to that of the unbranched compounds. Reducing the side chain in structure **(X)** to a two-carbon group destroys activity; most compounds with a single-carbon side chain are inactive, as are the related phenols. Active compounds are all substrates for decarboxylase and cause a fairly specific and slowly reversible competitive inhibition of it as a result of combination with the apoenzyme. Amides are less active than free acids, but chalcones, and flavones **(XI)** may

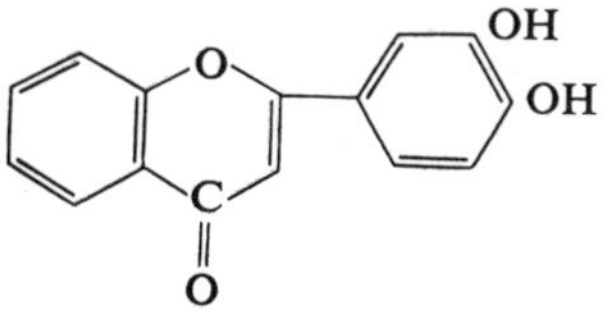

(XI)

be very active. Phenylpyruvic acid also retains some activity. Of the two hundred compounds examined in the study (*17*) the most potent proved to be 5-(3,4-dihydroxycinnamoyl)salicylic acid **(X)**, where $R = R_1 = OH$, $R_3 = R_4 = H$, and $R_2 = 4\text{-}OHC_6H_3CO_2H\text{-}3$, the salicylic acid residue. Many of the compounds were insoluble in water.

α-Methyl homologues of valine, leucine, serine, aspartic acid, and asparagine are known. Enzymic studies revealed strong inhibition of mammalian glutamic acid decarboxylase. -Meαthylmethionine is a potent inhibitor of the action of D-amino acid oxidase on phenylalanine and is also a methionine antagonist. Porter and his co-workers (*18*) found that DL-α-hydrazino-3,4-dihydroxyphenyl-α-methylpropionic acid is very potent, while having no effect on the MAO system; this type of study has been extended (*19*) to cover eleven related benzylhydrazines and benzyloxyamines of varying potency.*

* See also T. L. Sourkes, *Pharmacol. Rev.*, **18**, 53 (1966).

B. Actions and Mode of Action of α-Methyldopa (AMD)

The effects of administering AMD to animals and man are not in dispute. The decarboxylase of kidney (*20*) and other tissues is inhibited by the L isomer of the acid, and sympathetic vasomotor tone is reduced. These facts may be causally related. The blood pressure falls; AMD also acts centrally as a sedative and hypnotic. The acute pharmacological responses to administration of dopa and of 5-hydroxytryptophan, 5-HTP (*21*), are prevented. The urinary levels of metanephrine and normetanephrine rise, and that of homovanillic acid falls (*22*).

The content of 5-HT and of norepinephrine in brain and in peripheral tissue is reduced (*23*). With 5-HT this depletion is relatively short-lived and is proportional to the concentration of AMD, but with norepinephrine the depletion persists for several days (*24*). It has accordingly been suggested that AMD causes a slow and continuing release of catecholamine from tissue stores, in particular of norepinephrine from adrenergic nerves (*25*, *26*), which is then destroyed by catechol *ortho*-methyl transferase and MAO, and that this action is reinforced by a diminished capacity for reabsorption and binding of extra-cellular catecholamine (*27*). Whatever the precise mechanism, and there is no reason to deny that all of those described may play a part, there are both resemblances to and differences from the mode of action of guanethidine.

First, AMD merely reduces, but does not abolish, the effects of stimulating an adrenergic nerve (*28*, *29*). This reinforces the hypothesis that it acts as an antimetabolite (*17*, *30*) by producing α-methylnorepinephrine which is usually a weaker pressor agent than is norepinephrine (*31*). With α-methyl-*m*-tyrosine **(XII)** it is more certain that the end product metaraminol **(XIII)** is less active; **(XII)** is effective in reducing the blood pressure in man (*32*).

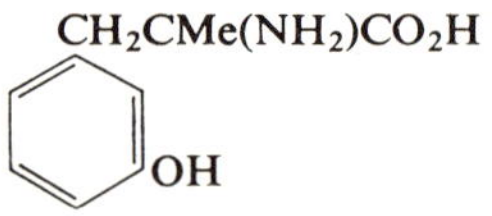

(XII)

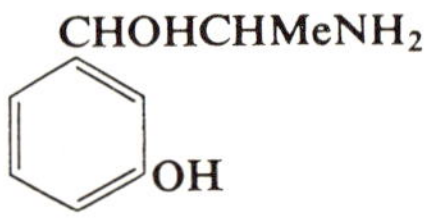

(XIII)

Second, AMD causes a substantial fall in the blood pressure of hypertensive patients when they are lying down, without reducing the renal blood flow. This is not so with guanethidine. Both drugs may cause bradycardia from blockade of the sympathetic accelerator supply to the heart; both cause some orthostatic hypotension, especially after exercise. It has been suggested that AMD reduces the cardiac output, but the evidence about this is conflicting (*33*, *34*). A reduction of extracellular fluid volume through concomitant diuretic therapy increases the hypotensive effect of AMD (*35*), but this is probably an additive effect, because a reduced circulating volume reduces the output from the heart. It has been suggested that AMD reduces the sensitivity of the tissues to circulating norepinephrine, but this is not so, although, like guanethidine, it reduces the effect of sympathomimetics, which act by the release of tissue catecholamine (*29*). It is also claimed (*36*), as a result of studies of renal and cardiac hemodynamics, that AMD has a direct action in relaxing arteriolar smooth muscle and thus in lowering peripheral vascular resistance. This would bring about a reduction in cardiac output.

AMD acts centrally as a depressant, causing sedation, drowsiness, and mental depression. In mice it reduces the toxicity of amphetamine (*37*), an action which is prevented by prior treatment with inhibitors of MAO. Nevertheless, the effects obtained are contradictory, as AMD is a direct antagonist of reserpine-induced depression (*38*, *39*) and causes great excitement in mice pretreated with these same inhibitors of MAO. AMD reduces the levels both of 5-HT and of norepinephrine in brain but does not increase the urinary output of 5-hydroxyindoleacetic acid, the usual metabolic end product of 5-HT (*40*).

The same temporal difference is found between the restoration of norepinephrine and 5-HT (*41*) as was found in the heart and other peripheral tissues. Vogt (*42*) concludes that AMD acts both as an inhibitor of dopa decarboxylase and as an antimetabolite, which is probably as near to the truth as we are likely to get. When taken by mouth some 50% of AMD is absorbed. The major portion of this is excreted in the urine within 48 hours, 24% as unchanged AMD and 64% as sulfate (*43*).

C. Blockade of Adrenergic Neurones

Blockade of adrenergic neurones arises from the action of drugs which block sympathetic pathways by causing a failure in the release of norepinephrine at nerve terminals. A clear distinction is to be drawn between these drugs, which have little effect on the action of circulating epinephrine or norepinephrine, and those causing postsynaptic sympathetic blockade, often called sympatholytics, which antagonize the action of extracellular epinephrine or norepinephrine on the relevant tissue, commonly a smooth-muscle cell. It is not our intention to attempt an exhaustive account of these drugs but, in keeping with the outlook of the volume as a whole, to try to deal only with such relations between pharmacodynamic action and chemical constitution as have emerged. In this area these relations are of distinctly limited scope.

D. Structure–Activity Relationships

The point of departure in the study of these substances, whose history is relatively short, is the work of Hey and Willey (*44*), who synthesized TM-10

(XIV). In association with Bain and his co-workers (*45*), it was shown that this compound abolished the effects of stimulating postganglionic adrenergic nerves. The powerful muscarinic effect of TM-10 diminished its potential

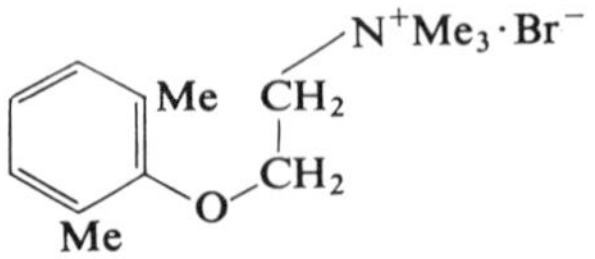

(XIV)

Xylocholine, TM-10

value as a therapeutic agent. Not surprisingly, however, its discovery led to synthesizing numerous related compounds with the primary aim of finding drugs free from the unwanted muscarinic activity. Of compounds structurally very close to TM-10 the corresponding 2,6-dichloro compound has been shown to be active. A *C*-methyl derivative of this compound **(XV)**, where

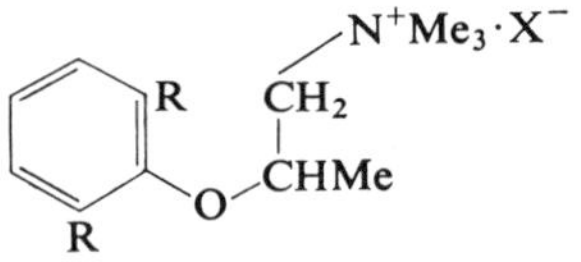

(XV)

R=Cl, is also active and free from muscarinic activity (*46*, *47*). The (+) isomer of **(XV)**, in which R is Me, was significantly more active than its enantiomer. In these compounds a large cationic head or larger substituents in the 2 or 6 position abolish activity.

The structural features of TM-10 which were preserved in the more successful developments were the ammonium pole and a phenyl or substituted phenyl group, but the geometrical relationship was not the same as in TM-10, whose aryl group and ammonium pole are separated by four bond distances (approximately carbon-carbon single-bond distances). Indeed, in the potent and rather specific benzyl quaternary ammonium compounds (*48*) this separation was reduced to two carbon-carbon bond distances, and the cationic head did not contain the trimethylammonio group N^+Me_3, but an ethyldimethylammonio group, N^+Me_2Et, or a 2-hydroxyethyldimethylammonio group,

$$N^+Me_2CH_2CH_2OH.$$

An *N*-benzyl-*N*-2-hydroxyethyl-*N,N*-dimethylammonium salt **(XVI)** was an early example of a drug more or less free from side effects, whereas the corresponding *N*-ethyl-*N,N*-dimethyl compound was more active but showed disadvantageously high toxicity and muscarinic activity. The structures of active compounds were, however, limited to cationic heads of the type N^+Me_3, N^+Me_2Et, and $N^+Me_2CH_2CH_2OH$. Whatever theory of the mode of action of this particular class of compound may be developed, it seems that it must accommodate the fact that only compounds having a cationic head of a limited size and complexity are effective. On the other hand, the quaternary nitrogen may become part of a nor-α-tropinium structure without loss of activity (see below).

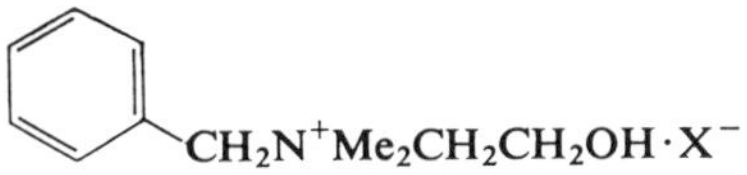

(XVI)

Recently Fielden et al. (*49*) described coumaran (2,3-dihydrobenzofuran) derivatives, such as those shown in structure **(XVII)** (SK&F 90, 109) and structure **(XVIII)**, where R = 7-Me (SK&F 90, 238), which are cyclic analogues

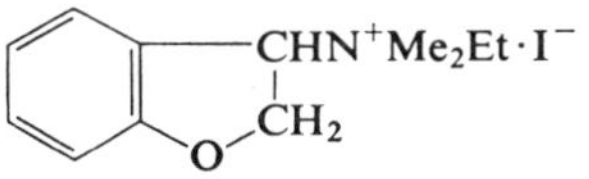

(XVII)

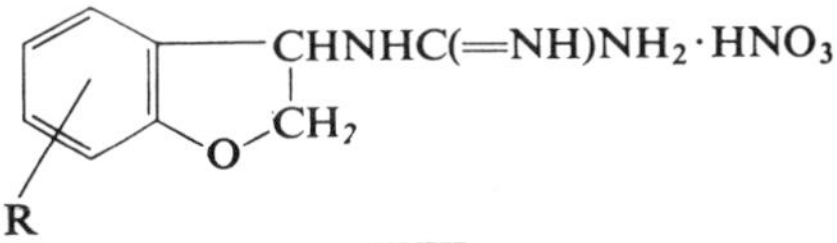

(XVIII)

of TM-10. These two examples show an activity in blocking adrenergic neurones that is of the same order as that of TM-10. The most active compound has structure **(XVIII)** with R = 5-Cl. All compounds with the guanidino side chain were active, whereas most of the others were inactive.*

The most important compound from the therapeutic viewpoint and the best investigated is bretylium, *N*-(2-bromobenzyl)-*N*-ethyl-*N*,*N*-dimethylammonium bromide or toluene-*p*-sulfonate **(XIX)** (*48*). Like other *ortho*-

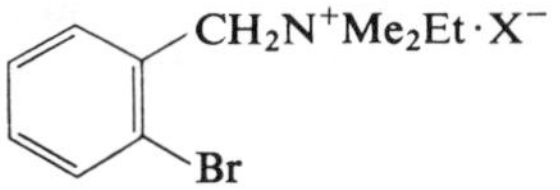

(XIX)

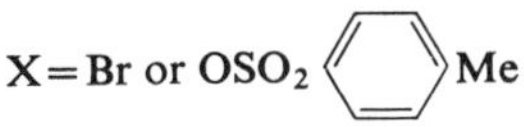

substituted compounds of this type it is virtually free from muscarinic activity. Variation of the *ortho* substituent from the electron-releasing methyl (comparable in size to bromine) through all four halogens (save fluorine,

* See also D. I. Barron et al., *Brit. J. Pharmacol.*, **25**, 534 (1965).

having the smallest size and relatively weak net polar effect) which are weakly electron-withdrawing, results in little or no change in activity, and apart from diminished duration of action the same is true when the *ortho* substituent is the powerfully electron-withdrawing nitro or trifluoromethyl group (*50*). It is noteworthy that replacement of the benzyl group in structure **(XVI)** by phenyl, α-methylbenzyl and, more interestingly, the isosteric 2-thenyl or 2-picolyl group led to inactive compounds (*51*). Compounds **(XX)** and **(XXI)**, however, showed moderate activity. Recently a group of nor-α-tropinium derivatives **(XXII)** which block adrenergic neurones have been reported

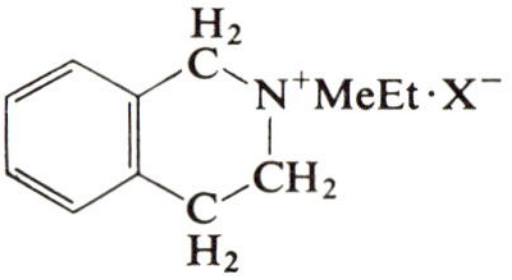

(XX)

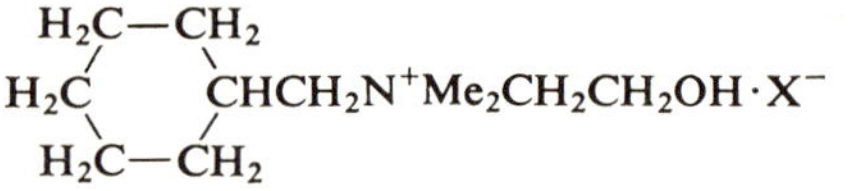

(XXI)

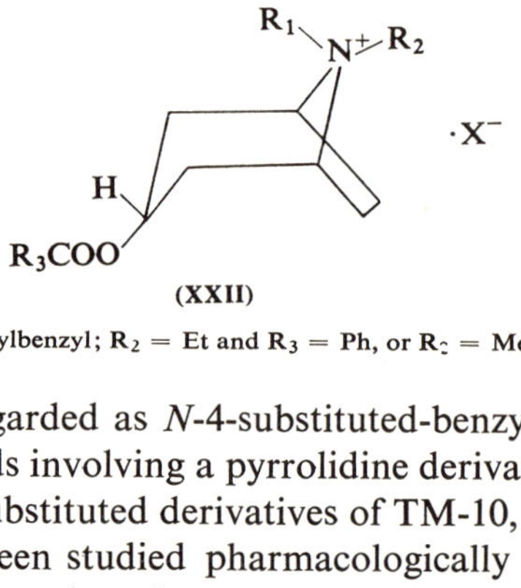

(XXII)

R_1 = 4-cyclohexylbenzyl; R_2 = Et and R_3 = Ph, or R_2 = Me and R_3 = *p*-tolyl

(*51*). These can be regarded as *N*-4-substituted-benzyl-*N*-ethyl- (or methyl-) ammonium compounds involving a pyrrolidine derivative.

A long series of 4-substituted derivatives of TM-10, prepared by Copp and his co-workers, has been studied pharmacologically by Boura and his co-workers (*53*). An ethoxycarbonyl, an acetyl, or a benzoyl group in the 4 position resulted in diminution or abolition of parasympathomimetic effects and often increased blocking of adrenergic neurones. The 4-benzoyl compound **(XXIII)**, which can be regarded as a benzophenone derivative, was very active

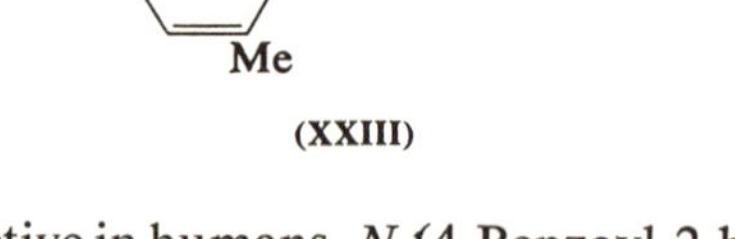

(XXIII)

in cats but much less active in humans. *N*-(4-Benzoyl-2-bromobenzyl)-*N*-ethyl-*N*,*N*-dimethylammonium salts, which combine the structural features of bretylium and of compound **(XXIII)**, as is often the case when this type of structural variation is studied, show only moderate activity. The most active compound derived from benzophenone was **(XXIV)**, in which the ammonium pole and the nearer benzene ring are separated by four carbon-carbon bond distances, as in TM-10.

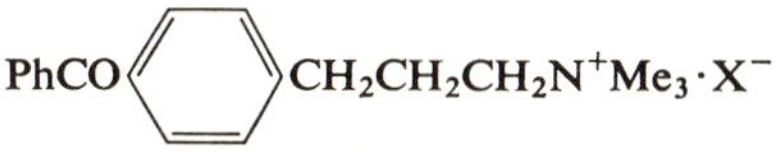

(XXIV)

Another group of compounds capable of adrenergic-neurone blockade, but which have structures only very tenuously connected with those previously discussed, are salts of derivatives of guanidine and related functional groups, that is, salts of amidoxime and amidine derivatives. Of these the most important is guanethidine **(XXV)** (*54*). Interest in these structures stemmed from the discovery that salts of the amidoxime derivative **(XXVI)** showed notable

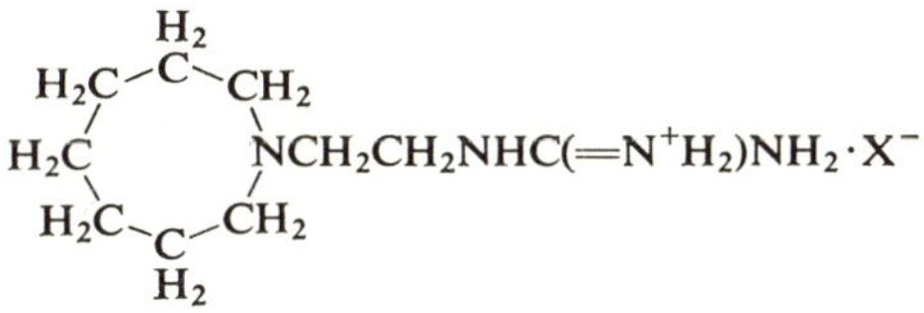

(XXV)

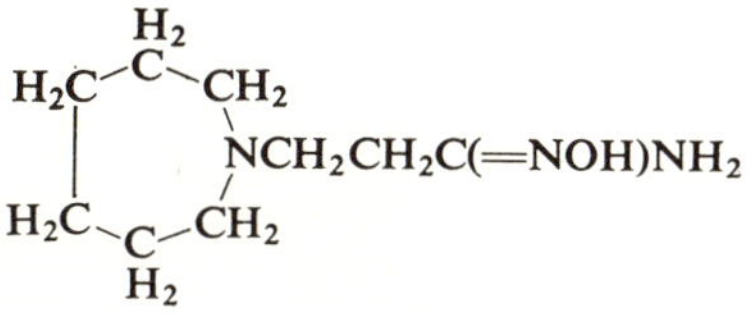

(XXVI)

antihypertensive activity in dogs; the presence of the amidoxime group and the seven-membered ring were soon shown to be necessary to the pharmacological action (*55, 56*). It was a natural step to the study of guanidine derivatives; maximal activity was shown with the eight-membered ring, and with a pair of methylene groups separating the guanidino group from the ring.

Amidine derivatives closely related to guanethidine and showing comparable activity are compounds **(XXVII)** and **(XXVIII)** with R = Me. Other values of

$$(CH_2)_nNCH_2CH_2C(=NH)NH_2$$

$n = 6$ or 7

(XXVII)

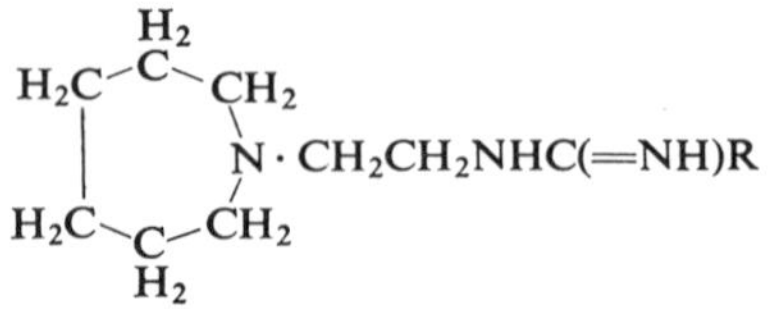

(XXVIII)

R gave relatively inactive compounds (*57*, *58*). Other active guanidine derivatives containing the *o*-bromo or chloro group (cf. bretylium) and aryloxy groups related to those of TM-10 and its congeners have been studied (*59*) without revealing any novel principles of structure–activity relationships. Short and his co-workers (*60*) have studied a further large group of guanidine derivatives and found that 1-[2-(4-methylpiperazino)-ethyl]guanidine trihydrochloride and 1-(2-diethylaminoethyl)-guanidine sulfate and its 3-methyl derivative were the most active compounds. These structures admit of very little change, such as homologation to give the 1-(3-diethylaminopropyl) analogue, without loss of activity. Hermansen (*61*) examined *N*-(2-guanidinoethyl)-hexahydrobenzo-[*d*]-azocine sulfate, which blocks adrenergic neurones without causing an initial rise in blood pressure. Augstein and Green (*62*)* reported on the efficacy of attaching cationic heads derived from guanidine, aminoguanidine, amidine, and amidoxime residues to the 2-phenoxyethylamine or the 2-aminoalkyl-1,4-benzodioxan residue, a process which, it was hoped, would increase the affinity of the compounds for sites of adrenergic action. Recent work by Najer et al. (*63*) deals with some *N*-2-guanidinoethylazaspiroalkanes, but no novel principles emerge from it.

The tenuous connection that these guanidine, amidoxime, and amidine derivatives have with the compounds discussed earlier in this section arise from their possession of a strongly basic functional group which will remain extensively protonated at biological pH. Consequently, these compounds will possess a positive pole in vivo, usually separated four or five bond distances from the nitrogen atom of a polyatomic quasi-alicyclic ring or three, four, five, or six bond distances from an aromatic ring. Brodie and his co-workers (*64*), in a brief study of the structural requirements for bretylium-like and guanethidine-like activity in guanidine derivatives, concluded that separation of the positive pole (protonated guanidine group or quaternary ammonium group) from a benzene ring by a single carbon atom gave rise to a bretylium-like effect, whereas a two-carbon separation was associated with a guanethidine-like effect. The tenuousness of the structural relations is clear: it rests on the universal possession of a positive pole, and the rest of the molecular structure has little in common, in the case of guanethidine and its immediate congeners, with the structures of the other classes of compounds.

* See also J. Augstein et al., *J. Med. Chem.*, **8**, 446 (1965).

E. Mechanism of Action

The mechanism of action of the adrenergic neurone blocking compounds has been the subject of detailed investigation.

TM-10 has various pharmacological effects, which include stimulation of autonomic ganglia, inhibition of amine oxidase activity, and neuromuscular blockade. These are weak or transient effects, but TM-10 has quite strong nicotinic and muscarinic cholinomimetic actions and is a powerful local anesthetic. Hey and Willey (*44*) suggested that the last property might account for the action of main interest, the failure of postganglionic nerves to respond to stimulation, which overtakes tissues one hour after exposure to this substance. Exley (*65*) demonstrated that this was not so and suggested as an alternative an interference with the biosynthesis of the adrenergic nerve transmitter, norepinephrine. The details of this controversy have been given by Bain (*45*). The major effect is probably due to multiple actions involving, primarily, depletion of the available store of norepinephrine in the neuronal terminal but, as Fielden et al. (*49*) point out in a recent discussion of this complex issue, the precise mode of action of drugs of this class has yet to be determined.

The main observed features of the mode of action of bretylium and guanethidine and their congeners are essentially similar to those of TM-10. The principal effect is a prolonged failure of tissues to respond to stimulation of postganglionic sympathetic nerves. It results from selective adsorption of the drug by the neurone (*66*).* It is apparently due to the combined inhibition of biosynthesis (*67*), prolonged slow release of the transmitter from its neuronal store, and blockade of the usual absorption of catecholamines from extracellular fluid (*68*, *69*).

Bretylium and guanethidine cause a transient rise in blood pressure when first administered. This may be due to a release of norepinephrine from nerve endings, to a direct action on arteriolar smooth muscle, sensitizing it to circulating catecholamine—that is, a postsynaptic effect (*70*)—or to inhibition of amine oxidase, which is a notable attribute of certain congeners of these compounds (*71*). It has been suggested that the hypotensive action of guanethidine is due in part to an effect on β receptors in the vascular musculature which is a postsynaptic site of action. The boundaries between the sites of action of the different categories of drug may not, therefore, be as clear as had once been thought (*72*).

Little account has been taken so far in this review of the opinion of Burn (*9*), that postganglionic "adrenergic" neurones are actually cholinergic, and that the acetylcholine released when they are stimulated exerts a nicotinic action similar to that found in the adrenal medulla and releases norepinephrine from

* See also B. B. Brodie et al., *Brit. J. Pharmacol.*, **25**, 171 (1965); R. A. Maxwell, *J. Pharmacol. Exptl. Therap.*, **148**, 320 (1965).

a neuronal store. There is much evidence for and against this attractive theory. If it proves correct, the action of these drugs may be inferred to be due wholly or partly to interference with this cholinergic function, an effect similar to that of a ganglion-blocking agent or a curariform relaxant, but exerted at a presynaptic intraneuronal subsynapse which is cholinoceptive and catecholamine-secretory. These ideas still have only the status of a hypothesis, but it is noteworthy that guanethidine has been shown to exert a curariform action on the neuromuscular junction (*73*).

In conclusion we note that the whole subject of the blocking agents of adrenergic neurones has recently been critically and comprehensively reviewed by Boura and Green (*74*).

9.3. POSTSYNAPTIC SYMPATHETIC BLOCKADE

A. Blockade of α-Receptors

1. STRUCTURE–ACTIVITY RELATIONSHIPS

a. Halogenoalkylamines

(1) *Congeners of Dibenamine*. A wealth of information is available on the subject of Dibenamine congeners but, whatever inferences are drawn, the limitations and complexity of the pharmacological observations should be strongly borne in mind. This is particularly important when quantitative pharmacological results are under consideration; indeed, these can at best form the basis of only qualitative relationships and theories.

The first lengthy account of the subject was given by Nickerson and Gump (*75*), whose list of requirements for an active compound, based on a survey of structure and activity in a considerable series of congeners of Dibenamine, $N(CH_2Ph)_2CH_2CH_2Cl$, may, with one or two amendments in the light of later discoveries, be summarized as follows. Certain requirements must be met: the compound must contain a tertiary amino group [see Section 9.3, A 1.a (2)], it must contain at least one 2-halogenoalkyl group capable of entering into aziridinium ion formation, it must include an unsaturated ring substituent attached to the amine in such a way as to allow resonance stabilization of the active intermediate aziridinium ion, and the ring substituents in benzyl derivatives, should not be out of the plane of the ring. The third requirement has been criticized (*76*) and, in the judgment of the present authors, is insecurely founded, but on the whole subsequent work has confirmed these requirements.

In 1956 the ground was again surveyed in a very detailed and comprehensive way by Ullyot and Kerwin (*77*). They recorded "specific data for all the compounds reported in the literature up to June 1952, and a number of unreported compounds." A detailed survey of structure–activity relationships up to that time was given. In 1962 Graham (*78*) again reviewed structure–activity relations in this field and noted that most of the compounds studied in the intervening period had been specially selected for their interest in relation to structure–activity theory. Only the more important features of the work up to that time will now be considered.

Graham assembled evidence to show that in a group of compounds of given carbon structure, such as that of the *N*-ethyl-*N*-(1-naphthylmethyl)-2-halogenoethylamines, variation of the halogen leads to antiepinephrine or antinorepinephrine activity according to the following order (*75*, *77*, *79*): $I \approx Br > Cl \gg F$. The observed changes in pharmacological activity stemming from this structural variation were as substantial as those stemming from more profound skeletal changes in the molecule. In particular, the fluoro compounds, which on both theoretical and experimental grounds were believed not to form aziridinium ions under conditions identical with, or similar to, those pertaining in vivo, had very little activity, if any. It has since been shown (*80*) that certain simple 2-fluoroethylamines, $FCH_2CH_2NH_2$ and $NH(CH_2CH_2F)_2$, do form the related aziridinium ion at measurable rates in basic deuterium oxide solution (the choice of solvent depended on the use of nuclear magnetic resonance measurements to study the reactions in question) at temperatures of 80 to 90°C. It would, however, imply a long and highly insecure extrapolation from these observations to suggest that simple fluoroethylamines or, for example, *N*-ethyl-*N*-(1-naphthylmethyl)-2-fluoroethylamine would give rise to significant amounts of aziridinium ion in vivo. Moreover, the suggestion made by the same authors, that "toxicity masks adrenergic blocking action" with these compounds, receives little support from the observed LD_{50} values, especially when it is noted that for a given family of halogeno compounds the fluoro compound is the least toxic but least active pharmacologically (*79*). Chapman and James (*76*) also showed that compounds which fulfilled other structural requirements were inactive because of the presence of an *N*-phenyl group and so had too weakly nucleophilic a nitrogen atom to enter into aziridinium ion formation.

If, relative to Dibenamine = 1, the activities of compounds of the type $ArCH_2NRCH_2CH_2Cl$, where R = alkyl, or the type $ArCH_2N(CH_2Ar)CH_2CH_2Cl$ are surveyed, they lie for the most part in the range 0.25 to 4.0 (*78*). Noteworthy exceptions are found with the compounds $PhOCH_2CHMeN(CH_2Ph)CH_2CH_2Cl$ (phenoxybenzamine) and $2\text{-}ClC_6H_4CH_2NEtCH_2CH_2Cl$, whose values are 20 and 15, respectively. The compound $Me_2NCH_2CH_2N(CH_2Ph)CH_2CH_2Cl$ is inactive, because it readily forms a piperazinium salt **(XXIX)** rather than an aziridinium salt, but the corresponding ω-dimethylaminopropyl compound is active: it forms the aziridinium salt **(XXX)** (*75*, *77*).

Replacement of a benzyl group by a phenethyl or a cinnamyl ($PhCH{=}CH{-}CH_2$) group has little effect on activity, but replacement by an α-methylphenethyl group (cf. phenoxybenzamine) doubles activity, and by a

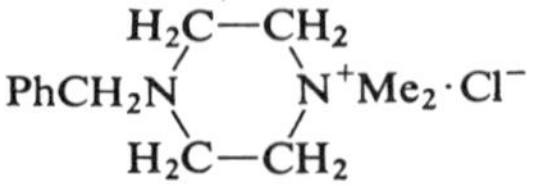

(XXIX)

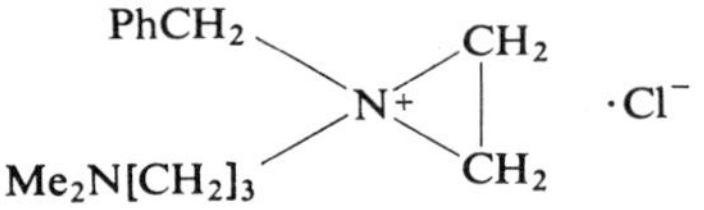

(XXX)

3,4-dihydroxy-(or dimethoxy-)α-methylphenethyl, giving **(XXXI)**, where $R{=}H$ or Me, results in a 5-fold increase. On the other hand, isosteric replacement of one or both benzyl groups by 2-thienyl decreases the activity ten times.

$$3,4\text{-}(RO)_2C_6H_3CH_2CHMeN(CH_2Ph)CH_2CH_2Cl$$

(XXXI)

$$PhOCH_2CHMeN(CH_2CH{=}CH_2)CH_2CH_2Cl$$

(XXXII)

$$2\text{-}EtC_6H_4OCH_2CHMeN(CH_2Ph)CH_2CH_2Cl$$

(XXXIII)

However, the *N*-(α-methylphenethyl)-*N*-2-thienyl compound shows a 10-fold increase in activity. *N,N*-Bis-(2-phenoxyethyl)-2-chloroethylamine, $(PhOCH_2CH_2)_2NCH_2CH_2Cl$, is more or less as active as Dibenamine, the replacement of one of its 2-phenoxyethyl groups by 2-phenoxyisopropyl resulting in a 20-fold increase in activity. Related compounds of high activity are those of structures **(XXXII)** and **(XXXIII)**, having relative activities of 15 and 10, respectively (*81*, *82*). Two other subgroups of compounds which have been much investigated and which show enhanced activity with $R{=}Et$ in each case are represented by structures **(XXXIV)** and **(XXXV)**. The former, with $R{=}Et$

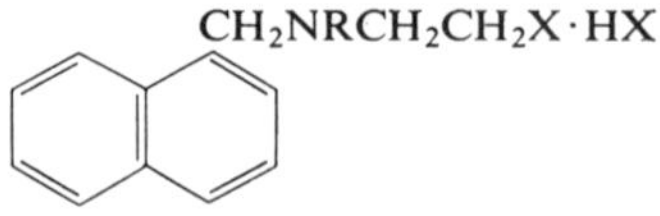

(XXXIV)*

* When $R{=}Et$ and $X{=}Br$, this is known as SY-28.

and X=Cl, has a relative activity of 10; the latter, with R=Et and X=Cl, a relative activity of 15. Isosteric replacement of the 1-naphthyl residue of structure **(XXXIV)** by a 3-thionaphthenyl residue reduces activity tenfold and, if R is $PhCH_2$, there is also a substantial reduction in activity. The influence of the variation of X (Cl, Br, or I) in compounds such as these has already been mentioned. Replacement of the 1-naphthyl residue of structure **(XXXIV)** by a 2-naphthyl group abolishes activity: the analogous 1-acenaphthenyl and 9-phenanthryl compounds are only two times more active than Dibenamine (*78*).

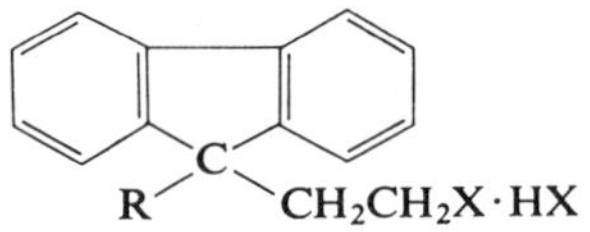

(XXXV)

In 1961 Schipper et al. (*83*) reported on "the synthesis and 'adrenolytic activity' of a series of *N*-substituted 2-chloromethyl- and 2,5-bis(chloromethyl)-pyrrolidines", and a few analogous derivatives of piperidine and tetrahydroisoquinoline. Although the *N*-substituted pyrrolidines bearing a single chloromethyl group were only weakly active by comparison with Dibenamine and phenoxybenzamine, 1-benzyl-2,5-bischloromethylpyrrolidine was "several hundred times" more effective than Dibenamine and had a considerably more favorable therapeutic index. The 1-butyl compound, however, was virtually inactive. The analogous 1-(2-phenoxyethyl)-, 1-(2-phenoxyisopropyl)-, and 1-(2-bromobenzyl)- compounds had activities very similar to that of Dibenamine, whereas the piperidine and tetrahydroisoquinoline derivatives were some ten or more times less active. The "dramatically enhanced 'adrenolytic' activity produced by the introduction of the second chloromethyl substituent" is discussed in terms of a possible "anchimeric assistance by the second chloromethyl group of nucleophilic attack by the receptor site" on an intermediate (and presumably pharmacologically active) aziridinium ion. The importance of the 1-benzyl group for activity over that of the 1-butyl group indicates that these compounds are essentially congeners of Dibenamine and conform to Belleau's "phenylethylamine" pattern [Section 9.3, A 1. a(4)].

An interesting new development due to Cignarella et al. (*84*) includes structures such as **(XXXVI)**. With X=Cl and Ar=Ph a compound 25 times

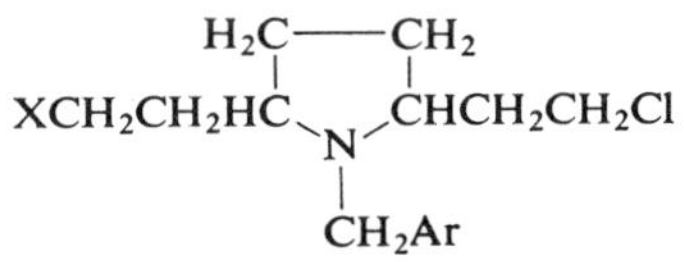

(XXXVI)

more active than phenoxybenzamine was obtained; with X=Cl and Ar=*o*-BrC_6H_4 the relative activity was 7.5; with X=OEt and Ar=Ph the relative activity was again 7.5.

(2) *Congeners of DMEA.* Hunt (*85*) first observed notable antiepinephrine activity in the first member of the series *N,N*-dimethyl-2-chlorophenethylamine (DMEA), and Ferguson and Wescoe (*86*) gave a full account of the pharmacology of this compound. They made the points that the blocking activity was of immediate onset and of short duration, and that the related aziridinium ion mediates all the actions of DMEA, and they noted the close structural relationship between agonist and antagonist in this case.

The synthesis and chemical properties of a large group of congeners of DMEA were first reported by Chapman and Triggle (*87*, cf. *88*). Graham and James (*89*) had previously given a full account of the pharmacology of a selection of the compounds. A further group of compounds was reported by Chapman et al. (*90*), and detailed pharmacological studies were published by Graham and Karrar (*91*).

The results assembled in Table 9.1 show that the most active of the compounds listed in it are some 200 times more active than Dibenamine and some ten times more active than phenoxybenzamine. Ferguson and Wescoe's observations of immediacy of onset and short duration of action have been confirmed. Significant activity is observed with certain secondary amino compounds (*87*, *89*) (numbers 14 and 18 in Table 9.1), a phenomenon only rarely observed among epinephrine antagonists of the halogenoethylamine series. Moreover, whereas *N,N*-dimethyl-β-hydroxyphenethylamine and the corresponding *N,N,N*-trimethylammonium compound are virtually inactive (*89*), *N,N*-dimethyl-2-bromo-1-phenylethylamine hydrobromide and *N,N*-dimethyl-2-bromophenethylamine hydrobromide, which yield the same aziridinium ion at almost the same rate in 1:1 aqueous acetone at 30°C, were equiactive within the limits of experimental error. It may be inferred that not only is the *N,N*-disubstituted aziridinium ion **(XXXVII)** capable of mediating the antiepinephrine activity, but so is the N-monosubstituted species **(XXXVIII)**, which will coexist in equilibrium with the conjugate base (an *N*-methylaziridine) in vivo.

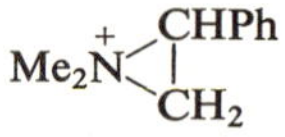

(XXXVII)

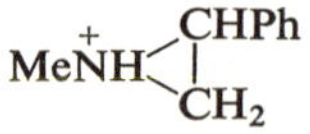

(XXXVIII)

It is also clear that a high level of activity is critically dependent on the nature of the *N*-alkyl groups. An increase in chain length beyond methyl and, particularly, a chain branching result in large decreases in activity, except for the *N,N*-diallyl compound and the 1-pyrrolidinyl compound. The replacement of one or both of the *N*-methyl groups necessary for high activity by

TABLE 9.1

Pharmacological Properties of some *N*-Mono- and *N*,*N*-Di-substituted 2-Chloro- (or bromo-) phenethylamine Hydrohalides, $C_6H_5CHYCH_2Z \cdot HY$

			ED_{50}, 10^{-6} mole/kg, for antagonism to	
No.	Z	Y	Epinephrine[a]	Norepinephrine[a]
	Dibenamine		7.7	10
	Phenoxybenzamine		0.28	0.55
1	NMe_2	Cl	0.046	0.1
2	$N(CH_2Ph)_2$	Cl	1.5	1.0
3	NMe_2	Br	0.035	0.056
4	NMeEt	Br	2.8	3
5	NEt_2	Br	5	1.8
6	N-*n*-Pr_2	Br	1	1.3
7	N-iso-Pr_2	Br	30	22
8	N-*n*-Bu_2	Br	4.4	4.5
9	$N(CH_2CH{=}CH_2)_2$	Br	0.03	0.03
10	Piperidino	Br	15	14
11	Morpholino	Br	4	4.5
12	1-Pyrrolidinyl	Br	0.05	0.08
13	$NMeCH_2Ph$	Br	2.4	1.7
14	NHMe	Br	0.6	0.5
15	NHEt	Br	100	80
16	NH-*n*-Pr	Br	very weak	very weak
17	NH-*n*-Bu	Br	very weak	very weak
18	$NHCH_2Ph$	Br	3	2.8

[a] Pressor test in the rat.

benzyl groups results in less diminution in activity than might be expected from size, but the *N*-benzyl compounds may owe their activity to a structural similarity to Dibenamine; see structures **(XXXIX)** and **(XL)**.

$$(PhCH_2)_2NCH_2CH_2Cl \cdot HCl$$

(XXXIX)

Dibenamine

$$(PhCH_2)_2NCH_2CHPhCl \cdot HCl$$

(XL)

In Table 9.2 results are assembled detailing the antiepinephrine activities of a series of *N*,*N*-dimethyl-2-bromophenethylamines with substituents (halogen

TABLE 9.2

Pharmacological Properties of some *N,N*-Dimethyl-2-bromo-2-(substituted-phenyl)ethylamine Hydrobromides and Related Compounds, 3-Z-4-$YC_6H_3CHBrCH_2NMe_2 \cdot HBr$ (*91*)

No.	Z	Y	ED_{50}, 10^{-6} mole/kg, for antagonism to: Epinephrine[a]	Norepinephrine[a]
1	H	Cl	0.002	0.002
2	H	Br	0.0006	0.0002
3	H	I	0.0006	0.0005
4	H	Me	0.0003	0.0007
5	H	Ph	0.030	0.030
6	F	H	0.030	0.032
7	Cl	H	0.0070	0.0071
8	Br	H	0.0050	0.0050
9	I	H	0.0040	0.0040
10	Me	H	0.0035	0.0030
11	Cl	F	0.0064	0.0064
12	Cl	Cl	0.0013	0.0013
13	Cl	Br	0.001	0.001
14	Br	F	0.0027	0.0027
15	Br	Cl	0.0012	0.0012
16	Br	Br	0.00045	0.00045
17	Br	Me	0.0003	0.0003
18	Me	F	0.0015	0.0015
19	Me	Cl	0.0011	0.0011
20	Me	Br	0.0006	0.0006
21	Me	Me	0.0005	0.0005
22	H	H	0.035	0.056

[a] Pressor test in the rat.

or methyl) in the 3 or 4 positions, or both, of the phenyl group. The more active members of this group of compounds, such as the 4-methyl, 4-bromo, or 4-iodo compounds or the 3-bromo-4-methyl compound, are some 10,000 times more active than Dibenamine (this activity is abolished by replacing the dimethylamino by the dicyclohexylamino group), and even the least active are about 100 times more active. We have here the most active antiepinephrine agents known. It may be mentioned in passing that both of the *N,N*-dimethyl-2-bromo-2-(1- or 2-naphthyl) analogues are more active than the parent compound, $PhCHBrCH_2NMe_2 \cdot HBr$. On the other hand, replacing the dimethylamino group of a 3,4-disubstituted phenyl compound by the larger morpholino or piperidino group causes a reduction in activity to a magnitude usually less than that of Dibenamine (*92*). Similarly, substituents in the 2 position of the phenyl group occasionally give rise to an activity (fluoro substituent) greater than that of Dibenamine, but usually it is noticeably less, possibly by as much as a factor of 100 (*93*).

(3) *Specificity.* It was initially assumed that 2-halogenoalkylamines exhibit a high degree of specificity in blocking the α receptors of norepinephrine. Various indications to the contrary have accumulated (for references see *78*). An attempt has been made to put this on a quantitative basis by recording an index of activity of drug antagonism, the pA_2 value, for three halogenoalkylamines which display widely varying antinorepinephrine potency in the popular pressor test, against a range of stimulants in one tissue. The results are shown in Table 9.3. SY-28 is a better antihistamine than norepinephrine antagonist; it is also a stronger antagonist of acetylcholine than the other two compounds. DMEA is 200 times stronger than Dibenamine in the pressor test, but not when in an equilibrium state on an isolated smooth muscle. These findings serve to reinforce the warning given in the opening paragraph of this section and to remind workers in the field of structure–activity relations, some of whom may not be deeply versed in biological studies, of the importance of drug affinity (*94*) to absolute potency and of the necessity of making comparative tests under rigidly controlled conditions with the same tissue before inferring a relation to molecular structure.

TABLE 9.3

Quantitative Drug Antagonism of Three Halogenoalkylamines[a]

pA_2 at 20 min[b] (vas deferens of guinea pig)					ED_{50}, μmole/kg (rat blood pressure)	
NE[b]	H[b]	3-HT[b]	Ach[b]	Brad[b]	NE[b]	2-Halogenoalkylamine
8.3	8.0	8.0	5.0	±	10.00[c]	Dibenamine
8.6[c]	9.2[c]	8.4	6.3	±	0.55[d]	SY-28
8.6	5.3	8.4	5.2	±	0.05[d]	DMEA

[a] Activities against the pressor action of norepinephrine in the spinal rat and against five stimulants of smooth muscle. SY-28 is a very powerful antihistamine, the figure confirming that of Graham and James (*89*). DMEA is weak. Atropine is $\approx$ 100 times more active than SY-28 against acetylcholine. All antagonize equally norepinephrine and dopamine. All may potentiate bradykinin in one concentration and antagonize it in higher concentration (*104*). The pA_2 is a measure of drug antagonism, the negative logarithm of the amount of antagonist (in moles) needed to reduce to its original value the effect of a double dose of the agonist.

[b] NE, norepinephrine: H, histamine; 3-HT, dopamine; Ach, acetylcholine; Brad, bradykinin.

[c] Nickerson and Gump (*75*).

[d] Graham and Karrar (*91*).

(4) *Theory of Drug–Receptor Interaction.* We now proceed to an exposition of a theory of drug–receptor interaction in this field due mainly to Belleau (*95*). Most of the facts assembled in this section concerning Dibenamine and its congeners appear to be capable of rational correlation in terms of this theory; a somewhat modified version of it with respect to DMEA and its congeners is due to the present authors (*90*) and independently to Triggle (*96*).

In 1958 Belleau (*95*) published a paper of profound theoretical importance for an understanding of the action of congeners of Dibenamine in blocking catecholamine α receptors. His theory is based squarely on a view, well known in the chemistry of N and S mustards and originally advanced by Nickerson and Gump (*75*) and strongly supported by Chapman and Graham and coworkers (see *78* for references), that not only do Dibenamine, its congeners, and many other 2-halogenoalkylamines, when liberated from their salts in aqueous solution, more or less rapidly and completely form the related aziridinium ion (well known as an alkylating agent), but also this ion (or one closely related to it and very readily formed from it) is the biologically active species. This view was supported by the isolation and characterization of crystalline aziridinium picrylsulfonates (*97*), which in favorable cases could be examined pharmacologically and shown to be highly active (*98*), and was supported also by a widely observed proportionality, where a suitable aziridinium salt could not be isolated, between the blocking activity and the chemically determined concentration of aziridinium ion (*99*, *100*). It is also worthy of emphasis that Dibenamine and its congeners, after an initial phase involving potentiation and competitive antagonism, produce an insurmountable blockade, which only reverts to surmountability when sufficient time has elapsed. It was a short and logical step, first taken by Nickerson and Gump (*75*), to ascribe the pharmacological effects of 2-halogenoalkylamines to the alkylation by the aziridinium ion of a nucleophilic group in the receptor, a similar idea having been also well developed in the biochemistry of N and S mustards. Harvey and Nickerson (*101*) claimed to have obtained evidence of the involvement of thiol groups of proteins in the alkylation; the status of their evidence was permissive rather than compelling. Belleau (*95*) advanced good reasons for favoring a carboxylate or phosphate anionic group (A in Figure 9.1) both as an essential binding site in the catecholamine α receptor for the protonated amino group of sympathomimetic agents and as one which would be readily alkylated by an aziridinium ion to yield a more or less readily hydrolyzable ester. Anchimeric assistance from appropriately placed groups was thought to occur in the hydrolysis. Alkylation would lead to "masking" of the receptor and blockade; hydrolysis, to "unmasking" and recovery. Thiol, hydroxyl, and amino groups are alkylated, giving intrinsically unreactive products, so enzymic dealkylation would have had to be postulated. In a later paper Belleau (*102*) favored the phosphate anionic group for A on

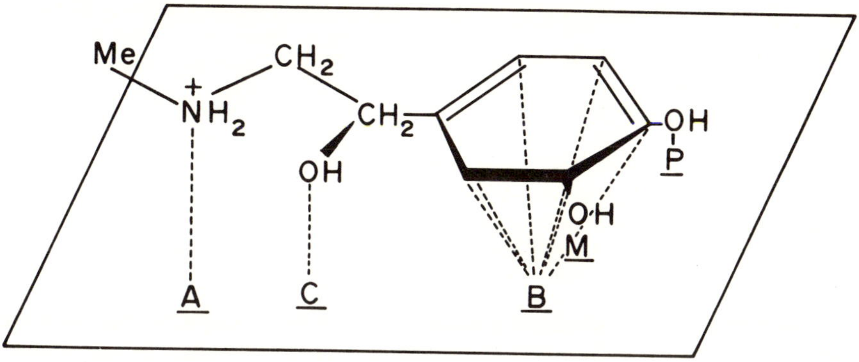

Fig. 9.1

the grounds that "phosphate esters of β-aminoalcohols are much more stable towards hydrolysis than carboxylate esters." This was thought to agree better with the long duration of the blockade produced by Dibenamine. Moreover, the lack of a difference in potency between norepinephrine completely labeled with deuterium on the α carbon ($3,4\text{-}(OH)_2C_6H_4CH(OH)CD_2NH_2$) and ordinary norepinephrine leads to the reasonable conclusion that "the binding of the ammonium function (positive pole) of noradrenaline by alpha-receptors does not concern the α-hydrogen atoms" (*103*). Evidence of a deuterium isotope effect in known substrates of MAO is provided, so α-deuterionorepinephrine apparently does not act as a substrate for MAO at the receptor level.

Graham and Katib (*104*) have provided evidence in favor of alkylation of a carboxylate group. They have shown that brief administration of trypsin to a tissue blocked by SY-28 results in partial or complete restoration of the sensitivity of the tissue to epinephrine or to norepinephrine. Trypsin-like enzymes are known to occur in blood and body fluids. If it may be assumed that trypsin is specific to certain amide bonds and to carboxylate ester linkages but is without action on phosphate ester linkages, then it seems that the establishment and reversal of blockade involve respectively, alkylation of a carboxylate group and hydrolysis of the ester formed.

In Figure 9.1 is shown a second binding site, B, responsible for the binding of the benzene ring in catecholamines. The interaction of a pressor drug with site A is supposed to "trigger an excitatory response," whereas site B "contributes mainly to efficacious binding of the drug." Other binding centers, P and M, are concerned with the catecholic hydroxyl groups, and a binding center (not shown) for the alcoholic hydroxyl group is also necessary, but this, it was asserted, had been shown by Lands (*105*) to be essentially associated with inhibitory responses. We shall discuss the importance of this site later in connection with a development of Belleau's theory which is necessary for an understanding of the behavior of the DMEA group.

Great importance was attached to the distance separating sites A and B and to the "phenylethylamine pattern," described as follows (*95*):

"Regardless of the nature of the functional groups, a given molecule will be considered potentially active either as an agonist or antagonist if it includes a group capable of interacting with site A and if one of the probable conformations allows this group to be located at approximately three interatomic distances away from a ring possessing aromatic character."

Presumably, carbon-carbon interatomic distance is implied here. A four-point contact (A, B, P, and M) of agonist or antagonist with the receptor was suggested: it is arguable that this should be a five-point contact; see Fig. 9.1. Enzyme studies have suggested that the catecholic hydroxyls undergo chelation with a metal, possibly magnesium, which itself is bound by chelation to the receptor surface.

Recognizing the carbonium ion character of the carbon atoms of the aziridinium ring, Belleau proposed that site A of the receptor, which binds the positive pole of an agonist, should be responsible, after initial interaction with the positive pole of the aziridinium ion, for the ultimately covalent binding of an aziridinium ring carbon atom (Figures 9.2 and 9.3). Aziridinium ring-opening then ensues, and the net result in Dibenamine congeners is the alkylation of A through the nucleophilic displacement of the β-halogen of the drug; "a more or less labile ester is produced." Further, the "phenylethylamine pattern" is destroyed. The rate of hydrolysis of the ester produced is determined by other factors, such as anchimeric assistance. The importance of the interaction of the benzene ring with B is strongly emphasized in relation to the transition from the arrangement of Figure 9.2 to that of Figure 9.3.

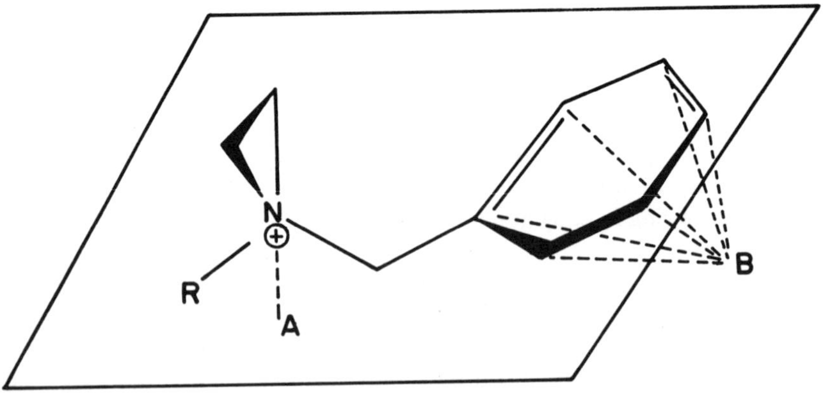

Fig. 9.2

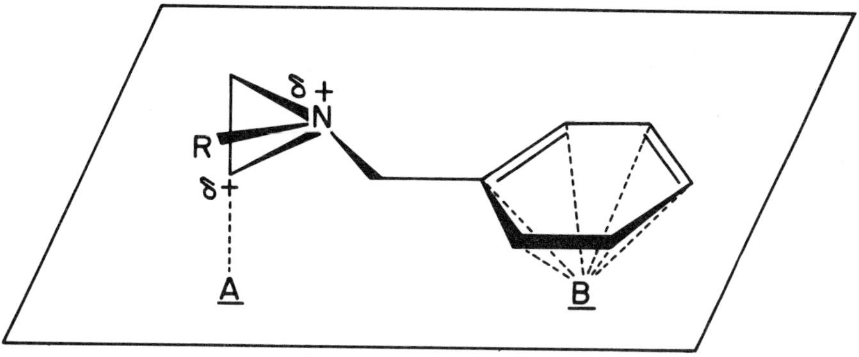

Fig. 9.3

It is inferred from the fact that the electron-releasing catecholic hydroxyl groups considerably strengthen agonist activity that a greater electron density in the benzene ring strengthens its interaction with B. Consequently, substituents in Dibenamine congeners having polar properties similar to those of hydroxyl groups ($+E$ and $\pm I$ effects) and being situated in the 3 or 4 position, or both of the benzene ring, provided their size is limited, should enhance activity. Because rotation of the ring can disorient a 3-substituent in relation to site M, a single substituent would be expected to be more effective in the 4 position. The data assembled in Table 9.4 show how successful the theory is qualitatively.

At first glance the phenoxyethylamine group of Dibenamine congeners $C_6H_5OCH_2CHRNR'CH_2CH_2Cl$, and the related aziridinium ion, C_6H_5O-$CH_2CHRN^+R'(CH_2)_2$, deviate from the "phenylethylamine" pattern. However, there is evidence (*106*) that a β-related oxygen atom facilitates the cyclization of the halogenoethylamine to aziridinium ion; the relevant activated complex (transition state) is shown in structure **(XLI)**.

Given the carbonium-like character of the aziridinium carbon atoms in the fully formed ion, an analogous $C^{\delta+}$–O interaction would also stabilize the ion.

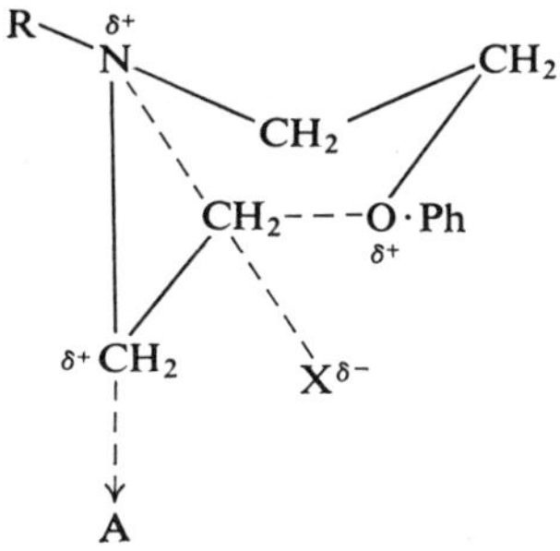

(XLI)

TABLE 9.4

Structure and Activity of Congeners of Dibenamine[a]

	Character of substituent	Compatibility[b] with P	Predicted activity	Observed range of activity
	$C_6H_5CH_2N(CH_2CH_2Cl)(C_2H_5)$			
Substituent in phenyl ring:				
1. 2-CH_3	$+I$		act.	act.
2. 2-OCH_3	$+E, -I$		act.	act.
3. 4-OCH_3	$+E, -I$	C	act.	inact.
4. 3-CF_3	$-I$		act.	act.
5. 3-Cl	$-I, +E$		act.	act.
6. 4-C_2H_5	$+I$	X	inact.	inact.
7. 4-Cl	$-I, +E$	doubtful	inact.	slight act.
8. 3,4-$(OCH_3)_2$	$+E, +E$	±C	slight act.	slight act.
9. 3,4-(OCH_2O)	$+E, +E$	C	act.	slight act.
	$(C_6H_5CH_2)_2NCH_2CH_2Cl$			
Substituent in one ring:				
10. 2-OCH_3	$+E$		act.	act.
11. 3-CF_3	$-I$		act.	slight act.
12. 3-I	$-I, +E$		act.	act.
13. 4-CH_3	$+I$	C	act.	act.
14. 4-OCH_3	$+E, -I$	C	act.	act.
15. 3,4-$(OCH_3)_2$	$+E, +E$	±C	act.	act.
16. 3,4-(OCH_2O)	$+E, +E$	C	act.	slight act.
Substituent in both benzyls:				
17. 2-CH_3	$+I$		act.	act.
18. 3-CH_3	$+I$		act.	act.
19. 3-CF_3	$-I$		act.	slight act.
20. 3-Cl	$-I, +E$		act.	slight act.
21. 4-CH_3	$+I$	C	act.	act.
22. 4-C_2H_5	$+I$	X	inact.	inact.
23. 4-OCH_3	$+E, -I$	C	act.	act.
24. 2,4-Cl_2	$-I, -I$	ring strongly deactivated	inact.	inact.
25. 3,4-Cl_2	$-I, -I$	ring strongly deactivated	inact.	inact.

[a] From Belleau (*95*); the observed data were taken from Ullyot and Kerwin's review (*77*). Significant activity is designated by act., and, unless otherwise noted, does not refer to the degree of activity.

[b] Absolute compatibility of a 4 substituent with site P, based on positive or negative effect of substituent on pressor activity of sympathomimetic amines. C, compatible; X, incompatible. In case of incompatibility at P the unsubstituted benzyl is considered to interact with site B.

Moreover, this conformation allows the point of attachment to A in the receptor to take up a position approximately three carbon-carbon bond distances from the benzene ring. The high blocking activity of compounds of the type of phenoxybenzamine, $PhOCH_2CHMeNEtCH_2CH_2Cl$, is understandable on this basis, as is the lack of activity of a hydrocinnamyl isostere, such as $PhCH_2CH_2CH_2NRCH_2CH_2Cl$. However, an analogous argument, dependent on the relations shown in structure **(XLII)**, accounts for the activity

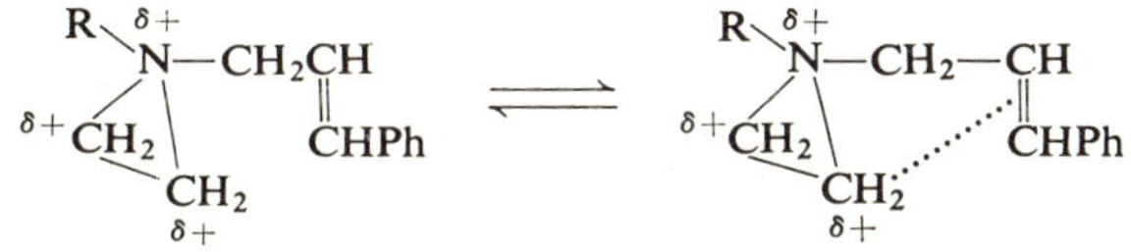

(XLII)

of the cinnamyl derivative, the π electrons of the olefinic bond having a role similar to that of lone-pair *p*-electrons of an oxygen atom. A satisfactory account also can be given of the effect of substituents in the phenyl ring of these phenoxy compounds. Unfortunately, an attempt (*102*) to obtain explicit experimental evidence in favor of this attractive hypothesis by measurement of rates of cyclization of compounds of the type *p*-$XC_6H_4O[CH_2]_2NEtCH_2$-CH_2Cl gave no evidence of a regular relation between rates of cyclization and the electron-releasing power of X and, consequently, of the ether-oxygen atom, as measured by the basicity of amines of the type *p*-$XC_6H_4O[CH_2]_2NEt_2$. The author (*102*) had to fall back on somewhat less specific conformational arguments.

Evidence in favor of the involvement of the folded conformation of structure **(XLI)** in the structure of aziridinium ions derived from phenoxyethyl compounds was obtained from the synthesis, effected by Belleau and Cooper (*107*), of rigid cyclic analogues of these compounds, viz. the *cis* and *trans* isomers of *N*-methyl-*N*-2′-phenoxycyclopentyl-2-chloroethylamine, **(XLIII)**, which yield

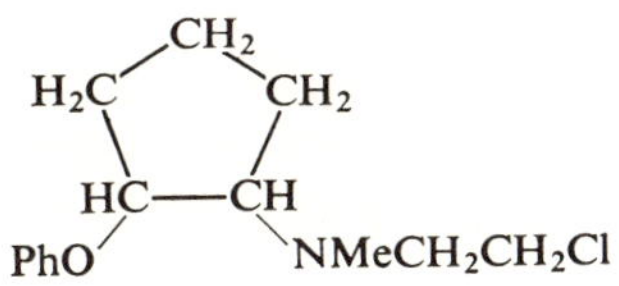

(XLIII)

aziridinium ions having the Newman projection formulae, **(XLIV)** and **(XLV)**. The pharmacological studies reported are extremely slender, but there seems to be evidence that these isomers are respectively approximately equipotent with, and more potent than, phenoxybenzamine.

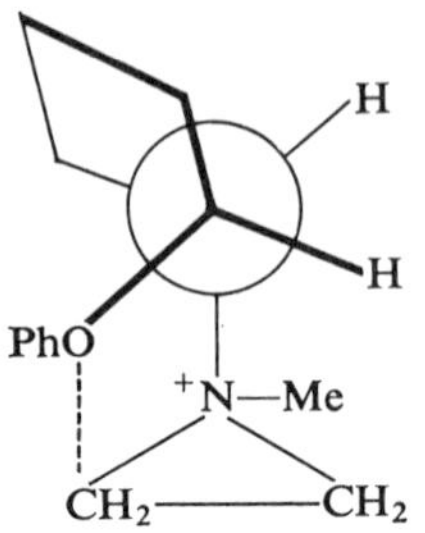

(XLIV)

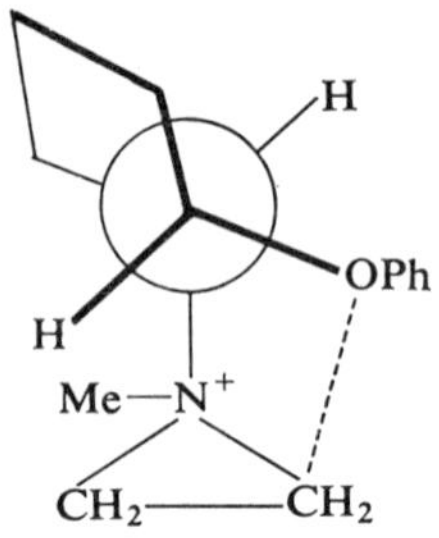

(XLV)

A satisfactory account of the blocking activity of 2-halogenoalkylamines containing condensed polynuclear aromatic residues, such as a 1-naphthylmethyl group in place of the benzyl groups of Dibenamine, can also be given in terms of an order of the electron-donating power of the aryl groups, for which independent evidence is available.

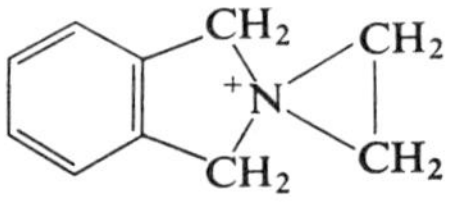

(XLVI)

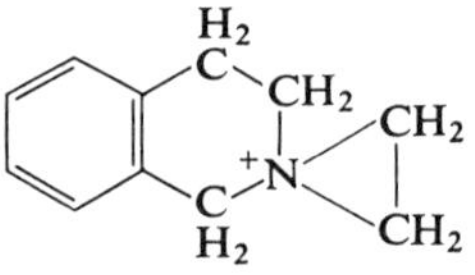

(XLVII)

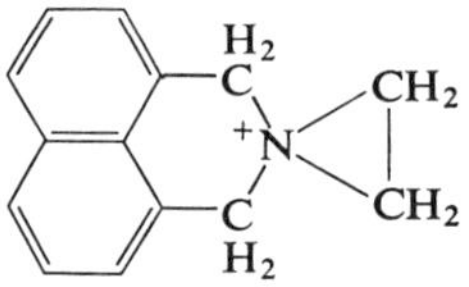

(XLVIII)

Spirocyclic aziridinium ions, structures **(XLVI)** to **(XLVIII)**, present some interesting features (*108*). In the parent 2-halogenoethylamine the structural analogy to Dibenamine and, hence, the "phenylethylamine" pattern are preserved, but the conformational rigidity of the ions apparently results in inactivity. However, this is not the case for structures **(XLIX)** and **(L)**; the former, for example, is among the most active *orally* effective compounds

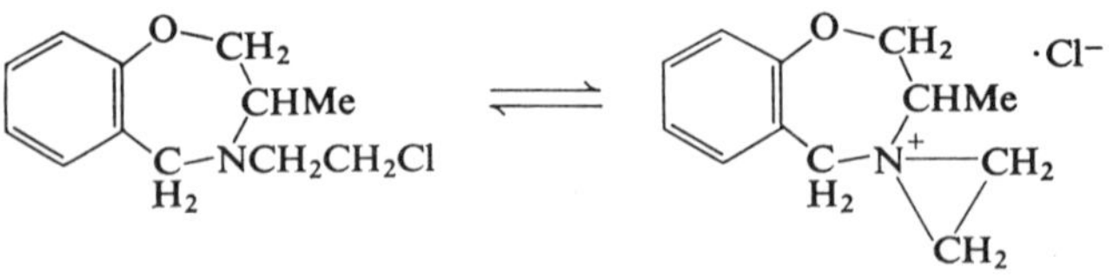

(XLIX)

known. Belleau (*108*) has advanced a conformational explanation of the differences between structures **(XLVI)** to **(XLVIII)** and structures **(XLIX)** and **(L)**, which depends on the greater conformational flexibility in the latter two.

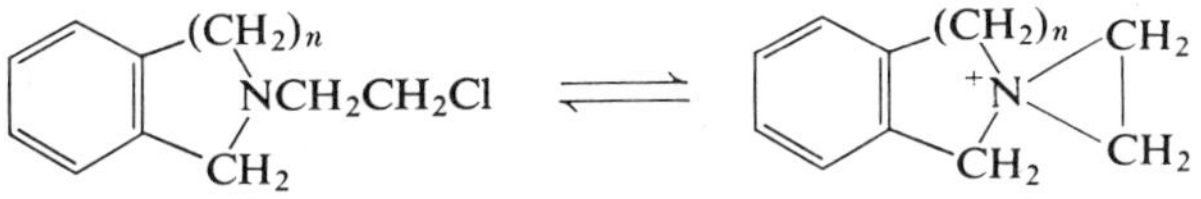

$n = 3$ or 4

(L)

In his 1958 paper Belleau (*95*) also offered an explanation of the structure–activity relations in the so-called DMEA series, $ArCHXCH_2NMe_2$, where X is Cl or Br and Ar is usually phenyl or substituted phenyl. This explanation has since been modified by Belleau himself (*103*) and more extensively by Chapman and his co-workers (*87*, *90*) and by Triggle (*96*).

Chapman and Triggle (*87a*) and Graham and Karrar (*91*) showed that, with the possible exception of the *N*,*N*-diallyl group, the *N*,*N*-dimethyl group was essential to high activity; for example, replacement of *N*,*N*-dimethyl by *N*,*N*-diethyl resulted in a 150-fold decrease in activity; by *N*,*N*-di-isopropyl, in an 850-fold decrease. *N*,*N*-Dibenzyl compounds had greater activity than expected on this basis but were regarded as Dibenamine congeners rather than true members of the DMEA group. For this reason subsequent work has been mainly concentrated on *N*,*N*-dimethyl compounds.

A few active compounds with secondary amino groups, such as $PhCHBr$-$CH_2NHMe \cdot HBr$ and $PhCHBrCH_2NHCH_2Ph \cdot HBr$, were discovered in this series. Liberation of the free bases from these salts would almost certainly give high yields of the corresponding tertiary aziridinium ions (protonated aziridines), in contrast to the usual quaternary ions. At physiological pH the protonated aziridines would be predominantly converted into the corresponding bases. Like epoxides (oxiranes), aziridines are alkylating agents, although they are less reactive than aziridinium ions, so the observed pharmacological properties are not entirely unexpected, provided the compounds possess a fundamental structure giving rise to high activity.

Chapman and Triggle (*87a*) demonstrated experimentally the rapid conversion of halogenoamines of the DMEA series into the corresponding aziridinium ions; similarly, the *N*,*N*-dimethyl-2-bromo-2-phenylpropylamine hydrobromide, $PhCMeBrCH_2NMe_2 \cdot HBr$, with its tertiary bromoalkyl group, had similar chemical reactivity to the secondary bromoalkyl analogue but was pharmacologically inactive. It appears that the moiety, ArCHBr, is essential to activity in these bromoalkylamines.

The observed activities of some twenty of these compounds are summarized in Table 9.5; see Graham and Karrar (*91*). The most active show a very high degree of activity ($\approx$ 10,000 times that of Dibenamine in the popular pressor test), appropriate substituents in the *meta* or *para* position of the phenyl group, or in both, being necessary for maximal activity. Except for fluoro compounds, *ortho*-substituted compounds are 100 to 1000 times less active than the corresponding *para* compounds (*94*). The observed order of activity may be summarized as follows: 3,4-disubstituted compound > *p*-compound > *m*-compound $\gg$ *o*-compound and, as substituents are varied, Me $\approx$ I > Br > Cl > F > Ph > H, whatever the position of substitution.

It is virtually certain that at physiological pH a 1,1-dimethyl-2-arylaziridinium ion will be rapidly and almost quantatively formed from the bromoethylamine, but Graham (*109*) has shown that in one case at least, that of SY-28, a significant proportion of the ion becomes attached to plasma proteins. There is also evidence that added egg albumin increases the rate of disappearance of the aziridinium ion in aqueous acetone (*110*). Nevertheless, a significant proportion and, it must be assumed, a more or less constant proportion of the aziridinium ion formed from the administered bromoethylamine must rapidly reach the α receptor of catecholamine. This particular point, however, requires fuller investigation than it has so far received, if our theorizing in this field is to be based as securely as possible. As in the case of many other compounds previously discussed, determinations of the relative antiepinephrine and antinorepinephrine activities of aged solutions of 1,1-dimethyl-2-(3,4-dibromophenyl)aziridinium bromide at successive points in time gave values which lay on the chemically determined curve showing the relative concentrations of the ion as a function of time. This is cogent evidence that the aziridinium ion or a species easily and directly obtained from it is responsible for the pharmacological activity. The most likely hypothesis in the light both of studies of the solvolysis of these aziridinium ions in 1:1 acetone and water at 37°C and of previous work is that the epinephrine antagonist in the form of the carbonium ion, **(LII)**, itself rapidly formed from the aziridinium ion, structure **(LI)**, reacts with a nucleophile, Y^-, in the receptor and so becomes attached to it.

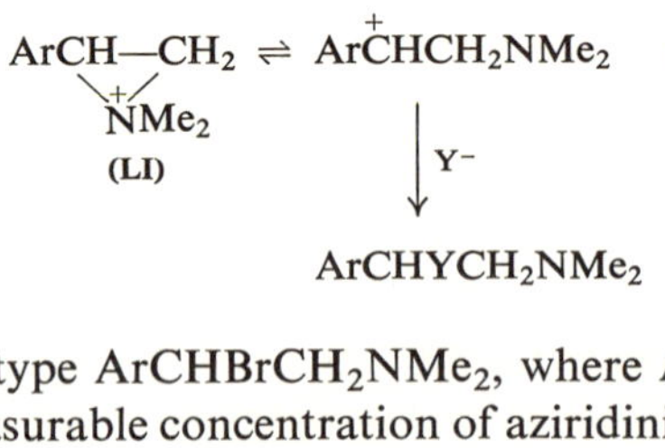

(LI) **(LII)** **(LIII)**

Compounds of the type $ArCHBrCH_2NMe_2$, where Ar is 1-naphthyl or 2-naphthyl, yield no measurable concentration of aziridinium ion in 1:1 acetone and water at 31°C (*87b*). These compounds were, however, significantly more

TABLE 9.5

Pharmacological Properties of some *N,N*-Dimethyl-2-bromo- (or chloro-) 2-(Ring-substituted)phenethylamine Hydrobromides and Related compounds[a]

3-Z,4-$YC_6H_3CHXCH_2NMe_2 \cdot HX$

No.	Z	Y	X	ED$_{50}$, moles × 10^{-9} per kg, for antagonism to: Epinephrine	Norepinephrine
1	F	H	Br	30.0±6.0	32.0±6.4
2	Cl	H	Br	7.0±1.4	7.1±1.4
3	Br	H	Br	5.0±1.2	5.0±1.2
4	I	H	Br	4.0±0.9	4.0±0.9
5	H	Cl	Br	2.1±0.3	2.1±0.3
6	H	I	Br	0.56±0.05	0.51±0.05
7	Cl	F	Br	6.4±1.1	6.4±1.0
8	Cl	Cl	Br	1.3±0.2	1.3±0.2
9	Cl	Br	Br	1.0±0.1	1.0±0.1
10	Br	F	Br	2.7±0.4	2.7±0.4
11	Br	Cl	Br	1.2±0.06	1.2±0.06
12	Br	Br	Br	0.45±0.02	0.50±0.02
13	Cl	Cl	Cl	2.8±0.3	2.8±0.3
14	Br	Br	Cl	0.9±0.1	0.9±0.09
15	Me	H	Br	3.5±0.9	3.0±0.9
16	Me	Me	Br	0.5±0.04	0.5±0.04
17	Br	Me	Br	0.3±0.01	0.3±0.01
18	Me	F	Br	1.5±0.3	1.5±0.3
19	Me	Cl	Br	1.1±0.07	1.1±0.07
20	Me	Br	Br	0.6±0.07	0.6±0.07
21	Me	Me	Cl	1.0±0.1	1.0±0.1
22	H	Ph	Br	30.0±4.1	30.0±4.0

[a] Antagonism to the action of epinephrine (given intravenously as hydrochloride) and of norepinephrine (given as hydrogen tartrate) on the blood pressure of groups of atropinized spinal rats pretreated with 5 mg/kg of hexamethonium bromide was measured. ED$_{50}$ values are doses of antagonist necessary to reduce by 50% the pressor response to a standard dose of catecholamine (1.0 μg/kg, or 0.005 μmole/kg). Antagonist administered intravenously as its hydrohalide, in saline or water.

active against epinephrine and norepinephrine than the parent compound, in which Ar was Ph. Because the solvolysis of the 1-naphthyl or 2-naphthyl derivative reached an apparent equilibrium when about 26 or 46% decomposition had occurred, the chemical observations were explained in terms of the rapid and reversible formation of a carbonium ion, $ArC^{+}HCH_2$-NMe_2, from the aziridinium ion. These somewhat anomalous pharmacological observations may be interpreted in terms of the formation at the receptor of the carbonium ion from circulating bromoethylamine, as in the scheme of structures **(LI)**–**(LIII)**. On this hypothesis the aziridinium ion, although involved in the formation of the structure **(LII)**, is not present in titratable amounts. On the other hand, compounds of the type $ArCRBrCH_2NMe_2$, where Ar = Ph and R = Me, Et, or i-Pr; Ar = 1-naphthyl and R = Me, show chemical behavior broadly similar to that of $ArCHBrCH_2NMe_2$ but are all virtually inactive against epinephrine and norepinephrine, so that it appears that in these cases the carbon structure of the bromoethylamine with its tertiary carbon atom attached to bromine precludes pharmacological activity.

This hypothesis is also strongly confirmed by the work of Belleau and Triggle (*111*), who have obtained the enantiomeric *N,N*-dimethyl 2-bromophenethylamine hydrobromides. The derived amines may confidently be expected to yield the related enantiomeric aziridinium ions by an internal S_N2 process and, therefore, without racemization but with inversion of configuration. The enantiomers produced an identical antiepinephrine response at the stereospecific receptor; this indicates forcibly that they attack the receptor through a common derived species which lacks molecular dissymetry, viz. the carbonium ion, structure **(LII)**. In Belleau's theory of the catecholamine α receptor (cf. Figure 9.1) A, B, C, M, and P are essential binding sites in the receptor for the positive nitrogen pole, the benzene ring, the alcoholic hydroxyl group, and the catecholic hydroxyls, respectively. Site C is only briefly mentioned by Belleau. In particular, he interprets the effect on activity of substituents in the benzene ring of an antagonist of epinephrine belonging to the Dibenamine series, in terms of the polar effects of the substituents and their consequences for the binding between the benzene ring and B, which binding is thought to be strengthened by an increase of electron density in the ring, the result being an increase in activity (cf. Figure 9.3). In Table 9.6 are listed for some DMEA-type compounds the values of Hammett's σ constants (*112*) as an index of polar effects, ED_{50} values against epinephrine and norepinephrine, and values of k, the initial first-order rate coefficient for solvolysis at 37°C in 1:1 acetone and water, as an index of the reactivity of the aziridinium ion and, presumably, of the derived carbonium ion. Polar effects on reactivity are very small: with σ ranging from -0.170 to $+0.391$ the values of k change by a factor of only 3. It is also clear that there is no regular relation between σ and ED_{50} values in general; indeed, compounds almost equiactive pharmacologically (such as Nos. 2 and 6) may have σ values of opposite sign. It is seen, however, that for any given *meta*- and *para*-substituted pair the compound which, according to the relevant σ value, has a substituent of greater electron-releasing or smaller electron-withdrawing

TABLE 9.6

Polar Effects of Substituents in and Some Pharmacological Properties of Ring-substituted *N,N*-Dimethyl-2-bromophenethylamine Hydrobromides

			ED_{50}, 10^{-9} mole/kg, for antagonism to		
No.	Substituent	Hammet's σ	Epinephrine	Norepinephrine	k,[a] min^{-1}
1	H	0.00	35.0	56.0	0.03
2	4-Me	−0.170	0.50	0.53	0.03
3	4-F	0.062	7.0	7.4	
4	4-Cl	0.224	2.1	2.1	0.01
5	4-Br	0.232	1.3	1.3	≈0.01[b]
6	4-I	0.250	0.56	0.51	
7	3-Me	−0.069	3.5	3.0	≈0.03[b]
8	3-F	0.337	30.0	32.0	
9	3-Cl	0.373	7.0	7.1	≈0.02[b]
10	3-Br	0.391	5.0	5.0	≈0.01[b]
11	3-I	0.352	4.0	4.0	

[a] At 37°C in 1:1 acetone and water (see text).
[b] Estimated from results for closely related compounds.

power, (the *para* isomer), is the more active. We conclude that polar effects do not play a dominant role in influencing the strength of attachment to the receptor and, hence, the ED_{50} values of the compounds of this series, but that they play a secondary role once the major effects have come into play. The major effect of substituents we regard as steric for reasons which will be set out.

Belleau has emphasized the "phenylethylamine pattern" in the interaction with the receptor of epinephrine and of antagonists of the Dibenamine series (cf. Figure 9.3). Recognizing the carbonium ion character of the carbon atoms of the aziridinium ring, he proposed that site A of the receptor, which binds the positive pole of epinephrine, should be responsible for the ultimately covalent binding of an ethyleniminium ring carbon atom in an antagonist of the Dibenamine series, the result being that the point of attachment to A and the benzene ring are separated by approximately three carbon-carbon single-bond lengths (Figure 9.3). It has often been assumed (e.g., *87a*) by analogy with the reactions of epoxides in neutral or basic media that an S_N2 ring opening would result in attack on the least substituted ring carbon atom. A more correct analogy may be made with the reactions of protonated epoxides, in which case even the S_N2 mechanism would lead to the same orientation of ring opening as the carbonium ion mechanism proposed above. It is clear, however, that whatever the orientation of ring opening of an ion of structure

(LI) at the receptor, the point of attachment (an aziridinium carbon atom) to A in the receptor could lie at a distance of at most only two carbon-carbon bond lengths from the benzene ring and that this distance would be more likely to be one bond length. Belleau initially accommodated this class of compound to his theory only by inadvertently including an oxygen atom in the receptor at A, as a comparison of Figures 9.3 and 9.4 shows.

Chapman and Triggle (*87a*) have prepared, and Graham and James (*89*) have examined, compounds of the type here under discussion, *N*,*N*-dimethyl-2-bromo-3-phenylpropylamine ($PhCH_2CHBrCH_2NMe_2 \cdot HBr$), and the corresponding 4-butylamine and 4-but-3-enylamine derivatives, $Ph(CH_2)_2CHBr$-$CH_2NMe_2 \cdot HBr$ and $PhCH{=}CHCHBrCH_2NMe_2 \cdot HBr$, respectively, in which the point of attachment of the antagonist to A in the receptor will be distant from the benzene ring by two or three carbon-carbon bond lengths in the first compound or three or four bond lengths in the second, depending on the orientation of ring opening of the aziridinium ion at the receptor. In the third compound the conjugation with the phenyl group of the carbonium carbon is preserved. None of these compounds shows any measurable activity, so for these and the reasons set out above a different hypothesis from that of Belleau concerning the mode of attachment of this class of antagonist to the receptor is necessary. In a more recent publication, Belleau (*108*) developed his earlier hypothesis by emphasizing for this class of compound the role of the "open" carbonium ion in the attachment of the antagonist to the receptor. He asserts that alkylating agents of the present series "are forced by the receptor to interact initially in the extended ionic form, thus respecting the optimal distance relationship between the phenyl ring and the nitrogen for initial interaction with the receptor." It is also proposed that the alkylation product is a phosphate ester, although experimental evidence of this from the synthesis of an appropriate model compound has not yet been obtained. It

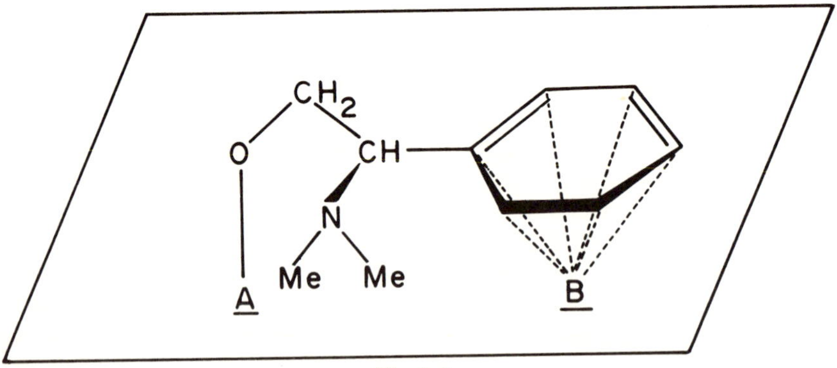

Fig. 9.4

must be pointed out, however, that the "optimal distance relationship" can be maintained only if the carbonium carbon of ion **(LII)** attaches itself, not to that part of the receptor which binds the ammonium pole of the agonist (A in Figure 9.1) but, as suggested below, to the binding site of the alcoholic hydroxyl group (C in Figure 9.1); cf. Belleau (*103*, p. 83). In this respect, therefore, antagonists of the present group must be regarded as differing distinctly from those of the Dibenamine group, in which the potentially positively charged carbon atom of the aziridinium ion, it is thought, becomes attached to A in the receptor. Indeed, it may be best to regard the *N*,*N*-dimethyl-2-aryl-2-halogenoethylamines as a group of antagonists distinct from the Dibenamine group by virtue of their great potency, short duration of action, surmountability, and different geometry of attachment to the receptor.

We believe that antagonists of this class attach themselves to the receptor in a manner quite similar to that of the agonists, as shown in Figure 9.5 (cf. Figure 9.1). Moreover, maximal activity is associated with substituents Y and Z, which are of about the same size as hydroxyl groups, their polarity playing only a secondary role. Further, any increase in size of the "cationic head" (Me_2NH^+ group) results in drastic reduction in activity, with the possible exception of the diallylamino group. The nature of the receptor must be such that it can accept readily and bind firmly a "cationic head" of a size no greater than that of Me_2NH^+, and groups at P and M of the size specified above. The main evidence in favor of this contention is to be found in the ED_{50} values listed in Tables 9.2 and 9.5. The highest activity is found with *p*-methyl, *p*-chloro, *p*-bromo, and *p*-iodo compounds and with 3,4-dichloro, -dibromo, and -dimethyl compounds. Now, it is likely that the catechol nucleus in epinephrine takes up the conformation shown in Figure 9.6 (*113*, *114*). Inspection of scale models reveals that the closest "match" in size is between chlorine and hydroxyl, and accordingly the *p*-chloro or 3,4-dichloro compounds might be

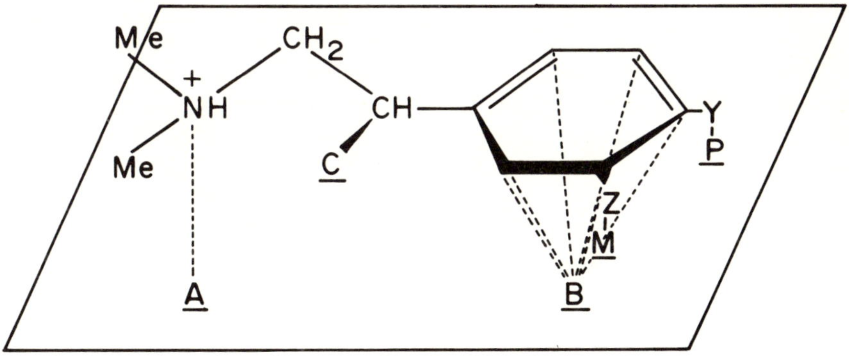

Fig. 9.5

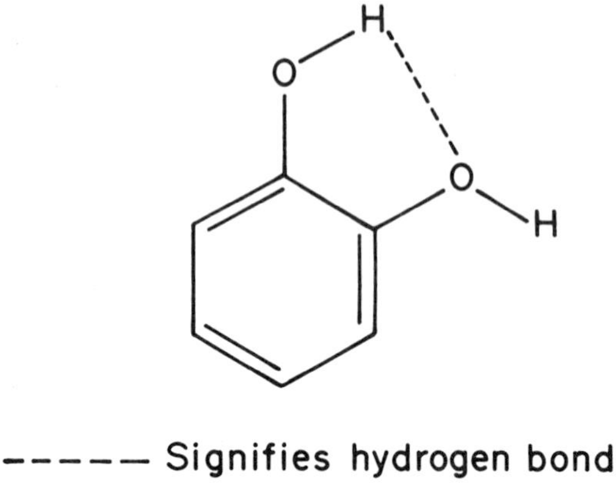

Fig. 9.6

expected to be the most active; in fact, the *p*-bromo, *p*-iodo, and *p*-methyl compounds have higher activity than the *p*-chloro compound, and the 3,4-dibromo higher than the 3,4-dichloro. With the methyl group some steric disadvantage may well be offset by a favorable polar effect, but the positive σ values of the *p*-halogens lie in the order I > Br > Cl, whereas the opposite order would be required to offset the steric factor. The greater activity of the *p*-monosubstituted compound than of the *m*-isomer is due partly to polar effects but also, as Belleau has suggested (*95*), to the fact that rotation of the phenyl group can provide a conformation in which the *m*-substituent does not interact with the appropriate site in the receptor, whereas this is not possible for the *p*-substituent. Despite Belleau's further elaboration of his views of the nature of the adrenergic receptor (*103*, pp. 92–93), in our judgment our knowledge of the nature of the receptor in relation to the interaction of the catecholic hydroxyl groups with it is not such that further discussion of the effect of substituents in the benzene ring of these antagonists is warranted.

However, we now emphasize the importance of the site C (Figures 9.1 and 9.5) associated with the binding of the alcoholic hydroxyl group of epinephrine and norepinephrine. This seems to us to have been underestimated in previous theories of antagonism to epinephrine. We propose the hypothesis that a group in the receptor at C can form a weak bond, probably a hydrogen bond, with the alcoholic hydroxyl group: weak, because abolition of this interaction, as in (+)-epinephrine or Epinine [$3,4\text{-}(OH)_2C_6H_3CH_2CH_2NHMe$], results in diminution but not abolition of activity (*115*). Any such group would be likely to react readily with a carbonium carbon to form a covalency, as indicated by the bond length in Figure 5, and this interaction is regarded as critical in establishing the necessary geometric relation of antagonist and receptor. The short duration of action suggests the formation of an ester grouping at C, in the splitting of which the dimethylamino group can assist and so increase the rate of regeneration of the receptor. Interaction of the carbonium carbon with site A is thought to be unlikely, as this almost abolishes interaction of the ring with B and interaction of X and Z with P and M.

b. Miscellaneous Compounds

Miscellaneous compounds include *N,N*-diethyl-2-phenoxyethylamine and some derivatives with substituents in the benzene ring (*116*), certain benzo-1,4-dioxan derivatives (*117*) of the general structure **(LIV)**, and the *bis*benzo-1,4-dioxan-2-ylmethyl derivative (*118*), structure **(LV)**. Optical resolution of

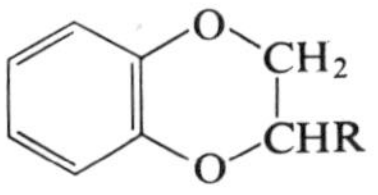

(LIV)

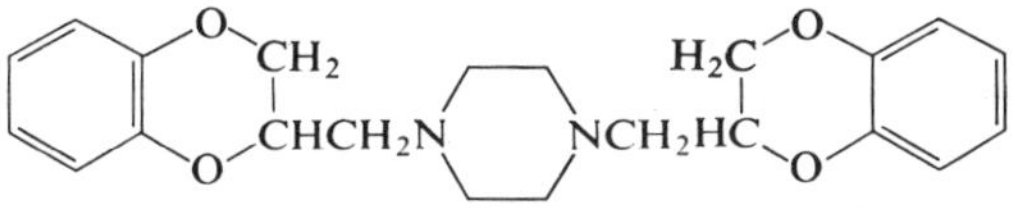

(LV)

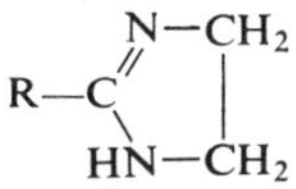

(LVI)

(LIV) with $R=CH_2NEt_2$ was accomplished by Trefouël, Trefouël and Dunant (*119*), the (−) isomer being more active than its enantiomer. Compound **(LV)** is the most active of this group.

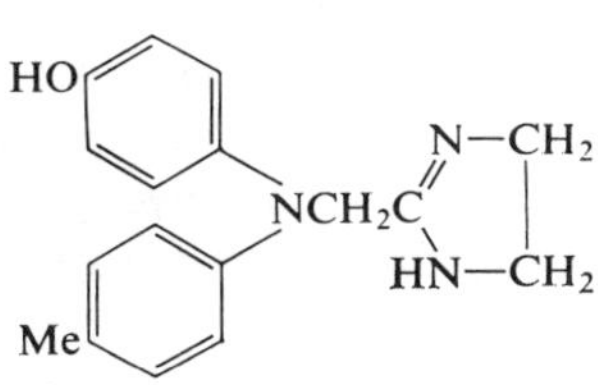

(LVII)

Certain 2-substituted imidazolines of the structure **(LVI)**, such as tolazoline ($R=PhCH_2$) or phentolamine, **(LVII)**, also appear to block α receptors, but their action is weak and easily reversible (*120*). Finally, among a series of dibenzazepines investigated by Randall and Smith (*121*) the most active compound, azapetine, **(LVIII)**, appears to be about as active as tolazoline.

None of these groups of compounds has received the intensive investigation to which the halogenoethylamines have been subjected. Little of significance has emerged in the study of their structure–activity relationships. It is very

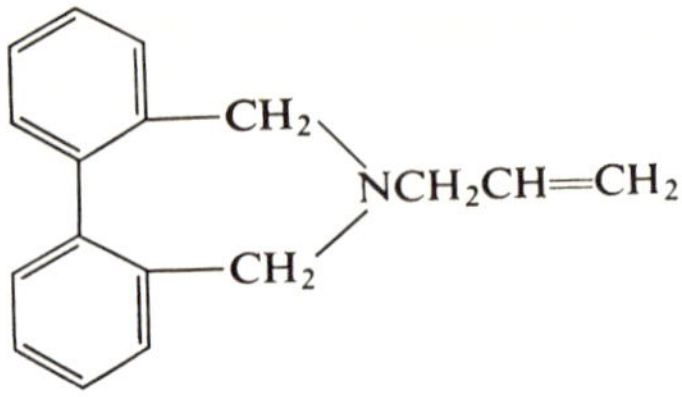

(LVIII)

probable that all the compounds are more or less monoprotonated at physiological pH, though this matter has not been thoroughly investigated, so that there probably are species containing a positive ammonium pole capable of interaction with site A in Belleau's model of the receptor (Figure 9.1), but nowhere is there a suggestion of conformity to the "phenylethylamine pattern." Moreover, there are substantial pharmacological dissimilarities between these compounds and the halogenoethylamines. We have confined ourselves to this very brief and incomplete account of these compounds, because their study has not yet shed much light on the relationships between chemical constitution and pharmacodynamic action.

B. Blockade of β-Receptors

Knowledge in this area is much less extensive and less coherent than in the area of blockade of α receptors and, in particular, structure–activity relations are less clear. Accordingly, the brief account which follows has been deliberately restricted to the main features of the subject as it stands at present.

The usually accepted evidence of activation of β receptors includes the relaxation of smooth muscle (for example, of arterioles, bronchioles, or uterus), the stimulation of cardiac muscle with increase in heart rate (positive chronotropic action) and force (positive inotropic action), and the rise in the concentration of free fatty acids in plasma, glycogenolysis and hyperglycemia. The order of potency of N-substituted derivatives of (±)-norepinephrine in producing these effects is as follows: *N*-cyclopentyl > *N*-isopropyl > other *N*-alkyl > epinephrine > norepinephrine. This order appears to be roughly correlated with the basic strength of the amine. Despite some assertions to the contrary, it appears that the actions listed above are not inhibited by blockers of α receptors (*122*).

1. HISTORY

It has been known since 1949 (*123*) that apparently effective postsynaptic blockade of α receptors, whether by surmountable or insurmountable antagonists, can apparently be reversed by administration of "noncatecholamine" sympathomimetic amines, such as ephedrine, but only during the last decade has it been realized that this phenomenon is due to a blockade of β receptors (*124*) resulting in the unmasking of a motor response dependent upon residual, unblocked α receptors. Structure–activity relations have lately been explored with a view to obtaining compounds capable of specifically blocking β receptors but free from α receptor-blocking properties or from the stimulant side effects consequent upon occupancy of either receptor.

2. STRUCTURE–ACTIVITY RELATIONSHIPS

In 1949 Aström (*123*) showed that only "noncatecholamine" sympathomimetics reversed an "established" blockade of α receptors. Levy and Ahlquist (*124*) examined some twenty compounds, mainly of this kind, and found that only ephedrine, PhCHOHCHMeNHMe, and methoxamine, 2,5-$(OMe)_2$-$C_6H_3CHOHCH_2NHMe$, could restore the pressor response to epinephrine in the dog, after doses of phenoxybenzamine which had reversed it. It was thought that methoxamine might displace phenoxybenzamine from the α receptor. The 3,4-dichloro analogue of isoproterenol, DCI,* was introduced by Powell and Slater (*125*), and the activity of related compounds was explored by Levy (*126*), who showed that the analogue, $ArCHOHCH_2NH$-i-Pr, had a duration of activity about five times longer than that of another analogue, $ArCHOHCH_2NH_2$, and that the order of potency placed the former first, the latter last, and a third analogue, $ArCHOHCH_2NHMe$, between them, when Ar was 3,4-$Cl_2C_6H_3$ in all of them. Replacement of the alcoholic hydroxyl group by chlorine in DCI and related compounds gave rise to blockade of α receptors (cf. Section 9.3, A 1.a), and it is clear that the hydroxyl group is essential for β-blocking activity. Some fluoro compounds, including *N*-isopropyl-2-(3,4-difluorophenyl)-2-hydroxyethylamine, were also studied and found to be less active than the corresponding chloro compounds.

Two important new series of β-blockers, actually or potentially clinically useful, have been described during the past few years. The 2-amino-1-arylethanol series, $ArCHOHCH_2NHR$, is notable for the compound pronethalol, *N*-isopropyl-2-amino-1-(2-naphthyl)ethanol, in which Ar is 2-naphthyl and R is isopropyl (*127*). The 1-amino-3-aryloxy-2-propanol series, $ArOCH_2CHOHCH_2NHR$, is likewise notable for the compound propanolol, *N*-isopropyl-1-amino-3-(1-naphthyloxy)-2-propanol, in which Ar is 1-naphthyl and R is isopropyl (*128*). Stock and Westerman (*129*) have given an account of the tissue distribution of another member of this series, *N*-isopropyl-1-amino-3-(*m*-tolyloxy)-2-propanol hydrochloride (*m*-$MeC_6H_4OCH_2CHOHCH_2NH$-i-Pr·HCl). Moreover, 4-(2-isopropylamino-1-hydroxyethyl)-methansulfonanilide (i-$PrNHCH_2CHOHC_6H_4NHSO_2Me$-4) and a related hydroxypropyl compound (*130*) and Segontin,† $Ph_2CHCH_2CH_2NHCHMeCH_2Ph$ (*131*),

* *N*-Isopropyl-2-(3,4-dichlorophenyl)-2-hydroxyethylamine.

† *N*-(3-phenyl-2-propyl)-1,1-diphenyl-3-propylamine.

have been reported as β-blockers. A compound Isoptin,* Ar·C(i-Pr)(CN)-$(CH_2)_3NMe(CH_2)_2Ar$, where Ar is 3,4-$(MeO)_2C_6H_3$, has been shown to have similar properties (*132*).

Howe (*133*) has given an account of the effect of varying the N-alkyl group in analogues of pronethalol. The facts are summarized in Table 9.7. It can be seen that the structural requirement for potency of the same order or greater than that of pronethalol is that R in 2-$C_{10}H_7CHOHCH_2NHR$ shall be of the form $CH_3CR_1R_2$, where $R_1=H$ or CH_3 and $R_2=(CH_2)_nH$ or $(CH_2)_nPh$, with $n=1$, 2, or 3. This requirement is very similar to that considered by Moed and his co-workers to be necessary in the isoproterenol series for sympathomimetic activity at β receptors (*134*). Dialkyl substitution at the nitrogen atom or quaternization of it is strongly unfavorable to β-blocking. The hydroxyl group is also essential for activity: replacing it by a methoxyl, thiol, or amino group or a hydrogen atom abolishes activity. Moreover, *R*-(−)-pronethalol is about 40 times more potent than its enantiomer (*133*, *135*): the absolute configuration indicated would be expected from the absolute configuration of *R*-(−)-isoprenaline (*136*) and has been confirmed by optical rotatory dispersion studies. Pronethalol is metabolized in the liver, and the products, mainly 2-naphthoic acid and 2-hydroxy-(2-naphthyl)acetic acid, are excreted in the urine. The clinical investigation of pronethalol has been hampered by undesirable side effects in man and a carcinogenic effect in mice. On the other

TABLE 9.7

N-Alkyl-2-amino-1-(2-naphthyl)ethanol Hydrochlorides, 2-$C_{10}H_7 \cdot CHOHCH_2NHR$

R	Potency	R	Potency
Et	<10	CH_2CH_2Ph	10
i-Pr	100[a]	$CHMeCH_2Ph$	50, 100
t-Bu	150	CMe_2CH_2Ph	100
n-Pr	10	$CH_2CH_2CH_2Ph$	60
CHMeEt	80	$CHMe(CH_2)_2Ph$	200, 400
$CHEt_2$	10	$CMe_2(CH_2)_2Ph$	100
CH_2-i-Pr	20	$CHMe(CH_2)_6Me$	5
n-Bu	10	$CHMe(CH_2)_3Ph$	100
CHMe-*n*-Pr	50		

[a] Pronethalol is given an arbitrary potency of 100.

* α-Isopropyl-α-(*N*-methyl-*N*-homoveratryl)-γ-aminopropyl-3,4-dimethoxyphenylacetonitrile.

hand, propanolol has been shown to have a therapeutic ratio about ten times that of pronethalol (*128*). At the time of writing there seems to be little published information about structure–activity relationships among analogues of propanolol.

In 1963 Corrodi et al. (*137*) reported on a series of substituted phenylethanolamines and phenylpropanolamines which block β receptors. The analogues of DCI in which nuclear chlorine atoms were replaced by methyl groups showed a somewhat greater activity than DCI and a positive inotropic effect, and the 4-monomethyl compound, 4-$MeC_6H_4CHOHCH_2NH$-i-Pr, behaved similarly. Propanolamine derivatives were substantially less active than the corresponding ethanolamine derivatives. Further work on the pharmacology and physicochemical relationships of the compounds is promised.

3. ACTION OF BLOCKERS OF β RECEPTORS

DCI is a weak sympathomimetic agonist: it occupies the β receptors of catecholamines, and this causes sufficient stimulation to give rise to undesirable side effects. The stimulation of cardiac muscle results in a positive inotropic response (*138*) and arrhythmia (*139*). Other effects are raised levels of sugar and lactic acid in blood (*140*) and mobilization of unesterified lipid (*141*). In the presence of more strongly adsorbed catecholamines it acts as a competitive antagonist (*142*). Thus, since its sympathomimetic efficacy is so much less than that of isoproterenol, the net effect is antagonism (*143*). This type of antagonism is sometimes called competitive dualism. Both pronethalol and propanolol are much less potent as agonists and more potent as antagonists than is DCI.

ACKNOWLEDGMENTS

We are indebted to Dr. R. Howe, Imperial Chemical Industries Ltd., Pharmaceuticals Division, for some of the information given in Section 9.3, B, 3.

REFERENCES

1. W. J. Chick, G. Irvine, J. D. Lever, and J. D. P. Graham, *J. Anat.* (*London*), **99**, 299 (1965).
2. S. Kaufman, *J. Biol. Chem.*, **234**, 2677 (1959).
3. P. Holtz, R. Heise, and K. Lüdtke, *Arch. Exptl. Path. Pharmakol.*, **191**, 87 (1938).
4. J. Axelrod, *Biochim. Biophys. Acta*, **45**, 614 (1960).
5. H. Blaschko, G. V. R. Born, A. D'Iorio, and N. R. Eade, *J. Physiol.* (*London*), **133**, 548 (1956).
6. T. Chruściel, in *Adrenergic Mechanisms* (J. R. Vane, G. E. W. Wolstenholme, and M. O'Connor, eds.), Churchill, London, 1960, p. 539.

7. U. S. von Euler, in *Adrenergic Mechanisms*, (J. R. Vane, G. E. W. Wolstenholme, and M. O'Connor, eds.), Churchill, London, 1960, p. 493.
8. J. Adams-Ray, H. Nordenstam, and J. Rhodin, *Acta Neuroveget.* (*Vienna*), **18**, 304 (1958).
9. J. H. Burn, *Brit. Med. J.*, **1**, 1623 (1951).
10. R. P. Ahlquist, *Am. J. Physiol.*, **153**, 586 (1948).
11. E. W. Sutherland and T. W. Rall in *Adrenergic Mechanisms* (J. R. Vane, G. E. W. Wolstenholme, and M. O'Connor, eds.), Churchill, London, 1960, p. 295.
12. B. Belleau, in *Adrenergic Mechanisms* (J. R. Vane, G. E. W. Wolstenholme, and M. O'Connor, eds.), Churchill, London, 1960, p. 223.
13. J. Axelrod, I. J. Kopin, and J. D. Mann, *Biochim. Biophys. Acta*, **36**, 576 (1959).
14. H. Blaschko, *Pharmacol. Rev.*, **4**, 415 (1952).
15. C. C. Porter, J. A. Totaro, and C. A. Stone, *J. Pharmacol. Exptl. Therap.*, **140**, 308 (1963).
16. O. Schales and S. S. Schales, *Arch. Biochem. Biophys.*, **24**, 83 (1949).
17. W. J. Hartman, R. I. Akawie, and W. G. Clark, *J. Biol. Chem.*, **216**, 507 (1955).
18. C. C. Porter, L. S. Watson, D. C. Titus, J. A. Totaro, and S. S. Byer, *Biochem. Pharmacol.*, **11**, 1067 (1962).
19. E. Hansson, R. M. Fleming, and W. G. Clark, *Intern. J. Neuropharmacol.*, **3**, 177 (1964).
20. T. L. Sourkes, *Arch. Biochem. Biophys.*, **51**, 444 (1954).
21. H. Dengler and G. Reichel, *Arch. Exptl. Pathol. Pharmakol.*, **234**, 275 (1958).
22. A. W. Stott and R. Robinson, *J. Pharm. Pharmacol.*, **15**, 773 (1963).
23. S. M. Hess, R. H. Connamacher, M. Ozaki, and S. Udenfriend, *J. Pharmacol. Exptl. Therap.*, **134**, 129 (1961).
24. C. C. Porter, J. A. Totaro, and C. M. Leiby, *J. Pharmacol. Exptl. Therap.*, **134**, 139 (1961).
25. A. Pletscher, W. P. Burkard, and K. F. Gey, *Biochem. Pharmacol.*, **13**, 385 (1964).
26. J. M. van Rossum and J. A. T. M. Hurkmans, *J. Pharm. Pharmacol.*, **15**, 493 (1963).
27. S. M. Hess, *Arch. Intern. Pharmacodyn.*, **138**, 584 (1962).
28. M. D. Day and M. J. Rand, *Brit. J. Pharmacol.*, **22**, 72 (1964).
29. C. A. Stone, C. A. Ross, H. C. Wenger, C. T. Ludden, J. A. Blessing, J. A. Totaro, and C. C. Porter, *J. Pharmacol. Exptl. Therap.*, **136**, 80 (1962).
30. M. D. Day and M. J. Rand, *Intern. J. Neuropharmacol.*, **3**, 173 (1964).
31. A. Sjoerdsma, A. Vendsalu, and K. Engelman, *Circulation*, **28**, 492 (1963).
32. D. Horwitz and A. Sjoerdsma, *Life Sci.*, **3**, 41 (1964).
33. R. Sannerstedt, E. Varnanskas, and L. Werko, *Acta Med. Scand.*, **171**, 75 (1962).
34. M. H. Weil, B. H. Barbour, and R. B. Chesne, *Circulation*, **28**, 165 (1963).
35. P. J. Cannon, R. T. Whitlock, R. C. Morris, M. Angers, and J. H. Laragh, *J. Am. Med. Assoc.*, **179**, 673 (1963).
36. G. Onesti, A. N. Brest, P. Novack, and J. H. Moyer, *Am. J. Cardiol.*, **9**, 863 (1962).
37. B. N. Halpern, C. Drudi-Baracco, and D. Bessirard, *Compt. Rend. Soc. Biol.*, **157**, 1421 (1963).
38. M. D. Day and M. J. Rand, *J. Pharm. Pharmacol.*, **15**, 631 (1963).
39. B. G. Benfey and D. R. Varma, *Brit. J. Pharmacol.*, **22**, 366 (1964).
40. D. F. Sharmons and S. E. Smith, *J. Neurochem.*, **9**, 403 (1962).
41. T. L. Sourkes, G. F. Murphy, B. Chavez, and M. Zielinska, *J. Neurochem.*, **8**, 109 (1961).
42. M. Vogt, *Brit. Med. Bull.*, **21**, 57 (1965).
43. R. P. Buhs, J. L. Beck, O. C. Speth, J. L. Smith, N. R. Trenner, P. J. Cannon, and J. H. Laragh, *J. Pharmacol. Exptl. Therap.*, **143**, 205 (1964).
44. P. Hey and G. L. Willey, *Brit. J. Pharmacol.*, **9**, 471 (1954); British Patent 765,850.

45. W. A. Bain in *Adrenergic Mechanisms* (J. R. Vane, G. E. W. Wolstenholme, and M. O'Connor, eds.), Churchill, London, 1960, p. 131.
46. R. A. McLean, R. J. Geus, R. J. Mohrbacher, P. A. Mattis, and G. E. Ullyot, *J. Pharmacol. Exptl. Therap.*, **129**, 11 (1960).
47. R. A. McLean, R. J. Geus, J. Pasternack, P. A. Mattis, and G. E. Ullyot, *J. Pharmacol. Exptl. Therap.*, **129**, 17 (1960).
48. A. C. A. Boura, F. C. Copp, and A. F. Green, *Nature*, **184**, BA70, (1959).
49. R. Fielden, A. M. Roe, and G. L. Willey, *Brit. J. Pharmacol.*, **23**, 486 (1964).
50. F. C. Copp, in *Advances in Drug Research*, Vol. 1 (N. J. Harper and A. B. Simmonds, eds.), Academic Press, New York, 1964, p. 164.
51. F. C. Copp in *Advances in Drug Research*, Vol. 1 (N. J. Harper and A. B. Simmonds, eds.), Academic Press, New York, 1964, p. 165.
52. M. Dóda, O. Fehér, L. György, and K. Nádor, *Brit. J. Pharmacol.*, **21**, 10 (1963).
53. A. L. A. Boura, G. G. Coker, F. C. Copp, W. G. Duncombe, A. R. Elphick, A. F. Green, and A. McCoubrey, *Nature*, **185**, 925 (1960).
54. R. A. Maxwell, R. P. Mull, and A. J. Plummer, *Experientia*, **15**, 267 (1959).
55. R. P. Mull, P. Schmidt, M. R. Dapero, J. Higgins, and M. J. Weisbach, *J. Am. Chem. Soc.*, **80**, 3769 (1958).
56. R. A. Maxwell, S. D. Ross, and A. J. Plummer, *J. Pharmacol. Exptl. Therap.*, **123**, 128 (1958).
57. R. P. Mull, R. H. Mizzoni, M. R. Dapero, and M. E. Egbert, *J. Med. Chem.*, **5**, 651 (1962).
58. A. L. A. Boura, F. C. Copp, and A. F. Green, *Nature*, **195**, 1213 (1962).
59. A. L. A. Boura, F. C. Copp, A. F. Green, H. F. Hodson, G. K. Ruffell, M. F. Sim, E. Walton, and E. M. Grivsky, *Nature*, **191**, 1312 (1961).
60. J. H. Short, U. Biermacher, D. A. Dunnigan, and T. D. Leth, *J. Med. Chem.*, **6**, 275 (1963).
61. K. Hermansen, *Acta Pharmacol. Toxicol.*, **20**, 201 (1963).
62. J. Augstein and S. M. Green, *Nature*, **201**, 628 (1964), cf. M. J. Davey and H. Reinert, *Brit. J. Pharmacol.*, **24**, 29 (1965).
63. (a) H. Najer, R. Giudicelli, and J. Sette, *Bull. Soc. Chim. France*, **1964**, 2572.
(b) H. Najer, R. Giudicelli, J. Sette, and J. Menin, *Bull. Soc. Chim. France*, **1965**, 204.
64. E. Costa, R. Kuntzman, G. L. Gessa, and B. B. Brodie, *Life Sci.*, **1**, 75 (1962).
65. K. A. Exley, *Brit. J. Pharmacol.*, **12**, 297 (1957).
66. A. L. A. Boura, W. G. Duncombe, R. D. Robson, and A. McCoubrey, *J. Pharm. Pharmacol.*, **14**, 722 (1962).
67. G. F. Abercrombie and B. N. Davies, *Brit. J. Pharmacol.*, **20**, 171 (1963).
68. H. J. Dengler, H. E. Spiegel, and E. O. Titus, *Nature*, **191**, 816 (1961).
69. G. Hertting, J. Axelrod, and R. W. Patrick, *Brit. J. Pharmacol.*, **18**, 161 (1962).
70. S. D. Gokhale and O. D. Gulati, *Brit. J. Pharmacol.*, **16**, 317 (1961).
71. F. F. Abboud and J. W. Eckstein, *Circulation Res.*, **11**, 788 (1962).
72. R. Kutzman and M. M. Jacobson, *J. Pharmacol. Exptl. Therap.*, **141**, 166 (1963).
73. W. W. Hofmann and A. P. Spivock, *Am. J. Med. Sci.*, **244**, 64 (1962).
74. A. L. A. Boura and A. F. Green, *Ann. Rev. Pharmacol.*, **5**, 183 (1965).
75. M. Nickerson and W. S. Gump, *J. Pharmacol. Exptl. Therap.*, **97**, 25 (1949); cf. M. Nickerson, *ibid.*, **95**, 27 (1949).
76. N. B. Chapman and J. W. James, *J. Chem. Soc.*, **1954**, 2103.
77. G. E. Ullyot and J. F. Kerwin in *Medicinal Chemistry*, Vol. 2 (F. F. Blicke and C. M. Suter, eds.), Wiley, New York, 1956, p. 234.

78. J. D. P. Graham, in *Progress in Medicinal Chemistry*, Vol. 2 (G. P. Ellis and G. B. West, eds.), Butterworth, London, 1962, p. 132.
79. J. D. P. Graham and G. P. Lewis, *Brit. J. Pharmacol.*, **8**, 54 (1953).
80. P. L. Levins and Z. P. Papanastassiou, *J. Am. Chem. Soc.*, **87**, 826 (1965).
81. W. S. Gump and E. J. Nikawitz, *J. Am. Chem. Soc.*, **72**, 3846 (1950).
82. M. Nickerson and G. M. Nomaguchi, *J. Pharmacol. Exptl. Therap.*, **101**, 379 (1951).
83. E. Schipper, W. R. Boehme, M. L. Graeme, E. Siegmund, and E. Chinery, *J. Med. Chem.*, **4**, 79 (1961).
84. G. Cignarella, G. Nathansohn, G. Bianchi, and E. Testa, *Gazz. Chim. Ital.*, **92**, 3 (1962).
85. C. C. Hunt, *J. Pharmacol. Exptl. Therap.*, **95**, 177 (1949).
86. F. C. Ferguson, Jr. and W. C. Wescoe, *J. Pharmacol. Exptl. Therap.*, **100**, 100 (1950).
87. N. B. Chapman and D. J. Triggle, *J. Chem. Soc.*, **1963**, (a) 1385, (b) 4835.
88. N. B. Chapman in *Adrenergic Mechanisms* (J. R. Vane, G. E. W. Wolstenholme, and M. O'Connor, eds.), Churchill, London, 1960, p. 270.
89. J. D. P. Graham and G. W. L. James, *J. Med. Chem.*, **3**, 489 (1961).
90. N. B. Chapman, K. Clarke, and R. D. Strickland, *Proc. Roy. Soc.* (*London*), **B163**, 116 (1965).
91. J. D. P. Graham and M. A. Karrar, *J. Med. Chem.*, **6**, 103 (1963).
92. R. M. Pinder, Ph.D. Thesis, Univ. of Hull, England, 1965.
93. D. J. Harvey, M.Sc. Thesis, Univ. of Hull, England, 1964.
94. E. J. Ariëns, *Arch. Intern. Pharmacodyn.*, **99**, 32 (1954).
95. B. Belleau, *Can. J. Biochem. Physiol.*, **36**, 731 (1958) and succeeding papers.
96. D. J. Triggle, *J. Theoret. Biol.*, **7**, 241 (1964).
97. J. F. Allen and N. B. Chapman, *J. Chem. Soc.*, **1960**, 1482.
98. J. D. P. Graham, *J. Med. Chem.*, **2**, 499 (1960).
99. J. D. P. Graham, *Brit. J. Pharmacol.*, **12**, 489 (1957).
100. J. D. P. Graham and G. P. Lewis, *Brit. J. Pharmacol.*, **9**, 68 (1954).
101. S. C. Harvey and M. Nickerson, *J. Pharmacol. Exptl. Therap.*, **109**, 328 (1953).
102. B. Belleau, *J. Med. Chem.*, **1**, 327 (1959).
103. B. Belleau, *Proceedings of the Symposium on Structure-Action Relationships, First International Congress of Pharmacology, Stockholm*, Vol. 7, Pergamon, New York, 1962, p. 75.
104. J. D. P. Graham and H. Al Katib, *Brit. J. Pharmacol.*, in press.
105. A. M. Lands, *Am. J. Physiol.*, **169**, 11 (1952).
106. B. Cohen, E. R. Van Artsdelen, and J. Harris, *J. Am. Chem. Soc.*, **70**, 281 (1948); **74**, 1875 (1952).
107. B. Belleau and P. Cooper, *J. Med. Chem.*, **6**, 579 (1963).
108. B. Belleau, *J. Med. Chem.*, **1**, 343 (1959).
109. J. D. P. Graham, *Recenti Progr. in Med.*, **28**, 488 (1960).
110. D. J. Triggle, Ph.D. Thesis, Univ. of Hull, England, 1959.
111. B. Belleau and D. J. Triggle, *J. Med. Chem.*, **5**, 636 (1962).
112. L. P. Hammett, *Physical Organic Chemistry*, McGraw-Hill, New York, 1940, p. 184.
113. M. M. Davies, *Trans. Faraday Soc.*, **34**, 1427 (1938).
114. Yu. S. Rozum, *Biokhimiya*, **17**, 476 (1952).
115. H. Blaschko, *Proc. Roy. Soc.* (*London*), **137B**, 310 (1950).
116. J. Levy and E. Ditz, *Arch. Intern. Pharmacodyn.*, **47**, 138 (1934).
117. (a) E. Fourneau and D. Bovet, *Arch. Intern. Pharmacodyn.*, **46**, 178 (1933).
(b) D. Bovet and P. Maderni, *Compt. Rend. Soc. Biol.*, **114**, 980 (1933).
(c) D. Bovet and A. Simon, *Arch. Intern. Pharmacodyn.*, **55**, 15 (1937).

118. (a) J. F. O'Leary, *Federation Proc.*, **12**, 355 (1953).
(b) R. P. Ahlquist, *Am. J. Physiol.*, **153**, 586 (1948).
(c) R. P. Ahlquist and B. Levy, *J. Pharmacol. Exptl. Therap.*, **127**, 146 (1959).
119. J. Trefouël, J. Trefouël and M. Dunant, *Bull. Sci. Pharmacol.*, **42**, 459 (1935).
120. (a) R. F. Furchgott, *Pharmacol. Rev.*, **7**, 183 (1955).
(b) G. Roberts, A. W. Richardson, and H. D. Green, *J. Pharmacol. Exptl. Therap.*, **105**, 466 (1952).
121. L. O. Randall and T. H. Smith, *J. Pharmacol. Exptl. Therap.*, **103**, 10 (1951).
122. M. Nickerson and G. C. M. Chan, *J. Pharmacol. Exptl. Therap.*, **133**, 186 (1961).
123. A. Aström, *Acta Physiol. Scand.*, **18**, 295 (1949).
124. B. Levy and R. P. Ahlquist, *J. Pharmacol. Exptl. Therap.*, **121**, 414 (1957).
125. C. E. Powell and I. H. Slater, *J. Pharmacol. Exptl. Therap.*, **122**, 480 (1958).
126. B. Levy, *J. Pharmacol. Exptl. Therap.*, **127**, 150 (1959).
127. (a) J. S. Stephenson, PH 137065; (b) United Kingdom Pat. 909, 357; (c) J. W. Black and J. S. Stephenson, *Lancet*, **1962-II**, 311.
128. (a) A. F. Crowther and L. H. Smith, United Kingdom Pat. Appl. 44357/62; (b) J. W. Black, A. F. Crowther, R. G. Shanks, L. H. Smith, and A. C. Dornhurst, *Lancet*, **1964-I**, 1080.
129. K. Stock and E. Westermann, *Biochem. Pharmacol.*, **14**, 227 (1965).
130. K. W. Dungan and P. M. Lech, *Federation Proc.*, **23**, 124 (1964).
131. (a) E. Lindner, *Verhandl. Deut. Ges. Inn. Med.*, **70**, 202 (1964); (b) E. Lindner, *Arch. Intern. Pharmacodyn.*, **146**, 475 (1963).
132. H. Haas, *Arzneimittel Forsch.*, **14**, 461 (1964).
133. (a) R. Howe, *Biochem. Pharmacol., Suppl.*, **12**, 85 (1963); (b) A. F. Crowther, R. Howe, and L. H. Smith, United Kingdom Pat. Appl. 46034/61.
134. H. D. Moed, J. van Dijk, and H. Niewind, *Rec. Trav. Chim.*, **74**, 919 (1955).
135. R. Howe, United Kingdom Pat. Appl. 33157/61.
136. P. Pratesi, A. La Manna, A. Campiglio, and G. Pagani, *Farmaco Ed. Sci.*, **15**, 3 (1960).
137. H. Corrodi, H. Persson, A. Carlsson, and J. Roberts, *J. Med. Chem.*, **6**, 751 (1963).
138. N. C. Moran and M. E. Perkins, *J. Pharmacol. Exptl. Therap.*, **124**, 223 (1958).
139. N. C. Moran, J. I. Moore, A. K. Holcomb, and G. Mushet, *J. Pharmacol. Exptl. Therap.*, **136**, 327 (1962).
140. R. S. McCutcheon, *J. Pharmacol. Exptl. Therap.*, **136**, 209 (1962).
141. G. G. Muir, D. A. Chamberlain, and D. T. Pedoe, *Lancet*, **1964-II**, 930.
142. R. C. de la Mata, M. Penna, and D. M. Aviedo, *J. Pharmacol. Exptl. Therap.*, **135**, 197 (1962).
143. B. Levy and R. P. Ahlquist, *J. Pharmacol. Exptl. Therap.*, **130**, 334 (1960).

CHAPTER 10

EFFECTS OF DRUGS ON THE AFFERENT NERVOUS SYSTEMS

CEDRIC M. SMITH

DEPARTMENT OF PHARMACOLOGY
STATE UNIVERSITY OF NEW YORK AT BUFFALO
BUFFALO, NEW YORK

10.1. INTRODUCTION

A. Definitions and Scope of Review

The information input to the central nervous system is received and transferred over the afferent, sensory, nervous system. The afferent system is composed of a variety of receptors, some more, some less, specialized in their responsiveness to alterations in the physical and chemical environment. The directness with which the inputs from exteroceptors and interoceptors are perceived varies markedly; for example, visual input is rather directly perceived, but input along some afferents from skeletal muscles or lungs are only exceptionally perceived directly.

It is an aphorism that *any* alteration in sensory input to the central nervous system, however small, produces some change in the function of that system and, therefore, a change in the output. Two extremes of "connectedness" between input and output may be considered: for example, the connection between visual input and central nervous system motor output is very "loose" and generally quite complex, whereas nociceptive input is very "tightly" connected to motor escape and autonomic output. Hence, the magnitudes of response to drug effects on sensory systems are a function not only of the local nervous disturbance but of the nature of the central nervous connections and the "significance" of that input. A variety of central sensory systems may be involved in a switching mechanism in limiting the input to only preselected appropriately channeled and temporally patterned nerve activity (*1*).

Afferent systems as sites of drug action may be considered under two categories, primary sites and secondary sites.

Drugs whose primary action is on other than sensory systems may also act on sensory nerve endings and afferent pathways. This possibility is stressed, because pharmacological analyses more and more involve the explanation of drug actions in terms of effects at many sites. A rational interpretation of drug effects thus involves both the quantitative delineation of drug actions at all the sites at which they induce effects and the determination, in terms of primary and secondary influences, of the significance of this information with respect to organismal function.

Such a synthesis of information can become extremely involved. One example should suffice. Chlorpromazine, via an action on the reticular formation or input thereto, produces a decrease in the efferent outflow to muscle spindles, with the consequence that the afferent inflow to reticular formation is decreased. It is, at the moment, extremely difficult to ascertain the significance of each of these steps in the production of the gross effects of chlorpromazine, except that the initiating action probably took place within the central nervous system.

A review of all drugs and all sensory systems is a monumental task; therefore, this review is limited to those systems best known to the author. The specialized chemosensory systems of olfaction and taste are not discussed in detail, because the major portion of the work in these areas is, in fact, the determination of structure–activity relationships. Several reviews of these systems have appeared recently (*1a–6*).

Only certain afferent systems and drug classes are considered herein. The choices have been in part arbitrary, and in part they reflect the fact that only a few systems have been sufficiently examined for responsiveness to compounds to permit any meaningful review of the relationships between chemical structure and biological activity.

Some reviews, which will be cited, have centered on compiling the literature on all drugs affecting certain sensory systems and discussing the sites and modes of actions. This chapter focuses on only selected aspects of such investigations.

B. Source and Nature of Information

1. A GENERALIZED SENSORY ENDING

Although sensory endings vary widely in their structure and associated tissues, it is useful for this discussion to present a generalized form. The ultimate sensory nerve structure is the bare nonmyelinated nerve axon, which either courses relatively freely among tissue cells, such as the bare endings in skin, or is enveloped in highly structured receptor components, such as the carotid chemoreceptor cells, muscle spindles, Pacinian corpuscles, or special sense organ receptors. This nonmyelinated nerve termination is the site of origin of the graded, local potentials generally referred to as generator potentials. Proximal to this is the electrically regenerative region, the site of origin of the propagated action potentials. In medullated fibers this regenerative region is the first node of Ranvier; in nonmedullated fibers the regenerative area is less well delineated.

2. DIRECT RECORDING OF AFFERENT NERVE ACTIVITY

The barriers to the penetration of drugs to sites of action include the blood vessel membrane, connective tissue, the nerve sheath (perineurium), Schwann cell membrane and cytoplasm (myelin sheath), and the nerve membrane itself. Local anesthetics and certain cholinergic compounds appear to act with greater ease on the regenerative region near the nerve ending than on the nerve trunk itself. This greater sensitivity frequently has been attributed to the fact that the diffusion barrier is less effective or thinner near the nerve terminations (see discussion by Paintal, *7*). Other possibilities exist, however. For example, the safety margin for transmission may be smaller in the fibers near their terminations; the "abortive" spike potentials from frog muscle spindle fibers near their terminations, recorded by Katz (*8*, *9*), are consistent with this suggestion. Further, variations in the relative permeability of a passive membrane sheath would not be expected to alter the concentration of an agent on either side at equilibrium, although the rates of diffusion might vary widely; Paintal (*7*) has described experiments with infusions of procaine that are consistent with this interpretation. In this connection, Lorente de No and Honrubia (*10*) recently proposed that nerve fibers of desheathed nerve trunks behave qualitatively differently from nerves in an intact trunk; in fact, they described desheathing as a demyelinating effect. It is commonly known that the concentrations of local anesthetics required to block the conduction of desheathed nerves are similar to those effective on sensory nerve preparations (0.01 to 0.2% of procaine), whereas ten times that amount may be required to block conduction in intact nerve trunks.

a. Recording from Individual Fibers

The most direct method of determining drug effects on afferent systems is to record the electrical activity of the afferent fiber or its end terminations. The afferent fiber yields propagated action potentials; the ending yields local, nonpropagated generator potentials. Ideally, one would have recordings of the behavior of a sufficient number of individual units, from which a histogram could be constructed describing the behavior of each unit in comparison with many similar units. This, of course, is rarely accomplished owing to the technical difficulties of isolating and recording from so many units in comparable circumstances.

Recording from single afferent fibers has been done rather routinely; large myelinated fibers are isolated by the teasing of a large peripheral nerve or dorsal root until single units are obtained. This technique, however, is extremely difficult with small myelinated or nonmyelinated C fibers, although a few investigators have succeeded, notably Iggo (see, for example, *11*). In any event, it is not yet sufficiently routine for a systematic analysis of a variety of drugs.

b. Recording from Multifiber Preparations

Asynchronous electrical activity of a number of fibers may be recorded from multifiber nerve filaments. The technique is relatively simple, but the analysis of the results is complicated. With either integration of electrical activity or counting of action potentials greater than some given magnitude the largest potentials are given the greatest weight. A large number of spontaneously active and unresponsive units may well mask an effect on a minor number of smaller fibers. As suggested, this technique is of little value in measuring the activity of C fibers, because the potentials generated are small with respect to the noise level of most biological amplifiers and because the activity of larger fibers will mask other activity.

A particularly useful technique for the determination of C-fiber activity is the occlusion procedure developed by Douglas and Ritchie (*12–16*). It is based on the fact that if one electrically stimulates a nerve trunk, such as the sural or vagus, and records the evoked compound action potential peripheral to the nerve near its termination, the magnitude of the evoked potential will be an inverse function of the activity in the nerves, which is propagated counter to the electrically evoked activity. Propagated activity originating in the peripheral sense organ will collide with the electrically evoked potential and thus be cancelled. By means of appropriate positioning of the stimulating and recording electrodes estimates of the average frequency of discharge along the C fibers may be made. It should be noted, however, that this provides only an overall assessment of the activity of all C fibers in a given conduction velocity range, which is expressed as an average frequency of all fibers.

c. Recording of Generator Potential Activity

The local summed activities of collections of sensory neurons may be recorded from some sensory systems with gross electrodes, such as the electro-olfactogram or electroretinogram, which are due, at least in part, to local nonpropagated generator potentials from a large number of sensory endings.

The effects of drugs other than local anesthetics and inorganic ions on the local generator potentials have been only rarely recorded; most agents altering afferent systems have yet to be examined for their effects on the generator and regenerative regions of the sensory nerve terminations. The inference of Paintal (*7*) that since local anesthetics have been shown to act primarily on the regenerative and not the generator region or the more proximal portions of the fiber, then other agents act at the same site, overlooks the fact that diffusion barriers may not be identical for all agents, nor can the mechanisms of action be assumed to be the same. Each agent will have to be examined explicitly to delineate its sites and mechanisms of action.

3. INDIRECT ASSESSMENT OF DRUG ACTION ON SENSORY RECEPTOR SYSTEMS

a. Induction or Alteration of Reflexes

By far the largest body of information on drug actions of sensory systems has been obtained by indirect means. The actions are inferred to take place when the effects of the agents on the effector and central nervous systems are excluded or when the sensory endings are exposed directly to the agent. The effect is monitored as the initiation of, or alteration in, reflex activity, such as the stimulation of respiration on exposure of the carotid-body circulation to cyanide or the drop in blood pressure induced by carotid-sinus baroreceptor activity.

This technique is particularly useful in ascertaining the reflex significance of drug effects at a given site, but it is hazardous to extrapolate such data. It remains to be shown for most systems what the nature of the relationships between changes in afferent activity and reflex alterations are. At the least the reflex response is a complex function of the change in frequency of afferent nerve activity, the numbers of afferent nerves involved, the specific afferent nerves involved, and the time course or rate of change of afferent activity. In addition one would expect distinct limits, such as a threshold for frequency or number of neurons activated and maximal inputs for given reflex outputs. In some systems, at least, excessive activation of sensory nerves may be associated with depression of the same reflex pathways that were activated with lesser afferent stimulations (for example, muscle spindle).

Thus, although reflexes induced by sensory stimulants may be useful for the routine examination of a series of agents and for ascertaining the reflex consequences of drug actions, the recording may be grossly misleading with respect to the precise effects of the agents on specific afferent fibers and the dose–effect relationships.

b. Induction of Perceptual Changes

As noted above, a large proportion of the afferent input is not directly perceived, but the recording of subjective responses may be a useful technique, particularly in the case of agents acting on exteroreceptors, such as the special senses or sensory receptors of the skin, cornea, mucous membranes, and teeth. It is beyond the scope of this review to do more than note the relevance of the well-developed field of psychophysics to the subjects under discussion and the ultimate necessity of establishing the correlations and information transfer functions between neural behavior and perception.

4. ANALYSES OF DRUG-INDUCED ACTIONS

As Paintal (*7*) has clearly outlined, drug effects on sensory endings may be of a variety of types including changes in threshold, stimulation, and depression and alterations in responses to appropriate stimuli. Some of the possible variations in response are depicted in Figure 10.1 as a function of intensity of stimulus.

It is clear that the linear curves presented in this figure are not the only possibilities. Furthermore, they do not take into account the dynamic characteristics of sensory processes. Such considerations drive home the fact that there are numerous simultaneous processes and that the response to a derangement of any of them may not always be readily predicted. The possibility of alternative types of curves reveals the tenuousness of any interpretation of site and mechanism based on the study of only one or two points on the theoretical curves.

It should be added that very few studies have been undertaken to determine the character of stimulus–response curves in the presence of drugs, yet this would seem to be one of the most reasonable things to do. In many experiments a determination of the whole curve would be extremely difficult because of the short duration of drug action. Even measuring responses to drugs under the conditions of two input magnitudes, no external input, and a less than maximal input can yield information that is helpful for differentiating the various types of drug action (Figure 10.2).

Certain inferences may be made regarding the site or mechanism of action of the drugs of Figures 10.1 and 10.2; see Table 10.1. It is clear from the tabulation that stimulus–response curves alone do not provide sufficient information for a decision on the sites of action; such data as the behavior of the generator potential itself and the response to an interposed antidromic

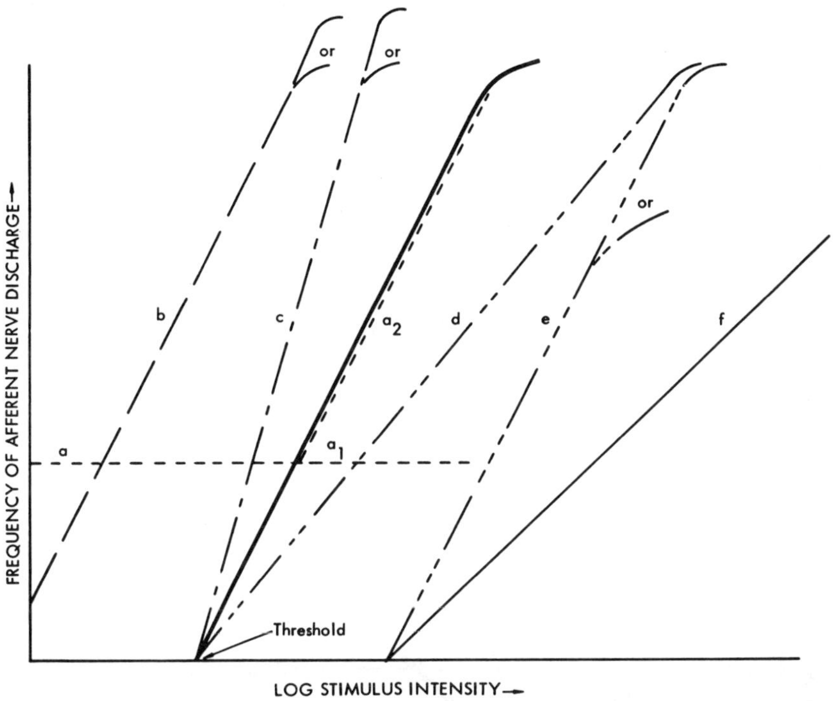

Fig. 10.1. Possible drug-induced alterations in the relationships between magnitude of natural stimulus input and frequency of discharge along afferent nerves. Solid-line control response shown as afferent discharge frequency linearly related within limits to the logarithm of the input stimulus. (a) Depicts drug effect of stimulation of afferent discharge with (a_1) a "desensitization" or depression of responsiveness of the ending to the natural stimulus or (a_2) no change in responsiveness of ending to natural stimulus. (b) Sensitization and stimulation with decrease in threshold but no change in slope. (c) Sensitization and stimulation with no change in threshold but increased responsiveness to natural stimulus. (d) Depression with no change in threshold, with or without change in maximal frequency. (e) Increase in threshold without change in responsiveness to natural stimulus. (f) Increase in threshold and decrease in responsiveness.

stimulus are required. Moreover, the crucial portions of the curve are those at threshold and low stimulus intensities. At these levels it may be particularly difficult to ascertain the presence or absence of depolarization of the generator region. One infers that the threshold is largely determined by the regenerative region, yet it seems equally likely that in some spontaneously active sensory systems the regenerative region is highly unstable and that minute changes in polarization of the generator membrane may cause alterations in discharge frequency.

Depressant drugs acting more centrally than the initial regenerative region

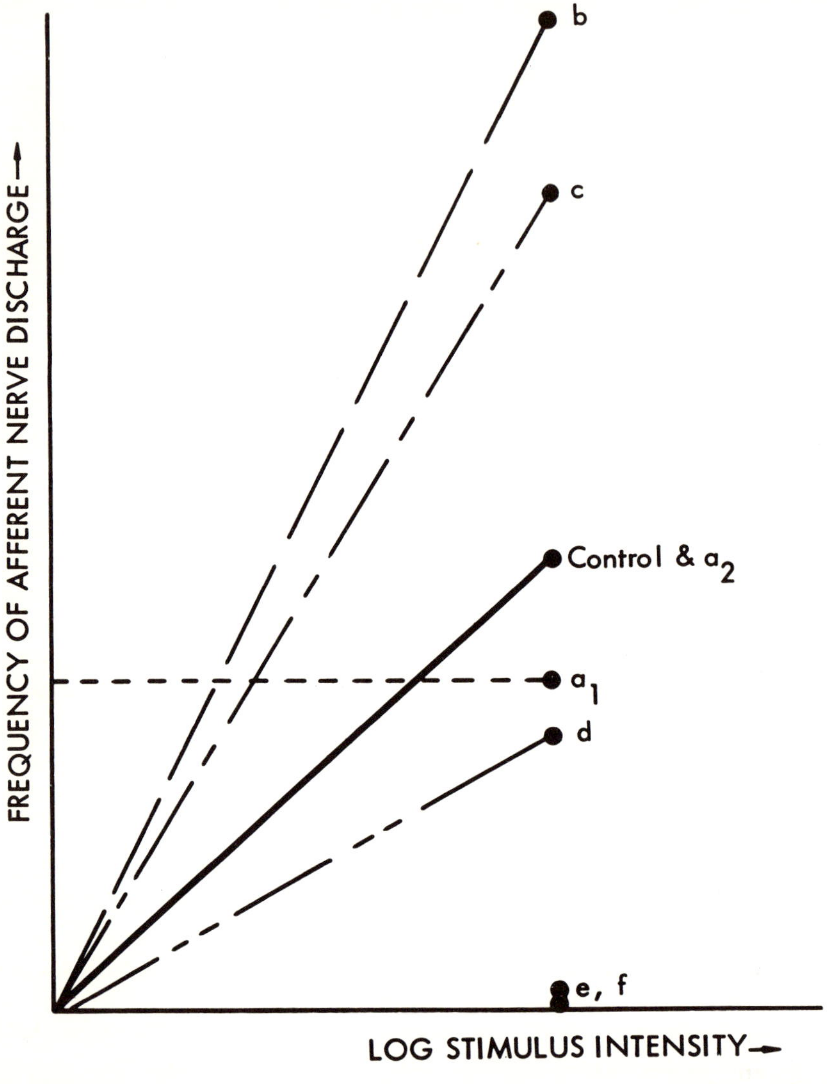

Fig. 10.2. Stimulus response characteristics of a sensory system assessed on the conditions of two input magnitudes, and one dose of each of drugs (a) to (f). It can be inferred from such a plot that drugs (a) and (b) stimulate alone; stimulation by (b) is more than additive with responses to natural stimuli; (c) increases the response to natural stimuli; whereas (d), (e), and (f) produce depression of varying degrees. (Points taken from curves of Fig. 10.1.)

would be expected to produce characteristic effects on a train of impulses. In low doses only certain of the impulses would drop out, leaving the intervals between the others relatively unaffected, that is, leaving a partial block of

TABLE 10.1

Site	Action	Expected alteration in stimulus–response curve
Generator region	Depolarize	b, assuming strictly additive with natural stimulus
Generator region	"Labilize"	c, plus perhaps shift in threshold
Generator region	"Stabilize"	e or f, depending on mechanism
Regenerative region	Depolarize	b, plus perhaps change in slope
Regenerative region	"Labilize"	c, plus perhaps shift in threshold
Regenerative region	"Stabilize"	d, e, or f, depending on mechanism

impulse transmission between the site of generation of the train and the recording site.

One of the major difficulties in quantitative analyses of drug actions is the fact that the true maximal activity analogous to that obtainable with isolated gut, muscle strips, or biochemical reactions can rarely, if ever, be ascertained in a sensory system. This is so because such stimuli usually produce evidence of irreversible changes and the appearance of irregular discharge patterns. Thus, many of the powerful analytic techniques for studying the kinetics of drug–receptor interactions, such as those reviewed by Ariëns (*17*) and Webb (*18*), are not readily employed.

Tachyphylaxis also complicates kinetic analyses. Words indicating a subsidence of effect on repeated exposure to an agent, such as *tachyphylaxis*, *desensitization*, *acute tolerance*, are used in this text interchangeably and without implying any mechanism underlying the phenomenon.

5. PRIMARY AND SECONDARY EFFECTS

All the sensory endings are embedded in tissues with which they are functionally connected. One of the major problems in all studies of drug effects on sense organs is the differentiation of the primary effects on the sensory nerve ending from the secondary effects on the surrounding tissues. For example, the excitation of carotid baroreceptors by adrenergic agents is probably the result of the vascular smooth-muscle contraction. The afferent endings in skeletal muscle spindles are directly coupled with specialized intrafusal fibers, which are probably activated by acetylcholine and succinylcholine. Less direct action seems possible, such as the actions of epinephrine and norepinephrine on sensory endings after their release induced by cholinergic agents or the stimulation of muscle sensory endings by potassium released from muscle by cholinergic agents (*19*). Many of the points raised in this general discussion have been illustrated recently in a series of papers by Eyzaguirre and co-workers (*19a–d*). These investigators also propose that in one sensory system, the carotid-body chemosensory organ, the mediation of the excitation by hypoxia or hypercarbia is through acetylcholine plus other substances. Finally, it can be stated that all sensory systems are either directly or indirectly modulated by efferent systems, and this must be kept in mind in determining sites and modes of action of substances influencing sensory nerve behavior.

10.2. STRUCTURE–ACTIVITY RELATIONSHIPS OF DRUGS AFFECTING SENSORY SYSTEMS

Two variables in structure–activity relationships exist, the drugs and the sensory endings, and there is no balance in the matrix in this presentation. Relatively few studies are pertinent to such considerations; the vast majority have analyzed one system or one drug of a class. This review will concentrate upon only certain studies which, in fact, provide some information on the relation of structure to activity, even though the experiments usually do not permit any inferences regarding the molecular "receptor" substance because the differences in activity may represent variations due to the presence of secondary sites of actions, to variations in rate of penetration, and to differences in mechanism or primary sites of action even within a chemically homologous series of compounds. Nevertheless, these data may be useful in the design of agents with new spectra of action. Emphasis will be given to groups of agents, such as choline esters, which have been tested on more than one system.

A. Carotid-Body Chemoreceptors

The large number of reports on the stimulation of carotid-body chemoreceptors with drugs have been reviewed by Heymans (*20*), Heymans and Neil (*21*), and Anichkov and Belen'kii (*22*). Physiologically, these carotid and aortic chemoreceptors are responsive to oxygen lack and carbon dioxide excess. The increase in frequency of the afferent nerve discharges is greater with both carbon dioxide excess and oxygen lack than with either alone; the same is true of the reflex increase in respiration. Probably the same units respond to both (*19b*, *23*). These units, furthermore, respond to a decrease in blood pressure such as that induced by hexamethonium or occlusion of the carotid artery proximally to the sinus.

Some general comments regarding the sensitivity of chemoreceptors are in order before considering in detail the effects of different classes of agents. Acidity stimulates, whereas alkalinity depresses, chemoreceptor activity. Cyanide has been known for years to be a very potent stimulus to carotid-body chemoreceptors; the response to cyanide is blocked by a prior exposure of the body to iodoacetate or a prior prolonged exposure to cyanide itself (and to fluoride, arsenite, malonate, or low glucose concentrations). The depressed responses may be restored by the administration of adenosine triphosphate. These experiments and a variety of others of a similar nature have led to the view that the sensory receptors are sensitive to certain anaerobic metabolites (reviewed *21*, *22*).

1. ACETYLCHOLINE AND CONGENERS

The stimulatory effects of acetylcholine (ACh) on carotid chemoreceptors have been demonstrated most often indirectly by recording the respiratory stimulation. That this respiratory stimulation is due to stimulation of the chemoreceptors was demonstrated by a variety of operative and blocking techniques (for example, *24–29*). Subsequently, the effect on chemoreceptors was monitored by recording from the afferent nerves themselves (for example, *19a–d*, *30–34*).

In spite of the great amount of work on the effects of ACh and congeners relatively little has been done that can be put within the framework of structure–activity relationships. With only one or two exceptions none of the studies reviewed have presented dose–effect curves. As has been noted, without such data it is extremely difficult to establish, except in a very gross sense, valid relationships between structure and activity in a series of compounds. Moreover, as will be seen throughout this discussion, there are a number of disagreements among different workers with respect to the activity of certain of the agents. At least some of the differences can be related to variations in technique or species of animal. In some instances the action potentials are recorded from the afferent nerves; in others, only the reflex response. The reflex response has proved to be quite useful in a variety of situations; however, it should not be forgotten that such responses are the sum result of a large number of different afferent inputs and that small changes in afferent activity from the carotid body may be offset by effects on baroreceptors, on ganglia, on vasomotor activity, etc. In some reports, too, it would appear that the investigators have been more concerned with finding data consistent with their pet hypothesis concerning the mechanism of generation of chemoreceptor potentials than with presenting an accurate account of the experiments themselves.

It seems operationally useful to make the generalization that the stimulation of carotid chemoreceptors by cholinergic substances is nicotinic in nature, rather than muscarinic, as detailed by Anichkov and Belen'kii (*22*). Of the monocholine esters, ACh and carbamoylcholine are the most effective stimulants. Philippot (*35*) and Schmidt and Comroe (*36*) found that acetyl-β-methylcholine was ineffective. Similarly, pilocarpine (*37*) has little stimulatory activity. A variety of trimethylammonium compounds are effective; these are reviewed in more detail below. Note should be made of those who have not found this generalization to hold. De Wispelaere (*38*) reported some stimulation of chemoreceptors with acetyl-β-methylcholine and β-methylcholine ethyl ether. Propionyl- and butyrylcholine are slightly less effective than ACh in inducing chemoreceptor nerve potentials, whereas benzoylcholine is one fifth to one tenth as active (*39*). The same investigators found that the thio analogues of ACh and butyrylcholine were more potent stimulants and longer lasting than the parent esters, as they are on autonomic ganglia (*40*).

In a recent extensive series of studies of carotid chemoreceptors in vitro the stimulatory effect of ACh was confirmed (*19b*; see also *19a, c, d*). The exposure of isolated carotid-body tissue to Locke's solution containing ACh (concentration, 10^{-6} to 5×10^{-5} w/v) elicited an initial marked increase in chemoreceptor afferent-nerve activity followed by subsidence within 2 to 4 minutes to almost the initial rate of discharge. When the ACh-containing solution was replaced with normal Locke's solution, the discharge again increased, subsequently to decline within minutes. The investigators concluded that the decrease following the initial activation is due to sensory-ending adaptation and not to "desensitization," since the responses to small injections of ACh during and after the sustained exposure to ACh were increased over control levels, rather than decreased. Further, the chemosensory discharge induced by interruption of the flow of Locke's solution was not affected during or after the exposure to "strong concentrations" of ACh. During exposure to a nitrogen atmosphere the responses to ACh were generally increased, although the *ratio* of frequency after ACh to the base-line control frequency was inversely related to the initial base-line frequency as altered by changing oxygen concentration in the bathing solution.

A variety of interesting observations in this series of investigations are outside the scope of this review. However, it should be stated that the investigators reinstate the hypothesis that ACh is one of the mediators of a chemosensory "synapse" in the carotid body. This reinstatement is based, essentially, on the following observations.

(1) ACh is present in the carotid body in sufficient concentrations.

(2) A chemoreceptor stimulatory substance is released from the carotid body during hypoxic or electrical stimulation (*19d*).

(3) The cholinergic blocking agents hexamethonium, tubocurarine, gallamine, and atropine initially increased the ongoing afferent chemoreceptor activity and that evoked by ACh; this excitation was followed by a depression of both types of activity (see below).

The authors argue from a number of points that during moderate natural stimulation a cholinergic mechanism may be responsible for chemoreceptor impulse initiation and that during strong stimulation the release of substances other than ACh may account for the failure of cholinergic blocking agents to block strong stimulation.

Philippot (*35*) surveyed a variety of choline and ACh derivatives for their effects on respiration when given intra-arterially to animals pretreated with atropine. Note that the atropine pretreatment may well have blocked any "muscarinic" effects of such agents; for example, the weak ganglion-stimulating activity of muscarine went undetected until experiments were carried out in the absence of any atropine premedication (*41*, *42*). ACh and carbamoylcholine were the most potent stimulants of respiration. Other agents with significant effects were acetyl-γ-homocholine and the methyl, ethyl, butyl, and vinyl ethers of choline. On the other hand, agents without significant effects on respiration included acetyl and carbamoyl-β-methycholine and the ethyl and methyl ethers of choline. Choline itself was approximately 1/50 as active as ACh and more active than acetyl-β-methacholine. Analogous derivatives of β-ethylcholine, β-propylcholine, and β-butylcholine were essentially inactive as respiratory stimulants.

On the other hand, alcohols can produce stimulation of carotid chemoreceptors, but they are orders of magnitude less potent than the corresponding quaternary ester derivatives. Liljestrand (*43*) examined the intra-arterial injection in cats of 1 to 3 ml of alcoholic solutions for their effects on blood pressure and respiration. Stimulation required 4 to 12% solutions with ethanol, whereas it required 1% with propyl alcohol, 0.4% with butyl, and 0.2% with amyl alcohol. Similar results were obtained from a recording of the action potentials in the chloralosed cat by Landgren et al. (*44*). For comparison, minimal effective concentrations of tetramethylammonium are of the order of a 1 μg/ml, whereas the most potent concentration of amyl alcohol examined was about 2 mg/ml, a potency ratio of 2000. Peculiarly, this excitation produced by alcohols was allegedly depressed by atropine, tubocurarine, hexamethonium, or decamethonium.

The order of potencies of the alcohols as chemoreceptor stimulants does not parallel their depolarizing activity on isolated frog nerve: methanol, ethanol and, to a lesser degree, propanol produce depolarization and block of conduction, whereas butanol, amyl, and higher alcohols cause hyperpolarization (*45*, *46*).

Arecoline, in contrast to pilocarpine, produces a reflex respiratory excitation when it is perfused through the isolated carotid sinus of the cat in a concentration of 10 μg/ml (*37*).

2. ALKYLAMMONIUM BASES

a. Tetramethylammonium

The present discussion of tetramethylammonium (TMA) is taken in large part from Anichkov and Belen'kii (*22*), whose book reports a large amount of Russian work not previously available in English translation.

As noted above, TMA is one of the most potent stimulants of the carotid chemoreceptors. The effective concentration is of the order of 1 μg/ml in a perfused carotid-body preparation. It is about one half as potent as nicotine (*47*); with prolonged perfusions of TMA the carotid chemoreceptors become insensitive to nicotine or ACh. Neither 1,1-dimethyl-4-phenylpiperazinium (DMPP) nor 4-*m*-(chlorophenylcarbamoyloxy)-2-butynyltrimethylammonium chloride (McN-A343) could be demonstrated by indirect means to produce significant stimulation of the aortic chemoreceptors of dogs (*47a*), whereas lobeline was quite effective. The effects of these two rather unusual ganglion stimulants on carotid chemoreceptors would be of great interest. DMPP is quite effective in stimulating muscle spindle afferents (see below).

b. Tetraethylammonium

The effects of tetraethylammonium (TEA) are not agreed upon by various investigators. TEA may inhibit the stimulation of chemoreceptor afferents produced by ACh and congeners. Moe et al. (*25*) were the first to demonstrate that TEA administered intravenously would block the respiratory stimulating actions of ACh, lobeline, and nicotine, whereas the responses to cyanide and to hypoxia were unaffected. Boelaert (*48*) in a short communication noted only that 1 to 10 mg/kg of TEA did not affect the sensitivity of carotid-body chemoreceptors. Heymans et al. (*49*) stated categorically that TEA given locally or intravenously did not alter the reflex responses to ACh or lobeline, although the figures they gave do show distinct depression of these responses with both TEA and hexamethonium. There seems little question that the action potentials induced in chemoreceptor nerves by ACh or lobeline were decreased or abolished after administration of TEA in the experiments of Budde et al.(*50*), Landgren et al. (*34*), and Dontas and Nickerson (*31*). Anichkov and Belen'kii (*22*) report in detail about experiments by Vedeneyeva (*51*) and by Dardynov (*52*) on the effects of TEA solutions perfused in the carotid-sinus preparation. In most of these experiments a solution of TEA of 100 mg/ml abolished the sensitivity of the carotid body to ACh, carbamoylcholine, and nicotine and in the remaining experiments reduced the sensitivity. At the same time, the reaction to cyanide was completely preserved. Also noted is the fact that the perfusion of TEA solutions alone frequently produced a transient stimulation of respiration.

TEA alone has a variety of interesting effects on the afferent activity from the carotid body and sinus. Landgren et al. (*34*) noted that the intra-arterial injection of 100 mg completely abolished the chemoreceptor potentials for 14 seconds. The intravenous injection of a similar amount reduced the responses to ACh or lobeline with little or no effect on the responses to hypoxia. Dontas and Nickerson (*31*) reported that TEA and some other ganglionic blocking agents injected intra-arterially depressed chemoreceptor activity, and they added the rather puzzling comment that quaternary and tertiary blocking agents usually increased chemoreceptor activity after a series of injections of such agents. They also noted that this occurred only when the receptors were partially blocked and the response to ACh was absent. Budde et al. (*50*) also found that intra-arterial injections of TEA produced a transient stimulation of chemoreceptor activity.

The recent studies of the carotid body in vitro of Eyzaguirre and co-workers (*19a–d*) appear to clarify some of these discordant results. In vitro TEA (or hexamethonium) initially or in low concentrations induces stimulation and augmentation of the responses to natural stimulation and ACh. On the other hand, larger doses of TEA or hexamethonium depress the responses to ACh and to natural stimulation. Eyzaguirre and Koyano (*19b*) appropriately emphasize that "the effectiveness of the blocking agent depends not only on the concentration used but also on the state of stimulation of the receptor." The responses to severe anoxia or large concentrations of sodium cyanide are not appreciably affected by cholinergic blocking agents. It should be noted, however, that a quantitative comparison of the different blocking agents and stimulants at all appropriate times and concentrations has yet to be carried out.

3. BISALKYLAMMONIUM COMPOUNDS

a. Hexamethonium

In a definitive study Douglas (*27*) determined that the intravenous administration of 20 mg/kg of hexamethonium would block the effects of ACh, lobeline, or nicotine on the chemoreceptors, as measured by the respiratory stimulation and increase in blood pressure induced by these stimulants injected intra-arterially. This large dose of hexamethonium did not alter the responses to cyanide or the increase in carotid chemoreceptor afferent discharge induced by ACh or lobeline, as assessed on the basis of reflex alterations in respiration and blood pressure. Intra-arterially administered hexamethonium has similar effects (*30*, *31*). By contrast, Heymans et al. (*49*) stated that hexamethonium, like TEA, does not block the reflex responses to ACh or lobeline; however, one of the figures illustrates the effects of hexamethonium administered locally around the carotid body, and there is a distinct depression of the effects of ACh. Dontas and Nickerson (*31*) have reported that hexamethonium itself would depress chemoreceptor activity. Byck (*53*) has reviewed these data and studied the subject by using dose–effect curves, with the result that it can be conclusively stated that the intravenous administration of hexamethonium depresses, but does not abolish, the reflex respiratory changes induced by nicotine; the doses of hexamethonium had no effect alone or produced an increase in the response to cyanide.

The depression by hexamethonium of the excitation of the carotid chemoreceptors produced by ACh, carbamoylcholine, nicotine, and cytisine have also been examined by Denisenko (*54*); the drugs were injected into the isolated carotid-sinus preparation, and the response of respiration was recorded. Hexamethonium, although blocking the effects of these cholinergic agents, did not influence the effects of potassium cyanide. The perfusion of the sinus by solutions of hexamethonium in concentrations of 10 mg/ml or more produced only a slight acceleration of respiratory rate, suggesting a moderate stimulation of the chemoreceptors.

Byck (*53*) suggested that hexamethonium alone increases the sensitivity of the chemoreceptors to cyanide. By contrast, Joels and Neil (*55*) reported briefly that hexamethonium depressed the afferent activity of chemoreceptors to all types of stimuli. Gollwitzer-Meier and Witzleb (*30*) found that hexamethonium in a dose of 100 μg to 1 mg injected intra-arterially produced depression of chemoreceptor afferent activity and also a blockade of the response to oxygen lack. In addition, the effects of lobeline and ACh were blocked. Pentamethonium, on the other hand, was reported to produce stimulation of the carotid chemoreceptors followed by depression; however, the stimulation was not evident when there was already a stimulation due to oxygen lack. Pentamethonium likewise produced an antagonism to lobeline. At least some of these apparently contradictory findings are related to differences in afferent activity detected directly rather than reflexly and to differences in dose, route, and time relationships of drug administration. Further studies will have to include an examination of the affinity and intrinsic activity of the various stimulants, such as nicotine, ACh, cyanide, hypoxia, etc.

b. Decamethonium

Relatively few studies have been done with this compound. Landgren et al. (*34*) reported that 2 mg of decamethonium injected intra-arterially abolished the chemoreceptor potentials induced by hypoxia in cats. Gollwitzer-Meier and Witzleb (*30*), on the other hand, found that decamethonium in doses of 1 to 20 μg produced no change in chemoreceptor afferent activity and no depression of the responses to lobeline. They noted that 50 μg injected intra-arterially produced respiratory paralysis by a neuromuscular block of the respiratory muscles.

Interestingly, Liljestrand (*56*) reported that decamethonium in concentrations of 0.5 to 1 mg/ml produced a depression of the taste afferents of the frog when applied topically, an effect also observed with tubocurarine.

c. Monocholine and Dicholine Esters of Dicarboxylic Acids

Landgren et al. (*34*) demonstrated that 50 μg of succinylcholine (SCh) injected intra-arterially produced a marked increase in the small and medium-sized potentials from sinus nerve afferents, which presumably were afferents from chemoreceptors. Larger concentrations, 1 to 2 mg, produced a "paralysis" of the chemoreceptor afferent discharge. The only other mention of SCh was that a dose of 20 μg given intra-arterially with occlusion of the carotid artery was sufficient to produce a stimulatory effect.

Anichkov and Belen'kii (*22*) present in detail the findings of Vishnyakov (*57*), who examined the effects of a variety of dicholine esters for their action on the isolated carotid sinuses, recording blood pressure and respiration. This work led to the examination of a variety of monocholine and dicholine esters of dicarboxylic acids (*58–60*).

Table 10.2 is taken from Rybolovlev (*60*) and is also reproduced by Anichkov and Belen'kii (*22*); unfortunately, it does not include SCh for comparison. The Russian workers were particularly interested in developing agents that would be useful as analeptics and thus desired to dissociate the muscular blocking activity of the compound from a stimulatory action on carotid chemoreceptors. Of particular interest in the table is the fact that the doses of all compounds required to produce changes in blood pressure were approximately one order of magnitude smaller than those required to produce respiratory excitation.

The monocholine compounds all had about the same potencies as respiratory stimulants, the side-chain length varying between 5 and 8. Rybolovlev (*60*) also compared bischoline esters for their effects on skeletal muscle, blood

TABLE 10.2

Nicotinomimetic Activities of Monocholine and Dicholine Esters of the Higher Homologues of Dicarboxylic Acids (*60*)

$ROCO(CH_2)_nOCOCH_2CH_2N^+(CH_3)_3 \cdot I^-$

Acid (*n*)	R	Doses giving equal effects, mg/kg: Pressor effect	Doses giving equal effects, mg/kg: Respiratory excitation
Pimelic acid (5)	$(CH_3)_3N^+CH_2CH_2 \cdot I^-$	0.005	0.03
Pimelic acid (5)	CH_3CH_2	0.005	0.04
Suberic acid (6)	$(CH_3)_3N^+CH_2CH_2 \cdot I^-$	0.002	0.005
Suberic acid (6)	CH_3CH_2	0.005	0.04
Azelaic acid (7)	$(CH_3)_3N^+CH_2CH_2 \cdot I^-$	0.004	0.02
Azelaic acid (7)	CH_3CH_2	0.005	0.04
Sebacic acid (8)	$(CH_3)_3N^+CH_2CH_2 \cdot I^-$	0.005	0.04
Sebacic acid (8)	CH_3CH_2	0.005	0.04

pressure, respiration, and lethality. The maximum ganglionic stimulating activity was present in the six-carbon compounds, that is, the suberic acid derivative. Similarly, the ability of the substances to cause an increase in respiration due to a stimulation of the carotid-sinus area was also maximal with the suberic acid compound. SCh was the most potent neuromuscular blocking agent in the series and, as mentioned by Dardymov and Ger (*52*), was approximately 10 times as potent as the suberic acid dicholine ester. The ethyldimethyl derivative of SCh was not markedly less potent as a curarizing compound than SCh itself, whereas the diethylmethyl derivative was approximately one third as active. On the other hand, the ethyldimethyl derivative of the suberic acid diester of choline was about one third as active a neuromuscular blocking compound as the parent choline ester with trimethylammonium. Likewise, the increase in blood pressure and the stimulation of respiration produced by the trimethylammonium suberic diester was markedly attenuated by the substitution of one ethyl for methyl on nitrogen. In the SCh series the replacement of the choline ester with a variety of other esters, such as methyl, hexyl, and isopropyl, resulted in a decrease in the neuromuscular blocking property. In contrast, the longer-chain esters exhibited greater stimulation of respiration and increases in blood pressure. Ethyl, methyl, propyl, butyl, and a variety of other alkyl esters were all about 10 to 20 times less active as neuromuscular blocking agents than SCh and 50 to 100 times more active as nicotinic agents with respect to causing an elevation in blood pressure and stimulation of respiration. In these series the same order of potency obtains for pressor responses as for respiratory excitation.

The sparse data of Landgren et al. (*34*) on SCh, showing that 50 μg was required for intra-arterial excitation of chemoreceptors, indicate that it is somewhat less potent than the choline diester of pimelic acid; this would fit the general trend observed by Rybolovlev (*60*).

The pharmacological properties of the most potent compound in the series, the suberic acid derivative, have appeared recently (*52*); the drug is given the name Corconium or subecholine. The addition of subecholine to the fluid perfusing the carotid sinus in situ led to profound respiratory stimulation. Subecholine was found to be some 10 times as active as cytisine which, as shown below, has approximately the same activity as nicotine. On intravenous injection subecholine and cytisine had approximately the same potency, presumably because the former may be hydrolized by plasma cholinesterase.

The respiratory stimulating action of subecholine was abolished by the prior administration of either TEA or hexamethonium. As noted above, Dardymov and Ger (*52*) also found that TEA alone produced some respiratory stimulation, whereas hexamethonium was much less effective in this regard. They cite Vedeneyeva (*51*), who also noted an initial stage of respiratory stimulation following TEA administration. The only other property of subecholine discovered was its ability to block neuromuscular transmission. Its neuromuscular blocking property was reported to be approximately 1/10 that of SCh, in agreement with previous studies. These investigators were unable to find any effect of subecholine on the respiratory center itself in animals under artifical respiration even at doses some 10 times the lethal dose. The margin between doses producing respiratory stimulation and those producing a lethal neuromuscular block is of the order of 1 to 750 on intravenous injection and 1 to 17.5 on subcutaneous injection.

The chemoreceptor stimulating effects of SCh are apparently not generally appreciated. In a recent paper, Stern et al. (*61*) examined the reflex consequences of stimulation of the carotid chemoreceptors with nicotine injected intra-arterially in doses of 50 μg/kg in 3 to 5 ml of solution. The same animal received continuously an intravenous drip of a solution of SCh at a rate of 1 to 2 mg/min. The question may be raised whether the SCh effects on chemoreceptors interacted with those which were presumed to be induced by nicotine.

d. Antagonism of the Chemoreceptor Stimulation Induced by Acetylcholine or Nicotine

The preponderance of data presented thus far indicates that ACh, nicotine, and lobeline actions on carotid chemoreceptors are very effectively blocked by the prior administration of hexamethonium, TEA, or pentamethonium, whereas decamethonium is probably inactive.

As discussed by Heymans (*20*) and Heymans and Neil (*21*), the numerous reports on the effects of atropine administered systemically are in general agreement that there is little influence on the subsequent chemoreceptor responses to ACh, nicotine, and lobeline. In fact, a large number of studies of these substances have been carried out in atropinized preparations in order to prevent the marked changes in cardiovascular function induced by the choline esters; this pretreatment would serve to mark any "muscarinic" effects of the compounds. The local application of atropine will, in fact, reduce the responsiveness of the carotid bodies to oxygen lack and carbon dioxide excess as well as to lobeline and ACh; this effect might well be expected from the local anesthetic properties of atropine, as pointed out by Heymans (*20*).

Landgren et al. (*34*) reported that 1 to 3 mg of atropine given intra-arterially depressed the chemoreceptor response to oxygen lack without affecting the baroreceptors and that it blocked the effects of 300 μg of lobeline. It is not quite clear from the description given, but it appears that a lower dose, 500 μg, of atropine given intra-arterially blocked the lobeline effect but not the response to oxygen lack. Further, Atanackovic and Dalgaard-Mikkelsen (*62*) demonstrated that the increase in blood pressure produced by ACh after large doses of atropine is due, at least in part, to the effects of ACh on the carotid bodies. Eyzaguirre and Koyano (*19b*) recently implied that atropine has the same qualitative effects, stimulation and depression, as *d*-tubocurarine and gallamine.

As might be anticipated from the fact that hexamethonium or TEA will block the effects of ACh, tubocurarine also is an effective blocking agent of these substances at the carotid chemoreceptors. Anichkov and Belen'kii (*22*) mention that Anichkov (*63*) demonstrated that perfusion of the sinus with curare reduced its sensitivity to ACh, but that the sensitivity to cyanide was retained. Landgren et al. (*34*) reported that 300 μg of "curarine" administered intra-arterially to the carotid sinus was effective in antagonizing 300 μg of lobeline and that there was less effect on the response to the oxygen lack than on the response to lobeline. They also stated that 100 to 3000 μg of "curarine" depressed the chemoreceptors for 7 to 8 seconds. Another curarine-like compound, *meso*-3,4-diphenylhexane-*N*,*N'*-bistrimethylammonium iodide, is discussed by Anichkov and Belen'kii (*22*). Perfusion of the carotid sinus with a solution containing this substance abolished the responsiveness of the chemoreceptors to ACh but did not alter its response to hypoxia (*64*).

As noted elsewhere in this review, a large number of these studies needs to be redone by recording from definitively identified afferent fibers of a variety of types with a standardized control of the perfusing fluid. The wide spectrum of sensitivity of the whole system to a variety of influences necessitates an exquisitely rigid control of extraneous influences. Just the pressure alone in the region of the carotid sinus body has distinct effects upon the afferent traffic; a drop in blood pressure produces an acceleration in the discharge of the afferent fibers (*23*, *65*). The reflex responses are clearly a complex function of a variety of inputs, and it seems inescapable in reading all these reports that smaller changes in afferent inflow may well be masked when only reflex changes in respiration are measured. Furthermore, the nature of a given drug effect is a function of the state of responsiveness of the chemoreceptor afferents themselves. As discussed in detail by Anichkov and Belen'kii (*22*) and Heymans and Neil (*21*), the exposure of the carotid bodies to any of a variety of stimulants will, in fact, depress the subsequent responsiveness of the neurons and the associated reflex connections to subsequent stimulation due to such things as oxygen lack; perfusion of the carotid sinus area with nicotine will depress the subsequent responsiveness to ACh. In many of the experiments reported it is not at all clear what the actual state of the chemoreceptor cells themselves is at a given instant in time: whether they are, in fact, firing, and whether the reflex response is decreased because of central components or the initial substance to which the cells are exposed is blocking the attachment of the second drug to its specific receptors (*19b*). A review of these more complicated experimental procedures is outside the scope of this chapter and would not significantly contribute to a discussion of structure–activity relationships except as they relate to the establishment of common sites of action of the different substances.

4. ANTICHOLINESTERASES

A variety of anticholinesterases have been examined for their actions, and much discussion has arisen over interpretation of the results (see summary, *19b*). In general, all these substances potentiate the actions of ACh without altering significantly the effects of nicotine or lobeline. In vitro, however, the action of physostigmine is to produce a variable degree of increase in chemosensory activity. The excitation is obtained consistently and to a greater degree in the presence of 5% CO_2 in O_2 than in the absence of CO_2. It was suggested that this was related to increased inactivation of cholinesterase in the presence of CO_2. The interaction between eserine effects and hypoxia was not discussed (*19b*). The interactions between these cholinesterases and oxygen lack will not be considered further.

It is actually rather surprising that there is as good agreement as there is between the reflex effects of a variety of drugs given into the carotid circulation and the action potential records taken from such nerves, because it is well known that electrophysiological techniques detect only the relatively large fibers and the nerves themselves contain large numbers of small and non-myelinated fibers. The reflex consequences of stimulation of each of these groups is well established as rather different (see, for example, *66*, *67*).

5. NICOTINE AND ITS ANALOGUES

Anichkov and Belen'kii (*22*) have reviewed a large amount of Russian work on the chemoreceptor stimulatory activity of nicotine and nicotine-like alkaloids and a variety of derivatives. The activities of these substances, from the data they give, are presented in Table 10.3 along with the chemical structures. As chemoreceptor stimulants, nicotine and cytisine are of approximately the same potency, and from other data it appears that their nicotinic effects on ganglia are of the same order of magnitude. In general, there is an interaction between the nicotine analogues and ACh, such that the response to ACh is decreased during the phase of depression that supervenes after the stimulatory effects of nicotine or cytisine. However, the response to carbon dioxide or cyanide also is frequently reduced. As has been mentioned, it is difficult to ascertain whether this is an interaction in the same pathway or whether it has something to do with excessive activity of the nerves themselves or the reflex connections. Krylov's experiments, quoted by Anichkov and Belen'kii (*22*), indicate that the administration of nicotine resulted in a loss of sensitivity of

TABLE 10.3

Potency of Nicotine Analogues as Stimulants of Respiration[a] (*22*)

Nicotine analogue	Minim. effect. concn. in carotid-sinus perfusate, $\mu g/ml$	Remarks
Nicotine 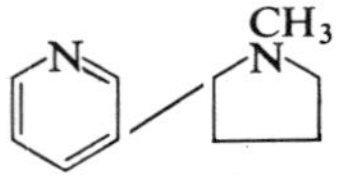	0.5	Nornicotine distinctly less potent; acetyl, amino, and amino acetyl derivatives all less potent, but some may have higher therapeutic index.
Anabasine (neonicotine) 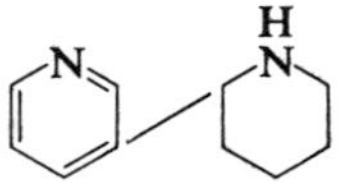	10.0	Methylanabasine less potent (but see nicotine); amino and acetylamino derivatives less potent.
Coniine 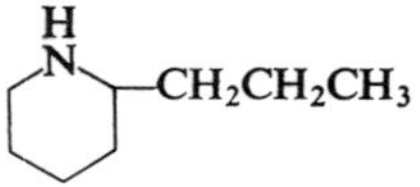	20.0	
Nikethamide 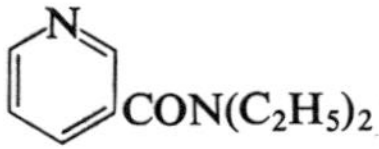		
Lobeline 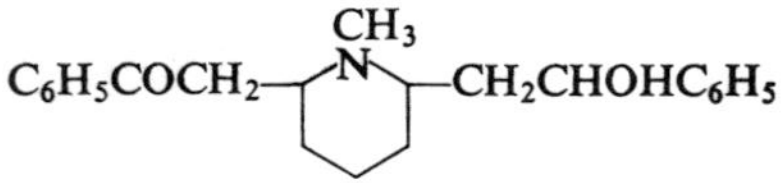	2.0	Norlobeline less effective; no side groups or symmetrical alcoholic or keto side groups 1/10 as active.
Cytisine 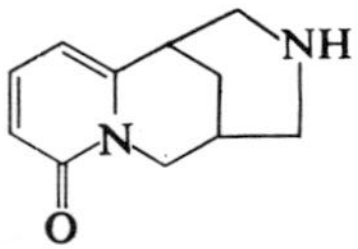	0.5	Therapeutic index twice that of lobeline; *N*-methyl derivative 1/20 as active as cytisine.
Tetramethylammonium $(CH_3)_4N^+Cl^-$	1.0	

[a] Both piperidine and trimethylamine have detectable stimulatory actions.

the chemoreceptors to ACh but a retention of their sensitivity to cyanide and to potassium.

As noted above, nicotine and cytisine have approximately the same potency; however, nornicotine is distinctly less potent than nicotine, whereas the *N*-methyl derivative of cytisine is only 1/20 as active as cytisine. A similar contradiction is found in a comparison of nicotine derivatives with those of anabasine. *N*-Methylanabasine is much less potent than anabasine itself, whereas nicotine is more potent than nornicotine. The acetyl, amino, and aminoacetyl derivatives of nicotine or anabasine are less potent than the parent compounds. However, Anichkov and Belen'kii point out that 2-acetylaminonicotine and the dextrorotatory 2-aminonicotine, although distinctly less potent than nicotine, may have larger therapeutic indices, that is, be more selective in their effects on the chemoreceptors than nicotine. The work of Arbuzov (*68*) pointed out that the levorotatory isomers of each of the pairs of amino or acetylamino-nicotine were more active than the dextrorotatory derivatives; the toxicity also was greater for the *levo* compounds. The relationship between activity and toxicity, however, varied with the different substances, and the compound with the "widest margin of safety" was the dextrorotatory 2-aminonicotine. As far as can be determined, no further work has been done with this substance.

Lobeline is an asymmetric compound with an alcohol and ketone side chain. The compound with both functions removed (lobelane) or the derivative with symmetrical hydroxyl (lobelanidine) or symmetrical ketone (lobelanine) side chains is each about 1/10 as active as lobeline itself, suggesting that, at least with lobeline, both of these oxygen-containing moieties are significant in determining potency. Further, two other related alkaloids, lobinine and isolobinine, have asymmetrical side chains, and both have powerful stimulating effects on respiration (see *40*, *69*).

Gorelik (*70*) and Mikhel'son et al. (*59*) discuss in detail the fact that lobeline and cytisine are ineffective respiratory stimulants when given by other than the intravenous route. One of the major reasons for this is that their pronounced central nervous system stimulatory activity overrides the peripheral effects. The authors emphasize the fact that the quaternary dicholine ester of suberic acid does not produce an effect centrally and is, therefore, a more usable agent for the clinical manipulation of respiration. They compared the effectiveness of lobeline, cytisine, and the dicholine ester of suberic acid on intravenous and subcutaneous administration in cat and man. The sensitivities of the cat and man, in milligrams per kilogram, to each of the three agents are said to be almost identical. Moreover, the subcutaneous doses of cytisine and the suberic acid derivative were approximately 10 times the intravenous dose, whereas the subcutaneous dose of lobeline required for respiratory stimulation was somewhat more than 10 times the intravenous dose; the subcutaneous administration of lobeline to man was complicated by the frequent occurrence of emesis.

Zeymal and Rybolovlev (*71*) reported on the quaternary derivatives of nicotine, arecoline, anabasine, and cytisine. Each of these agents produced a convulsion, whereas the quaternary analogues did not. Nicotine monomethiodide caused an increase of blood pressure and respiration in about 3 times the dose required for the tertiary base (1.7 times on a molar basis), although the lethal dose of the quaternary is quite similar to that of nicotine itself. Similar differences in potency were found with cytisine and its methylammonium derivative. The quaternary derivative of arecoline produced a drop in blood pressure, but the authors were able to demonstrate in atropinized animals an increase in nicotinic activity of the quaternary derivative of arecoline over that of the parent substance. The methiodide derivative of arecoline produced on intravenous injection (0.1 mg/kg) a stimulation of respiration that was shown to be due to an action at the carotid-sinus area. Presumably, analogous effects of quarternization of cytisine were obtained, although they were not described in detail.

As discussed by Anichkov and Belen'kii (*22*), sparteine and its dextrorotatory analogue, pachycarpine, are weak stimulants of ganglia and carotid-sinus chemoreceptors. Piperidine and trimethylamine also may produce weak stimulating actions on carotid bodies.

A variety of other agents have been found to influence carotid chemoreceptor activity. For example, Gollwitzer-Meier and Witzleb (*72*) obtained transient stimulation of chemoreceptors and saphenous-nerve skin receptors with a series of adrenergic blocking agents; moderately effective doses of Hydergin, phentolamine, Dibenamine, and tolazoline were 10 to 20, 33, 165 to 330, and 330 mg/kg, respectively. The responses to hypoxia, potassium, or lobeline were unaffected by these agents. It is doubtful that this stimulatory action is related to adrenolytic activity. A discussion of these and other agents is left to other types of reviews.

B. Baroreceptors of the Carotid Sinus and Aortic Arch

A rather wide variety of agents that have been found to cause activation or sensitization of carotid or aortic baroreceptor afferents includes cholinergic agents, TEA, adrenergic agents, vasopressin, adenosine triphosphate, and volatile anesthetics; those that produce depression include local anesthetics, papaverine, priscoline, sodium nitrite, and alcohols (reviewed *7*, *20*, *21*). The large majority of the investigations have involved the recording of reflex activity. Few studies have included a sufficient number of agents or doses of agents to provide data useful for a structure–activity correlation other than an over-all spectrum of sensitivity of the endings to various classes of agents.

The stimulatory actions of the adrenergic agents and the depression by relaxants of smooth muscle are probably best explained as secondary effects of the agents on the distensibility of carotid sinus wall (*7*, *20*, *21*), and they therefore will not be discussed further here.

The sensitization of baroreceptors by volatile anesthetics is particularly interesting, because it can be related to differences in the cardiovascular and respiratory effects of these agents (*73–75*). Paintal (*7*) stresses the fact that volatile anesthetics produce sensitization of the pressoreceptors followed by increased adaptation and, with high concentrations or prolonged exposure, depression. Sensitization of baroreceptors is not produced by nitrous oxide or cyclopropane (*76*), but these gases do sensitize pulmonary stretch receptors, perhaps because these are exposed to higher concentration directly through the airways (*7*).

At present, there are insufficient quantitative data on the anesthetics for further conclusions to be drawn about structure–activity relationships.

Even with respect to ACh and nicotine, it can be concluded only that the latter is probably appreciably more active than the former and that the stimulation and sensitization produced by them is antagonized by hexamethonium or tubocurarine but not by atropine (*77*). TEA also evokes an increased sensitivity of large and medium fibers from baroreceptors; hexamethonium is much less effective. Pentamethonium and pendiomide do not cause sensitization (*78*).

The question should be raised, however, of the degree to which stimulation or sensitization of baroreceptors by such agents tends to influence the reflex responses generally attributed to chemoreceptor activation. As noted earlier, there are, essentially, no quantitative comparisons of the changes in afferent-nerve activity produced by a series of chemoreceptor stimulants; the major quantitative studies have employed reflex endpoints. The fact that many of the substances, such as nicotine, also cause stimulation of receptors, which would partly oppose the reflex response from other receptor sites, imposes very serious limitations on the interpretability of the experiments. This is particularly true if it is assumed that the various agents employed will very probably exhibit somewhat different actions at the two sites.

The same problem exists with the veratrum alkaloids, many of which have been found to cause excitation of one or the other afferent nerve. Yet there are essentially no studies comparing a series of different veratrum alkaloids and other agents on the afferent-nerve activity of a given receptor. A large number of studies have been directed at delineating the sites and mechanisms of action of these agents and their relative potencies, but they are of extremely limited use in the present context, in view of the fact that the agents may exhibit markedly different spectra of action on different afferent systems, the central nervous system, skeletal muscle, and so forth (*79–85*).

C. Skeletal Muscle Spindle Afferents

1. EXCITANTS

a. Acetylcholine and Congeners

The study of the stimulation of the activity of afferent nerves from muscle spindles produced by cholinergic substances originated with the investigations of SCh (Granit et al., *86*) and of ACh (Hunt, *87*). These investigations were part of the then current interest in the function of the muscle spindle and of the small (gamma or fusimotor) motor nerve innervation of the specialized muscle fibers, the intrafusal muscle fibers, lying within the spindle.

The effects of drugs on the function of sensory nerves from spindles have been reviewed recently (*7*, *19*). For the present purposes attention will be directed largely to quaternary ammonium compounds and the mammalian spindle. Most of the work on frog spindles has already been reviewed, and the frog spindle differs significantly from the mammalian with respect to type of intrafusal muscle fiber and its innervation. Further, the tachyphylaxis to ACh exhibited by isolated frog muscle severely constrains any quantitative comparisons of agents' activities (*88*); the presence of such marked tachyphylaxis is apparently not generally appreciated and may account for some of the discrepancies in reported results (see, for example, review *7*).

To establish precise dose–effect curves and make quantitative comparisons of the potencies of drugs, the author and his colleagues adopted a technique for the intra-arterial injection of the test substances into the muscles in which the spindles under study were situated. This technique, coupled with the recording from a large number of individual afferents in each preparation, has permitted a detailed analysis of the effects of a large number of congeners on the afferent function of cat muscle spindles (*89–96*).

The afferent endings in the spindle are histologically of two classes: the primary, or annulospiral, endings and the secondary, or flower spray. The two types are correlated with the conduction velocities of the afferent fibers; the primary are the terminations of the larger, group Ia, fibers of faster conduction velocity, whereas the secondary are of group II.

ACh is a surprisingly weak stimulant of the fibers from both primary and secondary endings; intra-arterial doses of 10 to 160 μg are required. Moreover, the dose–response curve is quite flat (Figure 10.3). By contrast, SCh is a potent stimulant; effective doses range from 0.625 to 10 μg. Larger doses, 20 to 50 μg, produce a sustained, intense activation with subsequent erratic discharge activity and derangement in the response to subsequent doses of the agent. SCh produces markedly different amounts of excitation of different afferents. Verhey and Voorhoeve (*97*) reported that the afferents from secondary endings were much less sensitive to SCh than the primary. The subsequent studies of Albuquerque and Smith (*89*) confirmed and extended this observation with a

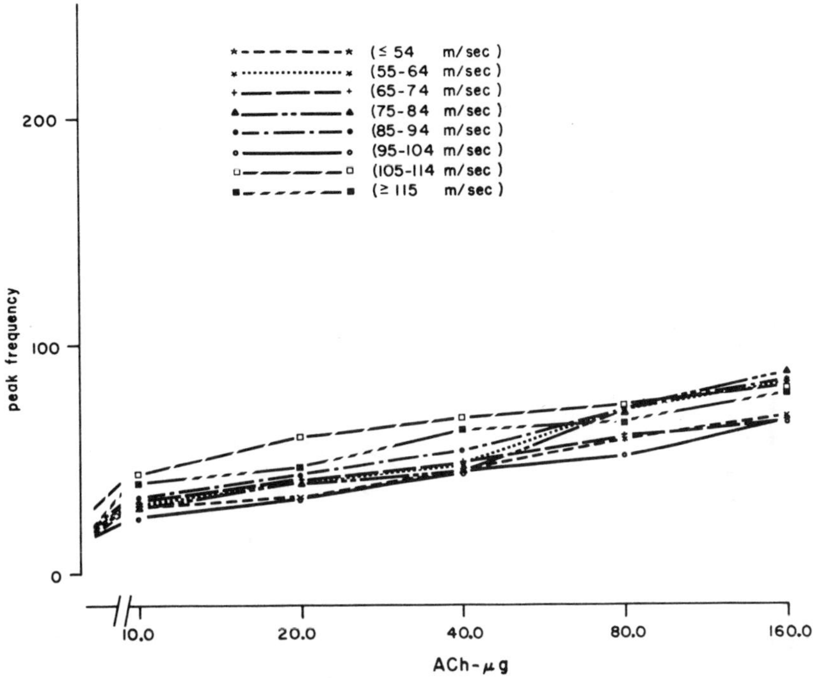

Fig. 10.3. Dose-effect curves for muscle spindle excitation produced by acetylcholine in five cats. Abscissa, dose of acetylcholine administered intra-arterially in micrograms plotted logarithmically. Ordinate, mean peak frequency in impulses per second attained with a given dose. The number of units in each group was: 5, 4, 2, 2, 4, 3, 4, 2 (⩽54 to ⩾115 m/sec, respectively). The range for all fibers with the largest dose of 160 μg was 53 to 88 impulses/sec. An increase in frequency was exhibited by all units with the lowest dose of 10 μg: the controls ranged from 10 to 38 impulses/sec; the average increase was 14 impulses/sec (*89*, *90*).

large number of afferents in the same and different cats. The degree of activation of the afferent fiber was found to be correlatable with its conduction velocity. Figure 10.4, taken from Albuquerque and Smith (*91*), illustrates the dose–effect curves for SCh on groups of fibers, combined according to conduction velocity. Not only are the fibers of faster conduction velocity more sensitive to all doses of SCh, but they exhibit dose–effect curves with steeper slopes than those of slower fibers. The curves of the faster fibers are clearly concave upwards, whereas the slower are approximately linear. No one simple transformation has been found that will permit the construction of linear dose–effect curves for all the agents for all fiber groups.

These examples of two drugs with similar stimulant effects illustrate the difficulties encountered in establishing meaningful generalizations regarding structure–activity relationships. Keeping in mind the differences in

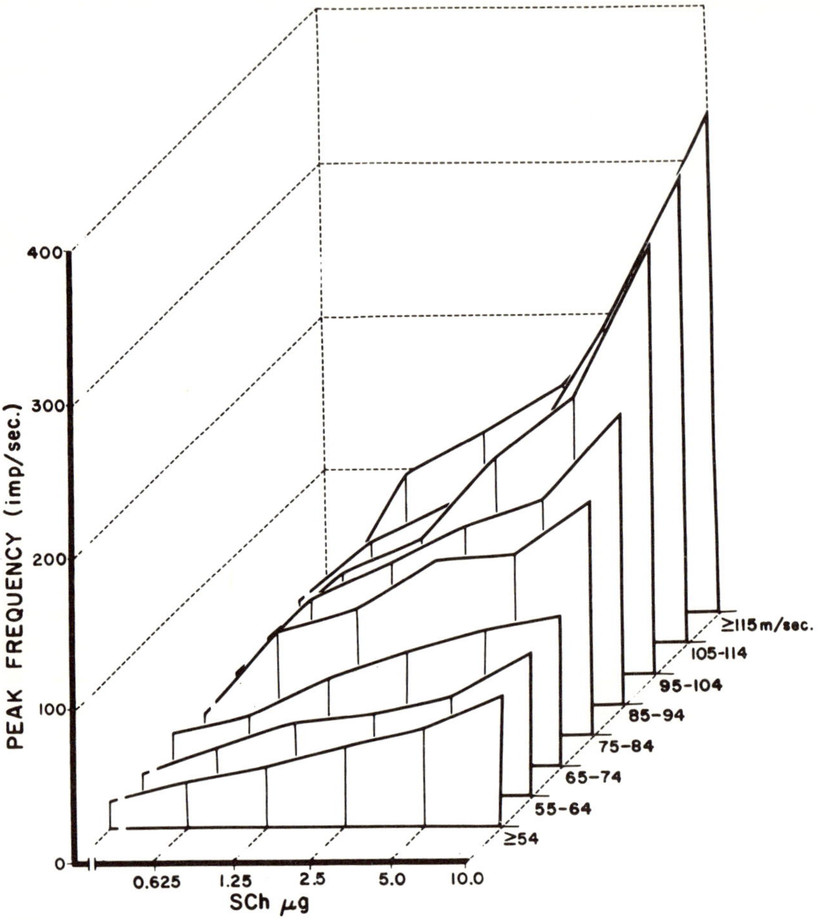

Fig. 10.4. Three-dimensional plot of peak frequency of afferent discharge as functions of dose of SCh and conduction velocity of the afferent fibers. *X* axis, dose of intra-arterially administered SCh plotted logarithmically. *Y* axis, mean peak frequency of muscle spindle afferents in impulses per second. *Z* axis, conduction velocity in meters per second. The fibers are grouped according to conduction velocity. The number of units in each group are 9, 7, 5, 2, 4, 7, 4, 6, (⩽54 to ⩾115 m/sec, respectively) (*91*, *92*).

dose–response curves, equivalent doses for ACh and SCh chlorides are approximately 160 and 0.625 μg for the fastest-conducting fibers and 160 and 5 to 10 μg, respectively, for the slower fibers.

Muscarine, in contrast, produces only a depression in the spontaneous activity of afferents from muscle spindles (*89*). The mechanism underlying this effect is unknown. Furthrethonium iodide is inactive (*97*).

Nicotine is one of the most potent stimulants of spindle afferent activity known. It also produces even more selective activation of the faster-conducting fibers than does SCh. In fact, 2.5 to 5 μg of SCh produces more activation of fibers from secondary endings than does 10 μg of nicotine, whereas the group of fastest-conducting fibers are slightly more affected by nicotine than by SCh (Figures 10.4 and 10.5). The dose–response curves of faster afferents to nicotine are steeper than those of comparable fibers to SCh.

The marked potency of nicotine prompted us to examine another ganglion stimulant, DMPP (1,1-dimethyl-4-phenylpiperazinium iodide). The pattern of the effects of DMPP more closely resembled those of SCh than of nicotine. The sensitivity of the fiber groups was a smoother function of conduction velocity than with either nicotine or SCh (Figure 10.6). On the slower-conducting units it was approximately as potent as SCh and more potent than nicotine. On the faster groups, however, it was somewhat less than half as potent as SCh (*90*, *91*).

Decamethonium, as noted by previous investigators (reviewed *19*), produced a long-lasting excitation. However, in contrast to nicotine or SCh, this excitation was not selective for the more rapidly conducting fibers. In fact, the faster afferents exhibited an initial acceleration in discharge, which was then interrupted by periods of little or no afferent activity. On the other hand, the afferents from the slower fibers exhibited a sustained high-frequency discharge (Figure 10.7). This effect on the slowly conducting fibers clearly indicates that the fibers from secondary endings are capable of discharging at rapid rates but do so only after decamethonium, and not after SCh, nicotine, DMPP, or ACh!

Monoquaternary compounds are also effective in stimulating the afferent endings of muscle spindles. TMA had effects on afferents from primary and secondary receptors similar to those of SCh, but it was approximately one third to one half as potent. TEA (1 to 2 mg, intra-arterially) failed to cause any excitation.

Pentamethonium and hexamethonium (1 to 2 mg, intra-arterially) were also inactive in evoking an excitation of spindle afferents. The doses were associated with changes in the mechanical muscle-twitch response to nerve stimulation: after TEA there was approximately a 20% increase and after pentamethonium and hexamethonium a 10 to 20% decrease.

An aromatic analogue of decamethonium, the bischoline ether of hydroquinone, also causes prolonged spindle afferent excitation (*98*). It is, however, distinctly less potent than decamethonium or SCh; 2 to 5 mg/kg given intravenously produces spindle excitation lasting up to one hour. The responses of the different spindle afferent fibers to this substance have not been examined. During the spindle excitation fusimotor neuromuscular transmission is still present, as is the response to muscle stretch. The monosynaptic reflex is depressed by these doses of the bischoline ether. The possibility of inducing

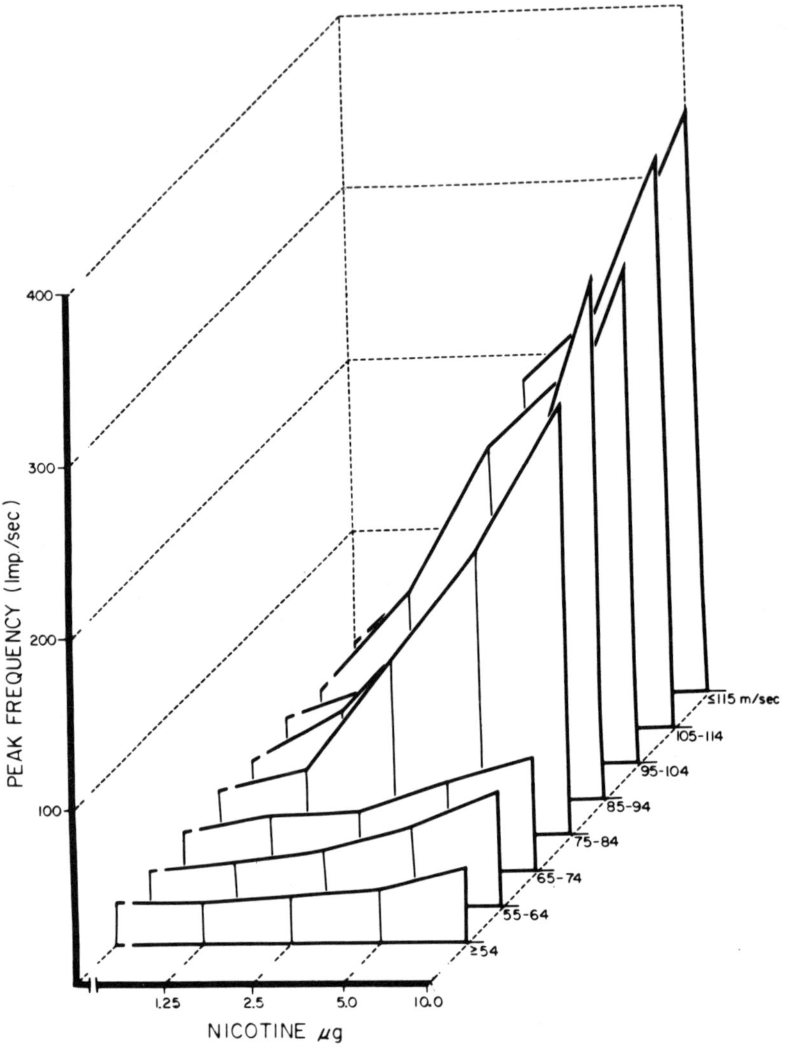

Fig. 10.5. Three-dimensional plot of peak frequency of afferent discharge as functions of dose of nicotine and afferent conduction velocity. *X* axis, dose of intra-arterially administered nicotine plotted logarithmically. *Y* axis, mean peak frequency in impulses per second attained with a given dose. *Z* axis, conduction velocity in meters per second. The number of units in each conduction velocity group were 5, 4, 2, 2, 4, 3, 4, 2 (≤54 to ≥115 m/sec, respectively) (*91*, *92*).

reflex depression in patients in doses that do not affect neuromuscular transmission is currently under investigation. Ginzel et al. (*99*, *100*) showed many years ago that it, as well as decamethonium, could depress the knee jerk in

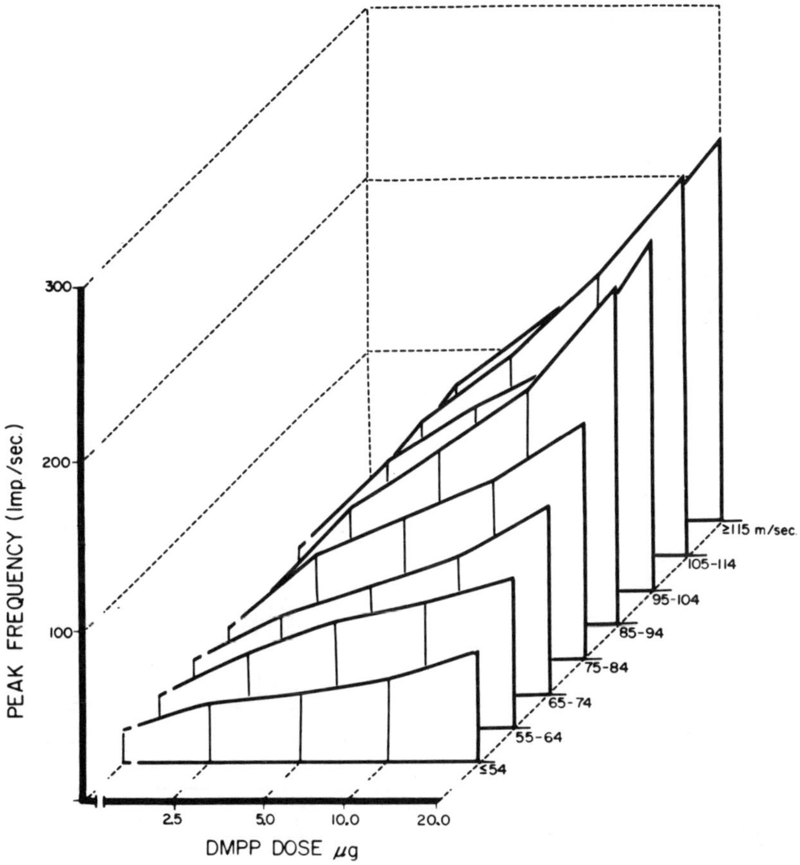

Fig. 10.6. Three-dimensional plot of peak frequency of 35 muscle spindle afferents as function of DMPP dose and afferent conduction velocities. Control frequency prior to any drug administration is plotted on the left of the graph. *X* axis, dose of intra-arterially administered DMPP plotted logarithmically. *Y* axis, mean peak frequency in impulses per second attained with the given dose of DMPP. *Z* axis, conduction velocity in meters per second. The afferent fibers are grouped according to conduction velocities. The number of fibers in each group were 6, 4, 4, 4, 3, 7, 5, 2 (≤54 to ≥115 m/sec, respectively). As examples of the magnitude of variability in each of the above groups the ranges of peak frequencies following a dose of 10 μg were 30–52, 68–72, 65–90, 80–135, 130–145, 113–170, 98–192, 130–150 impulses/sec for each group ≤54 through ≥115 m/sec, respectively (*91*, *92*).

doses that did not alter the muscle-twitch response to nerve stimulation. This selective effect on reflex and nerve stimulation-induced contractions could not be demonstrated with the stretch reflex of ankle extensors in decerebrate cats (*101*).

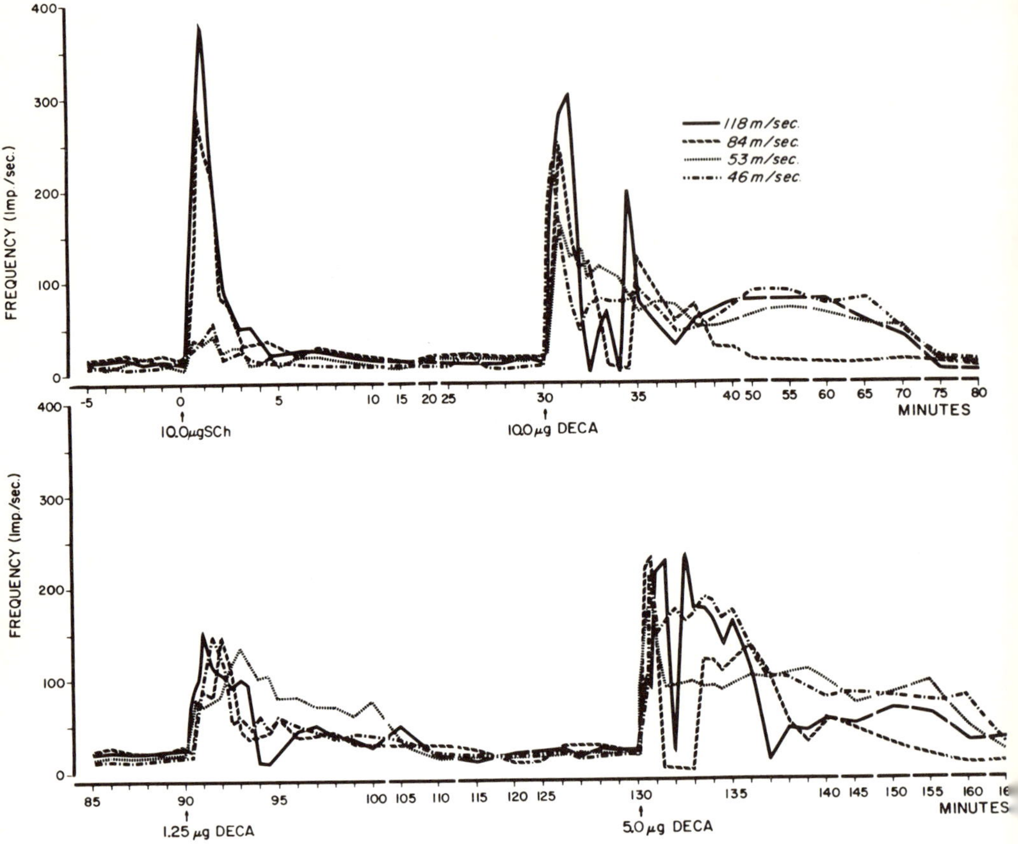

Fig. 10.7. Comparison of decamethonium and succinylcholine effects on skeletal muscle spindle afferents. Ordinate, frequency of afferent discharge in impulses per second; abscissa, time in minutes. Drugs injected intra-arterially. Various line patterns depict responses of different fibers; conduction velocity of afferent fibres indicated in meters per second (*93*).

Recent experiments have clarified the conditions under which spindle afferent excitation does produce reflex depression. In preparations in which the input to the lumbar cord is strictly limited to the muscle under study, SCh and nicotine given either to the muscle or intravenously produce a triphasic alteration in the homonymous monosynaptic reflex: a brief increase, a depression of 1 to 2 minutes, followed by an increase above control levels of 10 to 20 minutes (*93*, *96*, *102*). Decamethonium, on the other hand, produces only a depression of the monosynaptic reflex with a concomitant increase in the dorsal root reflex. It is to be noted that decamethonium excites group II fibers to the same extent as group Ia, whereas SCh excites primarily the Ia group. These findings, then, are close to what would be predicted from previous knowledge of the reflex connections of muscle afferents (*103*, *104*).

In contrast to the experiments just cited, in the numerous previous studies of Henatsch and his colleagues and Fujimori and Eldred, SCh was found to produce a depression of the monosynaptic reflex [reviewed and analyzed (*19*) and (*105*)]. This depression has been recently demonstrated to occur with SCh only in preparations in which the cord is not extensively deafferented, and so it appears to be due to heterosynaptically mediated influences (*96*). Further, the studies of Cook et al. (*105*) and Whitsel et al. (*95*) indicate that presynaptic inhibition is, at least in part, involved in this reflex depression. Henatsch (*106*) and Kato et al. (*107*) have discussed in detail this and other possible mechanisms of the stretch reflex depression consequent to spindle afferent excitation.

A more general lesson, however, is to be derived from these experiments. The reflex consequences of these changes in afferent input are directly related to the spectrum of afferent nerves from the spindle excited (SCh versus decamethonium) as well as to the degree to which other muscles are exposed to the agent. It seems safe to say that more is known of the specifics of drug effects on spindle afferents and the reflex effects of these alterations than is known of other afferent systems. These considerations raise further cautions concerning inferences about drug actions on specific afferent systems, when they are based solely on the initiation or modification of reflexes by a single dose of drug.

b. Antagonism to Spindle Excitation of Tubocurarine

The transmission from fusimotor nerve to intrafusal muscle is distinctly less sensitive to blocking by tubocurarine than the extrafusal neuromuscular system (*94*; reviewed *19*).

Tubocurarine pretreatment markedly decreases the responsiveness of muscle spindle afferents to stimulation by quaternary ammonium compounds. The tubocurarine-caused depression of the excitation of spindle afferents induced by SCh is not, however, directly proportional to the depression of extrafusal neuromuscular transmission (*108*). A significant depression of spindle responsiveness to SCh is shown by doses of tubocurarine that do not depress the muscle twitch on nerve stimulation. On the other hand, after doses of tubocurarine that completely abolish the muscle twitch SCh still causes detectable, although decreased, excitation of spindle afferent activity. Similar results were obtained with dihydro-β-erythroidine in place of tubocurarine. They are not unexpected in view of the fact that neuromuscular transmission is a threshold-dependent response and therefore essentially an all-or-none one at a given junction and that the spindle-stimulating effect of SCh is a graded function of the concentration. In other words, the dose–effect curve of the depression of neuromuscular transmission is much steeper than that of the depression of spindle response to SCh (see Figure 10.8).

The effects of a dose of tubocurarine that would block completely both intrafusal and extrafusal neuromuscular transmission were examined with respect to the responsiveness of afferents from primary and secondary receptors, to SCh, ACh, decamethonium, and nicotine.

With due regard to matching the responses, the interaction of these stimulants with pretreatment doses of tubocurarine sufficient to block fusimotor neuromuscular transmission can be summarized as follows (*94*):

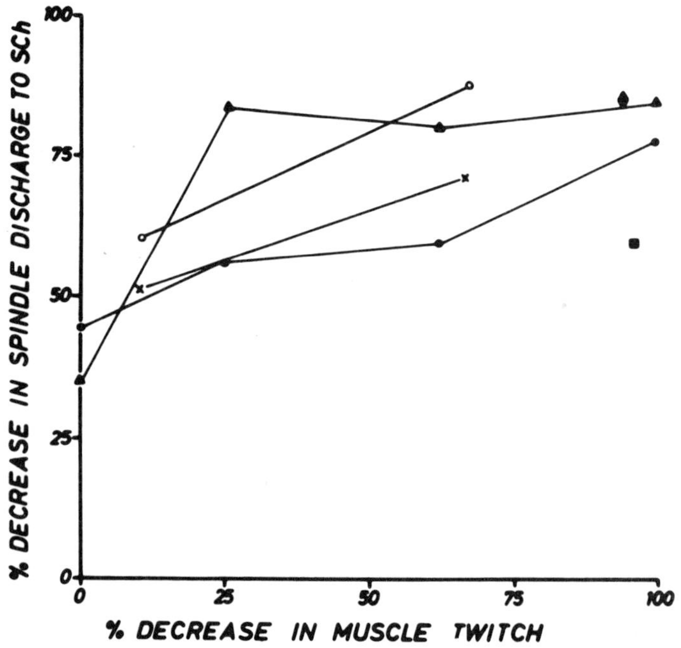

Fig. 10.8. Relationship of the depression of neuromuscular transmission and the depression of succinylcholine-induced spindle afferent stimulation produced by dihydro-β-erythroidine. Ordinate, per cent decrease induced by dihydro-β-erythroidine in the spindle stimulation to succinylcholine (SCh 0.25 mg/kg, intravenously); abscissa, per cent decrease induced by dihydro-β-erythroidine in the twitch contraction of triceps surae muscle to single shock nerve stimulation elicited every 10 sec. Dihydro-β-erythroidine administered in various doses (0.5 to 4 mg/kg, intravenously) and the response to nerve stimulation and SCh assessed and plotted against one another. Different symbols depict different spindle afferents and different experiments. Doses of dihydro-β-erythroidine which had no effect on the muscle twitch (ca. 0.5 mg/kg, intravenously) effectively reduced the response to SCh.

(1) The stimulation induced by nicotine, SCh, ACh, or decamethonium is antagonized by prior tubocurarine pretreatment.

(2) The effects of ACh or decamethonium on secondary as well as primary endings were almost always completely blocked by tubocurarine pretreatment sufficient to abolish fusimotor neuromuscular transmission.

(3) The depression by tubocurarine of responses to nicotine or SCh was generally less than 100% and there was little differentiation among receptor types.

The findings were interpreted as indicating that there were differences among agents with respect to the magnitude of antagonism by tubocurarine and that, with the exception of ACh and decamethonium, the stimulation of spindle afferents could not have been the sole result of the stimulant's presynaptic action at fusimotor nerve terminals, since such transmission was blocked.

The results may be taken to indicate further that the various structurally related compounds act at more than one site. Thus, statements of structure–activity relationships devolve on considerations of site or mechanism of action and not only on correlations among the structure and potency.

If the view is correct that these quaternary ammonium substances stimulating spindle afferent endings act at more than one site, then studies of the relationship between structure and activity can provide little information useful for inferring the nature or type of bonding with the receptor. The most plausible sites and mechanisms of action include the following: fusimotor nerve terminals, postsynaptic actions at intrafusal muscle end plate, action on the intrafusal muscle fiber membrane or muscle directly, actions on the afferent ending (the generator region or the first node), and effects secondary to the release from muscle of an excitatory substance such as potassium ion.

Indirect evidence suggests that ACh could act presynaptically but SCh not exclusively so (*89*). Smith and Eldred (*109*) have suggested that SCh probably does not act on the sensory ending, because it is inactive after the induction of intrafusal-fiber contracture by means of ryanodine. Many problems still remain. The differential activation of the endings of faster afferents may be related to their greater sensitivity to rate of change in length, but this cannot be unambiguously related to the time course of drug effects (*89*, *91*).

Of immediate interest would be the effects of infusions of the rapidly acting agents and the effects of drug-induced excitation on the responsiveness of the endings to the appropriate stimulus, muscle stretch, and the development of a useful isolated preparation for the quantitative assay of drugs affecting spindle function.

2. DEPRESSANTS

A few substances have been found to cause a depression of muscle spindle activity, but the number investigated has been so small that little regarding structure–activity relationships can be established.

So-called centrally acting muscle-relaxants may have, in addition to central effects, a depressant effect on muscle spindles. Mephenesin in intravenous doses that block polysynaptic reflexes also decreases tonic muscle spindle activity. In fact, the sustained activity with tonic muscle stretch is more susceptible to depression than is the response to phasic stretch (*110*). Procaine is somewhat more active, but the percent depression of tonic activity is not significantly different from that of phasic activity. Caramiphen produces only a slight depression, but this is complicated by a drop in systemic blood pressure, which tends to cause an increase in spindle afferent activity.

A triazine compound, 2,4-bis(diethylamino)-6-(2-phenylacetylhydrazino)-1,3,5-triazine, Ciba 28882-Ba (*111*), is a particularly potent depressant of spindle afferent activity. Abolition of afferent activity can be obtained with intravenous doses of 0.03 to 0.3 mg/kg (*110*). This triazine derivative produces effects on fusimotor outflow in even smaller doses, presumably acting centrally. Matsushita et al. (*112*, *112a*) have reported on a complex unsymmetrical bis-methonium compound, MI-65-S,* that also produces depression of spindle afferent activity, although fairly large doses are required, 3 mg/kg subcutaneously administered. This agent produces ataxia, incoordination, and flaccidity with retention of phasic flexor reflexes in the mouse, cat, dog, and monkey. Respiration is depressed and body temperature decreased. The only major effect discovered other than depression of muscle spindle afferent activity was a block of transmission through autonomic ganglia and a profound hypotension on intravenous administration to anesthetized animals. No effects on spinal reflex activity could be obtained, and there was no antagonism of strychnine in cats.

Interestingly, the dimethyl and diethylaminoethyl derivatives of MI-65-S produced moderate augmentation of spindle afferent activity. The tertiary derivatives were essentially inactive.

It is plausible that some of the peripheral depressant effects on sensory systems are the consequence of local anesthetic properties of the compounds. The data on even a series of local anesthetics are, however, insufficient as bases for such a suggestion. It might be expected, from the extensive studies of compounds with local anesthetic properties, that some agents would have more effect on spindle afferents than their local anesthetic potency assessed by other techniques would indicate. In this connection, the effects of systemically administered quaternary local anesthetics would be of great interest (see F, p. 564).

* 2-(3-Dimethylaminopropyl)-1,3,3*a*,4,9,9*a*-hexahydro-4,9-*O*-benzo-2*H*-benz(*f*)isoindole dimethiodide.

D. Pain Production: Effects of Substances on Skin and Exposed Blister Base

1. ACETYLCHOLINE AND CONGENERS

Keele and Armstrong (*113*) have reviewed the effects of a variety of ACh congeners and antagonists applied to the base of an experimentally induced blister of the skin. Table 10.4 has been prepared from their summary.

Of particular interest are the points that carbamoylcholine and nicotine were less potent than ACh and that methacholine and pilocarpine did not produce pain when applied to the blister base. These observations again suggest a nicotinic type of action, and the antagonism of ACh caused by tubocurarine and hexamethonium add further consistence. However, atropine is also effective in blocking ACh effects. Unfortunately, other classes of stimulants were not examined for possible antagonism caused by atropine. If its local anesthetic property were responsible for the antagonism of ACh effects, then a nonspecific antagonism of many pain-producing substances would be expected.

This spectrum of stimulating and blocking agents is not typical of either of the prototype systems, the autonomic ganglia or the skeletal muscle, in that decamethonium produces no excitation as it does with certain skeletal muscle, yet it is as effective a blocking agent of ACh as tubocurarine (*114*, *115*).

The fact that ACh is more potent on the blister base than carbachol or nicotine (whereas the reverse is true of a number of other receptors, such as carotid chemoreceptors and muscle spindle afferents) may be a reflection of the absence of appreciable cholinesterase activity in the blister base. Keele and

TABLE 10.4

Cholinergic Agents and Pain Production on Application to Exposed Blister Base (*113*)

	Effective concentration, g/ml	Caused pain	Antagonized pain produced by subsequent ACh
Acetylcholine	1×10^{-5} to 1×10^{-3}	+	−
Carbamoylcholine	1×10^{-4} (1/10 to 1/25 as potent as ACh)	+	− ?
Nicotine tartrate	$1\text{-}5 \times 10^{-4}$ (?1/10 as potent as ACh)	+	+
Methacholine	10^{-3}	−	~
Pilocarpine	10^{-3}	−	~
Decamethonium	ca. 10^{-5}	−	+
d-Tubocurarine	ca. 10^{-5}	−	+
Atropine	ca. 10^{-4}	−	+
Hexamethonium	ca. 10^{-3}	−	+

Armstrong (*113*) found that neostigmine application caused neither pain nor potentiation of ACh.

Keele and Armstrong (*113*) also detail the studies of Skouby (*114, 115*), in which on iontophoretic or intradermal application the pain threshold was reduced by ACh, methacholine, or neostigmine, whereas in their own studies methacholine was inactive even in concentrations 10 to 100 times greater than ACh. A unique finding in these studies (*113*) was that methacholine, decamethonium, and SCh, as well as ACh, could sensitize "pain" receptors to subthreshold concentrations of potassium chloride. Further, these sensitizing effects were allegedly antagonized by 0.5 to 2 mg of atropine administered orally or intramuscularly, by 50 to 100 mg administered locally, and by tubocurarine administered locally.

The results of Skouby are rather difficult to reconcile with those of Keele and Armstrong and with the effects of the same compounds on other sensory sites. At least part of the differences may be a consequence of the complex system employed, the assessment of activity on the basis of subjective responses, or the variations in the role of circulation and metabolizing enzymes in controlling the magnitude and duration of the response.

2. CAPSAICIN AND ANALOGUES

The active principle of pepper, capsaicin, causes stimulation and sensitization of a variety of sensory endings, including gustatory, warmth receptors, and pain receptors of mucous membranes. A number of analogues of capsaicin are known to possess pungent odors or the characteristic pepper taste and sensation or both. Capsaicin is *N*-vanillyldecylenoylamide **(I)**. The undecylenic

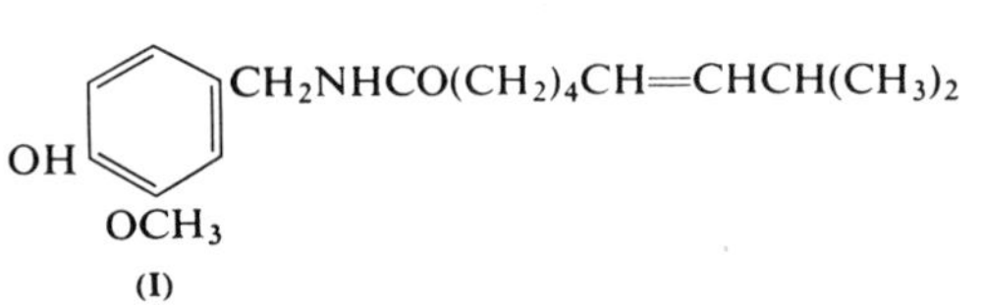

(I)

Capsaicin

acid analogue was shown many years ago to be active (*116*). The limited water solubility of capsaicin has made its systemic administration somewhat complicated: it is usually dissolved in a small amount of alcohol and is emulsified in water with the addition of a detergent, such as Tween 80. Capsaicin stimulates skin receptors for warmth and pain and perhaps others. If left in contact with the skin, a marked hyperemia and edema develops. In addition, there is a remarkable sensitization of the warmth receptors, even with small amounts (*5, 11*; reviewed *113*).

Toh et al. (*118*) have examined the blood pressure and respiratory reflex consequences of injections of capsaicin into a variety of vascular beds. Their experiments indicate that it can stimulate certain carotid baroreceptors in the neck, the afferents of which run in the vagus, receptors in heart and lungs, and receptors in muscle. No change was found in the blood flow through the isolated rabbit ear on the addition of capsaicin to the perfusing blood, whereas 0.1 μg/ml produced a contraction of the isolated guinea pig ileum (*119*). Coleridge et al. (*120*), Pórszász et al. (*121*), and Bevan (*122*) have confirmed and extended these findings on stimulation by capsaicin of receptors in the pulmonary vascular bed. Coleridge et al. (*120*), on the basis of recordings from vagal nerve filaments, concluded that capsaicin stimulated and sensitized pulmonary arterial baroreceptors; other receptors in the intrapulmonary arterial bed also were activated after capsaicin administration. The minor discrepancies among the reports on capsaicin from different investigators have been reviewed by Coleridge et al. (*120*).

Vanillyldecanoylamide was slightly more potent than capsaicin in causing alterations in blood pressure and respiration on intravenous administration, whereas vanillylamine and vanillylacetamide were ineffective (*118*). The eight-membered to ten-membered saturated or unsaturated carbon chain is apparently a necessary structural component (*117*). All of such compounds are notably pungent.

Of particular interest is the desensitization or tachyphylaxis that occurs with repeated injections or prolonged exposure to capsaicin. An acute desensitization occurs with many stimulants of afferent endings, such as ACh or nicotine. The phenomenon has been mentioned sporadically, but no detailed study has been made other than in the context of sensory adaptation.

Jancsó (*123*, *124*) and co-workers (*125*, *126*) and Pórszász and Jancsó (*127*, *128*) made an extended study of the desensitization to capsaicin with a number of very interesting findings. Desensitization to the lethal effects of capsaicin can be developed by administering progressively increasing doses, so that within hours the animals can tolerate without difficulty 30 to 40 times the originally acute lethal dose (*117*). Local skin desensitization has been demonstrated in man. After systemic "desensitization" in animals carried out over 2 to 5 days the irritation of the eye induced by a variety of topically applied agents is markedly decreased or abolished. The list of usually irritating substances allegedly without significant irritant effects after desensitization to capsaicin includes ammonia, chloroacetophenone, formaldehyde, nicotine, veratrine, allyl alcohol, and hypertonic glucose and saline, and also vanillyl ethylhexyl ketone, undecylenoyl piperidine, and methyl salicylate. The effects of mustard oil and formic acid presumably also are depressed, but the responses to pinching, heat, and electrical stimuli are unaltered.

The inflammatory responses to dextran, 48/80,* serotonin, and egg albumin

* For structure see Ref. *128a*.

were unaltered by capsaicin desensitization (*117*). Jancsó and co-workers directed their experiments toward elucidating the role of sensory nerves and axon reflexes in the generation of certain types of inflammatory responses, and as such the experiments are necessarily indirect, but they have made a very good case for the participation of nerve activity in the inflammatory response to a variety of irritants. The major assumption in their interpretations is that the desensitization to capsaicin is the result of its effects on nerves and a concomitant desensitization to a variety of chemical irritants.

The only direct evidence for this thesis has been presented by Pórszász and Jancsó (*127*), to the effect that the increase in the propagated potentials recorded from multifiber filaments of skin nerves in response to capsaicin, ACh, or histamine were absent in animals desensitized to capsaicin. On the other hand, in preparations acutely desensitized to nicotine by repeated injections at short time intervals the neural response to capsaicin was not altered, although that to ACh was abolished. Moreover, the neural responses to tactile and other stimuli were, at least grossly, unaltered by capsaicin desensitization. The afferent nerve impulses induced by the application of mustard on the skin were unaltered by capsaicin desensitization, although a pain response to topical mustard could not be elicited in the same animal.

Much more needs to be done in following up these interesting experiments. The following indicate the initial problems and point up areas of present gaps in knowledge: (1) the confirmation and precise quantitation of the generalized chemical desensitization produced by repeated capsaicin injections, (2) the determination of which sensory endings are activated or sensitized by capsaicin, (3) the examination of specific receptor–nerve systems with respect to development of desensitization, the responses to the appropriate stimulus and the spectrum of cross-tolerance to other chemical stimuli, and (4) the examination of an anatomically defined axon–reflex system with respect to capsaicin activation, desensitization, and cross-desensitization.

Jancsó (*117*) has noted that a number of analogues of capsaicin can also be used to elicit this desensitization, including the vanillyl, decanoyl, nonanoyl, or nonenoyl amides. The heptanoylamide has a "mild" desensitizing action; desensitization is also detectable with the proprioamide.

3. TRYPTAMINE DERIVATIVES

Keele and Armstrong (*113*) have summarized the structure–activity relationships of tryptamine derivatives with respect to their potencies as pain-producing agents when applied to an exposed blister base (Table 10.5). The effective concentration of 5-hydroxytryptamine (serotonin, 5-HT) is approximately 1×10^{-7} to 5×10^{-5} *M*.

Substitution of other moieties for the indole nucleus of 5-HT resulted in a

TABLE 10.5

Effects of Structural Changes in Tryptamine Molecule upon Pain-Producing Potency[a] (*113*)

Structural change	Relative potency
1. Changes in nucleus such as substitution of *p*-OHC_6H_4, $CH_2CH_2NH_2$, or $(CH_3)_2CHCH_2CH_2NH_2$ for 4-, 5-, 6-hydroxyindole nucleus	0.001
2. Alteration in chain length:	
Decrease by one unit, CH_2	0.001
Increase by one unit, CH_2	0.01
3. Substitution on indole nucleus (position):	
OH 4	10 to 20
5	50 to 100
6	2 to 4
Cl 5	5
OCH_3 5	2 to 4
6	1 to 2
CH_3 2	1
5	2
7	1 to 5
4. Side-chain substitution:	
α-Me	0.1
α,α-Me_2	0.1
β,β-Me_2	0.1
α-COOH, α-CH_2OH	0.1
N-Et; *N*-Bu; *N,N*-Me_2	0.1
N-acetyl	0.1
N-Me	10
Substitution in both indole nucleus and side chain, such as 5-OH, NMe	100 to 200

[a] Potency of tryptamine, 1.

loss of potency. On the other hand, all analogues containing substituents on the nucleus (hydroxyl, chloro, methyl, or methoxy) were equal to or more potent than tryptamine itself. Nevertheless, most of the alterations of the 5-HT structure resulted in a decrease in potency, except substitutions on the nucleus and *N*-methylation.

In general, as Keele and Armstrong point out, the orders of potencies of the various tryptamine congeners in producing pain and in causing smooth-muscle stimulation are in agreement. However, there are distinct divergencies: *N*-methyltryptamine is a more potent pain-producer than tryptamine but it is less active on smooth muscle (*129*), and the corresponding 5-hydroxy analogues differ, 5-HT being six times as potent on the rat's stomach as 5-hydroxy-*N*-methyltryptamine and the latter being the more potent pain-producer.

Tachyphylaxis to 5-HT and analogues made testing difficult, particularly of possible antagonists. Phenyldiguanide, which excites pulmonary receptors much as does 5-HT (see below), was found by Fastier et al. (*130*) to cause pain resembling that caused by 5-HT in its somewhat delayed onset. Exposure to phenyldiguanide depresses the response to 5-HT, but it leaves the response to histamine and potassium chloride unaffected.

Large doses of 5-HT (50 to 100 μg/kg, intravenous) are known to stimulate the pulmonary stretch receptors of cats and dogs (*131–133*) but not rabbits. Paintal (*7*) discusses the previous findings and suggests that 5-HT has an effect similar to that of veratrum alkaloids. Among other receptors whose medullated fibers are stimulated is the slowly adapting cutaneous pressure receptor (*134*). A variety of receptors with nonmedullated afferent fibers are excited by 5-HT, including gastric stretch receptors (*135*), on which it is five times more potent than phenyldiguanide, and gastric mucosal receptors, pulmonary deflation receptors and, probably, carotid baroreceptors.

The variability among types of receptors stimulated by 5-HT is puzzling. Further, the time course and potency of the substance relative to those of other agents vary widely. The possibility of indirect actions, such as smooth-muscle stimulation causing or contributing to the effect, confounds the interpretations of most of these experiments. The possibility of a direct effect of 5-HT on nonmyelinated fibers, analogous to that produced by ACh or nicotine, has yet to be explored. 5-HT is without effect on muscle spindle stretch receptors (*97*).

E. Drug Effects on Nonmyelinated Nerves

We have seen that cholinergic agents stimulate a wide variety of sensory receptors, and recent studies have demonstrated that ACh and congeners can affect nerves directly. The evidence of effects on myelinated fibers is disputed, but there is little question that ACh and congeners depolarize and block transmission of nonmyelinated fibers.

Armett and Ritchie (*136–139*) have examined in detail the effects of ACh and some analogues on the membrane potential and propagated spike of nonmyelinated mammalian nerve by the sucrose gap technique. ACh, carbamoylcholine, TMA, and nicotine each cause a depolarization and decrease in the compound evoked spike potential. The concentrations in the bath solution were quite large in comparison to those effective on intra-arterial injections in evoking trains of action potentials from nerve fibers and intact endings in vivo (*136*, *140*).

Table 10.6 summarizes the data on a comparison of cholinergic substances.

TABLE 10.6

Potency of Acetylcholine and Related Compounds on Nonmyelinated Nerve (*137*)

	Concentration required to reduce spike height, m*M*
Nicotine	0.6
Acetylcholine	1.7 to 16
Carbamoylcholine	1.7 to 16
Tetramethylammonium	1.5 to 5
Pilocarpine	3.7 (less effective than 1.7 m*M* acetylcholine)
Arecoline	5.2
Methacholine	Occasionally enhanced after-potential
Bethanechol	Ineffective

Nicotine is the most potent. ACh, carbachol, and TMA are approximately equipotent and one half to one third as active as nicotine. Pilocarpine and arecoline are distinctly less potent than the others, whereas methacholine and bethanechol were ineffective. In spite of the large concentrations required the spectrum of sensitivity reveals the "nicotinic" nature of the effects in analogy with the autonomic actions of these substances.

In line with this generalization, TEA had no effect alone in this preparation, but it did reduce the effect of ACh. Tubocurarine and hexamethonium in concentrations of 10^{-3} to 10^{-4} g/ml also blocked ACh actions. Atropine produced slight depressant effects alone and blocked ACh actions (*137*). The ACh effects were noted to be antagonized by choline or triethanolamine (*138*).

Of particular interest were the interactions between certain anticholinesterases and ACh. Only a very slight potentiation of ACh actions was found with the lowest concentrations of physostigmine and diisopropyl fluorophosphate, and the most striking action was the antagonism of the effects of ACh. This antagonism was observed with physostigmine, neostigmine, edrophonium, and diisopropyl fluorophosphate (*137*).

Further study of the interactions among these agents would be of interest, particularly with respect to ascertaining the degree to which ACh competes for given receptor sites as compared with a less direct antagonism. Armett and Ritchie (*138*, *139*) conclude that ACh produces a selective increase of permeability to sodium and calcium and that if potassium permeability is increased it is to a lesser extent than sodium permeability. This conclusion was based on examining the influences of changes in external ion composition; of note was the fact that a reduction in external Ca^{++} decreased the ACh-induced depolarization whereas replacement of sodium by calcium increased it.

F. Local Anesthetics

The qualitative effects of local anesthetics on sensory endings has been thoroughly reviewed by Paintal (*7*), and there are detailed references to previous studies of mechanism and nature of action. As Paintal points out, in spite of the fact that it has been long known that smaller fibers tend to be more susceptible to local anesthetics than larger ones, it is not known whether local anesthetics affect the sensory endings of fibers with small diameters more than those with large. The in vitro studies clearly indicate that the primary, or a major, site of local anesthetic action when the drug is given systemically is at the regenerative region (*7–9*, *141*). Larger concentrations are required for an action on the generator region, and the rate of penetration into nerve trunks appears to be generally slow. Thus, the nerve terminal on the first node or origin of regenerative propagated impulses is a major site of action of local anesthetics on sensory endings. Whether or not this represents the site of action of other agents affecting sensory endings remains to be seen; so far it is an attractive working hypothesis. Although this regenerative region is susceptible of depression from procaine or sodium in low concentration, it should not be forgotten that the generator region also is depressed by procaine, and with large concentrations effects at this site too must be anticipated.

Data relevant to structure–activity relationships in respect to local anesthetics have been collected largely by Zipf and his co-workers (*142–145*), who use the catchword *Endoanästhesie*, and by Bein (*146*). As is well known, many substances possess local anesthetic activity, and it has been amply demonstrated that the administration of agents into the vascular system can result in alterations in afferent inflow. A number of compounds are discussed in the section on muscle spindles in this chapter. Of pertinence here are the following questions on the degree of generalization possible.

(1) Are the actions of "local anesthetics" on any or all sensory systems correlatable with other measures of local anesthetic activity?

(2) What generalizations can be made in relation to chemical structure and depressant effects on one or more sensory systems?

(3) Are the differences in sensitivity among systems functions of the structure, the rate of onset and duration, the type of sensory ending, the size of afferent fiber, the pattern of sensory discharge, or other properties?

In a series of tropeines (*145*) there was not a perfect correlation between the anesthesia assessed on the rabbit cornea and the endoanesthesia of pulmonary stretch receptors of guinea pigs recorded electrophysiologically. However, the most potent local anesthetic (*N*-isopropylnor-α-tropine benzoate ester) was the second most potent depressant of lung stretch receptor activity. The most potent was *N*-isopropylnor-α-tropine benzilate ester. In this series of derivatives, although they were incomplete, the *N*-isopropyl group and the benzilate or benzoate ester groups were optimal over *N*-ethyl, methyl, allyl, or a variety of other acid esters of tropine.

A comparison of the depressant effects of a variety of agents on vagal afferent excitation induced by ACh, histamine, 5-HT, and veratridine (*146*) revealed that procaine (5 mg/kg, intravenous), benzonatate (Tessalon, 0.44 mg/kg), lidocaine (3.3 mg/kg), and dodecyl nonaethylenoxyde ether (3.8 mg/kg) effectively reduced or abolished the increased vagal activity from lung receptors induced by all agents. Tetracaine (0.7 mg/kg, intravenous) was effective against ACh-induced activity but not against histamine-induced activity. With the use of various blocking agents and by measuring respiratory excursions, it could be shown that the increased afferent activity induced by ACh and histamine was the result of bronchospasm. The doses of each of these endoanesthetics were approximately 1/10 to 1/6 of the LD_{50}.

Another example of the variations in order of potencies among local anesthetics in different test situations was presented by Bein and Bucher (*146*); similar data are given by Zipf (*142*) and Sell et al. (*148*). The series of compounds were compared with respect to 50% block of conduction in frog sciatic nerves, intradermal infiltration anesthesia, corneal surface anesthesia after intravenous administration, depression of afferent activity of lung afferents in rabbits, and depression of the flexor reflex in cats and rabbits. There was a rough correlation among the potencies with respect to depression of the flexor reflex of cats and rabbits, whereas there was a less obvious relationship between lung receptor afferent activity depression and depression of the flexor reflex and even less between any in vivo activity and the potency of the same compounds as depressants of nerve conduction. Furthermore, there were even greater discrepancies from a 1:1 correlation among conduction, infiltration, and surface anesthetic potencies.

The exceptions from correlation were clearly not referable simply to differences in lipoid solubility or diffusibility through such membranes as the nerve sheath or cornea. They can, however, be explained if one wishes to postulate three essentially unrelated aspects of each drug's actions, the significance of each aspect being different in each test: for example, diffusibility to site of action on nerve, rate of association with the drug receptor, rate of dissociation, and rate of destruction or vascular removal.

Assuming that these are the pertinent determinants of potency and time course of action, how can these properties be partitioned so that specific problems in structure–activity relationships can be attacked? In most instances the ratio of the rate of association to dissociation would be taken as a measure of the affinity of the drug for the receptor, which in the case of the depressants has not necessitated the postulation of a second "efficacy" factor analogous to "intrinsic activity" for excitatory agents.

A first step in unraveling these problems bearing directly on activity determination would be to define experiments in which each of these factors could be ascertained for two or more agents relatively uncomplicated by the presence of any other factor. Next the agents could be used to characterize various preparations. Such data in conjunction with multifactorial analyses and perhaps simple analogue simulation would permit the resolution of the contributions of each of these aspects to the total drug syndrome and, hence, to the rational design of agents with different properties.

The alternative to this suggestion of the confluence of many processes is that the agents differ markedly with respect to their activity or mechanism of action on different nerve tissues and that the characteristic activity of the nerves is differentially affected by various local anesthetics. To prove this, however, one would have to rule out the roles of other processes, such as diffusion differences, in the generation of observed potency variations.

Among the many factors is the possibility that fibers of different size react differently to various local anesthetics. The fact that the smaller fibers of slower conduction velocity are usually but not always (see *148a*) more sensitive to cocaine and procaine is, of course, well established, but the possibility that different degrees of relative sensitivity might be obtained with different agents has never been thoroughly investigated.

In perhaps the only study of its type, Kondo (*148b*) has demonstrated that the factors governing the conduction of an impulse through an area of nerve exposed to a local anesthetic include the prior frequency of nerve impulses, the number and frequency of impulses which have failed to be conducted through the partially blocked area, plus the number and frequency of impulses which have traversed the region.

The differences in spectrum of the effects of local anesthetic agents extend to other tissues as well. In a comparison of dodecyl polyethyleneoxide ether (DOR-9/3) and procaine the depression of the afferent activity of stretch receptors of the guinea pig caused by the former was accompanied by no electrocardiographic changes, whereas a comparable degree of depression caused by the latter was associated with marked cardiac toxicity (*144*); interestingly, this same report cites the fact that formalin edema is blocked by DOR-9/3.

DOR-9/3 and benzonatate (Tessalon) have recently been found to produce depression of afferent activity in nerves from lung stretch receptors, aortic baroreceptors, left and right atrial receptors, and groups Ia and II fibers from muscle spindles (*149*). The only differential noted was that the slowly adapting, tonically firing units tended to exhibit more marked depression for longer periods of time than the more rapidly adapting units.

As noted above, local anesthetics characteristically antagonize readily the stimulatory effect of veratrine or veratramine. Two unusual substances, α-fagarin and α-allocryptopin, block the stimulation of vagal afferents induced by veratrine and also the arrhythmia induced by aconitine (*150*), but the statement is made that these substances alone are without effect on afferent activity.

The discussion of the difficulties of accurate assay techniques for local anesthetics has been succinctly summarized by Barlow (*151*, pp. 41, 42, 60–77). After a detailed consideration of the many studies of various structures exhibiting some type of local anesthetic activity Barlow concludes rather pessimistically that "the usefulness of local anesthetics on mucous surface, at nerve-endings, and in the spinal cord cannot really be related to chemical structure or even physicochemical properties."

The vast literature on local anesthetic assays on the cornea or intradermal wheal could be construed as germane to the present review. This author has nothing new to contribute to the many excellent reviews (e.g., *81*, *151*, *152*).

Currently used test methods are, in general, quite adequate for indicating possible clinical usefulness, as Barlow says, but they only rarely provide information useful for establishing the mechanism of action or the relation between molecular action and chemical structure. In some series of substances there is agreeable correlation among potencies of compounds and test objects (*153*), but in others there is not. Some compounds are very active on the cornea and relatively inactive when injected intradermally, and of many substances the reverse is true (e.g., procaine).

Quaternary compounds may be as active as the parent tertiary derivative (*154–156*). In the series tested the benzyl quaternary tended to be more active than the methyl quaternary, but with cocaine and cinchocaine derivatives on infiltration both the methyl- and benzylammonium derivatives were approximately equipotent and somewhat less potent than the tertiary base. When tested for conduction anesthesia the benzyl derivative was consistently more potent than the methyl analogue. These quaternary derivatives are another example of the fact that generalizations do not always hold; these compounds deserve further study, particularly with respect to their effects on sensory endings upon systemic administration.

One other point is that a variety of agents may be evoking their activity via a relatively selective block of given nerve fibers or endings; an example is the selective effects on adrenergic nerve endings of choline 2,6-xylyl ether (*157*, *158*).

It is generally assumed that the local anesthetics have a common mode of action, but this may be open to question. Certainly, experiments demonstrating common qualitative effects on threshold generation of propagated potentials, sodium and potassium permeabilities, and so forth have not been done. Certain investigators, moreover, have suggested that procaine cation (*159*) and the quaternary methyl derivative of procaine may produce block by membrane depolarization rather than stabilization as is more commonly stated (*160*).

10.3. CONCLUSION

This review has focused on two facets. The techniques and problems in establishing meaningful structure–activity relationships for drug effects on afferent endings have been discussed generally, and certain of the nerve and afferent receptor systems and classes of drugs for which there are sufficient data to begin a quantitative analysis of the relation of structure to activity have been considered. With respect to stimulatory cholinergic agents, the afferent systems behave as though they were nicotinic rather than muscarinic and more like ganglionic synapses than nerve-muscle junctions of skeletal muscles. Muscarine or acetyl-β-methacholine have proved to be quite impotent or lacking in stimulant effect entirely, whereas nicotine is generally effective. But the order of potency among the "cholinergic" agents in the different systems varies widely, a fact which is partly attributable to variations in the method of drug administration or in the amounts of cholinesterase present. Many of the agents are presumed to act on the regenerative region of the first node or the region adjacent to the nerve ending itself, but this has not been demonstrated with any of the agents except the local anesthetics.

In spite of the limited sample of drugs and sensory endings considered there is no question that structure–activity studies will become truly meaningful only with the recording of the reactions of specific endings and afferent nerves to drug actions assessed quantitatively over wide dose ranges. An analysis of sites of action for each agent becomes mandatory with the realization that the activation of the ending or afferent fiber can be achieved by a variety of means, many of which are the result of drug actions on tissues other than the nerve or ending itself.

The vast majority of experiments have entailed the examination of reflexes or changes in perception upon the systemic or local administration of a drug. Such analyses of the alterations in reflexes produced by an agent are necessary and useful in the determination of the spectra of sites of action of an agent in the whole organism, but they provide only inferential information of very limited value on agents' effects on a sensory receptor system.

Thus, progress in this field is dependent upon the determination of dose–effect relationships of a variety of drugs on populations of different types of sensory receptor and nerve. The subject is not esoteric, in that many frequently used drugs are now known to alter sensory input. It remains to be determined how extensive the phenomenon is and whether it can be turned to predictive ends, such as to the design of agents with specific actions on one type of afferent receptor.

ACKNOWLDGEMENTS

Research was supported by USPHS grant NB-0973. A portion of this report was prepared during the tenure of a position as staff scientist at the Institute for Defense Analyses, Arlington, Virginia.

REFERENCES

1. R. Melzack and P. D. Wall, *Science*, **150**, 971 (1965).
1a. M. G. J. Beets in *Molecular Pharmacology*, Vol. II (E. J. Ariëns, ed.), Academic, New York, 1962, pp. 3–54.
2. "Recent Advances in Odor: Theory, Measurement, and Control," *Ann. N.Y. Acad. Sci.*, **116**, 357 (1964).
3. R. H. Wright, *The Science of Smell*, Allen & Unwin, London, 1964.
4. E. S. Hodgson in *Physiology of Insecta*, Vol. I (M. Rockstein, ed.), Academic Press, New York, 1964, Chap. 9, pp. 363–396.
5. R. W. Moncrieff, *The Chemical Senses*, Leonard Hill, London, 1951.
6. Y. Zotterman, ed., *Olfaction and Taste*, Pergamon, London, 1963.
7. A. S. Paintal, *Pharmacol. Rev.*, **16**, 341 (1964).
8. B. Katz, *J. Physiol. (London)*, **111**, 248 (1950).
9. B. Katz, *J. Physiol. (London)*, **111**, 261 (1950).
10. R. Lorente de Nó and V. Honrubia, *Proc. Natl. Acad. Sci., U.S.*, **52**, 1142 (1964).
11. A. Iggo, in *Pain and Itch-Nervous Mechanisms* (G. E. W. Wolstenholme and M. O'Connor, eds.), Churchill, London, 1959, pp. 41–56.
12. W. W. Douglas and J. M. Ritchie, *J. Physiol. (London)*, **138**, 19 (1957).
13. W. W. Douglas and J. M. Ritchie, *J. Physiol. (London)*, **139**, 385 (1957).
14. W. W. Douglas and J. M. Ritchie, *J. Physiol. (London)*, **139**, 400 (1957).
15. W. W. Douglas and J. M. Ritchie in *Pain and Itch-Nervous Mechanisms* (G. E. W. Wolstenholme and M. O'Connor, eds.), Churchill, London, 1959, pp. 26–39.
16. W. W. Douglas and J. M. Ritchie, *Physiol. Rev.*, **42**, 297 (1962).
17. E. J. Ariëns, ed., *Molecular Pharmacology*, Vols. I & II, Academic Press, New York, 1964.
18. J. L. Webb, *Enzyme and Metabolic Inhibitors*, Vol. I, Academic Press, New York, 1963.
19. C. M. Smith, *Ann. Rev. Pharmacol.*, **3**, 223 (1963).
19a. C. Eyzaguirre and H. Koyano, *J. Physiol. (London)*, **178**, 385 (1965).
19b. C. Eyzaguirre and H. Koyano, *J. Physiol. (London)*, **178**, 410 (1965).
19c. C. Eyzaguirre and H. Koyano, *J. Physiol. (London)*, **178**, 438 (1965).
19d. C. Eyzaguirre, H. Koyano, and J. R. Taylor, *J. Physiol. (London)*, **178**, 463 (1965).
20. C. Heymans, *Pharmacol. Rev.*, **7**, 119 (1955).
21. C. Heymans and E. Neil, *Reflexogenic Areas of the Cardiovascular System*, Churchill, London, 1958.
22. S. V. Anichkov and M. L. Belen'kii, *Pharmacology of the Carotid Body Chemoreceptors*, Pergamon, London, 1963.
23. C. Eyzaguirre and J. Lewin, *J. Physiol. (London)*, **159**, 222 (1961).
24. A. Schweitzer and S. Wright, *Quart. J. Exptl. Physiol.*, **28**, 33 (1938).
25. G. K. Moe, L. R. Capo, and B. R. Peralta, *Am. J. Physiol.*, **153**, 601 (1948).
26. G. Liljestrand, *Acta Physiol. Scand.*, **24**, 225 (1951).
27. W. W. Douglas, *J. Physiol. (London)*, **118**, 373 (1952).
28. C. Heymans, J. J. Bouckaert, S. Farber, and F. J. Hsu, *Arch. Intern. Pharmacodyn.*, **54**, 129 (1936).
29. S. V. Anichkov, V. V. Zakusov, A. I. Kuzmetsov, and N. G. Polyakov, *Physiol. J. (USSR)*, **21**, 809 (1936); cited in Ref. *22*.
30. K. Gollwitzer-Meier and E. Witzleb, *Arch. Ges. Physiol.*, **256**, 381 (1953).
31. A. S. Dontas and M. Nickerson, *Federation Proc.*, **13**, 37 (1954).
32. U. S. von Euler, G. Liljestrand, and Y. Zotterman, *Acta Physiol. Scand.*, **1**, 383 (1941).
33. S. Landgren, E. Neil, and Y. Zotterman, *Acta Physiol. Scand.*, **25**, 24 (1952).
34. S. Landgren, G. Liljestrand, and Y. Zotterman, *Acta Physiol. Scand.*, **26**, 264 (1952).

35. E. Phillipot, *Arch. Intern. Pharmacodyn.*, **57**, 357 (1937).
36. C. F. Schmidt and J. H. Comroe, Jr., *Physiol. Rev.*, **20**, 115 (1940).
37. N. G. Polyakov-Stanevich, *Sci. Papers Kirov Mil. Med. Acad.*, **17**, 143 (1938); cited in Ref. 27.
38. H. DeWispelaere, *Arch. Intern. Pharmacodyn.*, **56**, 363 (1937).
39. G. Liljestrand and Y. Zotterman, *Acta Physiol. Scand.*, **31**, 203 (1954).
40. D. Bovet and F. Bovet-Nitti, *Structure et Activité Pharmacodynamique des Médicaments du Systéme Nerveux Végetatif*, S. Karger, New York and Basel (1948).
41. I. Sanghvi, S. Murayama, C. M. Smith, and K. R. Unna, *J. Pharmacol. Exptl. Therap.*, **142**, 192 (1963).
42. L. Gyermek, E. B. Sigg, and E. Bindler, *Am. J. Physiol.*, **204**, 68 (1963).
43. G. Liljestrand, *Acta Physiol. Scand.*, **29**, 74 (1953).
44. S. Landgren, G. Liljestrand, and Y. Zotterman, *Arch. Exptl. Pathol. Pharmakol.*, **219**, 185 (1953).
45. J. Berney and J. Posternak, *Helv. Physiol. Pharmacol. Acta*, **14**, C5 (1956).
46. J. E. P. Toman, *Pharmacol. Rev.*, **4**, 168 (1952).
47. S. N. Asratyan, *Physiol. J.* (*USSR*), **24**, 33 (1938); cited in Ref. *22*.
47a. M. Penna and D. M. Aviado, *Arch. Intern. Pharmacodyn.*, **140**, 269 (1962).
48. R. E. Boelaert, *Arch. Intern. Pharmacodyn.*, **75**, 417 (1948).
49. C. Heymans, A. L. Delaunois, L. Martini, and P. Janssen, *Arch. Intern. Pharmacodyn.*, **96**, 209 (1953).
50. H. Budde, K. Donat, and E. Witzleb, *Arch. Intern. Pharmacodyn.*, **100**, 479 (1955).
51. Z. I. Vedeneyeva, *Physiol. J.* (*USSR*), **37**, 732 (1951); cited in Refs. 22 and 52.
52. I. V. Dardymov and B. A. Ger, *Farmakol. Toksikol.*, **26**, 661 (1963); *Federation Proc.*, **23**, T917 (1964).
53. R. Byck, *Brit. J. Pharmacol.*, **16**, 15 (1961).
54. P. P. Denisenko, *Gangliolytics and Agents Blocking Neuromuscular Synapses*, Leningrad, 1958; cited in Ref. *22*.
55. N. Joels and E. Neil, *J. Physiol.* (*London*), **164**, 11 (1962).
56. G. Liljestrand, *Pharmacol. Rev.*, **6**, 73 (1954).
57. S. M. Vishnyakov, *Pharmacol. Toxicol.* (*USSR*) (*English Transl.*), **15**, 3, 14 (1952).
58. I. V. Dardymov and R. S. Rybolovlev, *Bull. Exptl. Biol. Med.* (*USSR*) (*English Transl.*) **40**, 41 (1955); cited by Anichkov and Belen'kii (*22*).
59. M. Ya. Mikhel'son, R. S. Ryboloblev, A. M. Gorelik, and I. V. Dardymov in *The Physiological Role of Acetylcholine and the Search for New Medicinal Drugs* (M. Ya, Mikel'son, ed.), The Leningrad Medical Institute, I. P. Pavlov, 1957 (pp. 468–501 in. translation of Joint Publications Research Service of U.S. Dept. of Commerce).
60. R. S. Rybolovlev in *The Physiological Role of Acetylcholine and the Search for New Medicinal Drugs* (M. Ya. Mikhel'son, ed.), The Leningrad Medical Institute, I. P. Pavlov, 1957 (pp. 390–420 in translation of Joint Publications Research Service of U.S. Dept. of Commerce).
61. S. Stern, R. E. Ferguson, and E. Rapaport, *Am. J. Physiol.*, **206**, 1189 (1964).
62. D. Atanackovic and Sv. Dalgaard-Mikkelsen, *Acta. Physiol. Scand.*, **22**, 77 (1951).
63. S. V. Anichkov, *Physiol. J.* (*USSR*), **33**, 267 (1947); cited in Ref. *22*.
64. A. I. Mitrofanov, *Bull. Exptl. Biol. Med.* (*USSR*), **7**, 60 (1957); cited in Ref. *22*.
65. S. Landgren and E. Neil, *Acta Physiol. Scand.*, **23**, 152 (1951).
66. C. Eyzaguirre and K. Uchizono, *J. Physiol.* (*London*), **159**, 268 (1961).
67. W. W. Douglas and W. Schaumann, *J. Physiol.* (*London*), **132**, 173 (1956).
68. S. Ya. Arbuzov, *Pharmacol. Toxicol.* (*USSR*) **8**, 22 (1945); cited in Ref. *22*.
69. R. Pannier and J. Backer, *Arch. Intern. Pharmacodyn.*, **70**, 110 (1945).

70. A. M. Gorelik in *The Physiological Role of Acetylcholine and the Search for New Medicinal Drugs* (M. Ya. Mikhel'son, ed.), The Leningrad Medical Institute, I. P. Pavlov, 1957 (pp. 452–467 in translation of Joint Publication Research Service of U.S. Dept. of Commerce).

71. E. V. Zeymal and R. S. Rybolovlev in *The Physiological Role of Acetylcholine and the Search for New Medicinal Drugs* (M. Ya. Mikhel'son, ed.), The Leningrad Medical Institute, I. P. Pavlov, 1957 (pp. 421–451 in translation of Joint Publication Research Service of U.S. Dept. of Commerce).

72. K. Gollwitzer-Meier and E. Witzleb, *Arch. Ges. Physiol.*, **259**, 499 (1954).

73. D. Whitteridge and E. Bülbring, *J. Pharmacol. Exptl. Therap.*, **81**, 340 (1944).

74. D. Whitteridge, *Brit. Med. Bull.*, **14**, 5 (1958).

75. T. J. Biscoe and R. A. Millar, *J. Physiol. (London)*, **173**, 24 (1964).

76. J. D. Robertson, A. A. B. Swan, and D. Whitteridge, *J. Physiol. (London)*, **131**, 463 (1956).

77. J. Diamond, *J. Physiol. (London)*, **130**, 513 (1955).

78. A. S. Dontas, *Federation Proc.*, **13**, 37 (1954).

79. L. C. Weaver, W. R. Jones, and S. M. Kupchan, *J. Pharm. Sci.*, **51**, 1144 (1962).

80. W. Flacke, *J. Pharmacol. Exptl. Therap.*, **141**, 230 (1963).

81. A. M. Shanes, *Pharmacol. Rev.*, **10**, 59, 165 (1958).

82. A. S. Paintal, *J. Physiol. (London)*, **135**, 486 (1957).

83. J. M. Benfòrado, W. Flacke, C. R. Swaine, and W. Mosimann, *J. Pharmacol. Exptl. Therap.*, **130**, 311 (1960).

84. S. M. Kupchan, N. Gruenfeld, and N. Katsui, *J. Med. Chem.*, **5**, 690 (1962).

85. H. Kurihara, *Japan. Circulation J.*, **28**, 219 (1964).

86. R. Granit, S. Skoglund, and S. Thesleff, *Acta. Physiol. Scand.*, **28**, 134 (1953).

87. C. C. Hunt, *Federation Proc.*, **11**, 75 (1952).

88. C. M. Smith, *Arch. Intern. Pharmacodyn.*, **127**, 369 (1960).

89. E. X. Albuquerque and C. M. Smith, *J. Pharmacol. Exptl. Therap.*, **146**, 344 (1964).

90. E. X. Albuquerque and C. M. Smith, *Pharmacologist*, **6**, 168 (1964).

91. E. X. Albuquerque and C. M. Smith, *J. Pharmacol. Exptl. Therap.*, **149**, 320 (1965).

92. E. X. Albuquerque and C. M. Smith, *Pharmacologist*, **7**, 187 (1965).

93. E. X. Albuquerque and B. Whitsel, *Federation Proc.*, **24**, 267 (1965).

94. C. M. Smith and E. X. Albuquerque, *Pharmacologist*, **6**, 168 (1964).

95. C. M. Smith, E. Xavier, and J. Grossie, *Federation Proc.*, **23**, 234 (1964).

96. B. L. Whitsel, E. X. Albuquerque, and C. M. Smith, *Pharmacologist*, **7**, 187 (1965).

97. B. A. Verhey and P. E. Voorhoeve, *Acta Physiol. Pharmacol. Neerl.*, **12**, 23 (1963).

98. D. Langrehr and H. D. Henatsch, *Arch. Exptl. Pathol. Pharmakol.*, **243**, 407 (1962).

99. K. H. Ginzel, H. Klupp, H. Stormann, and G. Werner, *Arzneimittel-Forsch.*, **2**, 271 (1952).

100. K. H. Ginzel, H. Klupp, H. Stormann, and G. Werner, *Arch. Exptl. Pathol. Pharmakol.*, **218**, 308 (1953).

101. C. M. Smith, A. V. Budris, and J. W. Paul, *J. Pharmacol. Exptl. Therap.*, **136**, 267 (1962).

102. P. E. Voorhoeve and B. A. Verhey, *Acta Physiol. Pharmacol. Neerl.*, **12**, 12 (1963).

103. C. C. Hunt and E. R. Perl, *Physiol. Rev.*, **40**, 538 (1960).

104. P. B. C. Matthews, *Physiol. Rev.*, **44**, 219 (1964).

105. W. A. Cook, Jr., D. R. Neilson, Jr., and J. M. Brookhart, *J. Neurophysiol.*, **28**, 290 (1965).

106. H. D. Henatsch in *Symposium on Muscle Receptors* (D. Barker, ed.), Hong Kong Univ. Press, Hong Kong, 1962, pp. 67–80.

107. M. Kato, H. Takamura, and B. Fujimori in *Symposium on Muscle Receptors* (D. Barker, ed.), Hong Kong Univ. Press, Hong Kong, 1962, p. 31–42.

108. C. M. Smith and H. J. Kaese, *Arch. Exptl. Pathol. Pharmakol.*, **243**, 320 (1962).
109. C. M. Smith and E. Eldred, *J. Pharmacol. Exptl. Therap.*, **131**, 237 (1960).
110. J. Grossie and C. M. Smith, *Arch. Intern. Pharmacodyn.*, **159**, 288 (1965).
111. H. J. Bein and H.-U. Fehr, *Brit. J. Pharmacol.*, **19**, 375 (1962).
112. A. Matsushita, N. Yanagisawa, and H. Shimazu, *J. Pharmacol. Exptl. Therap.*, **147**, 343 (1965).
112a. A. Matsushita, *Jap. J. Pharmacol.*, **14**, 434 (1964).
113. C. A. Keele and D. Armstrong, "Substances Producing Pain and Itch," *Physiological Society of London Monographs*, Arnold, London, 1964.
114. A. P. Skouby, *Acta Physiol. Scand.*, **24**, 174 (1951).
115. A. P. Skouby, *Acta Physiol. Scand.*, **29**, 340 (1953).
116. W. Heubner, *Arch. Exptl. Pathol. Pharmakol.*, **107**, 129 (1925).
117. N. Jancsó, *Bull. Millard Fillmore Hosp.* (Buffalo, N.Y.), **7**, 53 (1960).
118. C. C. Toh, T. S. Lee, and A. K. Krang, *Brit. J. Pharmacol.*, **10**, 175 (1955).
119. E. Göres and F. Jung, *Acta Biol. Med. Ger.*, **3**, 41 (1959).
120. H. M. Coleridge, J. C. G. Coleridge, and C. Kidd, *J. Physiol.* (*London*), **170**, 272 (1964).
121. J. Pórszász, G. Such, and K. Pórszász-Gibiszer, *Acta Physiol. Acad. Sci. Hung.*, **12**, 189 (1957).
122. J. A. Bevan, *Circulation Res.*, **10**, 792 (1962).
123. N. Jancsó, *Acta. Physiol. Acad. Sci. Hung.*, *Suppl.*, **11**, 11 (1957).
124. N. Jancsó, *Acta Physiol. Acad. Sci. Hung.*, *Suppl.*, **12**, 15 (1958).
125. N. Jancsó and A. Jancsó-Gábor, *Arch. Exptl. Pathol. Pharmakol.*, **236**, 142 (1959).
126. N. Jancsó, A. Jancsó-Gábor, and I. Takáts, *Acta Physiol. Acad. Sci. Hung.*, **19**, 113 (1961).
127. J. Pórszász and N. Jancsó, *Acta Physiol. Acad. Sci. Hung.*, **16**, 299 (1959).
128. J. Pórszász, *Acta Physiol. Acad. Sci. Hung.*, **15**, 291 (1959).
128a. R. Baltzly, J. S. Buck, E. J. De Beer, and F. J. Webb, *J. Am. Chem. Soc.*, **71**, 1301 (1949).
129. J. R. Vane, *Brit. J. Pharmacol.*, **14**, 87 (1959).
130. F. N. Fastier, M. A. McDowall, and H. Waal, *Brit. J. Pharmacol.*, **14**, 527 (1959).
131. J. A. Schneider and F. F. Yonkman, *Am. J. Physiol.*, **174**, 127 (1953).
132. J. A. Schneider and F. F. Yonkman, *J. Pharmacol. Exptl. Therap.*, **111**, 84 (1954).
133. S. R. Kottegoda and J. C. Mott, *Brit. J. Pharmacol.*, **10**, 66 (1955).
134. N. Fjällbrant and A. Iggo, *J. Physiol.* (*London*), **156**, 578 (1961).
135. A. S. Paintal, *J. Physiol.* (*London*), **126**, 271 (1954).
136. C. J. Armett and J. M. Ritchie, *J. Physiol.* (*London*), **152**, 141 (1960).
137. C. J. Armett and J. M. Ritchie, *J. Physiol.* (*London*), **155**, 372 (1961).
138. C. J. Armett and J. M. Ritchie, *J. Physiol.* (*London*), **165**, 141 (1963).
139. C. J. Armett and J. M. Ritchie, *J. Physiol.* (*London*), **165**, 130 (1963).
140. G. L. Brown and J. A. B. Gray, *J. Physiol.* (*London*), **107**, 306 (1948).
141. J. Diamond, J. A. B. Gray, and D. R. Inman, *J. Physiol.* (*London*), **142**, 382 (1958).
142. H. F. Zipf in *Lokalanästhesie und Lokalanästhetika* (H. Killian, ed.), Georg Thieme Verlag, Stuttgart, 1959, pp. 138–149.
143. H. F. Zipf and K. Hansen, *Arch. Exptl. Pathol. Pharmakol.*, **242**, 284 (1961).
144. H. F. Zipf and P. Reichertz, *Arch. Exptl. Pathol. Pharmakol.*, **231**, 96 (1957).
145. H. F. Zipf, E. Ch. Dittmann, and H. Marquardt, *Arzneimittel-Forsch.*, **13**, 1097 (1963).
146. H. J. Bein and K. Bucher, *Helv. Physiol. Pharmacol. Acta*, **15**, 55 (1957).
147. Z. Hansen and H. F. Zipf, *Arch. Exptl. Pathol. Pharmakol.*, **240**, 253 (1960).
148. R. Sell, E. Lindner, and H. Jahn, *Arch. Exptl. Pathol. Pharmakol.*, **234**, 164 (1958).
148a. J. E. P. Toman, *Pharmacol. Rev.*, **4**, 168 (1952).

148b. T. Kondo, *Japan J. Physiol.*, **5**, 274 (1955–56).
149. D. Langrehr, *Arch. Exptl. Pathol. Pharmakol.*, **245**, 427 (1963).
150. R. Meier and H. J. Bein, *Arch. Exptl. Pathol. Pharmakol.*, **215**, 119 (1952).
151. R. B. Barlow, *Introduction to Chemical Pharmacology*, Wiley, 2nd ed., 1964.
152. S. Weidling and C. Tegnér, *Progr. in Med. Chem.*, **3**, 332–398 (1963).
153. K. H. Beyer, A. R. Latven, W. A. Freyburger, and M. P. Parker, *J. Pharmacol. Exptl. Therap.*, **93**, 388 (1948).
154. K. Nádor, F. Herr, Gy. Pataky, and J. Borsi, *Nature*, **171**, 788 (1953).
155. L. Gyermek, *Nature*, **171**, 788 (1953).
156. F. Herr, K. Nádor, Gy. Pataky, and J. Borsi, *Arch. Exptl. Pathol. Pharmakol.*, **217**, 447 (1953).
157. K. A. Exley, *Brit. J. Pharmacol.*, **12**, 297 (1957).
158. P. Hey and G. L. Willey, *Brit. J. Pharmacol.*, **9**, 471 (1954).
159. R. Straub, *Arch. Intern. Pharmacodyn.*, **107**, 414 (1956).
160. J. C. Skou, *J. Pharm. Pharmacol.*, **13**, 204 (1961).

AUTHOR INDEX

Numbers in parentheses are reference numbers and indicate that an author's work is referred to although his name is not cited in the text. Numbers in italics show the page on which the complete reference is listed.

C

D

H

W

SUBJECT INDEX

N

Q